Rare Lung Diseases

This book aims to be a complete guide to diagnose, manage, and treat rare lung diseases encountered by practicing pulmonologists and trainees. It extensively covers the "more common" of the rare lung diseases, categorizing them based on developmental lung anomalies in adults, airway disorders, diffuse parenchymal lung diseases, neoplasms, rare vascular disorders, and other miscellaneous conditions. This comprehensive review facilitates the study and understanding of this complex and diverse set of disorders, focusing on differential diagnosis, evidence-based discussions of management algorithms, and thoughtful analysis of treatment options.

Key Features

- Reviews multiple rare lung diseases, including those acquired congenitally to be expressed in old age
- Enriched with case studies and illustrations to guide respiratory physicians and trainees to devise an effective treatment plan
- Focuses on concerned investigations, with a section on the role of new procedures in management

Rare Lung Diseases

A Comprehensive Clinical Guide to Diagnosis and Management

Edited by

Sujith V. Cherian, MD, FCCP
Associate Professor of Medicine
Divisions of Critical Care, Pulmonary and Sleep Medicine
University of Texas Health–McGovern Medical School
Houston, Texas

Anupam Kumar, MD, FCCP
Assistant Professor of Medicine
Director, Interstitial Lung Disease Clinic
Divisions of Pulmonary and Critical Care Medicine
Baylor College of Medicine
Houston, Texas

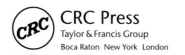

CRC Press is an imprint of the
Taylor & Francis Group, an **informa** business

First edition published 2023
by CRC Press
6000 Broken Sound Parkway NW, Suite 300, Boca Raton, FL 33487-2742

and by CRC Press
4 Park Square, Milton Park, Abingdon, Oxon, OX14 4RN

CRC Press is an imprint of Taylor & Francis Group, LLC

© 2023 Taylor & Francis Group, LLC

This book contains information obtained from authentic and highly regarded sources. While all reasonable efforts have been made to publish reliable data and information, neither the author[s] nor the publisher can accept any legal responsibility or liability for any errors or omissions that may be made. The publishers wish to make clear that any views or opinions expressed in this book by individual editors, authors or contributors are personal to them and do not necessarily reflect the views/opinions of the publishers. The information or guidance contained in this book is intended for use by medical, scientific or health-care professionals and is provided strictly as a supplement to the medical or other professional's own judgement, their knowledge of the patient's medical history, relevant manufacturer's instructions and the appropriate best practice guidelines. Because of the rapid advances in medical science, any information or advice on dosages, procedures or diagnoses should be independently verified. The reader is strongly urged to consult the relevant national drug formulary and the drug companies' and device or material manufacturers' printed instructions, and their websites, before administering or utilizing any of the drugs, devices or materials mentioned in this book. This book does not indicate whether a particular treatment is appropriate or suitable for a particular individual. Ultimately it is the sole responsibility of the medical professional to make his or her own professional judgements, so as to advise and treat patients appropriately. The authors and publishers have also attempted to trace the copyright holders of all material reproduced in this publication and apologize to copyright holders if permission to publish in this form has not been obtained. If any copyright material has not been acknowledged, please write and let us know so we may rectify in any future reprint.

Except as permitted under U.S. Copyright Law, no part of this book may be reprinted, reproduced, transmitted, or utilized in any form by any electronic, mechanical, or other means, now known or hereafter invented, including photocopying, microfilming, and recording, or in any information storage or retrieval system, without written permission from the publishers.

For permission to photocopy or use material electronically from this work, access www.copyright.com or contact the Copyright Clearance Center, Inc. (CCC), 222 Rosewood Drive, Danvers, MA 01923, 978-750-8400. For works that are not available on CCC please contact mpkbookspermissions@tandf.co.uk

Trademark notice: Product or corporate names may be trademarks or registered trademarks and are used only for identification and explanation without intent to infringe.

Library of Congress Cataloging-in-Publication Data

Names: Cherian, Sujith V., editor. | Kumar, Anupam, MD, editor.
Title: Rare lung diseases : a comprehensive clinical guide to diagnosis and management / edited by Sujith V Cherian, Anupam Kumar.
Description: First edition. | Boca Raton, FL : CRC Press, 2023. | Includes bibliographical references and index. | Summary: "This book aims to be a complete guide to diagnose, manage and treat rare lung diseases encountered by practicing pulmonologists and trainees. This comprehensive review facilitates the study and understanding of this complex and diverse set of disorders, focusing on differential diagnosis and evidence-based discussions of management algorithms"-- Provided by publisher.
Identifiers: LCCN 2022043144 (print) | LCCN 2022043145 (ebook) | ISBN 9780367544560 (hardback) | ISBN 9780367544553 (paperback) | ISBN 9781003089384 (ebook)
Subjects: MESH: Lung Diseases | Rare Diseases
Classification: LCC RC756 (print) | LCC RC756 (ebook) | NLM WF 630 | DDC 616.2/4--dc23/eng/20220919
LC record available at https://lccn.loc.gov/2022043144
LC ebook record available at https://lccn.loc.gov/2022043145

ISBN: 9780367544560 (hbk)
ISBN: 9780367544553 (pbk)
ISBN: 9781003089384 (ebk)

DOI: 10.1201/9781003089384

Typeset in Warnock
by KnowledgeWorks Global Ltd.

DEDICATIONS

To my parents who taught by example the value of hard work, perseverance, and dedication; to my wife, Elena for her constant support and encouragement, my children Eva, Sasha, and Isaac who constantly bring happiness and cheer in my journey, and to all the patients to whom I will forever remain indebted.

— **Sujith V. Cherian**

To my dearest parents, wife Aparna, children Sapna and Sanjay, teachers, and the countless patients for whom I dedicate this book — this publication is an acknowledgment of their lives and daily struggles.

— **Anupam Kumar**

CONTENTS

Foreword ix
Preface xi
Editors xiii
Contributors xv

1 Introduction 1
  Sujith V. Cherian and Anupam Kumar

2 Developmental Lung Anomalies in Adults 3
  Oriana Salamo, Logan Hostetter, Alberto A. Goizueta, Daniel Ocazionez-Trujillo, and Sujith V. Cherian

PART A: RARE GENETIC LUNG DISEASES

3 Genetic Infiltrative Lung Diseases 15
  Isabel C. Mira-Avendano

4 Alpha-1 Antitrypsin Deficiency 20
  Vickram Tejwani and James K. Stoller

PART B: RARE AIRWAY DISORDERS

5 Benign Central Airway Disorders 33
  Prince Ntiamoah and Laura K. Frye

6 Bronchiolitis 42
  Bilal F. Samhouri and Jay H. Ryu

7 Allergic Bronchopulmonary Aspergillosis (ABPA) 51
  Sunjay R. Devarajan and Nicola A. Hanania

PART C: RARE PULMONARY VASCULAR DISEASES

8 Pulmonary Arteriovenous Malformations (PAVMs) and Hereditary Hemorrhagic Telangiectasia (HHT) 57
  Minkyung Kwon, Daniil Gekhman, Carlos Rojas, and Augustine Lee

9 Diffuse Alveolar Hemorrhage (DAH) Syndromes 63
  Gaurav Manek and Rendell W. Ashton

10 Pulmonary Veno-Occlusive Disease and Pulmonary Capillary Hemangiomatosis 70
   Dana Gross, Akhilesh Padhye, Roberto Barrios, and Sandeep Sahay

PART D: RARE DIFFUSE PARENCHYMAL LUNG DISEASES

11 Pleuroparenchymal Fibroelastosis (PPFE) 77
   Bhavna Seth and Sonye K. Danoff

12 Immunoglobulin G4-Related Lung Disease 85
   Lauren Abplanalp, Hira Iftikhar, and Girish B. Nair

13 Eosinophilic Lung Diseases 91
   Nauman A. Khan and Sujith V. Cherian

14 Hard Metal Lung Disease and Other Rare Occupational Lung Diseases 101
   Matthew Zheng, Robert M. Marron, and Sameep Sehgal

15 Adult Pulmonary Alveolar Proteinosis 110
   Katherine Richards, Anupam Kumar, and Tisha Wang

PART E: RARE DIFFUSE CYSTIC LUNG DISEASES

16 Lymphangioleiomyomatosis 116
   Rosa M. Estrada-Y-Martin

17 Lymphocytic Interstitial Pneumonia and Associated Cystic Lung Diseases 125
   Evelyn Lynn, Liam Jeremiah Chawke, Aurelie Fabre, David J. Murphy, and Cormac McCarthy

vii

18	Birt–Hogg–Dubé Syndrome	132
	Stephan A. Reyes and Rosa M. Estrada-Y-Martin	
19	Pulmonary Langerhans Cell Histiocytosis and Other Histiocytic Lung Diseases	137
	Maryam Kaous, Bihong Zhao, and Isabel C. Mira-Avendano	

PART F: RARE PULMONARY NEOPLASMS

20	Primary Pulmonary Lymphoproliferative Neoplasms	145
	Bibi Aneesah Jaumally, Khalid Mohamed Ahmed, and Saadia A. Faiz	
21	Diffuse Idiopathic Pulmonary Neuroendocrine Cell Hyperplasia	153
	Amitha M. Avasarala, Sameer K. Avasarala, Sanjay Mukhopadhyay, Subha Ghosh, and Atul C. Mehta	
22	Pulmonary Amyloidosis	160
	Parijat Sen and Said Chaaban	
23	Primary Tracheal Tumors	168
	Moiz Salahuddin and Carlos A. Jimenez	

PART G: RARE PLEURAL DISORDERS

24	Unusual Causes of Pleural Effusion	177
	Niranjan Setty, Nai-Chien Huan, and Rajesh Thomas	
25	Thoracic Endometriosis	194
	Ravi Kanth Velagapudi and John P. Egan	
26	Tumors of the Pleura	199
	Nai-Chien Huan and Rajesh Thomas	

Index 212

FOREWORD

It is the first week of March 2022, as I write this foreword. The pandemic of COVID-19 seems to be waning after more than two years of unrelenting misery and desperation. The enormous toll this scourge has taken is yet to be fully understood. It was a week before observed Rare Disease Day on February 28, 2022, a day dedicated to "raising awareness and generating change for the 300 million people worldwide living with a rare disease, their families and carers." On Rare Disease Day, many events occur across the globe and people connect. Rare diseases have a severe impact on affected patients and families as well as posing a heavy burden on society. Those with rare diseases likely suffered disproportionately through the COVID-19 pandemic, adding to their sense of isolation.

In the United States, rare (orphan) disease is defined as a disease or condition affecting fewer than 200,000 persons, but the definition varies across the globe with the average prevalence threshold of 40 to 50 cases per 100,000 persons. Because there are more than 6,000 rare diseases, an estimated 25 million people are affected in the United States alone. Although some rare diseases may be recognized promptly, correct diagnosis often takes years, exposing patients to harm from numerous diagnostic procedures, progression of disease, and inappropriate treatments. Even when diagnosed, patients with rare diseases may be faced with a lack of effective therapy.

In years past, rare diseases were often considered unlikely to be a productive focus for research by policy makers and funding agencies. However, remarkable progress has been made in the understanding of many of these rare diseases in recent years, although even basic understanding is lacking in others. In some cases, this scientific progress has led to new effective treatments. Examples of this progress among pulmonary disorders include sirolimus therapy for lymphangioleiomyomatosis (LAM), a disorder thought to be nearly always fatal not many years ago, and granulocyte-macrophage colony-stimulating factor (GM-CSF) therapy for pulmonary alveolar proteinosis (PAP). Much of this advance has involved identification of genetic causes of rare diseases with innovative approaches and technologies. Elucidation of underlying molecular mechanisms has led to targeted treatments, as in LAM and PAP. In addition, discoveries achieved in rare diseases have led to important insights into the pathogenic mechanisms underlying more common diseases, and thus, to new targets for therapies.

The progress achieved in the understanding of rare diseases has been made possible not only by technologic innovations, genomic revolution, and skilled scientists, but also patient/family advocacy groups whose energy and participation have not only raised the awareness for rare diseases but also research funding. Patients are the ones who are intimately familiar with the effects of rare diseases and their perspective has helped guide the researchers and clinicians in their investigative endeavours though collaborative partnerships.

One of the difficulties patients with rare diseases face is delayed diagnosis since many clinicians may have never encountered these diseases. From the clinician's perspective, the diagnosis of rare or unusual diseases is to consider a broad differential diagnosis in the initial diagnostic assessment, since failure to diagnose rare diseases generally results from not having considered the diagnosis in the first place. It also helps to recognize the characteristic patterns of presentation associated with these disorders.

Thus, it is hoped that this book provides state-of-the-art reviews on a variety of rare lung diseases to facilitate timely diagnosis and appropriate management of patients affected with these disorders. The rapid pace of scientific advances in recent years has fueled hope and optimism that more effective therapies will continue to be identified that will result in meaningful improvements in the lives of patients with rare lung diseases. I wish to express my gratitude and congratulations to the editors, Drs. Sujith V. Cherian and Anupam Kumar, and the authors for their contributions to this inspiring work.

Jay H. Ryu, MD
Consultant, Division of Pulmonary and Critical Care Medicine
Dr. David E. and Bette H. Dines Professor of Pulmonary
and Critical Care Medicine
Mayo Clinic College of Medicine and Science
Rochester, Minnesota

PREFACE

Patients with respiratory disorders have an inherent disadvantage in that irrespective of the type of lung disease, their symptoms are often nonspecific and presentation is delayed. Within respiratory disorders, patients with rare lung disorders are probably the most "orphaned" due to a marked delay in securing a diagnosis, relative lack of knowledge in the physician community, and a paucity of effective treatment modalities. From the research standpoint, these conditions pose a challenge to gain a comprehensive understanding due to the inability to recruit adequate number of patients and a lack of appropriate funding, as opposed to the more common respiratory ailments. While no specific definition exists for rare lung disorders, they are a markedly heterogeneous group of lung disorders that are characterized by distinct clinical presentation, radiographic features, and natural history. There is no reliable data on the epidemiology of rare lung diseases, but they all share the common trait of being universally appreciated but notoriously under-recognized. In terms of classification, rare lung disorders can be either primary (mainly involving the lung as a sole or dominant manifestation) or secondary (lung involvement secondary to rare systemic causes). They may also be classified based on underlying pathogenesis (i.e., genetic, or iatrogenic causes) or the primary site of involvement within the respiratory system (airways, parenchyma, vasculature, and pleura).

The primary objective of this book is to provide a concise review of the clinical features, natural history, diagnosis, and management of the most appreciated rare lung disorders. The topics that have been included in the book are broadly classified into selected rare genetic, airway, vascular, parenchymal, cystic, neoplastic, and pleural disorders. Within these broad topics, we have included conditions we thought the clinical community may be most keen to know, and where treatment could make a difference for the patient. We have omitted rare pulmonary infections, pulmonary vasculitis, and drug-related toxicities.

Our hope is that readers of this book will find it to be a contemporary review of the rare pulmonary disorders discussed, but at the same time, handy and engaging. The book focuses on the clinical aspects of these conditions. We thank the contributors to this textbook who are experts in their respective fields and those with a keen interest in the topic they have written. We would also like to thank the editorial staff of the publishing house for keeping us focused on the timeline and for their assistance at every stage of the book design.

Sujith V. Cherian, MD, FCCP
Anupam Kumar, MD, FCCP

EDITORS

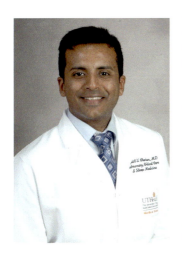

Sujith V. Cherian, MD, FCCP, is Associate Professor of Internal Medicine, in the Divisions of Critical Care, Pulmonary and Sleep Medicine at the University of Texas Health–McGovern Medical School, Houston. He developed a keen interest in rare lung diseases during his training, with several publications focusing on rare lung diseases. He teaches medical students, residents, and clinical fellows on several topics, including rare lung diseases, for which he has received several teaching awards and was recently inducted into the Academy of Master Educators at UT Health. He frequently talks at grand rounds, seminars, and has been invited to present at both local, national, and international conferences. Dr. Cherian is an elected fellow of the American College of Chest Physicians (ACCP) and is a member of several national and international pulmonary organizations including the World Organization of Bronchology and Interventional Pulmonology and the American Association of Bronchology and Interventional Pulmonology. He holds several leadership positions in the ACCP and serves on the editorial board of several journals including *CHEST* and *Shanghai Chest*. Furthermore, he is section editor of *Occupational and Environmental Lung Diseases in Current Pulmonology Reports* and serves as a peer reviewer for several leading respiratory journals worldwide.

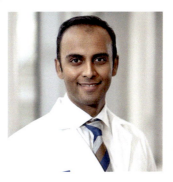

Anupam Kumar, MD, FCCP, is an Assistant Professor of Medicine in the Division of Pulmonary and Critical Care Medicine at Baylor College of Medicine, Houston, Texas. He is also the Director of the Interstitial Lung Diseases (ILD) Clinic at Baylor College of Medicine. His areas of expertise include interstitial lung diseases, acute respiratory distress syndrome (ARDS), and lung transplantation. Within interstitial lung diseases, he has an affinity for rare lung disorders, particularly cystic lung diseases and pulmonary alveolar proteinosis. He has published on various topics of interstitial lung diseases in leading journals in the field of respiratory medicine and popular online educational resources such as UpToDate.com. He is a recipient of the Distinguished Educator Award in Pulmonary Medicine by the American College of Chest Physicians (ACCP). He is a peer reviewer for several respiratory medicine journals and serves on the editorial board of a few of them. Dr. Kumar is an active member of the Lung Transplant Steering Committee of ACCP and holds the designation of Fellow of the American College of Chest Physicians (FCCP).

CONTRIBUTORS

Lauren Abplanalp
Division of Pulmonary and Critical Care
Oakland University William Beaumont School of Medicine
Royal Oak, MI

Khalid Mohamed Ahmed
Divisions of Critical Care, Pulmonary and Sleep Medicine
University of Texas Health–McGovern Medical School
Houston, TX

Rendell W. Ashton
Department of Pulmonary, Critical Care and Sleep Medicine
Respiratory Institute
Cleveland Clinic
Cleveland, OH

Amitha M. Avasarala
Department of Medicine
University of Pittsburgh Medical Center (Mercy)
Pittsburgh, PA

Sameer K. Avasarala
Department of Pulmonary, Critical Care and Sleep Medicine
Case Western Reserve University School of Medicine
Cleveland, OH

Isabel C. Mira-Avendano
Divisions of Critical Care, Pulmonary and Sleep Medicine
University of Texas Health–McGovern Medical School
Houston, TX

Roberto Barrios
Houston Methodist Hospital
Houston, TX

Said Chaaban
Interstitial Lung Disease Program
Division of Pulmonary and Critical Care
University of Kentucky
Lexington, KY

Liam Jeremiah Chawke
Department of Respiratory Medicine
St. Vincent's University Hospital
Dublin, Ireland

Sujith V. Cherian
Divisions of Critical Care, Pulmonary and Sleep Medicine
University of Texas Health–McGovern Medical School
Houston, TX

Sonye K. Danoff
Department of Pulmonary and Critical Care Medicine
School of Medicine
Johns Hopkins University
Baltimore, MD

Sunjay R. Devarajan
Department of Pulmonary, Critical Care and Sleep Medicine
Baylor College of Medicine
Houston, TX

John P. Egan
Department of Pulmonary and Critical Care Medicine
Spectrum Health–Michigan State University College of Human Medicine
Grand Rapids, MI

Rosa M. Estrada-Y-Martin
Divisions of Critical Care, Pulmonary and Sleep Medicine
University of Texas Health–McGovern Medical School
Houston, TX

Aurelie Fabre
Department of Histopathology
St. Vincent's University Hospital
Department of Medicine
University College
Dublin, Ireland

Saadia A. Faiz
Department of Pulmonary Medicine
University of Texas MD Anderson Cancer Center
Houston, TX

Laura K. Frye
Division of Respiratory, Critical Care, and Occupational Pulmonary Medicine
University of Utah
Salt Lake City, UT

Daniil Gekhman
Department of Pulmonary, Critical Care and Sleep Medicine
Baylor College of Medicine
Houston, TX

Subha Ghosh
Department of Thoracic Radiology
Cleveland Clinic
Cleveland, OH

Alberto A. Goizueta
Department of Pulmonary Medicine
University of Texas MD Anderson Cancer Center
Houston, TX

Dana Gross
Division of Pulmonary and Critical Care Medicine
University of Miami Hospital
Miami, FL

Nicola A. Hanania
Department of Pulmonary, Critical Care and Sleep Medicine
Ben Taub Hospital
Baylor College of Medicine
Houston, TX

Logan Hostetter
Department of Internal Medicine
Divisions of Critical Care, Pulmonary and Sleep Medicine
University of Texas Health–McGovern Medical School
Houston, TX

Nai-Chien Huan
Department of Respiratory Medicine
Sir Charles Gairdner Hospital
Perth, Australia
and
Department of Respiratory Medicine
Queen Elizabeth Hospital
Kota Kinabalu, Malaysia

Hira Iftikhar
Division of Pulmonary and Critical Care
Oakland University William Beaumont School of Medicine
Royal Oak, MI

Bibi Aneesah Jaumally
Division of Pulmonary, Allergy and Critical Care Medicine
University of Alabama
Birmingham, AL

Carlos A. Jimenez
Department of Pulmonary Medicine
University of Texas MD Anderson Cancer Center
Houston, TX

Maryam Kaous
Divisions of Critical Care, Pulmonary and Sleep Medicine
University of Texas Health–McGovern Medical School
Houston, TX

Nauman A. Khan
Department of Internal Medicine
Divisions of Critical Care, Pulmonary and Sleep Medicine
University of Texas Health–McGovern Medical School
Houston, TX

Anupam Kumar
Divisions of Pulmonary and Critical Care Medicine
Baylor College of Medicine
Houston, TX

Minkyung Kwon
Department of Pulmonary, Critical Care and Sleep Medicine
Baylor College of Medicine
Houston, TX

Augustine Lee
Department of Pulmonary Medicine
Mayo Clinic
Jacksonville, FL

Evelyn Lynn
Department of Respiratory Medicine
St. Vincent's University Hospital
Dublin, Ireland

Gaurav Manek
Department of Pulmonary, Critical Care and Sleep Medicine
Respiratory Institute
Cleveland Clinic
Cleveland, OH

Robert M. Marron
Department of Thoracic Medicine and Surgery
Temple University Hospital
Philadelphia, PA

Cormac McCarthy
Department of Respiratory Medicine
St. Vincent's University Hospital
Department of Medicine
University College
Dublin, Ireland

Atul C. Mehta
Lerner College of Medicine
Respiratory Institute
Cleveland Clinic
Cleveland, OH

Sanjay Mukhopadhyay
Pulmonary Pathology
Cleveland Clinic
Cleveland, OH

David J. Murphy
Department of Radiology
St. Vincent's University Hospital
Dublin, Ireland

Girish B. Nair
Division of Pulmonary and Critical Care
Oakland University William Beaumont School of Medicine
Royal Oak, MI

Prince Ntiamoah
Department of Pulmonary, Critical Care and Sleep Medicine
Respiratory Institute
Cleveland Clinic
Cleveland, OH

Daniel Ocazionez-Trujillo
Department of Diagnostic and Interventional Imaging
University of Texas Health–McGovern Medical School
Houston, TX

Akhilesh Padhye
Department of Internal Medicine
Houston Methodist Hospital
Houston, TX

Stephan A. Reyes
Department of Internal Medicine
Divisions of Critical Care, Pulmonary and Sleep Medicine
University of Texas Health–McGovern Medical School
Houston, TX

Katherine Richards
Department of Pulmonary, Critical Care and Sleep Medicine
Baylor College of Medicine
Houston, TX

Carlos Rojas
Department of Radiology
Mayo Clinic
Scottsdale, AZ

Jay H. Ryu
Division of Pulmonary and Critical Care Medicine
Mayo Clinic
Rochester, MN

Sandeep Sahay
Division of Pulmonary, Critical Care and Sleep Medicine
Houston Methodist Hospital
Houston, TX

Moiz Salahuddin
Department of Pulmonology
Aga Khan University
Karachi, Pakistan

Oriana Salamo
Department of Internal Medicine
Divisions of Critical Care, Pulmonary and Sleep Medicine
University of Texas Health–McGovern Medical School
Houston, TX

Bilal F. Samhouri
Division of Pulmonary and Critical Care Medicine
Mayo Clinic
Rochester, MN

Sameep Sehgal
Department of Pulmonary Medicine
Cleveland Clinic
Cleveland, OH

Parijat Sen
Division of Pulmonary and Critical Care
University of Kentucky
Lexington, KY

Bhavna Seth
Department of Pulmonary and Critical Care Medicine,
Johns Hopkins University
Baltimore, MD

Niranjan Setty
Department of Respiratory Medicine
Sir Charles Gairdner Hospital
Perth, Australia

James K. Stoller
Cleveland Clinic
Cleveland, OH

Vickram Tejwani
Department of Pulmonary, Critical Care and Sleep Medicine
Respiratory Institute
Cleveland Clinic
Cleveland, OH

Contributors

Rajesh Thomas
Department of Respiratory Medicine
Sir Charles Gairdner Hospital
School of Medicine
University of Western Australia
Institute for Respiratory Health
Perth, Australia

Ravi Kanth Velagapudi
Department of Pulmonary & Critical
 Care Medicine
Spectrum Health–Michigan State
 University College of Human Medicine
Grand Rapids, MI

Tisha Wang
Department of Medicine
UCLA Division of Pulmonary, Critical
 Care, and Sleep Medicine
Los Angeles, CA

Bihong Zhao
Department of Pathology and Laboratory
 Medicine
University of Texas Health–McGovern
 Medical School
Houston, TX

Matthew Zheng
Department of Thoracic Medicine and
 Surgery
Temple University Hospital
Philadelphia, PA

1

INTRODUCTION

Sujith V. Cherian and Anupam Kumar

Contents

Introduction 1
Patient resources 1
Future directions 1
References..2

Introduction

Although not precisely known, approximately 1.2–2.5 million patients within the United States and 1.5–3 million patients within Europe are estimated to have rare lung diseases (RLDs) (1). Rare diseases have been defined numerically within the United States, as occurring less than 1 person in 200,000 people. However, RLDs are frequently undiagnosed, misdiagnosed, and typically associated with protracted delays in diagnosis. This is attributable to a multitude of factors such as lack of specificity of symptoms, paucity of data, deficiency of knowledge, and a lack of standardized guidelines for diagnosis. A 2005 EURORDIS survey of 5,980 patients with eight different rare diseases showed that 25% of patients had a delay of 5–30 years from first symptoms to a final diagnosis. Misdiagnosis was reported at 40%, and unnecessary interventions including inappropriate surgery and inappropriate medical therapy were performed in 16% and 33% patients, respectively. Furthermore, at least 18% of respondents felt they were "rejected" by their physician because of disease complexity or associated symptoms (2). Such delays have a significant negative impact on the quality of life of the patient. Furthermore, a timely diagnosis will obviate the need for additional tests, ineffective treatments, and potentially reduce hospitalizations—all of which can considerably mitigate the burden of healthcare expenditure per patient (3).

There is substantial heterogeneity among the various conditions that are categorized together as RLDs. Some RLDs, such as idiopathic pulmonary fibrosis and idiopathic pulmonary hypertension (not addressed in this publication) are more common than the other (e.g., developmental anomalies of the lung), while some primarily affect the lung (pulmonary alveolar proteinosis, pulmonary alveolar microlithiasis) as opposed to other conditions where the lung is only one of the organs involved (neurofibromatosis, lipid storage diseases). Furthermore, some diseases may be gender specific (lymphangioleiomyomatosis in women) (3). Thus, RLDs, by virtue of their rarity and heterogeneity, remain a diagnostic challenge for the pulmonology community.

Historically, clinical research in RLDs has been limited due to several reasons: (1) reluctance within the pharmaceutical industry to invest in RLDs due to the potentially low probability of investment returns from expected sales of the products, (2) lack of resources (e.g., databases and registries), (3) absence of a research community focusing on RLDs, and (4) difficulty with recruiting adequate number of patients into clinical trials due to the rarity of these entities (4). Over the last three decades, however, several new policies have come in to effect that have been initiated to promote clinical research in these diseases, such as the "Orphan Drug Act," which was developed to finance rare drug research and to develop new treatments for these patients. Prior to 1980, there were less than 10 products (treatments and devices for management of rare diseases) within the market, while over the last 30 years, there have been more than 400 such products within the market (5). Multicenter randomized controlled trials have been considered the gold standard of obtaining evidence on the efficacy of management approaches in any disease condition, but as stated above, with the rarity of these lung conditions, it is not possible in most cases, particularly the rarer entities. In these settings, alternate research modifications by investigators such as crossover, sequential, and adaptive study approaches (6) have been attempted with reasonable success rates. Moreover, focusing on clinically meaningful endpoints that predict survival (such as forced vital capacity, diffusing capacity for carbon monoxide), instead of mortality, may augment research recruitment and completion in the field of rare lung diseases (7).

Patient resources

Several well-established patient support organizations have emerged with a focus on RLDs. Both nationally and internationally, these organizations have been crucial in the education and support of patients and their families, fund raising, and encouragement of patients to enroll in clinical trials. Within the United States, a nonprofit network of patient organizations, healthcare providers, and individuals focusing on RLDs is the National Organization of Rare Diseases (NORD). Similarly, within Europe, the European Organization of Rare Diseases exists (Table 1.1). The goal of such organizations has been to maximize resources, with coordination of research efforts to promote international collaboration in the specialty of rare diseases. Starting registries as part of the international collaborative effort has been an asset not only for patient recruitment in clinical trials but also to help in the conduct and development of several epidemiological studies (3, 4).

Future directions

Substantial progress has been made in the field of RLD within the last decade. This is the result of the concerted and collaborative efforts of clinician scientists, patient organizations, and pharmaceutical companies. Several of these disorders such as lymphangioleiomyomatosis (8) and pulmonary arterial hypertension (9) have witnessed well-conducted studies resulting in the

DOI: 10.1201/9781003089384-1

TABLE 1.1: A Few Important Web Resources for Patients with Rare Lung Diseases (Not Fully Inclusive)

Orphanet: http://www.orpha.net

National Organization for Rare Disorders (NORD): http://www.rarediseases.org

Office of Rare Disease Research, US National Institutes of Health: http://www.rarediseases.info.nih.gov

Rare Diseases Clinical Research Network, US National Institutes of Health: http://rarediseasesnetwork.epi.usf.edu

International Rare Disease Research Consortium: http://www.irdirc.org

Pulmonary Fibrosis Foundation: http://www.pulmonaryfibrosis.org

Hereditary Hemorrhagic Telangiectasia: https://curehht.org/

Pulmonary Alveolar Proteinosis: https://www.papfoundation.org/

WASOG (World Association of Sarcoidosis and Other Granulomatous Disorders)— includes several national sites: http://www.wasog.org/patient_societies.htm

Endometriosis foundation of America: www.endofound.org

Hermansky-Pudlak Syndrome Network: http://www.hermansky-pudlak.org

The Lymphangioleiomyomatosis (LAM) Foundation: http://www.thelamfoundation.org

Pulmonary Hypertension Association: http://www.phassociation.org, http://www.phaeurope.org, http://www.phacanada.ca/en, http://www.phassociation.uk.com

---

development of novel treatment strategies with important clinical implications. Thus, research in these RLDs has resulted in them not being "orphan" anymore. While this represents only a handful of RLDs, there is an imminent need to extend the research efforts toward other RLDs. This requires a devoted effort toward education of pulmonologists (both in community and academic setting), establishment of dedicated referral centers to help take care of these patients, and promoting development of registries that enroll patients with RLDs. This will help lay the foundation for robust clinical studies to be performed worldwide with downstream reduction in patient morbidity and improvement in their quality of life.

References

1. Haffner ME, Whitley J, Moses M. Two decades of orphan product development. Nat Rev Drug Discov. 2002;1(10):821–5.
2. Survey of the Delay in Diagnosis for 8 Rare Diseases in Europe ('EURORDISCARE 2') [Internet]. 2007 [cited 01-24-2022]. Available from: https://www.eurordis.org/publication/survey-delay-diagnosis-8-rare-diseases-europe-%E2%80%98eurordiscare2%E2%80%99.
3. Spagnolo P, du Bois RM, Cottin V. Rare lung disease and orphan drug development. Lancet Respir Med. 2013;1(6):479–87.
4. Spagnolo P adBR. The Challenges of Clinical Research in Orphan Diseases. In: V Cottin, J-F Cordier, L Richeldi, editors. Orphan Lung Diseases: A Clinical Guide to Rare Lung Diseases. London: Springer-Verlag; 2015. p. 5–15.
5. Victory for a rare alliance. Lancet Respir Med. 2013;1(6):423.
6. Buckley BM. Clinical trials of orphan medicines. Lancet. 2008;371(9629):2051–5.
7. du Bois RM, Weycker D, Albera C, Bradford WZ, Costabel U, Kartashov A, et al. Forced vital capacity in patients with idiopathic pulmonary fibrosis: Test properties and minimal clinically important difference. Am J Respir Crit Care Med. 2011;184(12):1382–9.
8. McCormack FX, Inoue Y, Moss J, Singer LG, Strange C, Nakata K, et al. Efficacy and safety of sirolimus in lymphangioleiomyomatosis. N Engl J Med. 2011;364(17):1595–606.
9. Humbert M, Sitbon O, Simonneau G. Treatment of pulmonary arterial hypertension. N Engl J Med. 2004;351(14):1425–36.

2

DEVELOPMENTAL LUNG ANOMALIES IN ADULTS

Oriana Salamo, Logan Hostetter, Alberto A. Goizueta, Daniel Ocazionez-Trujillo, and Sujith V. Cherian

Contents

Introduction 3
Embryology of the lung and vasculature 3
Developmental lung anomalies in adults 4
Conclusion 13
References 13

KEY POINTS

- Developmental lung anomalies (DLAs) are structural defects arising from an aberrant embryologic process with an estimated incidence between 30 and 42 cases per 100,000 people.
- Although DLAs are usually discovered antenatally or in early childhood, they may be diagnosed later in adulthood.
- DLAs may present with nonspecific respiratory complaints or are found incidentally on chest imaging.
- DLAs are classified into three broad categories: bronchopulmonary, vascular, or combined lung and vascular anomalies.
- Careful radiological evaluation along with adequate knowledge of these rare entities helps clinch the diagnosis in most cases.
- Management of asymptomatic cases is not well-defined and controversial, while in symptomatic cases, surgical resection is required in the majority of DLAs.

Introduction

Developmental lung anomalies (DLAs) are structural defects arising from an aberrant embryologic process, accounting for 5–18% of all congenital abnormalities, with an estimated incidence between 30 and 42 cases per 100,000 (1). Most DLAs are typically discovered early in life, commonly prenatally during routine maternofetal ultrasound, or identified in the neonatal period or early childhood. However, a considerable number of patients with a DLA go unnoticed until later in life, representing a diagnostic challenge for the clinicians (2). While a significant number of DLAs in the adult population are asymptomatic and incidentally found on chest imaging, others may present with nonspecific respiratory complaints, such as cough, wheezing, or frequent lower respiratory tract infections, to more severe disease, such as pneumothorax, high-output heart failure, malignant transformation, or even life-threatening bleeding (3). Given its wide range of symptoms and no distinctive clinical characteristics, the recognition of DLAs relies on the identification of exclusive radiologic features to elucidate the diagnosis within the appropriate clinical context. Certainly, any thoracic asymmetry in the absence of previous surgeries or trauma, as well as any intrathoracic focal cystic or solid mass, or any well-defined hyperlucency, should raise suspicion for an underlying DLA in the right clinical context. As a result, it is imperative to raise awareness of DLAs in the adult population given the wide spectrum of symptoms and radiologic findings on chest imaging, including plain radiographs, ultrasonography (US), computed tomography (CT), and magnetic resonance imaging (MRI).

Overall, DLAs are a heterogenous group of disorders that can be classified into three broad categories: bronchopulmonary, vascular, or combined lung and vascular anomalies (4). Bronchopulmonary anomalies originate from an insult to the lung bud, an embryological endodermal structure that develops into the airways and the lung parenchyma, while vascular anomalies are caused by aberrant angiogenesis (5). Unfortunately, there is limited information regarding DLAs in the adult population since most of the available literature is focused in the pediatric setting or is presented as a radiological review. Knowledge of the incidence, clinical presentation, radiological appearance, and possible complications is of paramount importance for the pulmonologist given its wide-ranging clinical spectrum and implications in patient mortality and morbidity with delays in diagnosis. In this review, we provide insight into DLAs, briefly discussing the embryologic development of the lung and its vasculature while highlighting the most common anomalies in the adult population.

Embryology of the lung and vasculature

DLAs with abnormalities in anatomy are better understood by reviewing the embryology that gives rise to these structures.

The fetal lung begins to form at four weeks' gestation from the ventral foregut by creating an out pouching referred to as the lung bud; the development of which is dependent upon retinoic acid from surrounding mesodermal cells. The lung bud continues development via tracheoesophageal ridge formation separating the dorsal portion of the foregut forming the esophagus and the

DOI: 10.1201/9781003089384-2

ventral respiratory diverticulum, which comprise the trachea and lung buds. During the fifth week of development, the bronchial buds form the left and right main system bronchi with further division into three secondary bronchi on the right and two secondary bronchi on the left. The bronchi undergo sequential divisions creating the segmental bronchi of the adult lung. Further lung maturation is divided into three prenatal phases and a postnatal phase. The pseudoglandular period occurs during weeks 5–16, where tertiary bronchi divide to form terminal bronchioles. This is followed by the canalicular period (16–26 weeks) where terminal bronchioles form respiratory bronchioles and alveolar ducts. The third embryonic phase is the terminal sac period (26 weeks–birth) where primitive alveoli are formed and encounter capillaries. A fourth phase of maturation occurs during the postnatal period (8 months–childhood) where alveoli continue to propagate capillary bed contacts (6, 7). The pleural cavity is created by the visceral pleura arising from mesoderm surrounding the outside of the lung buds and parietal pleura is derived from somatic mesoderm of the body wall; the combination of which surrounds the mediastinal cavity and the lungs creating the intrapleural space (6, 7). Pulmonary veins arise from the posterior left atrium and connect with the veins of the lung bud. The primitive pulmonary artery arises as a major branch budding off the sixth aortic arch and while in close contact with the airways divides into the arterial system during lung bud formation and the pseudoglandular division phases. The highly sequential divisional phases of forming the lungs create ample opportunity for division malformations involving a coalescence of vasculature and parenchymal structures (6, 7).

Developmental lung anomalies in adults

Bronchopulmonary anomalies
Pulmonary agenesis, aplasia, and hypoplasia
Pulmonary agenesis (PA), initially described by De Pozze in 1673, is a rare DLA that arises from an abnormal development of the primitive lung bud, with an estimated incidence between 0.003 and 0.009% (8). The exact etiology of PA is still unknown; however, vitamin A and folate deficiency, genetic factors, and intrauterine viral infections have been proposed factors that can affect the normal development of the lung (9). Left-sided PA is found in 70% of the cases, and it usually has a better prognosis when compared to right-sided PA. Moreover, patients with right-sided PA (Figure 2.1) generally have mediastinal shift and malrotation of the carina, leading to venous return impairment and recurrent pulmonary infections (9). Around 50% of patients with PA have associated congenital anomalies, such as heart disease (patent ductus arteriosus, patent foramen ovale, tetralogy of Fallot, total anomalous pulmonary venous return), gastroesophageal anomalies (tracheoesophageal fistulas, duodenal atresia), and skeletal malformations. Most patients with PA and associated congenital anomalies are diagnosed prenatally or earlier in life, while those with isolated PA can remain asymptomatic until adulthood. Recurrent respiratory tract infections are commonly seen in adult patients with PA.

PA was originally classified into three groups according to the developmental stage of the primitive lung bud by Schneider in 1912 and was later modified by Boyden in 1955. Type 1 (agenesis) is a complete absence of lung and bronchus with no vascular supply, type 2 (aplasia) is a rudimentary bronchus with complete absence of pulmonary parenchyma (Figure 2.1), while type 3 (hypoplasia) is the presence of variable amounts of bronchial tree, pulmonary parenchyma, and supporting vasculature (10). On chest radiographs, PA can be seen as a radiopaque hemithorax with ipsilateral mediastinal shift and contralateral compensatory overinflation. Chest CT helps to visualize the rudimentary bronchus, while pulmonary angiography confirms the absence of the ipsilateral pulmonary vasculature. Conservative management is recommended for asymptomatic patients. For those with recurrent infections, bronchial stump resection is advised.

Congenital bronchial atresia
Congenital bronchial atresia (CBA) is a rare congenital anomaly more frequently seen in males, with an estimated prevalence of 1.2 cases per 100,000 (11). It consists in a focal interruption of a proximal bronchus, resulting in a cul-de-sac termination at a lobar, segmental, or subsegmental level, with preservation of the distal bronchial tree (12). The etiology of CBA has yet to be fully elucidated. Currently, there are two theories of pathogenesis: the first one proposes a disconnection between the terminal end of the bronchial bud and primitive bronchial cells, while the second one suggests a repetitive vascular insult resulting in focal ischemia (13). CBA is characterized by an obliterated

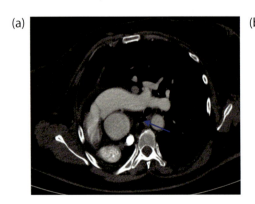 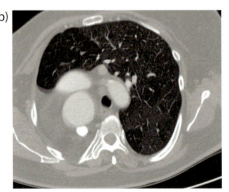

FIGURE 2.1 Pulmonary aplasia. (a–b) Axial CT images in soft tissue and lung windows demonstrating complete absence of the right pulmonary artery and agenesis of the right lung in a 56-year-old man. There is rightward mediastinal shift with compensatory hyperinflation of the left lung, which crosses the midline. Note the presence of rudimentary bronchus, consistent with pulmonary aplasia. (Reprinted from Cherian SV, Kumar A, Ocazionez D, Estrada-Y-Martin RM, Restrepo CS. Developmental lung anomalies in adults: A pictorial review. Respir Med. 2019;155:86–96. With permission from Elsevier.)

Developmental Lung Anomalies in Adults

bronchus, which is usually filled with mucus often resulting in a mucocele, with overexpansion of the normally developed distal parenchyma. The left upper lobe bronchus, specifically the apicoposterior segment, is the most frequently involved, followed by the right upper, middle, and lower lobes (3). CBA has been associated with other DLA, such as congenital lobar emphysema, congenital pulmonary airway malformation, and pulmonary sequestration (14).

CBA is usually diagnosed in early childhood, and it is rarely discovered later in life. In adults, CBA is typically asymptomatic, but can also present as recurrent postobstructive pneumonia, pneumothorax from spontaneous rupture of the hyperinflated lung, or degradation of the pulmonary parenchyma as a long-term complication. On chest x-ray, CBA appears as a perihilar mucocele, which is a well-defined circular opacity, with surrounding hyperlucency secondary to overexpansion and air trapping of the adjacent lung (3). Rarely, an air-fluid level can also be seen on imaging. Chest CT is the modality of choice since it allows better visualization of the mucocele, which is characterized as a distended, cylindrical, soft tissue opacity, typically described as a "finger-in-glove" appearance, and adjacent areas of hypoattenuated lung parenchyma (Figure 2.2) (13). Differential diagnosis should include endobronchial tumors, foreign body, or inflammatory strictures. The pathognomonic "blind-ending bronchus" is a bronchoscopic finding only present in approximately 50% of patients with this DLA. There are no current guidelines for the management of patients with CBA, but conservative management is recommended for asymptomatic patients. However, surgical

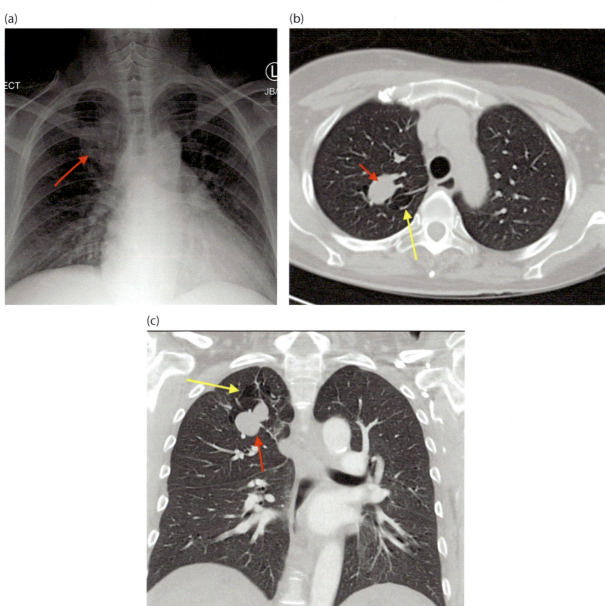

FIGURE 2.2 Congenital bronchial atresia. (a) Chest x-ray in a 51-year-old woman showing a right lobular opacity in the upper lobe found incidentally. (b) Chest CT in axial view showing the mucocele (red arrow) along with adjoining hyperlucent lung parenchyma (yellow arrow) consistent with bronchial atresia. (c) Coronal views showing the cylindrical "finger-in-glove" appearance of the mucocele (red arrow) along with hyperlucent lung parenchyma consistent with air trapping (yellow arrow).

resection is necessary for patients with recurrent and severe infections, for those with significant architectural compromise, or when malignant lesions cannot be excluded (15).

Bronchogenic cysts

Bronchogenic cysts (BCs) are considered a foregut malformation resulting from an abnormal budding of the developing tracheobronchial tree (3). Most BCs are in the mediastinum (65–90%), specifically in the subcarinal, followed by hilar, and paratracheal regions, while the remaining are found in the lung parenchyma, usually in the lower lobes (Figure 2.3) (5). Interestingly, BCs found in atypical locations, such as intracardiac, intramedullary, and retroperitoneal, have been reported (16–18). The cysts are typically solitary, unilocular, and thin-walled, lined by ciliated epithelium with bronchial mucus glands, surrounded by smooth muscle and cartilage (5). Most cysts are sealed without a communication with other structures. However, a small proportion of BCs have a patent connection with the airway, allowing the bacteria to enter the cavity, increasing the risk for frequent infections (2).

Most BCs are asymptomatic and incidentally found on chest imaging, especially when they are in the mediastinum. Conversely, patients with BCs can also develop symptoms depending on their size and location. The most frequent presentation is fever, chest pain, and productive cough, which represents recurrent lower respiratory tract infections, commonly seen in patients with bronchial communications (19). Around 45% of patients with BCs have complications, such as mass effect on the esophagus or main airway, pneumothorax, or rupture of the cyst into adjacent structures, especially the trachea, pleural, and pericardial cavity (20, 21). On chest x-ray, BCs are typically described as a well-rounded, soft tissue density, usually located in the subcarinal region, causing the main stem bronchi to be widened. Chest CT is the imaging of choice, and it usually demonstrates a cystic lesion with water attenuation in 50% of cases depending on the amount of proteinaceous content, with minimal or absent wall enhancement after contrast administration (2). It is also common to find displacement of the esophagus or main airway caused by extrinsic compression. Differential diagnosis of an infected BC should include lung abscess, hydatid cyst, fungal and mycobacterial infections, as well as malignancies.

Management of asymptomatic patients with BCs is a matter of debate. Most of the available recommendations are by thoracic surgeons, recommending the excision of the cysts because of their high risk for developing complications later in life, including malignant transformation (3). However, there are no large case series of asymptomatic patients with long-term follow-up to recommend against a conservative approach. On the other hand, the management of symptomatic patients is more straightforward. Surgical resection, via thoracoscopy or open approach, is generally preferred. Bronchoscopy with the endobronchial ultrasound (EBUS) for drainage has also been performed in patients that are considered high-risk surgical candidates (22).

Congenital lobar overinflation

Congenital lobar overinflation (CLO), also known as congenital lobar emphysema, is a DLA almost exclusively seen in neonates, more commonly in males, with an estimated incidence of 1 in 20,000–30,000 live births (23). CLO is characterized by hyperinflation of one or more segments of the lung with compression of adjacent structures. Left upper lobe, followed by right middle, and right upper lobe are the most frequently involved, with the lower lobes being rarely affected (24). The etiology of CLO remains unclear, and a definitive cause cannot be recognized in 50% of patients. Airway obstruction leading to air trapping can be classified into intrinsic and extrinsic causes in patients with CLO. An incomplete or defective cartilage formation causing bronchial wall weakening predisposes the airway to collapse, resulting in a "ball-valve" obstruction with subsequent air trapping as an example of intrinsic compression seen in 25% of cases (3). Furthermore, redundant mucosal folds, granulomas, and mucus plugging, which can be found in 25% of patients, are also considered intrinsic in nature (25). Extrinsic compression leading to significant air trapping can be seen in subjects with intrathoracic masses or vascular anomalies, such as anomalous pulmonary venous return or pulmonary artery sling. Interestingly, 12–20% of patients with CLO have concomitant congenital heart disease.

Patients with CLO may be asymptomatic until early adulthood. The magnitude of the affected lobe with emphysema, the compression of adjacent structures, and the extent of mediastinal shift determines the severity of the symptoms. Patients may present with gradual dyspnea, or sudden onset of chest pain and significant shortness of breath raising concerns for pneumothorax. It is frequent to find normal pulmonary function tests in

(a) 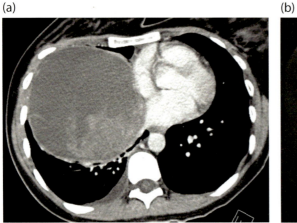 (b)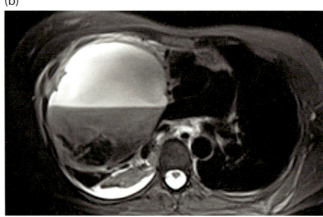

FIGURE 2.3 Infected intrapulmonary bronchogenic cyst. (a) Axial CT image demonstrates a cystic lesion in the right upper lobe with internal high-density components. (b) Axial T2W MRI demonstrating the cystic structure to contain fluid/fluid levels with internal hypointense foci.

Developmental Lung Anomalies in Adults

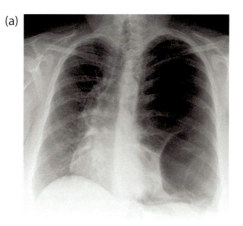 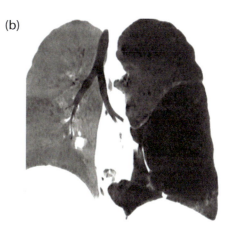

FIGURE 2.4 Congenital lobar overinflation. (a) Frontal chest x-ray demonstrating left upper lobe hyperinflation, hyperlucency and mass effect and rightward mediastinal shift consistent with congenital lobar overinflation. (b) Coronal minimum intensity (MinIP) demonstrate hyper-expansion of the left upper lobe with CLO in the left lower lobe. (Reprinted from Cherian SV, Kumar A, Ocazionez D, Estrada-Y-Martin RM, Restrepo CS. Developmental lung anomalies in adults: A pictorial review. Respir Med. 2019;155:86–96. With permission from Elsevier.)

asymptomatic patients or those with mild symptoms. However, typical obstruction is frequently seen in those with moderate to severe disease. Classic findings of overinflation and air trapping are seen on conventional chest x-rays and chest CT, such as flattening of the ipsilateral diaphragm, increased volume of the affected lobe, attenuated vascular markings (Figure 2.4), and mediastinal shift, with compression and atelectasis of the contralateral lung (26). Chest CT and chest MRI can be useful for demonstrating intrinsic or extrinsic causes of airway obstruction. Ventilation/perfusion commonly shows decreased ventilation and perfusion of the affected lobe. Bronchoscopy is generally not necessary for the diagnosis of CLO, but when performed, it can demonstrate the source of the intrinsic compression.

CLO can mimic a variety of congenital and acquired syndromes. Furthermore, differential diagnosis should include congenital pulmonary airway malformations, localized pulmonary interstitial emphysema, bullous emphysema, pneumothorax, airway obstruction secondary to foreign body, congenital bronchial atresia, bronchogenic cyst, endobronchial tumors, as well as Swyer–James–MacLeod (SJM) syndrome (3). SJM, also known as hyperlucent lung syndrome, is a rare disease characterized by localized hyperinflation with associated decreased vascularity, usually seen as a complication of postinfectious bronchiolitis obliterans. Management of asymptomatic patients is generally conservative, since clinical and radiological improvement over time has been reported in previous case series (1). Lobectomy of the affected lobe is the treatment of choice for symptomatic patients. After surgical resection of the compromised lobe, patients tend to have an excellent postoperative course and overall long-term prognosis.

Congenital pulmonary airway malformation

Congenital pulmonary airway malformation (CPAM), formerly known as congenital cystic adenomatoid malformation, are a rare heterogeneous cystic and noncystic group of anomalies largely diagnosed prenatally or within the first 2 years of life, with an estimated incidence of 1 in 25,000–35,000 pregnancies, comprising up to 25% of all DLA. CPAM arises from a defective bronchial tree development with a robust overgrowth of the primary bronchioles, resulting in cystic dilations of the airways. CPAM was first described by Chin and Tank in 1949, and since then, multiple classifications have been proposed, with the most recent one reviewed by Stocker in 2008, which consists in five categories (0–4) based on its histological characteristics (3, 27). Notably, CPAM types 1 and 2 have been described in adults, while the remaining are exclusively seeing in the pediatric setting. Interestingly, type 2 has been associated with other congenital defects, such as congenital heart disease, esophageal cysts, intestinal atresia, as well as concomitant DLA. The etiology of CPAM remains unknown; however, mutations altering thyroid transcription factor-1 (TTF-1) and hamartomatous growths have been proposed mechanisms (28).

The majority of patients with CPAM are diagnosed in utero or early in life. Nevertheless, adult patients with CPAM can be incidentally diagnosed on chest imaging, or can present with a wide spectrum of symptoms, such as frequent respiratory tract infections involving the same area of the lung, dyspnea, hemoptysis, or pneumothorax (29). Rarely, patients can present with air embolism or malignant transformation, such as pleuropulmonary blastoma or adenocarcinoma (30). CT of the chest is the imaging of choice, and it usually shows cystic lesions, either solitary or as a conglomerate (Figure 2.5), with associated areas of consolidation, representative of underlying infection (1). Interestingly, around 44% of patients have lower lobe lung lesions, and the vast majority are unilateral. Air trapping with flattening of the ipsilateral diaphragm and contralateral compensatory shift of the mediastinum can also be seen. Less frequently, a biopsy is often necessary to rule out underlying malignancy since persistent inflammation secondary to recurrent infections may alter the anatomy and classic radiological findings. Differential diagnosis should include bronchopulmonary sequestration, congenital lobar overinflation, and cystic bronchiectasis. For symptomatic patients, lobectomy is generally recommended. On the other hand, management for asymptomatic patients with CPAM continues to be controversial. Given their high inflammatory state, mostly driven by persistent and recurrent infections, with subsequent risk for malignant transformation, most authors advocate for the resection of the affected lung parenchyma (3).

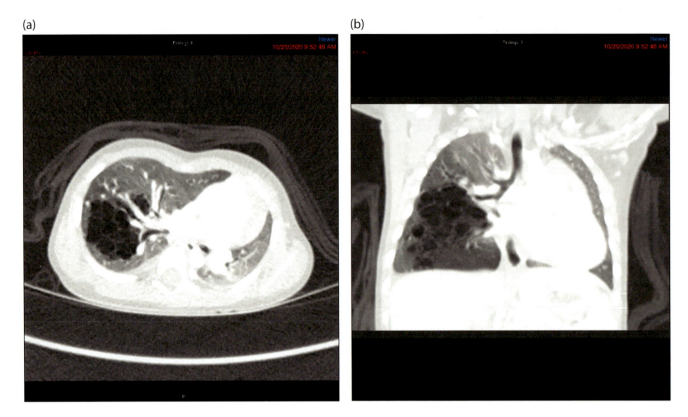

FIGURE 2.5 Congenital pulmonary airway malformation (CPAM). Chest CT in axial view (a) and coronal view (b) demonstrating coalescence of cystic opacities in the right lower lobe. Thoracoscopic lobectomy done showed lesional tissue with ciliated columnar epithelium and cytoplasmic mucin lining airways larger than the alveoli consistent with CPAM type 1. (Images courtesy of Stephen Machniki MD, Dept. of Radiology, Lenox Hill Hospital, Northwell Health, New York.)

Tracheal bronchus

Tracheal bronchus (TB) is a rare congenital anomaly that consists of an ectopic bronchus that arises from the trachea and is directed to the upper lobes. This DLA is more frequently seen in men, with a prevalence of 0.1–2% for the right TB and 0.3–1% for the left TB (31). The etiology of TB remains unclear, but it is likely secondary to an abnormal migration or selection during embryogenesis. TB is more frequently found within 2–6 cm from the carina and can present as a supernumerary bronchus if the remaining bronchial tree has a normal development, or considered a displaced bronchus if the right upper lobe bronchus has only two segmental branches. TB may coexist with other congenital anomalies, such as trisomy 21, congenital diaphragmatic hernia, and lobar emphysema (32, 33).

Patients with TB are usually asymptomatic and discovered as an incidental finding on chest imaging or bronchoscopy; however, they can present with cough, dyspnea, recurrent pneumonia, or hemoptysis (31). Occasionally, malignancies arising from the TB have been reported, such as carcinoid tumors and squamous cell carcinoma (34). Previous case reports have described accidental TB intubation, representing a challenge for the anesthesiologists and intensivists during endotracheal intubation. Conservative management is recommended for asymptomatic patients. On the other hand, for symptomatic patients, especially those with recurrent lower respiratory tract infections or those with localized bronchiectasis, pulmonary hygiene and antibiotic therapy is generally recommended. Furthermore, surgical resection of the affected lobe is advised for those who do not respond to medical therapy.

Tracheal diverticulum

Tracheal diverticulum (TD) is a rare benign outpouching of the tracheal wall, with an estimated incidence of 1% in the adult population. TD can be classified into two subgroups: congenital or acquired (35). Congenital TD arises from an endodermal differentiation defect and consists of a full-thickness tracheal wall invagination, which includes the respiratory epithelium, smooth muscle, and cartilage. Congenital TD is more common in males, is usually encountered on the right posterolateral side of the trachea in 97% of cases, 4–5 cm below the vocal cords or above the carina, and generally has a small neck opening. On the other hand, acquired TD can result from a surgical complication, secondary to tracheomalacia, or can also be seen in patients with longstanding increased intraluminal tracheal pressure. Histologically, acquired TD consists of a single-layer invagination, spearing the smooth muscle layer and cartilage, can be seen at any level of the airway, and generally has a wide neck opening.

Patients with TD are commonly asymptomatic and incidentally diagnosed on chest imaging. However, persistent cough, stridor, dyspnea, odynophagia, hoarseness, and hemoptysis have been reported (36). Patients can also present with frequent respiratory tract infections that can progress into a paratracheal abscess. Less frequently, TD can be diagnosed after endotracheal intubation as a result of its perforation and subsequent pneumomediastinum formation. CT of the chest is the imaging of choice. A thin-walled pouch filled with air located in the paratracheal region is generally pathognomonic of TD (37). CT can also help differentiate congenital from acquired TD based on its location, neck size opening diameter, and the presence or absence of cartilage.

Developmental Lung Anomalies in Adults

Differential diagnosis should include Zenker's diverticulum laryngocele, pharyngocele, and lung bullae. An asymptomatic patient can be managed conservatively. For those presenting with respiratory tract infection, antibiotics, mucolytics, and chest physiotherapy are warranted. Surgical resection is generally recommended for those with recurrent infections, especially for those patients with paratracheal abscess presenting with respiratory distress (38).

Accessory cardiac bronchus

Accessory cardiac bronchus (ACB), initially described by Brock in 1946, is a rare congenital anomaly of the tracheobronchial tree, where a supernumerary bronchus arises from the inferomedial wall of the right main bronchus or bronchus intermedius (31). Rarely, ACB originates from a left bronchus, and it generally has a diameter of 8–9 mm and a length of 12 mm (39). Histologically, it consists of normal respiratory mucosa and submucosa with cartilage within the bronchial wall (40). Most cases of ACB consist of a blind end; however, 30% of patients have associated undeveloped lung parenchymal tissue. ACB can be an isolated anomaly or may be associated with other DLA, such as tracheal bronchus, as well as congenital heart diseases.

The majority of patients with ACB are asymptomatic and incidentally diagnosed on chest imaging. Patients can also present with cough and hemoptysis. Recurrent pneumonia may also be seen in symptomatic patients since the blind-ending ACB may serve as a potential reservoir for infections (5). Less frequently, patients can present with empyema or malignant transformation. ACB cannot be visualized on chest x-rays, hence chest CT is the imaging of choice. CT chest shows a supernumerary bronchus that runs medially and caudally toward the heart. Conservative management, including antibiotics and mucolytics, are recommended for acute infections. Furthermore, surgical resection is advised for patients with recurrent pneumonias.

Vascular anomalies
Proximal interruption of a central pulmonary artery

Absence of a single pulmonary artery is a rare abnormality but may be an isolated congenital abnormality presenting in adulthood. This malformation occurs during the embryonic stage when one of the sixth aortic arches fails to develop, and thus the main pulmonary artery is unable to erupt from the arch (3, 41). Absence of a single pulmonary artery alone tends to be opposite of the aortic arch and pulmonary blood flow to the affected side will be supplemented through collaterals. Of note, while the proximal portion is interrupted the hilar and distal portions of correlating pulmonary artery are still present as these portions arise from the primitive ductus from the innominate or subclavian arteries (1). The affected lung will tend to be hypoplastic, but venous return is normal. When the left pulmonary artery is affected, it is usually in combination with other significant developmental abnormalities such as tetralogy of Fallot and is typically not seen in isolation (1, 2).

CT is the most elucidating imaging modality showing early termination of the main pulmonary artery within 1 cm of its origin. The lung may appear as hypoplastic compared to the opposite lung and 3D CT reconstructions can be used to map the associated collateral supplying vessels (1–3). Depending on the overall compensation in adults, they tend to be minimally symptomatic but may present with dyspnea and impaired exercise tolerance alone (3, 42, 43). Adults with proximal interruption of the pulmonary artery may also manifest symptoms due to pulmonary hypertension and can lead to hemoptysis, dyspnea, and right heart failure. Medical management of pulmonary hypertension is the mainstay of treatment unless life-threatening complications are found that require revascularization. Often times, these malformations may be revascularized in childhood (1, 44).

Anomalous origin of the left pulmonary artery

Anomalous origination of the left pulmonary artery (LPA) is secondary to absence of the left sixth aortic arch. In the abscess of the left sixth aortic arch, the left pulmonary artery develops collateral origination from the right pulmonary artery during early embryologic formation (1–3). Anomalous left pulmonary arteries appear as loop as it traverses around the trachea to its insertion into the left lung, thus giving the appearance of a "sling" (Figure 2.6) (2). Anomalous LPAs are typically designated as a type 1 or type 2 pulmonary artery sling. In type 1 PA, slings result in compression of the anterior esophagus, the posterior trachea, and the right main stem bronchus due to the course of the LPA (1–3, 44). Type 2 slings result in an inferiorly displaced "T-shaped" carina resulting in tracheal stenosis due to complete cartilaginous rings. Up to 50% of patients with type 2 slings are also associated with heart defects (2).

Findings may be present on chest x-ray with a paratracheal mediastinal mass, right main stem bronchus compression, right lung hyperinflation due to bronchus compression, and deviation of mediastinal structures (5). These malformations may be easily demonstrated on chest CT (2). Anomalous LPA malformations may be asymptomatic and typically do not require intervention. In cases where symptomatic compression of the trachea or bronchi occur, surgical decompression of the sling may improve symptoms (42, 44).

Anomalous pulmonary venous drainage/partial anomalous pulmonary venous return (PAPVR)

Venous malformation occurs at various locations with the main result causing venous blood to be drained into systemic circulation facilitating a left-to-right shunt. These shunts tend to

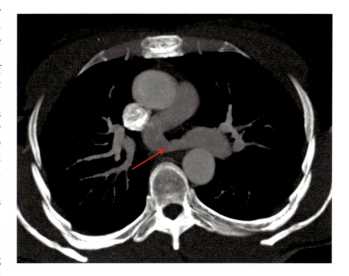

FIGURE 2.6 Pulmonary artery sling. Axial contrast enhanced CT image in a 30-year-old man demonstrating the left pulmonary artery arising from the right pulmonary artery and coursing in between the trachea and esophagus consistent with a pulmonary sling. Note that there is tracheal narrowing. (Reprinted from Cherian SV, Kumar A, Ocazionez D, Estrada-Y-Martin RM, Restrepo CS. Developmental lung anomalies in adults: A pictorial review. Respir Med. 2019;155:86–96. With permission from Elsevier.)

occur at a population prevalence of 0.4–0.7% (3, 5, 45). Venous malformations tend to be small resulting from a portion of pulmonary veins failing to separate from the cardinal veins (2). The most common form of this shunting is a result of left upper lobe pulmonary vein draining into the innominate vein (4, 45). Right chest pulmonary venous drainage malformations include pulmonary veins connecting with the left atrium, vena cava, azygous vein, or the coronary sinus (2, 3). This anomalous drainage is also typically found in isolation of other cardiac malformations. Other forms of anomalous venous drainage are associated with an atrial septal defect in up to 90% of cases (2).

Chest radiography is limited in presentation and if present may show signs of pulmonary hypertension such as an enlarged atria and pulmonary artery branches (Figure 2.7). Otherwise, MR is the preferred imagining modality to identify anomalous venous insertions as MR may quantify the degree of shunt if present (2). Patients with pulmonary hypertension due to left-to-right shunt and right-sided venous drainage are more likely to be symptomatic compared to left-sided malformations (3, 45). Treatment can be achieved with surgical resection or embolization and is indicated in symptomatic pulmonary hypertension causing right heart failure, or recurrent pneumonia (46).

Pulmonary vein varix

A pulmonary vein varix typically is found at the connection of the pulmonary veins to the left atrium; the insertion of which results in a focal dilation of the vein. A varix may be congenital or acquired as result of long-standing pulmonary hypertension or increased left atrial pressure due to mitral valve disease. A varix may present as a mediastinal mass on chest radiography and can be easily differentiated from an arteriovenous malformation with contrast enhanced chest CT. Management consists of treating underlying pulmonary hypertension and rarely need intervention unless the varix is complicated by rupture or intraluminal thrombi (2, 3, 47, 48).

Pulmonary arteriovenous malformations

Pulmonary arteriovenous malformation (AVM) results from a fistulous connection between pulmonary veins and arteries, without a capillary bed, resulting in an intrapulmonary right-to-left shunt. These malformations arise due to lack of division and formation of the typical capillary bed. Hereditary hemorrhagic telangiectasia or also known as Osler–Weber–Rendu syndrome are responsible for most cases of multiple AVM. Patients may be asymptomatic but common symptoms include dyspnea, hypoxemia, or hemoptysis due to ruptures. If shunting represents greater than 20% of cardiac output the classic triad of dyspnea, cyanosis and clubbing may be seen (4). Due to the arterial venous nature, these patients are also at risk of paradoxical embolisms involving the arterial system including stroke (3, 45, 49).

AVM may appear on chest radiography as a nodular opacity but contrast enhanced echocardiography demonstrating an intrapulmonary shunt is more sensitive (Figure 2.8). If an intrapulmonary shunt is demonstrated, multidetector computed tomography (MDCT) can characterize the size and nature of these AVMs. Treatment is indicated for symptomatic AVMs with a history of hemoptysis, embolisms, or persistent hypoxemia. Treatment includes embolization therapy for AVM of >2 cm or with feeding vessels >3 mm (1, 4). Surgical resection may also be indicated for larger, more complex lesions (3, 45).

Cystic hygroma

Cystic hygroma (CH) in the lung are a collection of lymphatic vessels that become dilated forming cysts. CH are notable for variable locations and often present as a soft-tissue fluid-filled mass. On chest x-ray, they may present as a mediastinal mass and on MDCT,

(a)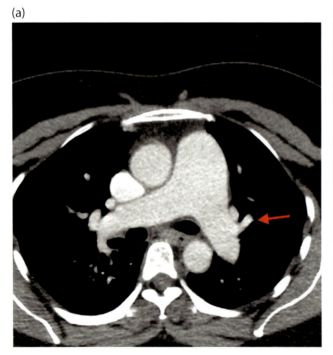

(b)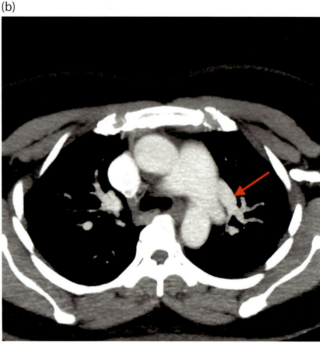

FIGURE 2.7 Partial anomalous pulmonary venous return. Chest CT scans in axial view (a) of a 59-year-old woman referred for pulmonary artery enlargement. Careful review showed the anomalous upper lobe pulmonary vein drain into the pulmonary artery (red arrow). Notice the enlarged pulmonary artery. This is better seen on the lower cuts of the CT image (b). A 2D echocardiogram subsequently revealed normal pulmonary artery pressures.

Developmental Lung Anomalies in Adults

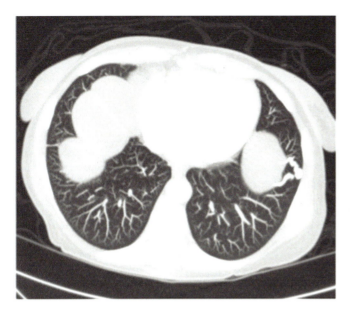

FIGURE 2.8 Pulmonary arteriovenous malformation. Chest CT scans with intravenous contrast on axial view in a 46-year-old patient presenting with hypoxemia revealing an arteriovenous malformation in the left lower lobe.

hygromas are a fluid-filled mass that do not enhance with contrast compared to vascular structures. Often, these lesions are asymptomatic. Postobstructive pneumonias may be present, and based on symptoms surgical evaluation may be appropriate (6).

Combined pulmonary parenchymal-vascular anomalies

Hypogenetic lung syndrome

Hypogenetic lung syndrome (HLS) is also known in the literature as congenital venolobar syndrome and scimitar syndrome. HLS is a form of anomalous pulmonary venous drainage associated with underdevelopment of the lung (5). The first case of anomalous pulmonary venous drainage into the inferior vena cava was in 1836 by Cooper (50). These anomalies most often occur on the right side and are characterized by hypoplastic lung, anomalous pulmonary venous return to the inferior vena cava, and a small or absent ipsilateral pulmonary artery. The affected lung will be abnormally undersized and can include anomalies of the right bronchial tree including diverticula. Less commonly, cases of the right bronchial tree distribution mirroring the left side bronchial tree have been described (5). The most distinctive finding of HLS is the anomalous pulmonary venous return to the inferior vena cava below the right hemidiaphragm. Although this is the most common drainage connection, it may connect to the supradiaphragmatic inferior vena cava, hepatic vein, portal vein, azygos vein, coronary sinus, or right atrium. In addition, other bronchopulmonary, cardiac, and skeletal anomalies have been described combined with HLS including bronchopulmonary sequestration, dextrocardia, scoliosis, and hemivertebrae (51).

Approximately 30–40% of HLS cases that present after infancy are discovered incidentally on chest radiography performed for an unrelated reason. The remaining 60–70% of patients present with complications related to pulmonary hypertension or hypoplastic lung such as fatigue and dyspnea or recurrent pneumonia and hemoptysis, respectively (52). The chest radiography is often diagnostic and characterized by a small hyperlucent affected lung, hyperinflated unaffected lung with consequential mediastinal shift to the affected side, abnormal arrangement of the pulmonary arteries, and the anomalous pulmonary vein traveling below the diaphragm connecting with the inferior vena cava. A distinctive finding of HLS on chest radiograph is that the anomalous pulmonary vein appears as a curvilinear tubular opacity that parallels the right heart border (Figure 2.9) (5, 51). The appearance of this specific finding has been compared to a Turkish dagger called the *scimitar*, which was first described by Halasz, giving this syndrome its name (53).

The management of HLS usually depends on the severity of pulmonary hypertension and the degree of left-to-right shunt. Right heart catheterization is often used to establish these variables and subsequent interventions (54). In a series of 122 patients

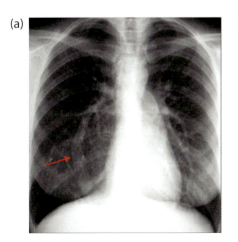
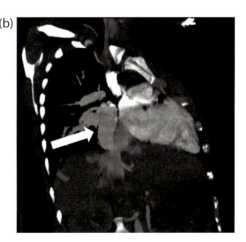
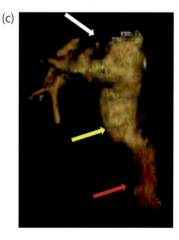

FIGURE 2.9 Hypogenetic lung syndrome/Scimitar syndrome: (a) PA chest x-ray in a 30-year-old woman showing characteristic curvilinear density in the right lower lobe (arrow) related to anomalous pulmonary venous drainage. (b) Coronal (MPR) CT images that demonstrate a scimitar vein draining into the IVC (white arrows). (c) 3D volume rendered image that demonstrates a pulmonary vein (white arrow) draining into the scimitar vein (yellow arrow), which finally terminates in the IVC (red arrow). (Reprinted from Cherian SV, Kumar A, Ocazionez D, Estrada-Y-Martin RM, Restrepo CS. Developmental lung anomalies in adults: A pictorial review. Respir Med. 2019;155:86–96. With permission from Elsevier.)

who were diagnosed with HLS after infancy, if patients did not have pulmonary hypertension and their left-to-right shunt was less than 50% (100 of 122) they remained asymptomatic (55). Surgical intervention is indicated in patients with pulmonary hypertension resulting in right heart failure and/or left-to-right shunt greater than 50%. Recurrent pulmonary infections of the affected lung are also an indication for surgical intervention (52, 54, 55).

Bronchopulmonary sequestration

A bronchopulmonary sequestration (BPS) is described as a mass of nonfunctioning lung tissue that is not in normal continuity with the tracheobronchial tree due to anomalous branching during development (56). This area of lung tissue retains the embryonic systemic arterial supply without any connection to the normal pulmonary artery circulation (5). This anomalous bronchopulmonary vascular formation was first described by Pryce and is one of the most common DLAs found antenatally (56). BPS can be subclassified into either intralobar or extralobar sequestration based on the pleural involvement and venous drainage of the anomalous lung structure (5). Again, both intralobar sequestration (ILS) and extralobar sequestration (ELS) are most commonly supplied by the systemic arterial circulation from separate branches of the thoracic or abdominal aorta but other systemic arteries including the intercostals, subclavian, celiac, splenic, and coronary arteries have been described (57, 58). Radiographically, BPS is typically found in the lower lobes of the lung with less than 5% of cases present in the upper lobes but other locations have been reported. The sequestration usually appears as a well-demarcated homogenous opacity in the posterior medial aspect of the left lower lung along the diaphragm.

ILS represents an estimated 75% of all BPS and is characterized by the lack of its own separate pleural investment and venous drainage into the pulmonary veins (5). A congenital abnormality is the most commonly accepted etiology of this finding but acquired origins have been suggested (59–61). ILS is commonly an incidental finding during an unrelated chest radiograph and approximately 15% of all cases remain asymptomatic throughout adulthood (62, 63). Symptomatic ILS typically presents as an adolescent or in early adulthood with up to half presenting after 20 years old (64). Patients will present with recurrent infection and, less frequently, hemoptysis (62, 65, 66). Although there is no direct connection between the normal tracheobronchial tree and the sequestrated lung, the development of recurrent infections is thought to be due to the ability of bacteria to access the sequestrated lung through the pores of Kohn allowing colonization with the inability to properly drain these areas resulting in recurrent infections (64). Additionally, persistent infections within the sequestration can form new connections to the normal tracheobronchial tree (5). Rarely, ILS has been reported to be complicated by the development of a malignancy including lung carcinoma and fibrous mesothelioma (67–69).

ELS represents approximately 25% of all BPS and is characterized by having its own pleural investment separate from the normal pleura of the lung and venous drainage that connects with the systemic circulation (5). The most common location for the pulmonary drainage of the sequestration to connect is the azygous and hemi-azygous veins. ELS is usually found during the first 6 months of infancy during evaluation of other congenital anomalies including diaphragm defects, heart defects, and communications to the foregut (3). In adulthood, ELS is an incidental finding during unrelated chest imaging in an estimated 10% of cases (63). Recurrent infections are the most typical presentation of ELS in adulthood but cases of hemothorax have been reported (70). Congenital pulmonary airway malformation has been associated with 50% of ELS cases and are termed hybrid lesions (1, 71).

Radiographically, ILS is seen within the left lung 60% of the time and usually in the posterior segment of the lower lobes but can be found in either lung or in the upper lobes (63). ELS most frequently presents in the lower left hemithorax (Figure 2.10) along the medial hemidiaphragm in 63–77% of cases but other locations including the mediastinum and retroperitoneum have

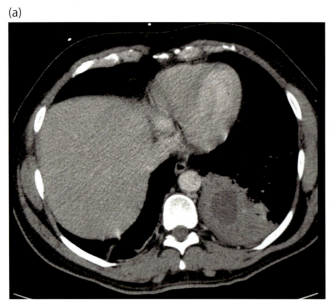
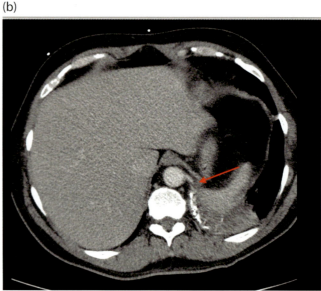

FIGURE 2.10 Bronchopulmonary sequestration. Chest CT scans in axial view of a 45-year-old man who presented with fever and pleuritic chest pain, which shows a necrotizing consolidative opacity in the left lower lobe (a). Images enhanced with intravenous contrast (b) highlight the systemic arterial supply (red arrow) from the aorta consistent with intra-lobar bronchopulmonary sequestration.

been reported (64, 72, 73). The sequestration will appear as a mass or cavity with or without air fluid levels and can have surrounding opacities suggestive of a cyst or pneumonia. Additional findings described are overinflation of the adjacent lung parenchyma suggesting air trapping. A good differential is important including lung abscesses, necrotizing pneumonia, and mycetomas for proper workup and diagnosis. Particularly, special attention should be directed at the presence of systemic arterial supply, pulmonary venous drainage, and the presence of pleural borders. CT angiography is the radiographic technique of choice due to the inconsistency of the conventional CT to distinguish systemic arterial supply (64, 74). Management of BPS, both ILS and ELS, usually involves surgical intervention including even the asymptomatic patient with incidentally discovered BPS (53, 62, 64, 72). This reasoning is recommended based on the development of complications from BPS if left untreated.

Conclusion

DLAs encompass a rare heterogenous group of disorders with unique manifestations but the ability to mimic other thoracic pathology frequently lead to a misdiagnosis. Our understanding and advancements in radiology have allowed us to diagnose increasing numbers of DLAs, but they remain a diagnostic challenge for the untrained clinician. The significance of an accurate diagnosis lies in the potential of these anomalies to cause complications including recurrent infections, respiratory failure, bleeding, malignancy, and even death, which can typically be prevented with timely intervention and early diagnosis. Awareness of the wide spectrum of congenital lung anomalies in adults is imperative for inclusion into the differential of adult pulmonary disorders and their management.

References

1. Lee EY, Dorkin H, Vargas SO. Congenital pulmonary malformations in pediatric patients: Review and update on etiology, classification, and imaging findings. Radiol Clin North Am. 2011;49(5):921–48.
2. Thacker PG, Rao AG, Hill JG, Lee EY. Congenital lung anomalies in children and adults: Current concepts and imaging findings. Radiol Clin North Am. 2014;52(1):155–81.
3. Cherian SV, Kumar A, Ocazionez D, Estrada YMRM, Restrepo CS. Developmental lung anomalies in adults: A pictorial review. Respir Med. 2019;155:86–96.
4. Trotman-Dickenson B. Congenital lung disease in the adult: Guide to the evaluation and management. J Thorac Imaging. 2015;30(1):46–59.
5. Zylak CJ, Eyler WR, Spizarny DL, Stone CH. Developmental lung anomalies in the adult: Radiologic-pathologic correlation. Radiographics. 2002;22 Spec No:S25–43.
6. Berrocal T, Madrid C, Novo S, Gutierrez J, Arjonilla A, Gomez-Leon N. Congenital anomalies of the tracheobronchial tree, lung, and mediastinum: Embryology, radiology, and pathology. Radiographics. 2004;24(1):e17.
7. Sadler TW, Langman J. Langman's Medical Embryology. 12th ed. Philadelphia: Wolters Kluwer Health/Lippincott Williams & Wilkins; 2012. xiii, 384 p.
8. Kumar P, Tansir G, Sasmal G, Dixit J, Sahoo R. Left pulmonary agenesis with right lung bronchiectasis in an adult. J Clin Diagn Res. 2016;10(9):OD15–OD7.
9. Kaya O, Gulek B, Yilmaz C, Soker G, Esen K, Akin MA, et al. Adult presentation of symptomatic left lung agenesis. Radiol Case Rep. 2017;12(1):25–8.
10. Kisku KH, Panigrahi MK, Sudhakar R, Nagarajan A, Ravikumar R, Daniel JR. Agenesis of lung — A report of two cases. Lung India. 2008;25(1):28–30.
11. Hutchison MJ, Winkler L. Bronchial Atresia. Treasure Island (FL): StatPearls; 2021.
12. Traibi A, Seguin-Givelet A, Grigoroiu M, Brian E, Gossot D. Congenital bronchial atresia in adults: Thoracoscopic resection. J Vis Surg. 2017;3:174.
13. Wang Y, Dai W, Sun Y, Chu X, Yang B, Zhao M. Congenital bronchial atresia: Diagnosis and treatment. Int J Med Sci. 2012;9(3):207–12.
14. Langston C. New concepts in the pathology of congenital lung malformations. Semin Pediatr Surg. 2003;12(1):17–37.
15. Gipson MG, Cummings KW, Hurth KM. Bronchial atresia. Radiographics. 2009;29(5):1531–5.
16. Fukada Y, Endo Y, Nakanowatari H, Kitagawa A, Tsuboi E, Irie Y. Bronchogenic cyst of the interatrial septum. Fukushima J Med Sci. 2020;66(1):41–3.
17. Chen F, Marx S, Zhang C, Cao J, Yu Y, Chen D. Intramedullary bronchogenic cyst in the foramen magnum region accompanied with syringomyelia: A case report and literature review. Medicine (Baltimore). 2019;98(5):e14353.
18. Piton N, Gobet F, Werquin C, Landreat A, Lefebvre H, Pfister C, et al. Retroperitoneal bronchogenic cyst. Ann Pathol. 2012;32(4):267–70.
19. Sarper A, Ayten A, Golbasi I, Demircan A. Isin E. Bronchogenic cyst. Tex Heart Inst J. 2003;30(2):105–8.
20. Suen HC, Mathisen DJ, Grillo HC, LeBlanc J, McLoud TC, Moncure AC, et al. Surgical management and radiological characteristics of bronchogenic cysts. Ann Thorac Surg. 1993;55(2):476–81.
21. Aktogu S, Yuncu G, Halilcolar H, Ermete S, Buduneli T. Bronchogenic cysts: Clinicopathological presentation and treatment. Eur Respir J. 1996;9(10):2017–21.
22. Dhand S, Krimsky W. Bronchogenic cyst treated by endobronchial ultrasound drainage. Thorax. 2008;63(4):386.
23. Demir OF, Hangul M, Kose M. Congenital lobar emphysema: Diagnosis and treatment options. Int J Chron Obstruct Pulmon Dis. 2019;14:921–8.
24. Sadaqat M, Malik JA, Karim R. Congenital lobar emphysema in an adult. Lung India. 2011;28(1):67–9.
25. Thakral CL, Maji DC, Sajwani MJ. Congenital lobar emphysema: Experience with 21 cases. Pediatr Surg Int. 2001;17(2–3):88–91.
26. Kumar B, Agrawal LD, Sharma SB. Congenital bronchopulmonary malformations: A single-center experience and a review of literature. Ann Thorac Med. 2008;3(4):135–9.
27. Ch'In KY, Tang MY. Congenital adenomatoid malformation of one lobe of a lung with general anasarca. Arch Pathol (Chic). 1949;48(3):221–9.
28. Baral D, Adhikari B, Zaccarini D, Dongol RM, Sah B. Congenital pulmonary airway malformation in an adult male: A case report with literature review. Case Rep Pulmonol. 2015;2015:743452.
29. McDonough RJ, Niven AS, Havenstrite KA. Congenital pulmonary airway malformation: A case report and review of the literature. Respir Care. 2012;57(2):302–6.
30. Smith JA, Koroscil MT, Hayes JA. Congenital pulmonary airway malformation in the asymptomatic adult: A rare presentation. Respir Med Case Rep. 2018;25:280–1.
31. Ghaye B, Szapiro D, Fanchamps JM, Dondelinger RF. Congenital bronchial abnormalities revisited. Radiographics. 2001;21(1):105–19.
32. Findik S. Tracheal bronchus in the adult population. J Bronchology Interv Pulmonol. 2011;18(2):149–53.
33. Nicolaou N, Du Plessis A. Squamous carcinoma arising from a true tracheal bronchus: Management and case report. Int J Surg Case Rep. 2015;6C:256–8.
34. Patrinou V, Kourea H, Dougenis D. Bronchial carcinoid of an accessory tracheal bronchus. Ann Thorac Surg. 2001;71(3):1034–5.
35. Chaudhry I, Mutairi H, Hassan E, Afzal M, Khurshid I. Tracheal diverticulum: A rare cause of hoarseness of the voice. Ann Thorac Surg. 2014;97(2):e29–31.

36. Tanrivermis Sayit A, Elmali M, Saglam D, Celenk C. The diseases of airway-tracheal diverticulum: A review of the literature. J Thorac Dis. 2016;8(10):E1163–E7.
37. Goo JM, Im JG, Ahn JM, Moon WK, Chung JW, Park JH, et al. Right paratracheal air cysts in the thoracic inlet: Clinical and radiologic significance. Am J Roentgenol. 1999;173(1):65–70.
38. Lin H, Cao Z, Ye Q. Tracheal diverticulum: A case report and literature review. Am J Otolaryngol. 2014;35(4):542–5.
39. Ghaye B, Collard P, Pierard S, Sluysmans T. CT presentation of left-sided accessory cardiac bronchus. Diagn Interv Imaging. 2018;99(12):827–8.
40. McGuinness G, Naidich DP, Garay SM, Davis AL, Boyd AD, Mizrachi HH. Accessory cardiac bronchus: CT features and clinical significance. Radiology. 1993;189(2):563–6.
41. Castaner E, Gallardo X, Rimola J, Pallardo Y, Mata JM, Perendreu J, et al. Congenital and acquired pulmonary artery anomalies in the adult: Radiologic overview. Radiographics. 2006;26(2):349–71.
42. Berdon WE, Baker DH, Wung JT, Chrispin A, Kozlowski K, de Silva M, et al. Complete cartilage-ring tracheal stenosis associated with anomalous left pulmonary artery: The ring-sling complex. Radiology. 1984;152(1):57–64.
43. Ten Harkel AD, Blom NA, Ottenkamp J. Isolated unilateral absence of A pulmonary artery: A case report and review of the literature. Chest. 2002;122(4):1471–7.
44. LaBelle MF, Rainer WG, Ratzer E, Miller KB. Surgical repair of pulmonary artery sling in an adult. Ann Thorac Surg. 2010;90(3):1009–11.
45. Porres DV, Morenza OP, Pallisa E, Roque A, Andreu J, Martinez M. Learning from the pulmonary veins. Radiographics. 2013;33(4):999–1022.
46. Fragata J, Magalhaes M, Baquero L, Trigo C, Pinto F, Fragata I. Partial anomalous pulmonary venous connections: Surgical management. World J Pediatr Congenit Heart Surg. 2013;4(1):44–9.
47. Palkar A, Shah R, Greben C, Talwar A. Pulmonary venous varix. Am J Respir Crit Care Med. 2015;192(12):e59.
48. Vaz N, Vollmer I, Perea RJ. Pulmonary venous varix: A rare entity imitating arteriovenous malformation. Arch Bronconeumol. 2016;52(11):562–3.
49. Dillman JR, Yarram SG, Hernandez RJ. Imaging of pulmonary venous developmental anomalies. Am J Roentgenol. 2009;192(5):1272–85.
50. Schramel FM, Westermann CJ, Knaepen PJ, van den Bosch JM. The scimitar syndrome: Clinical spectrum and surgical treatment. Eur Respir J. 1995;8(2):196–201.
51. Woodring JH, Howard TA, Kanga JF. Congenital pulmonary venolobar syndrome revisited. Radiographics. 1994;14(2):349–69.
52. Najm HK, Williams WG, Coles JG, Rebeyka IM, Freedom RM. Scimitar syndrome: Twenty years' experience and results of repair. J Thorac Cardiovasc Surg. 1996;112(5):1161–8; discussion 8–9.
53. Halkic N, Cuénoud PF, Corthésy ME, Ksontini R, Boumghar M. Pulmonary sequestration: A review of 26 cases. Eur J Cardiothorac Surg. 1998;14(2):127–33.
54. Ramirez-Marrero MA, de Mora-Martin M. Scimitar syndrome in an asymptomatic adult: Fortuitous diagnosis by imaging technique. Case Rep Vasc Med. 2012;2012:138541.
55. Dupuis C, Charaf LA, Brevière GM, Abou P, Rémy-Jardin M, Helmius G. The "adult" form of the scimitar syndrome. Am J Cardiol. 1992;70(4):502–7.
56. Pryce DM. Lower accessory pulmonary artery with intralobar sequestration of lung; A report of seven cases. J Pathol Bacteriol. 1946;58(3):457–67.
57. Biyyam DR, Chapman T, Ferguson MR, Deutsch G, Dighe MK. Congenital lung abnormalities: Embryologic features, prenatal diagnosis, and postnatal radiologic-pathologic correlation. Radiographics. 2010;30(6):1721–38.
58. Hilton TC, Keene WR, Blackshear JL. Intralobar pulmonary sequestration with nutrient systemic arterial flow from multiple coronary arteries. Am Heart J. 1995;129(4):823–6.
59. Stocker JT. Sequestrations of the lung. Semin Diagn Pathol. 1986;3(2):106–21.
60. Uppal MS, Kohman LJ, Katzenstein AL. Mycetoma within an intralobar sequestration. Evidence supporting acquired origin for this pulmonary anomaly. Chest. 1993;103(5):1627–8.
61. Eustace S, Valentine S, Murray J. Acquired intralobar bronchopulmonary sequestration secondary to occluding endobronchial carcinoid tumor. Clin Imaging. 1996;20(3):178–80.
62. Frazier AA, Rosado de Christenson ML, Stocker JT, Templeton PA. Intralobar sequestration: Radiologic-pathologic correlation. Radiographics. 1997;17(3):725–45.
63. Savic B, Birtel FJ, Tholen W, Funke HD, Knoche R. Lung sequestration: Report of seven cases and review of 540 published cases. Thorax. 1979;34(1):96–101.
64. Cooke CR. Bronchopulmonary sequestration. Respir Care. 2006;51(6):661–4.
65. Rubin EM, Garcia H, Horowitz MD, Guerra JJ. Fatal massive hemoptysis secondary to intralobar sequestration. Chest. 1994;106(3):954–5.
66. Miller EJ, Singh SP, Cerfolio RJ, Schmidt F, Eltoum IE. Pryce's type I pulmonary intralobar sequestration presenting with massive hemoptysis. Ann Diagn Pathol. 2001;5(2):91–5.
67. Hekelaar N, van Uffelen R, van Vliet AC, Varin OC, Westenend PJ. Primary lymphoepithelioma-like carcinoma within an intralobular pulmonary sequestration. Eur Respir J. 2000;16(5):1025–7.
68. Bell-Thomson J, Missier P, Sommers SC. Lung carcinoma arising in bronchopulmonary sequestration. Cancer. 1979;44(1):334–9.
69. Paksoy N, Demircan A, Altiner M, Artvinli M. Localised fibrous mesothelioma arising in an intralobar pulmonary sequestration. Thorax. 1992;47(10):837–8.
70. Avishai V, Dolev E, Weissberg D, Zajdel L, Priel IE. Extralobar sequestration presenting as massive hemothorax. Chest. 1996;109(3):843–5.
71. Conran RM, Stocker JT. Extralobar sequestration with frequently associated congenital cystic adenomatoid malformation, type 2: Report of 50 cases. Pediatr Dev Pathol. 1999;2(5):454–63.
72. Rosado-de-Christenson ML, Frazier AA, Stocker JT, Templeton PA. From the archives of the AFIP. Extralobar sequestration: Radiologic-pathologic correlation. Radiographics. 1993;13(2):425–41.
73. Baker EL, Gore RM, Moss AA. Retroperitoneal pulmonary sequestration: Computed tomographic findings. Am J Roentgenol. 1982;138(5):956–7.
74. Rappaport DC, Herman SJ, Weisbrod GL. Congenital bronchopulmonary diseases in adults: CT findings. Am J Roentgenol. 1994;162(6):1295–9.

PART A
Rare Genetic Lung Diseases

3

GENETIC INFILTRATIVE LUNG DISEASES

Isabel C. Mira-Avendano

Contents

Genetic infiltrative disorders of the lung	15
Pulmonary alveolar microlithiasis	15
Neurofibromatosis	16
Dyskeratosis congenita	16
Hermansky–Pudlak syndrome	18
Conclusion	18
References	19

KEY POINTS

- Genetic infiltrative lung diseases are characterized not only by lung involvement but multisystemic manifestations.
- Some of these conditions may have higher incidence of malignancies in diseases such as neurofibromatosis and dyskeratosis congenita due to increased oncogene expression.
- Hermansky–Pudlak syndrome and dyskeratosis congenita are rare reasons for usual interstitial pneumonia in a young population.
- Neurofibromatosis may be associated with lung cysts and hence should be considered as a possible differential in cystic lung diseases.
- Pulmonary hypertension due to multifactorial mechanisms can complicate neurofibromatosis and Gaucher and Niemann–Pick disease.
- A multidisciplinary approach with the participation of a pulmonologist, chest radiologist, lung pathologist, and geneticist is needed for a better approach to these patients.

Genetic infiltrative disorders of the lung

Out of the estimated 7,000 rare diseases worldwide, 80% of these diseases are genetic in origin, of which at least 5–10% affect the lung. These may affect the lung in isolation, or the lung may be one of the organs involved within a systemic disorder. Inheritance may be monogenic (single defective gene) or may involve genetic polymorphism. Most infiltrative disorders of the lung involve multiple genes, and several factors including environmental interaction play a part in the development of lung manifestations. Within this spectrum, no established treatment has been defined in most of these conditions (1). Early recognition is essential, and lung transplantation should be a consideration given the young age of most affected individuals. This chapter will focus on some of the genetic infiltrative disorders of the lung, their clinical and radiological manifestations, and management.

Pulmonary alveolar microlithiasis

Pulmonary alveolar microlithiasis (PAM) is a rare autosomal recessive disorder explained by the inability of alveolar epithelial type 2 cells to clear phosphorus ions from the alveolar space, leading to microlith (calcium phosphate deposits) or calcospherite formation in the extracellular fluid with the result of intra-alveolar accumulation of it (2, 3). It is caused by inactivating mutations in the gene encoding a sodium-dependent phosphate cotransporter (SLC34A2, Npt2b, NaPi-2b) (4).

Most patients are asymptomatic, being diagnosed after incidental finding of abnormal radiologic tests. Most cases present with slow progression (over 10–20 years) of dyspnea, dry cough, and in some cases weight loss. Clubbing is present in most patients with advanced disease, and pneumothorax has been seen as a complication (4). The average age at the time of diagnosis is 40 years. There is no sex predilection. It has been reported in all continents, but mostly in Europe and Asia, particularly in Turkey and China (4).

Advanced radiologic changes are seen in the setting of minimal clinical manifestations (clinic-radiologic dissociation). The sandstorm sign, which consists of diffuse, scattered bilateral areas of micronodular calcifications, distributed mostly over middle and lower lobes, is characteristic of PAM and can be seen either in the chest x-ray (CXR) or chest computed tomography (CT) (Figure 3.1). The vascular tree and borders of the heart and diaphragm are often obscured ("vanishing heart" phenomenon). A linear radiolucency at the pleural boundaries abutting the heart, diaphragm, and pleura on HRCT is also characteristic, referred to as the "black pleural sign." This characteristic imaging finding is likely secondary to the development of subpleural cystic changes, as reported in cross-sectional imaging and pathologic specimens (2, 3). This pattern can also be observed in mediastinal window images because calcification is present along the interlobular septa (3–5).

Diagnosis of PAM is often possible with history and characteristic imaging patterns, which may obviate the need for lung biopsy. However, a definitive diagnosis requires the demonstration of microliths, which are periodic acid-Schiff positive calcareous concentric lamellae around a central nucleus

DOI: 10.1201/9781003089384-3

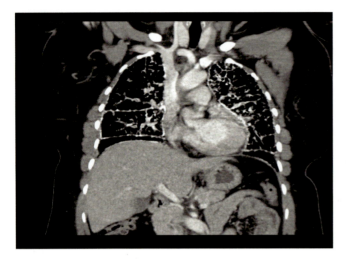

FIGURE 3.1 Pulmonary alveolar microlithiasis: Chest CT in coronal view showing calcification extending along the fissures and interlobular septal thickening in a 35-year-old woman with PAM.

with an amorphous or granular aspect (Figure 3.2) that may be seen even in expectorated sputum (3, 4). Otherwise, bronchoscopy with broncho-alveolar lavage (BAL) and transbronchial biopsies usually suffices with a reasonable yield and safety profile (3).

Treatment of PAM is not well defined, and most therapies have proven to be ineffective. Repeated bronchoscopy with serial lavages has been tried with minimal success. Moreover, corticosteroids, and calcium-chelating agents such as etidronate have been attempted with little to no success except for isolated case reports. Lung transplantation remains the only possible treatment for end-stage lung disease with no recurrences reported (3). Thus, in patients with either right heart failure or severe hypoxemic respiratory failure, lung transplantation should be considered (4).

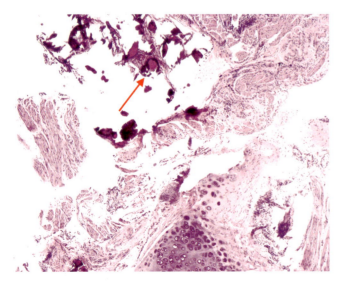

FIGURE 3.2 Transbronchial biopsies in the same patient showing intra-alveolar microlith consistent with PAM.

Neurofibromatosis

Neurofibromatosis (NF) is an autosomal dominant disorder, although up to 50% of cases arise sporadically due to spontaneous mutations. It is characterized by multiorgan involvement with compromise of skin, central and peripheral nervous system, bone, and eyes. NF type 1 (NF1), formerly known as von Recklinghausen disease, is associated with the *NF1* gene located on the long arm of chromosome 17 (at locus 17q11.2), whose protein product, neurofibromin, is a negative regulator of the proto-oncogene Ras, which explains the higher incidence of malignancies (6) including coexistence of different neoplastic tumors in the same patient (7, 8), along with rare cases of primary lung carcinosarcoma and primary lung rhabdomyosarcoma (9).

The manifestations of the disease increase in frequency and severity with age, with full criteria eventually recognized by the age of 10 years (10). Ninety-five percent of patients develop café au lait macules, neurofibromas, and Lisch nodules, and up to 70% have axillary or inguinal freckling.

Ras proteins play a central role in cell differentiation and growth, which is correlated with the development of neurofibroma-type tumors, which are benign in nature. The loss of neurofibromin seems to accelerate the production of those Ras proteins, which may also cause increased fibroblast production and then higher risk for interstitial lung disease (11). Moreover, proliferation and migration of endothelial cells cause pronounced pulmonary arterial remodeling and uniform wall thickening in cases associated with pulmonary hypertension (12).

The more common findings are subcutaneous and skin nodules, with rates of cystic changes and emphysema in the lung approximately 15 and 18%, respectively (Figure 3.3 a and b) (13, 14). The presence of emphysema seems to be related to a positive smoking history (13–15). Mediastinal masses are present in 15% of cases; 50% correspond to neurofibromas, but cases of malignant peripheral nerve sheath tumors and meningoceles have been reported (13, 16, 17). In small case series, clinical symptoms and abnormal pulmonary function tests were correlated with radiologic findings (14, 15).

Pulmonary hypertension (PH) associated with NF is categorized as group 5 (unclear and/or multifactorial mechanisms). There is female predominance and the reported cases have developed late in the course of the disease, with a median age at diagnosis of 57 years (12, 18, 19). Pulmonary capillary hemangiomatosis has been described, and questions about a relatively high prevalence of pulmonary veno-occlusive disease have been raised, given the development of respiratory failure following the initiation of vasodilators (20). There is a limited response to specific PH therapies, which prompts consideration for a quick referral to lung transplantation centers (19).

Dyskeratosis congenita

Dyskeratosis congenita (DC) is a congenital syndrome, secondary to short telomeres characterized by premature aging and bone marrow failure (21). Clinically, it presents with abnormal skin pigmentation, nail dystrophy, and oral leukoplakia (Figures 3.4 a and b). Similar telomere mutations have been documented in adults with idiopathic pulmonary fibrosis (22). These telomere-mediated disorders are now recognized as syndromes of telomere shortening, characterized by manifestations in multiple organs with the highest morbidity and mortality related to failure of the bone marrow, liver, and lung (21, 23, 24).

Pulmonary fibrosis (Figure 3.4c) develops in a proportion of patients with DC, and lung function decline may be detected

Genetic Infiltrative Lung Diseases 17

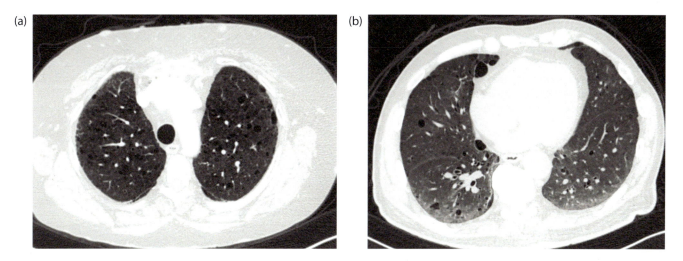

FIGURE 3.3 (a) Neurofibromatosis: Chest CT in axial view of a patient with neurofibromatosis with extensive cigarette smoking history showing the presence of emphysema in upper lobes. (b) Chest CT in axial view of the same patient showing the presence of cysts, reticular opacities, and paraseptal emphysema in the lower lobes—typical findings of neurofibromatosis.

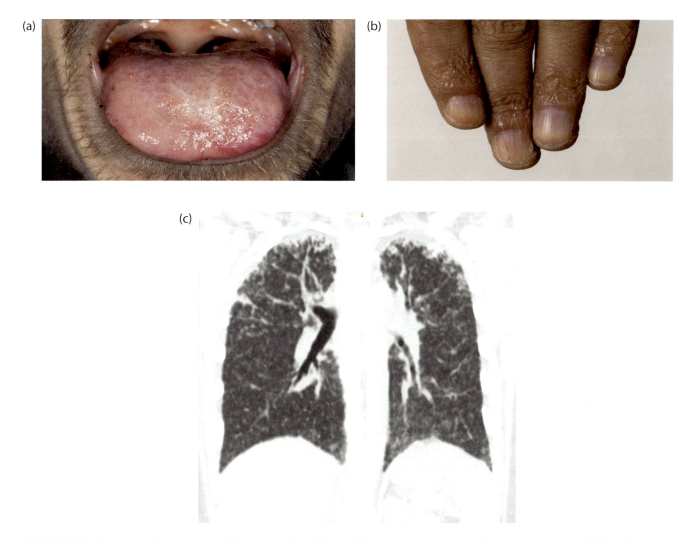

FIGURE 3.4 Dyskeratosis congenita: (a) Presence of oral leukoplakia in a patient with dyskeratosis congenita. (b) Nail dystrophy changes in the same patient with dyskeratosis congenita. (c) Chest CT in the same patient with dyskeratosis congenita showing upper lobe predominant honeycombing and pulmonary fibrosis.

early in life, usually associated with cytopenias and the onset of bone marrow failure (23).

Histopathologic findings on lung biopsy include interstitial fibrosis with pneumocyte hypertrophy, intra-alveolar foamy macrophages, and honeycombing, while radiologic findings have been characterized as atypical usual interstitial pneumonia (UIP) with frequent involvement of the middle and upper lobes (23, 25). No effective therapies exist for this disorder and lung transplantation should be considered in most cases.

Hermansky–Pudlak syndrome

Hermansky–Pudlak syndrome (HPS) is a rare autosomal recessive genetic disorder. Puerto Rico has the highest prevalence of HPS, with 1 in 1,800 in the northwest of the island, representing 50% of cases globally, most of them subtypes 1 and 3 (26, 27).

The HPS genes encode proteins that form complexes termed "biogenesis of lysosome-related organelles complexes (BLOCs)," which are critical regulators of protein trafficking to lysosome-like organelles, such as melanosomes and platelet dense granules, thus explaining many of the syndrome manifestations. The *HPS1* gene product is a component of BLOC3, and *HPS1* mutations cause highly penetrant pulmonary fibrosis (27, 28). Ten subtypes have been recognized; among them, HPS-1, HPS-2, and HPS-4 are associated with pulmonary fibrosis and generally manifest with more severe disease in general (26).

The diagnosis of HPS, regardless of the type, includes albinism and a functional platelet disorder resulting from a storage pool deficiency. Other manifestations include strabismus, nystagmus, and transillumination of the iris.

As in IPF, HPS-related pulmonary fibrosis is characterized by a UIP pattern (Figure 3.5) but, with the presence of giant lamellar body formation in alveolar epithelial type 2 cells (29). Basically, in all cases of HPS-1, pulmonary fibrosis is diagnosed around the fourth decade of life, with an average survival following the onset of pulmonary fibrosis of 10 years. The chest CT presents greater frequency of ground-glass opacities, more common subpleural thickening, and generally less honeycombing (30).

The role of antifibrotic therapies such as pirfenidone or nintedanib in HPS-associated pulmonary fibrosis is not well-established (31). Some patients have successfully received lung transplant, despite the bleeding diathesis. Indeed, it is advised to avoid unnecessary transfusions in these patients, to prevent alloimmunization that would decrease transplant options (28).

Conclusion

Genetic infiltrative disorders of the lung represent a large spectrum of disorders with complex pathogenesis, diverse clinical manifestations, and unique histopathologic and radiological features. Apart from the diseases outlined, several other diseases exist (Table 3.1). A high index of suspicion is required along with adequate knowledge of these rare entities to make a confident diagnosis of these disorders. Further research and international collaboration will provide insights into these disorders and help to identify markers of the diseases and potential targets for therapeutic intervention. Lung transplantation currently remains the only treatment option for several of these diseases.

TABLE 3.1: Other Rare Genetic Disorders Associated with Lung Involvement

Disorder	Characteristics
Niemann–Pick Disease	Lysosomal Storage Disease: There is an acid sphingomyelinase deficiency, resulting in accumulation of sphingomyelins into different organs, including the lungs. Type A is fatal during infancy. Type B is associated with milder disease. Lung compromise is frequently incidentally discovered in adults through abnormal chest CT findings—which manifests as basal predominant ILD (32).
Gaucher Disease	Lysosomal Storage Disease: Associated with deficient activity of the lysosomal enzyme glucosidase with accumulation of glucosylceramide. Gaucher cells (lipid laden macrophages) accumulate into different organs. Three subtypes are recognized, with pulmonary involvement seen in Type 1. Clinical ILD develops in <5% of cases; however, PFT abnormalities with decreased FRC, DLCO, and TLC is seen in up to 65% of patients (33). Hepatopulmonary syndrome and pulmonary hypertension can develop (32).
Familial Pulmonary Alveolar Proteinosis	Mutation of granulocyte-macrophage colony-stimulating factor characterized by accumulation of lipo proteinaceous material into distal airspaces (34).
Cutis Laxa	Abnormality in elastic fibers, causing abnormal skin (loose, redundant), vascular abnormalities, and pulmonary emphysema (35).
Marfan Syndrome	Disorder of the connective tissue, which results in aortic root dilation, ectopia lentis and emphysematous/bullous changes, and spontaneous pneumothorax (36).

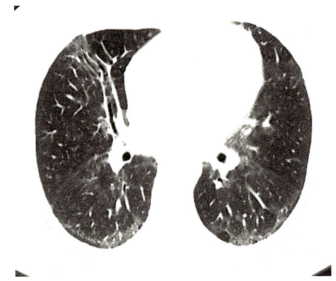

FIGURE 3.5 Hermansky–Pudlak syndrome. Chest CT in axial view showing traction bronchiectasis and reticular opacities consistent with pulmonary fibrosis in a patient with Hermansky–Pudlak syndrome.

References

1. Spagnolo P, Grunewald J, du Bois RM. Genetic determinants of pulmonary fibrosis: Evolving concepts. Lancet Respir Med. 2014;2(5):416–28.
2. Ferreira Francisco FA, Pereira e Silva JL, Hochhegger B, Zanetti G, Marchiori E. Pulmonary alveolar microlithiasis. State-of-the-art review. Respir Med. 2013;107(1):1–9.
3. Saito A, McCormack FX. Pulmonary alveolar microlithiasis. Clin Chest Med. 2016;37(3):441–8.
4. Castellana G, Castellana G, Gentile M, Castellana R, Resta O. Pulmonary alveolar microlithiasis: Review of the 1022 cases reported worldwide. Eur Respir Rev. 2015;24(138):607–20.
5. Raju S, Ghosh S, Mehta AC. Chest CT signs in pulmonary disease: A pictorial review. Chest. 2017;151(6):1356–74.
6. Casal A, Rodriguez-Nunez N, Martinez-Alegria A, Candamio S, Alvarez J, Valdes L. Neurofibromatosis type i with lung involvement in a cancer patient. Pulmonology. 2018;24(4):269–71.
7. Karoui S, Debbabi A, Serghini M, Haouet S, Fenniche S, Chraiet N, et al. Coexistence of a malignant stromal tumor of the stomach with an adenocarcinoma of the lung in a patient with neurofibromatosis type 1. Tunis Med. 2012;90(3):264–6.
8. Przybylik-Mazurek E, Palen J, Pasternak-Pietrzak K, Sowa-Staszczak A, Brzozowska-Czarnek A, Hubalewska-Dydejczyk A. Coexistence of neurofibromatosis type 1 with multiple malignant neoplasia. Neuro Endocrinol Lett. 2018;39(3):149–55.
9. Choi JS, Choi JS, Kim EJ. Primary pulmonary rhabdomyosarcoma in an adult with neurofibromatosis-1. Ann Thorac Surg. 2009;88(4):1356–8.
10. Gutmann DH, Aylsworth A, Carey JC, Korf B, Marks J, Pyeritz RE, et al. The diagnostic evaluation and multidisciplinary management of neurofibromatosis 1 and neurofibromatosis 2. JAMA. 1997;278(1):51–7.
11. Alves Junior SF, Zanetti G, Alves de Melo AS, Souza AS, Jr., Souza LS, de Souza Portes Meirelles G, et al. Neurofibromatosis type 1: State-of-the-art review with emphasis on pulmonary involvement. Respir Med. 2019;149:915.
12. Montani D, Coulet F, Girerd B, Eyries M, Bergot E, Mal H, et al. Pulmonary hypertension in patients with neurofibromatosis type 1. Medicine (Baltimore). 2011;90(3):201–11.
13. Ueda K, Honda O, Satoh Y, Kawai M, Gyobu T, Kanazawa T, et al. Computed tomography (CT) findings in 88 neurofibromatosis 1 (NF1) patients: Prevalence rates and correlations of thoracic findings. Eur J Radiol. 2015;84(6):1191–5.
14. Oikonomou A, Vadikolias K, Birbilis T, Bouros D, Prassopoulos P. HRCT findings in the lungs of non-smokers with neurofibromatosis. Eur J Radiol. 2011;80(3):e520–3.
15. Zamora AC, Collard HR, Wolters PJ, Webb WR, King TE. Neurofibromatosis-associated lung disease: A case series and literature review. Eur Respir J. 2007;29(1):210–4.
16. Bourgouin PM, Shepard JO, Moore EH, McLoud TC. Plexiform neurofibromatosis of the mediastinum: CT appearance. AJR Am J Roentgenol. 1988;151(3):461–3.
17. Tonsgard JH, Kwak SM, Short MP, Dachman AH. CT imaging in adults with neurofibromatosis-1: Frequent asymptomatic plexiform lesions. Neurology. 1998;50(6):1755–60.
18. Carrascosa MF, Larroque IC, Rivero JL, Garcia JA, Hoz MC, Ares MA, et al. Pulmonary arterial hypertension associated with neurofibromatosis type 1. BMJ Case Rep. 2010;2010: bcr0520102961.
19. Jutant EM, Girerd B, Jais X, Savale L, O'Connell C, Perros F, et al. Pulmonary hypertension associated with neurofibromatosis type 1. Eur Respir Rev. 2018;27(149).
20. Chaddha U, Puscas I, Prosper A, Ganesh S, Yaghmour B. A 63-year-old woman with neurofibromatosis type 1 and pulmonary hypertension with worsening hypoxemia. Chest. 2017;152(4): e89–e93.
21. Armanios M. Syndromes of telomere shortening. Annu Rev Genomics Hum Genet. 2009;10:4561.
22. Moore C, Blumhagen RZ, Yang IV, Walts A, Powers J, Walker T, et al. Resequencing study confirms that host defense and cell senescence gene variants contribute to the risk of idiopathic pulmonary fibrosis. Am J Respir Crit Care Med. 2019;200(2): 199–208.
23. Sorge C, Pereboeva L, Westin E, Harris WT, Kelly DR, Goldman F. Pulmonary complications post hematopoietic stem cell transplant in dyskeratosis congenita: Analysis of oxidative stress in lung fibroblasts. Bone Marrow Transplant. 2017;52(5): 765–8.
24. Du H, Guo Y, Ma D, Tang K, Cai D, Luo Y, et al. A case report of heterozygous TINF2 gene mutation associated with pulmonary fibrosis in a patient with dyskeratosis congenita. Medicine (Baltimore). 2018;97(19):e0724.
25. Dvorak LA, Vassallo R, Kirmani S, Johnson G, Hartman TE, Tazelaar HD, et al. Pulmonary fibrosis in dyskeratosis congenita: Report of 2 cases. Hum Pathol. 2015;46(1):147–52.
26. Huizing M, Malicdan MCV, Wang JA, Pri-Chen H, Hess RA, Fischer R, et al. Hermansky-Pudlak syndrome: Mutation update. Hum Mutat. 2020;41(3):543–80.
27. Vicary GW, Vergne Y, Santiago-Cornier A, Young LR, Roman J. Pulmonary fibrosis in Hermansky-Pudlak syndrome. Ann Am Thorac Soc. 2016;13(10):1839–46.
28. El-Chemaly S, Young LR. Hermansky-Pudlak syndrome. Clin Chest Med. 2016;37(3):505–11.
29. Harada T, Ishimatsu Y, Nakashima S, Miura S, Tomonaga M, Kakugawa T, et al. An autopsy case of Hermansky-Pudlak syndrome: A case report and review of the literature on treatment. Intern Med. 2014;53(23):2705–9.
30. Bin Saeedan M, Faheem Mohammed S, Mohammed TL. Hermansky-Pudlak syndrome: High-resolution computed tomography findings and literature review. Curr Probl Diagn Radiol. 2015;44(4):383–5.
31. O'Brien KJ, Introne WJ, Akal O, Akal T, Barbu A, McGowan MP, et al. Prolonged treatment with open-label pirfenidone in Hermansky-Pudlak syndrome pulmonary fibrosis. Mol Genet Metab. 2018;125(1–2):168–73.
32. Devine MS, Garcia CK. Genetic interstitial lung disease. Clin Chest Med. 2012;33(1):95–110.
33. Kerem E, Elstein D, Abrahamov A, Bar Ziv Y, Hadas-Halpern I, Melzer E, et al. Pulmonary function abnormalities in type I Gaucher disease. Eur Respir J. 1996;9(2):340–5.
34. Garcia CK, Raghu G. Inherited interstitial lung disease. Clin Chest Med. 2004;25(3):421–33.
35. Urban Z, Gao J, Pope FM, Davis EC. Autosomal dominant cutis laxa with severe lung disease: Synthesis and matrix deposition of mutant tropoelastin. J Invest Dermatol. 2005;124(6):1193–9.
36. Tun MH, Borg B, Godfrey M, Hadley-Miller N, Chan ED. Respiratory manifestations of Marfan syndrome: A narrative review. J Thorac Dis. 2021;13(10):6012–25.

4

ALPHA-1 ANTITRYPSIN DEFICIENCY

Vickram Tejwani and James K. Stoller

Contents

Introduction 20
History of AATD 20
Epidemiology of alpha-1 antitrypsin deficiency 21
Genetics and pathogenesis of alpha-1 antitrypsin deficiency..21
Clinical features of alpha-1 antitrypsin deficiency...24
Treatment of alpha-1 antitrypsin deficiency 27
Augmentation therapy 27
Lung transplantation 27
Lung volume reduction in alpha-1 antitrypsin deficiency...28
Emerging therapies for alpha-1 antitrypsin deficiency 28
References..28

KEY POINTS

- AATD remains under-recognized despite multiple guideline recommendations for AAT level testing in all individuals with fixed airway obstruction.
- Alpha-1 antitrypsin augmentation therapy in appropriately selected individuals slows progression of emphysema as assessed by CT densitometry.
- A number of novel therapies are under study that demonstrate promise; they vary in their pharmacologic pathways and how they address the pathophysiology of AATD.

Introduction

Alpha-1 antitrypsin deficiency (AATD) is an autosomal codominant condition that predisposes to chronic obstructive pulmonary disease (COPD), liver disease (including cirrhosis and hepatocellular carcinoma), and panniculitis, and is associated with anticytoplasmic antibody (C-ANCA) positive vasculitis (1–4). Based on an estimated United States prevalence of 100,000 for the most severe deficient variant, so-called PI*ZZ, AATD is characterized as a rare disease by Food and Drug Administration (FDA) criteria. Still, AATD is highly under-recognized, with fewer than 10,000 of the estimated 100,000 Americans currently diagnosed (5). For example, AATD individuals often experience long diagnostic delays (i.e., 5–8 years) between experiencing the first symptoms of AATD and initial diagnosis and may see many healthcare providers before being tested for AATD and diagnosed (5–9).

This chapter reviews AATD. After an initial discussion of the epidemiology of AATD, the pathobiology and genetics are reviewed. Clinical manifestations, risk factors, and other disease associations with AATD are discussed next. Finally, testing strategies are reviewed, followed by an evidence-based discussion of treatment, both currently available and emerging therapies.

History of AATD

The first description of AATD demonstrates Pasteur's quote that "chance favors the prepared mind" (10). In 1963, Carl Bertill-Laurell was a senior protein chemist working at the Lund University in Sweden. While conducting a quality control activity involving serum protein electrophoresis (SPEP) samples submitted to his laboratory, he noted that five of the samples lacked a strong band in the alpha-1 region of the SPEP. It was known in 1963, the date of the first publication describing AATD by Laurell and Eriksson (10), that a protein called alpha-1 antitrypsin (AAT) comprised the majority of the alpha-1 region of the SPEP. Laurell called upon Sten Eriksson, then a trainee at Malmo, to investigate the specimens and the circumstances surrounding them. As described to one of the coauthors (JKS), Eriksson noted that several of the specimens came from patients he was following in his longitudinal clinic and that several had early onset of emphysema and a family history of same. Thus, out of this serendipitous collaboration between a senior protein chemist and a then junior trainee came the first report of AATD in 1963 (10). Six years later in 1969, Harvey Sharp, a pediatric gastroenterologist in Minneapolis, Minnesota, who was caring for children with end-stage liver disease, first described cirrhosis in association with AATD (11).

In the approximately 60 years since the first description of AATD, substantial strides have been made in understanding the AAT molecule and the condition, including characterizing the protein as a 394 amino acid glycoprotein, locating and sequencing the gene (which is on the long arm of chromosome 14), characterizing the protein folding and trafficking through the hepatocyte, as well as describing the natural history of individuals with severe deficiency of AATD in the National Heart Lung and Blood Institute Registry of Individuals with AATD and other studies. Discovery is ongoing as AATD is perhaps the best developed example of a COPD endotype, with substantial progress in strategies to detect affected individuals and to treat AATD, including novel genetic approaches.

Epidemiology of alpha-1 antitrypsin deficiency

Prevalence estimates for AATD have been determined in two ways: by direct counting in population-based screening studies and by indirect estimates using genetic epidemiologic surveys (5). Population-based studies have been performed by screening an unselected group of individuals, i.e., all comers irrespective of any clinical features that might suggest AATD. Alternately, case-finding or targeted detection is conducted by testing individuals who have clinical features that suggest consideration of AATD (e.g., emphysema, family history of COPD or cirrhosis, etc.).

The largest available population-based screening study for AATD was conducted in Swedish newborns between November 1972 and September 1974 and included 95% of all of Swedish newborns during that period (12). Sveger et al. detected 120 severely deficient individuals (i.e., PI*ZZ and 2 PI*Z), demonstrating a prevalence of severe deficiency of AAT of 1 per 1,639 live births (12). In the second largest population-based screening study, O'Brien et al. screened 107,038 newborns in Oregon and identified 21 newborns with homozygous deficient genotypes (PI*ZZ or PI*Z Null) and 11 cases with variant genotypes (including PI*MZ, PI*SZ, and unspecified others), indicating a prevalence of 1 per 5,097 live births with severe deficiency of AAT (13). Extrapolating the results of the Oregon study to the U.S. population of approximately 330 million, there are an estimated 65,000 Americans with severe deficiency of AAT.

Severe deficiency is defined as having AAT serum levels that fall below a "protective threshold" value (i.e., the serum AAT value below emphysema risk rises) which is widely considered to be 11 micromolar (or 57 mg/dl) (1, 4). At the same time, the utility of this value has been challenged by its nonassociation with pulmonary risk in PI*SZ individuals (14) and by early studies suggesting that raising serum (and lung levels) of AAT above this threshold offers incremental protection against inflammation (15).

In data from 514 worldwide cohorts (69 countries throughout 11 geographic regions of the world), de Serres et al. estimated the global prevalence of PI*ZZ, PI*SZ and PI*SS individuals as 3.4 million; when extrapolated to the world population in 2015 (7.3 billion versus 4.4 billion in 2002 when the study was published), the prevalence of AATD individuals was estimated at 5.64 million (16, 17). de Serres et al. showed considerable variability in AATD prevalence among different ethnic groups, with the highest gene frequency for the Z allele recorded among individuals of Northern European descent (16–18). Conversely, AATD is very uncommon in Asian countries such as China and Indonesia. PI*S$_{iiyama}$ is the most common variant identified in Japan. Severe AATD is uncommon among African Americans and Hispanic Americans living in the United States, comprising 0.5% and 7.8%, respectively, of PI*ZZ individuals in the United States. In contrast, the S allele is relatively common with ~10% of Hispanic Americans carrying the PI*MS genotype (19).

Given that AATD occurs in all examined populations, substantial evidence in three lines of reasoning shows that AATD is under-recognized. First, surveys of practicing physicians show that only a minority test for AATD. For example, in a study of German and Italian family physicians, internists, and pulmonologists, Greulich et al. showed that only a third of the physicians reported testing for AATD testing (20). In the same study, while most (92%) of the surveyed German pulmonologists reported doing targeted testing for AATD, only 54% of the Italian pulmonologists tested for AATD. Furthermore, only a small minority (18 and 25%, respectively) reported testing all COPD patients for AATD (as suggested in the guidelines from the American Thoracic Society and European Respiratory Society [1] and many other guidelines [21]).

Further evidence of under-recognition is that epidemiologic studies consistently show that only a small minority of AATD individuals are recognized across a range of countries. Table 4.1 reviews the low frequencies of detected individuals across a variety of countries, all less than 21% and most substantially lower.

The third line of evidence showing under-recognition is that affected individuals frequently experience long delays, averaging 5–8 years (Table 4.2) (5–9, 20, 22), between the onset of initial symptoms and first diagnosis. Also, AAT deficient individuals typically see multiple healthcare providers before initial diagnosis, with little evidence that the diagnostic delay intervals from various estimates over time have shortened over nearly two decades of observations (5, 8). Because delay in diagnosis is associated with worsened clinical status at the time of initial diagnosis (22), enhancing early detection of affected individuals is imperative.

Genetics and pathogenesis of alpha-1 antitrypsin deficiency

Alpha-1 antitrypsin deficiency is inherited as an autosomal codominant condition. The AAT protein is coded by the SERPINA1 gene, located on the long arm of chromosome 14 (14q31-32.3), and contains 6 introns, 4 coding (2, 3, 4, and 5), and 3 noncoding (1a, 1b, and 1c) exons. Over 150 AAT allele variants have been described to date (1, 3, 4, 23).

Alpha-1 antitrypsin variants are named according to the PI (protease inhibitor) nomenclature that describes patterns of AAT protein expression, designated as the AAT "phenotype." Accordingly, the variants are named based on their band migration position in an isoelectric pH (4–5) gradient on gel electrophoresis—an older testing method—from "A" for anodal variants to "Z" for slower migrating variants. For example, PI*MM, the most common and normal AAT type indicates homozygosity for the wild type M allele (2). In contrast, PI*ZZ describes individuals who are homozygous for the severe deficiency Z allele; they comprise the majority (95%) of those with clinical disease associated with AATD (24).

In contrast to the phenotype, the AAT genotype refers to the specific allelic combination of an individual as detected by allele-specific gene amplification tests or other gene sequencing techniques. For example, a PI*MM individual has a wild type whole gene nucleotide sequence. In contrast, an individual with the PI*ZZ genotype has a single nucleotide polymorphism (guanine to adenosine) that results in a single amino acid substitution (of lysine for glutamic acid) at position 342 on the 394 amino acid AAT glycoprotein (Figure 4.1) (23).

In the context that severe deficiency of AAT predisposes to both COPD and to liver disease, including fibrosis and cirrhosis, the pathogenesis of lung and liver disease are linked but different (1, 3). Specifically, emphysema results from a "toxic loss of function" of AAT in the lung, in which deficiency of AAT depletes the lung's antiprotease screen, exposing the alveoli to unopposed

TABLE 4.1: Prevalence of Specific AATD Phenotypes in Selected Population Screening Studies

Main Language Origin*

First Author (Ref)	Year	Location	Subject Population	Number Screened	ZZ	SZ	MZ	SS	MS
Western Slavic									
Kaczor (107, 108)	2007	Poland	Random sample	859	0	0	2.10	0.12	3.26
Uralic									
Saris (109)	1972	Finland	College	664	0.15	—	5.12	—	—
Northern Germanic									
Sveger (110)	1979	Sweden	Military recruits	11,128	0.04	0.08	0.03	—	—
Dahl (111)	2002	Denmark	Random sample	9,187	0.07	0.11	4.90	0.13	5.00
Western Germanic									
Hoffman (112)	1976	Netherlands	Population survey	1,474	0.07	0.07	2.24	0	2.84
Dijkman (113)	1980	Netherlands	Newborns	95083	0.03	—	—	0.04	—
Kimpen (114)	1988	Belgium	Newborns	10,329	0.06	0.12	0.97	0.01	0.88
Cook (115)	1975	United Kingdom	Population survey	5,588	0.04	0.21	2.02	0.32	7.19
Webb (116)	1973	New York	Population survey	500	0	0	3.6	0.2	6
Lieberman (117)	1976	California	High school	1,841	0	0.27	1.85	0.05	6.90
Evans (118)	1977	New York	Newborns	1,010	0	0	1.19	0.89	3.07
Morse (119)	1977	Arizona	Population survey	2,944	0.07	0.20	3.0		7.1
O'Brien (120)	1978	Oregon	Newborns	107,038	0.02	0.01	—		
Dykes (121)	1984	Minnesota	Blood donors	904	0	—	2.77	0.22	4.09
Silverman (122)	1989	Missouri	Blood donors	20,000	0.04	0.01	0.01		
Spence (123)	1993	New York	Newborns	11,081	0.03	0.05	0.53	0.01	0.09
Eastern Romanic									
Klasen (124)	1978	Italy	Outpatients	202	0	0	1.98	0	4.95
Corda (125)	2011	Italy	Town screening	817	0.12		5.6	0.12	6.3
Western Romanic									
Goedde (126)	1973	Spain	Population survey	576	—	—	1.04	—	22.7
Spínola (127)	2009	Madeira	Volunteers	200	0	1	4	3	29
Spínola (128)	2010	Cape Verde	Volunteers	202	0	0	0.5	1.49	3.5
Afro-Asiatic									
Vandeville (129)	1973	Zaire	Population survey	132	0	0	0	0	0
Massi (130)	1977	Somalia	Newborns	347	0.86	0.28	0.28		2.59
Aljarallah (131)	2011	Saudi Arabia	Volunteers	158	0	3.8	2.53	1.9	
Altaic									
Harada (132)	1977	Japan	Blood donors	856	0	0	0.23	0	0.23

Source: From reference (133), with permission.

* Classification is based on the notion that linguistic phyla align with genetic clusters, reflecting their common origins.

TABLE 4.2: Diagnostic Delay Interval for Alpha-1 Antitrypsin Deficiency

Authors	Publication Year	Country	Diagnostic Delay in Years (mean ± SD or median, IQR)
Stoller et al. (7)	1994	United States	7.2 ± 8.3
Stoller et al. (8)	2005	United States	5.6 ± 8.5
Campos et al. (6)	2005	United States	8.3 ± 6.9
Kohnlein et al. (9)	2010	Germany	6
Greulich et al. (20)	2013	Germany	7 (13)
		Italy	6 (11)
Tejwani et al. (22)	2019	United States	5 (12)

proteolytic damage (2–4, 25). Various proteases—including neutrophil elastase, cysteinyl protease, and various matrix metalloproteinases—when unopposed, can threaten the integrity of lung elastin, which provides structural integrity and elasticity. Neutrophil elastase (NE), which is contained within the primary granules of polymorphonuclear leukocytes, represents a major proteolytic threat that is increased when neutrophils traffic to the lung as during inflammation, e.g., cigarette smoking, dust exposure, etc.

Alpha-1 antitrypsin is a member of the SERPIN (**ser**ine **p**rotease **in**hibitor) family of protease inhibitors (2–4, 25–27) and is the major antiprotease at the alveolar level, providing >90% of the antiprotease screen there; AAT binds neutrophil elastase avidly, neutralizing NE in a 1:1 stoichiometric ratio by binding to and

Alpha-1 Antitrypsin Deficiency 23

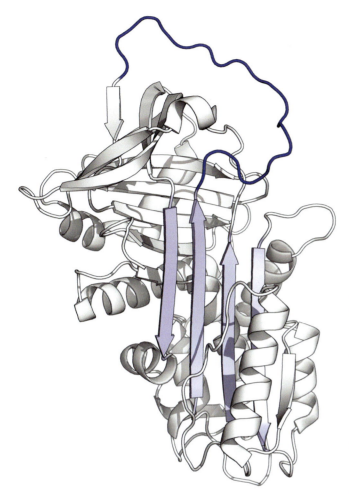

FIGURE 4.1 Alpha-1 antitrypsin glycoprotein.

cleaving the reactive site of AAT, catapulting NE in a mousetrap-like mechanism (Figure 4.2).

Depletion of serum levels of AAT causes downstream depletion of lung AAT levels, notably in the lung interstitium where elastin comprises the lung matrix and provides lung elasticity. Destruction of elastin in the alveolar walls results in wall degradation and loss of alveolar wall tethering, causing the airflow obstruction that is the physiologic signature of emphysema.

In contrast to the "toxic loss of function" that causes emphysema in the lung, liver disease in AATD results from a "toxic gain of function," in which a conformational abnormality of some AAT variants (e.g., Z, M_{malton}, S_{iiyama}, King's [Table 4.3]) (4) cause the variant AAT to fold abnormally, promoting polymerization and resultant accumulation within the hepatocyte. These polymers form the periodic acid-Schiff (PAS)-positive diastase-resistant eosinophilic globules that are characteristic (but not pathognomonic) of these AAT deficiency genotypes (Figure 4.3). Polymers form in a process called loop-sheet polymerization in which amino acid substitutions at strategic positions along the primary 394 amino acid structure of the AAT molecule destabilize regions of the molecule, promoting insertion of regions of adjacent AAT molecules into a neighboring AAT molecule (26). Polymerization overwhelms the usual protein trafficking and clearance mechanisms of the hepatocyte (e.g., autophagy) (28–30), causing AAT to accumulate intracellularly and a cascade of events that can produce liver fibrosis and cirrhosis. The toxic accumulation of AAT within the hepatocyte causes serum and therefore lung levels of AAT to be low.

Because the pathogenesis of lung and liver disease in AATD are different, some individuals experience primarily emphysema, other cirrhosis alone, and some both. While determinants of clinical expression are incompletely understood, known risk factors for emphysema include cigarette exposure and occupational dust exposure (31); risk factors for liver disease include male gender, age >50 years, obesity, diabetes, and the metabolic syndrome (4, 32, 33).

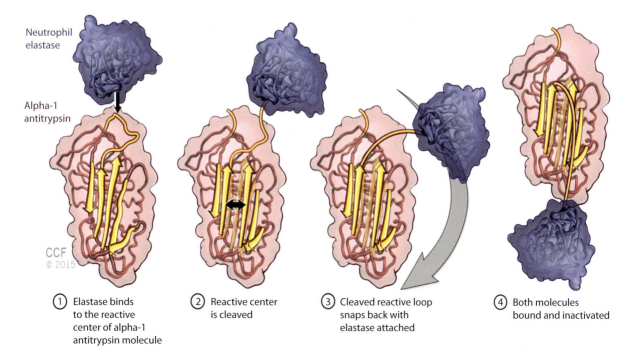

FIGURE 4.2 Mechanism of neutrophil elastase (blue) binding to alpha-1 antitrypsin (pink). Cleavage of the reactive loop releases steric energy in the AAT molecule, catapulting neutrophil elastase to the opposite end of the AAT molecule in a mousetrap-like mechanism.

TABLE 4.3: Selected PI Variants with Characteristics Including Type of Mutation, Cellular Defect, and Disease Association

PI Allele	Type of Mutation (rs Number)	Cellular Defect	Disease Association
Normal Alleles			
M1V	Val213	None	Normal
M1A	Ala213	None	Normal
M2	Arg101His on M3	None	Normal
M3	Glu376Asp on M1V	None	Normal
M4	Arg101His on M1V	None	Normal
Christchurch	Glu363Lys	None	Normal
V$_{munich}$	Asp2Ala on M1V	None	Normal
Deficiency Alleles	Glu264Val on M1V (rs17580)		
S	Glu342Lys on M1A (rs28929474)	IC Degradation	Lung
Z*	Phe52del on M2 (rs775982338)	IC Accumulation	Lung, liver
M$_{malton}$	Ser53Phe on M1V (rs55819880)	IC Accumulation	Lung, liver
S$_{iiyama}$	Pro369Leu on M1A	IC Accumulation	Lung
M$_{heerlen}$	Leu41Pro on M1V (rs28931569)	IC Degradation	Lung
M$_{procida}$	Gly67Glu on M1V (rs28931568)	IC Degradation	Lung
M$_{mineral\ springs}$*		IC Degradation	Lung
Null Alleles			
Q0$_{granite\ falls}$	Tyr160Ter on M1A (rs267606950)	No mRNA	Lung
Q0$_{bellingham}$	Lys217Ter on M1V (rs199422211)	No mRNA	Lung
Q0$_{ludwigshafen}$	Ile92Asn on M2	Disrupted tertiary structure	Lung[†]
Q0$_{hongkong-1}$	2-bp del Leu318 fs334ter on M2 (rs1057519610)	IC accumulation	Lung[†]
Q0$_{isola\ di\ procida}$	17 kb del on M2	Truncated protein IC Accumulation No mRNA	Lung
Dysfunctional Alleles			
F	Arg223Cys on M1V	Defective NE inhibition	Lung
Pittsburgh	Met358Arg (rs121912713)	Antithrombin 3 activity	Bleeding diathesis
M$_{mineral\ springs}$*	Gly67Glu on M1V (rs28931568)	Defective NE inhibition	Lung
Z*	Glu342Lys on M1A (rs28929474)	Defective NE inhibition	Lung, liver

Source: Adapted by permission from BMJ Publishing Group Limited from DeMeo DL and Silverman EK. Thorax 2004;59:259–264; and from Online Mendelian Inheritance in Man (OMIM®), Johns Hopkins University, Baltimore, MD. 7/04/2011: http://omim.org/entry/107400.

Abbreviations: IC: intracellular; bp: base pair(s); NE: neutrophil elastase, del: deletion; fs: frame shift; ter: terminal codon.

* Note that M$_{mineral\ springs}$ and Z have dysfunctional characteristics described based on altered rates of association and inhibition of neutrophil elastase, as well as deficiency characteristics.
† Although liver disease is theoretically possible in these null variants associated with IC accumulation, there are no reports of liver disease perhaps because of their rarity.

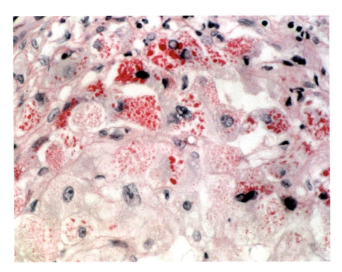

FIGURE 4.3 PAS-positive diastase-resistant globules in hepatocytes in a liver biopsy from a PI*ZZ individual.

To date, more than 150 variants of AAT have been described and are characterized as normal variants, deficiency variants, null variants, and dysfunctional variants (Table 4.3). In addition to the deficient variants that are characterized by intra-hepatocyte accumulation of mutant AAT, other deficient variants are characterized by enhanced degradation of intra-hepatocyte AAT without significant polymer accumulation (e.g., S variants) (4). Dysfunctional variants are characterized by various functional abnormalities, including lessened avidity to bind neutrophil elastase (e.g., Z and F variants) (34) and assuming an antithrombin function, causing a bleeding diathesis (e.g., Pittsburgh variant).

Clinical features of alpha-1 antitrypsin deficiency

Pulmonary manifestations of AATD are emphysema, chronic bronchitis, and bronchiectasis (1–4). The extrapulmonary manifestations are liver disease (e.g., chronic hepatitis, cirrhosis, and hepatocellular carcinoma) and less commonly, panniculitis

(35, 36) and vasculitis (especially anticytoplasmic antibody-associated vasculitis) (37–40). Other disease associations have been suggested but are less well-established, including gallbladder disease (41); glomerulonephritis; celiac disease; lung, colorectal, and bladder cancers; aneurysmal and aortic disease (42, 43); and pancreatitis.

Lung disease

Features suggestive of AATD-associated emphysema are occurrence in non- or minimal smokers, early onset (i.e., in the fourth and fifth decades of life), panacinar pathology (44), and disproportionate emphysematous involvement of the lung bases (Figure 4.4) (45). However, performing testing for AATD only when "classic" features are present will lead to under-recognition, given that most AATD patients present with the more usual signs and symptoms of COPD. As a specific example, the presence of upper lobe emphysema in a 65-year-old smoker should not exclude testing for AATD. As evidence, of the 1,129 participants in the NHLBI Registry of Individuals with Severe Deficiency of AAT, 81% had smoked and symptoms included usual features of COPD: dyspnea (84%), usual cough (42%), usual phlegm (46%), and wheezing with upper respiratory infections (76%) (24). Individuals with AATD may not present with distinctive features and may look phenotypically just like individuals with "usual" COPD. Therefore, to avert under-recognition, guidelines suggest testing all COPD patients for AATD (1, 21).

Given the unopposed proteolytic activity in AATD, an association with chronic bronchitis and bronchiectasis is biologically plausible. In a survey of individuals with AATD, 40% reported a diagnosis of chronic bronchitis (46). Also, AATD individuals with abnormal lung function are more likely to have a chronic bronchitis history than those with normal lung function (24). Based on a study of computed tomography scans from 74 individuals with AATD, bronchiectasis was identified in 95% of individuals with AATD (47). The same study found clinically significant bronchiectasis in 27% of participants, whereas the prevalence is estimated at 1% in the NHLBI Registry (24). Therefore, in patients with bronchiectasis and no other evident etiology (e.g., cystic fibrosis, hypogammaglobulinemia, mucociliary dysfunction, etc.), testing for AATD is recommended (1).

Liver disease

Liver disease associated with AATD may manifest as neonatal hepatitis, cirrhosis, and hepatocellular carcinoma. The Z and M_{malton} alleles are most commonly associated with liver disease given they are characterized by intra-hepatocyte polymerization of AAT protein (4, 32). Although S_{iiyama}, King's alleles, and other rare genotypes are known to cause intra-hepatocyte polymerization, their association with clinical liver disease is uncertain (48, 49). The ATS/ERS guideline on AATD recommends testing for AATD in all individuals "with unexplained liver disease, including neonates, children, and adults, especially the elderly."

Panniculitis

The association between panniculitis and AATD was first described by Warter et al. in 1972 and has since been multiply observed in case series and in various genotypes, including PI*ZZ, PI*SZ, PI*SS, and PI*MS. Panniculitis is an uncommon feature of AATD, occurring in ~1 per 1,000 AAT deficient individuals and it is unclear if it has a higher prevalence in AATD compared to non-AATD COPD (50). However, the finding of Z-type polymers in the skin of a PI*ZZ patient with panniculitis and the dramatic clinical response to intravenous augmentation therapy suggest that deficiency of AAT may be causal. In fact, panniculitis is widely considered to be an off-label indication for augmentation therapy. Painful, weepy cutaneous nodules are characteristic, sometimes necrosing (Figure 4.5) and commonly occurring at sites of trauma. Diagnosis is typically made by deep excisional biopsy. Individuals with panniculitis may also manifest a pan-serositis (51).

Vasculitis

AATD has also been shown to be associated with C-ANCA positive vasculitis, first reported in in 1993. Although studies since then have demonstrated over-representation of abnormal AAT genotypes among individuals with antibody-positive vasculitis (38, 52, 53), more recent studies of AATD have not identified an increased prevalence of vasculitis among individuals with AATD (40, 50). Therefore, earlier guideline recommendations notwithstanding, testing all patients with vasculitis for AATD may not be appropriate, although the presence of panniculitis should prompt consideration of AATD (1).

Natural history of alpha-1 antitrypsin deficiency

The long-term natural history of AATD has been best characterized by following individuals identified at birth in the aforementioned Swedish and Oregon population-based screening studies (12, 13). Follow-up of the Swedish cohort (which tested 200,000 consecutive newborns) to age 41 has indicated that 41-year-old never-smoking PI*ZZ individuals have normal lung function and no excess emphysema on CT scan compared with normal

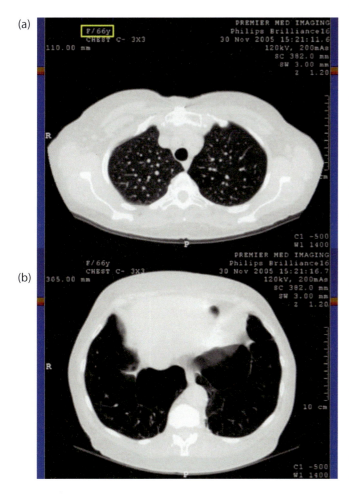

FIGURE 4.4 CT images of a patient with PI*ZZ AATD, demonstrating disproportionate basilar distribution of emphysematous change. (a) Apical cut. (b) Basal cut.

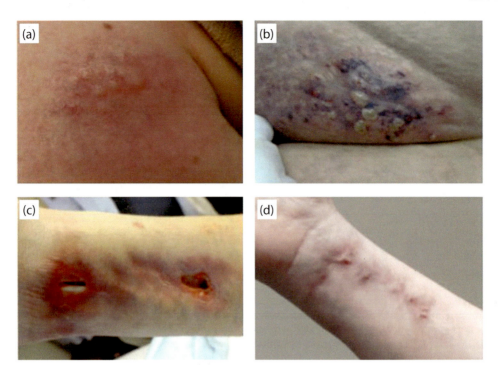

FIGURE 4.5 Panniculitis in patients with alpha-1 antitrypsin deficiency: (a) Violaceous nodule with overlying grouped yellowish pseudovesicles and telangiectasias on the right shoulder. (b) Erythematous, violaceous nodules on the left Mons pubis with fat-like projections and ulcerations. (c) Erythematous, violaceous nodules and plaques on the right volar wrist with marked ulcerations. (d) Complete healing was documented within 3 weeks of initiating intravenous augmentation therapy. (Reproduced with permission from Elsensohn AN, Curtis JA, Secrest AM, et al. Alpha-1 antitrypsin deficiency panniculitis presenting with severe anasarca, pulmonary embolus and hypogammaglobulinaemia. Br J Dermatol. 2015;173(1):289–291.)

age/gender-matched peers (54). In contrast, the few PI*ZZ ever smokers demonstrated a lower transfer factor and significantly more emphysema on CT scan than normal (PI*MM) never smokers. Data from the NHLBI Registry indicate that, on average, AATD individuals experience more rapid decline in FEV_1 decline than normal (24); among never smokers in the Registry, the average rate of FEV_1 decline was 67 mL/year and among ex-smokers, the rate was 54 mL/year, both exceeding the general age-related FEV_1 decline rates of approximately 20–25 mL/year in never smoking, normal adults. Among the few current smokers in the Registry, the rate of FEV_1 decline was even higher at 109 mL/year (55).

Rates of FEV_1 decline over time have been shown to vary by Global Obstructive Lung Disease (GOLD) strata; PI*ZZ individuals with GOLD Stage II COPD lose lung function faster than individuals with either milder or more severe degrees of airflow obstruction (56). As with COPD in general, exacerbations in AATD individuals are associated with worsened clinical status. In one series, 54% of 265 PI*ZZ individuals experienced an exacerbation over the first year of follow-up and 18% of these were frequent exacerbators (≥3 exacerbations/year) (57).

Finally, severe deficiency of AAT can be fatal. Specifically, in the NHLBI Registry, the overall mortality rate at 5 years of follow-up was 18.6%, approximately 3% per year (55). In keeping with the known adverse prognostic effect of low FEV_1, 36% of individuals entering the Registry with FEV_1 values less than 15% predicted died by 3 years in contrast to a 2.6% 3-year mortality rate among individuals with baseline FEV_1 greater than 50% predicted. Causes of death in Registry participants were emphysema in 72% and cirrhosis in 10% (58), which were the only causes of death more frequent than in age and gender-matched individuals. In a series of PI*ZZ never smokers (59), deaths attributed to cirrhosis accounted for 28% of deaths and deaths due to emphysema reduced to 45%, indicating that never smokers may escape risks related to early emphysema but more frequently develop clinically significant cirrhosis later in life.

Diagnosing alpha-1 antitrypsin deficiency

Available strategies to detect AATD include determining the serum AAT level, most frequently done by a turbidometric assay (nephelometry), in which normal serum levels generally range from 100–220 mg/dl or 20–53 micromolar (2–4, 27, 60). Other available tests include phenotyping, most commonly performed by isoelectric focusing, which can identify different band patterns associated with different alleles (Figure 4.6). Genotyping involves determining which AAT alleles are present, most frequently by using polymerase chain reaction probes that target the S and Z alleles and, in some laboratories, the F and I alleles. When clinical suspicion is high, characteristically when a low serum AAT level is not explained by the phenotype or genotype results, (34) definitive testing by gene sequencing may be needed.

Guidelines frequently recommend testing for both the AAT serum level and the genotype (21). Serum levels alone may be inadequate because AAT is an acute phase reactant, so that serum levels in many genotypes rise in acute inflammatory states, though minimally so in PI*ZZ. Also, the F allele is uniquely associated with a preserved AAT serum level but impaired binding avidity for neutrophil elastase, so that a normal serum level could miss the diagnosis in PI*FF individuals, however uncommon (34).

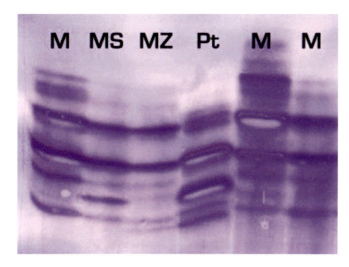

FIGURE 4.6 Isoelectric focusing showing different band patterns of different alleles.

Testing is commonly available in hospital laboratories or as send-outs to commercial laboratories. Furthermore, free test kits, some assessing 14 AAT alleles (61), are widely available from manufacturers of drugs for AATD as well as from the Alpha-1 Foundation in the so-called Alpha Coded Testing (ACT) trial (62). The latter offers users a free, home-based confidential test kit that is provided and processed by the University of Florida. The ACT allows patients to be tested without a physician order and has also facilitated allied health providers, such as respiratory therapists, recommending testing in appropriate clinical circumstances, e.g., when patients demonstrate fixed airflow obstruction on performing spirometry in the pulmonary function laboratory (5, 60). Other strategies to enhance testing have included providing prompts to physicians when their patients show fixed airflow obstruction on pulmonary function tests (both through an electronic medical record and in printed pulmonary function reports (63, 64), opt-out testing for AAT in the electronic medical record for guideline-appropriate candidates (65), and issuing reminders to patients to seek testing when seeking prescriptions for COPD-specific medications (66).

Treatment of alpha-1 antitrypsin deficiency

Treatment of COPD due to AATD is similar to treatment of "usual" COPD, with mainstays of smoking cessation, long-acting bronchodilators, preventive vaccinations, pulmonary rehabilitation, supplemental oxygen if indicated, and lung transplantation for advanced disease. Lung volume reduction surgery (LVRS) confers less advantage in AATD than in "usual" COPD, with the sparse available experience showing a shorter duration and smaller magnitude of FEV_1 increase following LVRS (67, 68). Currently, the available specific therapy for those with AATD-associated emphysema is called augmentation therapy, the intravenous infusion of pooled human plasma-derived AAT (69).

Augmentation therapy

Four augmentation therapy drugs have been approved by the FDA for treating individuals with emphysema due to AATD, the first of which was introduced in 1987. All four drugs have achieved registration by demonstrating biochemical efficacy, i.e., that the weekly infusion of 60 mg/kg of pooled human plasma-derived AAT raised and maintained serum levels of AAT above the serum protective threshold value of 11 micromolar or 57 mg/dl throughout the dosing interval.

Aggregate results of three randomized controlled trials of augmentation therapy have shown that treatment slows the progression of emphysema as assessed by CT densitometry, with little current definitive evidence that augmentation therapy lessens exacerbation frequency, enhances functional status, or quality of life, or prolongs survival (70, 71).

Augmentation therapy is indicated for individuals with emphysema due to severe deficiency of AAT, with an FDA-approved dose of 60 mg/kg weekly. Alternate dosing intervals (e.g., 120 mg/kg every other week) have been prescribed in clinical practice (24), and although the clinical significance is uncertain, the pharmacokinetics of every other week dosing indicates that serum AAT levels fall below 11 micromolar toward the end of the dosing interval (72). Augmentation therapy is generally well-tolerated, with only mild and infrequent side effects and very few patients experiencing side effects severe enough to prompt discontinuation (73, 74).

The cost of augmentation therapy is high (~$100,000 yearly), with cost-effectiveness studies showing that the quality-adjusted life-years (QALY) associated with augmentation therapy exceeds the usual criterion of $50,000 per QALY (75).

Augmentation therapy is not recommended for PI*MZ heterozygotes who may have COPD (if they smoke) (76), based on the absence of any supportive evidence of efficacy for heterozygotes and the biologic implausibility of benefit for such individuals; PI*MZ heterozygotes rarely have serum levels below the serum protective threshold value of 11 μM.

For PI*SZ heterozygotes, ~10% of such individuals may have serum levels below 11 μM, and PI*SZ smokers may develop emphysema (77, 78). Data from Franciosi et al. suggest that the risk of emphysema among PI*SZ individuals is unrelated to whether their serum level exceeds or falls below the protective threshold value (14). Although no randomized trials specifically address the efficacy of augmentation therapy in PI*SZ, the authors' practice is to offer augmentation therapy to selected PI*SZ individuals with emphysema.

Lung transplantation

Alpha-1 antitrypsin deficiency accounts for ~5% of lung transplantations performed in the United States according to the Registry of the International Society for Heart and Lung Transplantation. AATD patients with COPD ($n = 2,187$) had better long-term survival compared to those with "usual" COPD ($n = 9,616$) (survival half-life 6.1 versus 5.2 years, $p = 0.01$) (79). However, outcomes vary considerably across individual centers, likely reflecting local variation in candidate selection and practice (80–84). Although a survival benefit of lung transplantation is not established for COPD in general, a case-control study has suggested improved long-term survival in the subset with AATD-associated COPD. Tanash and colleagues matched 83 severe AATD COPD patients who underwent lung transplantation with 70 control cases (AATD COPD patients who did not undergo transplantation selected from the Swedish national AATD registry) (85). The estimated median survival time was 11 years (95% CI 9–14 years) in transplant recipients versus 5 years (95% CI 4–6 years) in controls. This is in contrast to findings from another natural history study of lung transplant recipients with "usual" COPD (231 patients) versus AATD-associated COPD (45 patients) at the Cleveland Clinic (86). While the overall rate of decline in FEV_1 slope and survival did not differ between the two groups, a trend toward worse early post–lung transplantation survival was observed in the AATD group. Criteria for lung transplantation in lung transplantation resemble those for COPD in general with attention to the specific comorbidities that may accompany AATD (e.g., cirrhosis with possible of hepatopulmonary syndrome, portopulmonary hypertension).

Lung volume reduction in alpha-1 antitrypsin deficiency

Results of the National Emphysema Treatment Trial have shown that in carefully selected subsets, lung volume reduction surgery (LVRS) for COPD can confer significant physiologic, functional, and survival benefits. Data regarding the efficacy of LVRS for individuals with AATD are more limited and generally less favorable; the improvement in FEV_1 following LVRS was smaller in AATD individuals and the duration of FEV_1 rise post-LVRS was shorter-lived (67, 68, 87–89). Guidelines from the ATS/ERS regarding LVRS state: "The scant evidence regarding the efficacy of LVRS (with possible resection of lower lobes) in individuals with AAT deficiency suggests that improvement in dyspnea, lung function, and functional status is possible. However, well-studied, robust selection criteria for ideal candidates remain elusive and the duration of lung volume reduction surgery benefit appears shorter than individuals with AAT-replete COPD."

Given the promise of reversibility and lower postprocedure morbidity and mortality, bronchoscopic lung volume reduction by inserting one-way endobronchial valves has been studied in a small number of AATD individuals and has shown some benefit for lung function and symptom burden but has associated procedural complications (90, 91). Taken together, we advise caution regarding lung volume reduction surgery for AATD. Although more study is needed, endoscopic lung volume reduction with deployment of endobronchial valves may offer a viable alternative for treatment, particularly as a bridge to lung transplantation.

Emerging therapies for alpha-1 antitrypsin deficiency

Many promising lines of research are under way regarding new treatment strategies for AATD, both regarding the pulmonary and hepatic sequelae. Direct delivery of AAT to the lung via inhalational therapy has been shown to be feasible and safe (Table 4.4) (92, 93). Thus far, clinical improvement has not been observed (94), though additional studies are planned to assess this. Gene therapy with exogenous transfer of DNA coding for normal AAT is being attempted through various delivery mechanisms (95–97).

A variety of other emerging treatment strategies are being explored in early phase studies currently. These wide-ranging approaches include: inhibiting intra-hepatic polymerization of AAT (98, 99), promoting hepatic secretion of AAT (100, 101), prolonging the serum half-life of AAT by pegylation (102) or by designing recombinant AAT proteins (103), interfering with mutant (and native) AAT production by small interfering mRNA, enhancing intra-hepatic degradation of mutant AAT by stimulating autophagy (e.g., by carbamazepine [104] or rapamycin [105]), doubling the delivered dose of intravenous augmentation therapy, administering "corrector" molecules that restore the liver's ability to secrete AAT with acute phase reactivity, and administering oral neutrophil elastase inhibitors (106).

Taken together, the future treatment landscape of AATD is bright, with promising approaches that will change the current treatment paradigm of augmentation therapy and offer alternative approaches. Further research will explicate the efficacy and practicality of these emerging options.

TABLE 4.4: Emerging Therapies for Alpha-1 Antitrypsin Deficiency

Treatment Approach	Examples
Augmentation therapy approaches	New routes of administration (e.g., inhaled, continuous infusion)
	New agents (e.g., recombinant yeast-derived alpha-1 antitrypsin, dimer AAT)
	Alternative dosing (e.g., 120 mg/kg/week)
Oral neutrophil elastase inhibitors	ATALANTA trial (134)
Prevention of polymer formation	Small peptides that insert into Z molecule preventing polymerization (135)
Elastin protection	Inhaled hyaluronic acid (136)
Hepatic secretagogues	4-phenylbutyrate (137)
Enhance autophagy	Carbamazepine, rapamycin (104, 105)
Gene therapy	Adeno-associated virus and other vectors with intramuscular, intrapleural, or whole limb perfusion delivery
Small interfering mRNA to lessen expression of the Z molecule	RNA interference to lessen AAT accumulation in liver (138)
Human-induced pluripotent stem cell lines (hIPSCs)	Generation of transgene-free lung disease-specific pluripotent stem cells (139)
Corrector molecule	Small molecule to increase AAT levels (106)
Gene editing	CRISPR approaches in murine models (140)

References

1. American Thoracic Society, European Respiratory Society. American Thoracic Society/European Respiratory Society statement: Standards for the diagnosis and management of individuals with alpha-1 antitrypsin deficiency. Am J Respir Crit Care Med. 2003;168(7):818–900. doi:10.1164/rccm.168.7.818
2. Hatipoglu U, Stoller JK. Alpha-1 antitrypsin deficiency. Clin Chest Med. 2016;37(3):487–504. doi:10.1016/j.ccm.2016.04.011
3. Greene CM, Marciniak SJ, Teckman J, et al. α1-Antitrypsin deficiency. Nat Rev Dis Prim. 2016;2:16051. doi:10.1038/nrdp.2016.51
4. Strnad P, McElvaney NG, Lomas DA. Alpha-1 antitrypsin deficiency. N Engl J Med. 2020;382(15):1443–55. doi:10.1056/NEJMra1910234
5. Stoller JK. Detecting alpha-1 antitrypsin deficiency. Ann Am Thorac Soc. 2016;13 Suppl 4:S317–25. doi:10.1513/AnnalsATS.201506-349KV
6. Campos MA, Wanner A, Zhang G, Sandhaus RA. Trends in the diagnosis of symptomatic patients with alpha-1 antitrypsin deficiency between 1968 and 2003. Chest. 2005;128(3):1179–86. doi:10.1378/chest.128.3.1179
7. Stoller JK, Smith P, Yang P, Spray J. Physical and social impact of alpha-1 antitrypsin deficiency: Results of a survey. Cleve Clin J Med. 1994;61(6):461–7.
8. Stoller JK, Sandhaus RA, Turino G, Dickson R, Rodgers K, Strange C. Delay in diagnosis of alpha-1 antitrypsin deficiency: A continuing problem. Chest. 2005;128(4):1989–94. doi:10.1378/chest.128.4.1989

9. Kohnlein T, Janciauskiene S, Welte T. Diagnostic delay and clinical modifiers in alpha-1 antitrypsin deficiency. Ther Adv Respir Dis. 2010;4(5):279–87.
10. Laurell Eriksson, A CB. The electrophoretic alpha-1 globulin pattern of serum in alpha-1 antitrypsin deficiency. Scand J Clin Lab Invest. 1963;15:132–40.
11. Sharp HL, Bridges RA, Krivit W, Freier EF. Cirrhosis associated with alpha-1-antitrypsin deficiency: A previously unrecognized inherited disorder. J Lab Clin Med. 1969;73(6):934–9.
12. Sveger T. Liver disease in alpha1-antitrypsin deficiency detected by screening of 200,000 infants. N Engl J Med. 1976;294(24):1316–21. doi:10.1056/nejm197606102942404
13. O'Brien ML, Buist NR, Murphey WH. Neonatal screening for alpha1-antitrypsin deficiency. J Pediatr. 1978;92(6):1006–10.
14. Franciosi AN, Carroll TP, McElvaney NG. SZ alpha-1 antitrypsin deficiency and pulmonary disease: More like MZ, not like ZZ. Thorax. 2021;76(3):298–301. doi:10.1136/thoraxjnl-2020-215250
15. Campos MA, Geraghty P, Holt G, et al. The biological effects of double-dose alpha-1 antitrypsin augmentation therapy. A pilot clinical trial. Am J Respir Crit Care Med. 2019;200(3):318–26. doi:10.1164/rccm.201901-0010OC
16. de Serres FJ. Worldwide racial and ethnic distribution of alpha-1 antitrypsin deficiency: Summary of an analysis of published genetic epidemiologic surveys. Chest. 2002;122(5):1818–29.
17. de Serres FJ, Blanco I. Prevalence of α1-antitrypsin deficiency alleles PI*S and PI*Z worldwide and effective screening for each of the five phenotypic classes PI*MS, PI*MZ, PI*SS, PI*SZ, and PI*ZZ: A comprehensive review. Ther Adv Respir Dis. 2012;6(5):277–95. doi:10.1177/1753465812457113
18. Luisetti M, Seersholm N. Alpha1-antitrypsin deficiency. 1: Epidemiology of alpha-1 antitrypsin deficiency. Thorax. 2004;59(2):164–9.
19. de Serres FJ, Blanco I, Fernández-Bustillo E. Ethnic differences in alpha-1 antitrypsin deficiency in the United States of America. Ther Adv Respir Dis. 2010;4(2):63–70. doi:10.1177/1753465810365158
20. Greulich T, Ottaviani S, Bals R, et al. Alpha-1 antitrypsin deficiency – diagnostic testing and disease awareness in Germany and Italy. Respir Med. 2013;107(9):1400–8. doi:10.1016/j.rmed.2013.04.023
21. Attaway A, Majumdar U, Sandhaus RA, Nowacki AS, Stoller JK. An analysis of the degree of concordance among international guidelines regarding alpha-1 antitrypsin deficiency. Int J Chron Obstruct Pulmon Dis. 2019;14:2089–2101. doi:10.2147/COPD.S208591
22. Tejwani V, Nowacki AS, Fye E, Sanders C, Stoller JK. The impact of delayed diagnosis of alpha-1 antitrypsin deficiency: The association between diagnostic delay and worsened clinical status. Respir Care. 2019;64(8):915–22. doi:10.4187/respcare.06555
23. Brantly M, Nukiwa T, Crystal RG. Molecular basis of alpha-1 antitrypsin deficiency. Am J Med. 1988;84(6A):13–31.
24. McElvaney NG, Stoller JK, Buist AS, et al. Baseline characteristics of enrollees in the National Heart, Lung and Blood Institute Registry of alpha-1 antitrypsin deficiency. Alpha-1 antitrypsin Deficiency Registry Study Group. Chest. 1997;111(2):394–403.
25. Carrell RW, Lomas DA. Alpha-1 antitrypsin deficiency–a model for conformational diseases. N Engl J Med. 2002;346(1):45–53.
26. Lomas DA, Mahadeva R. Alpha-1 antitrypsin polymerization and the serpinopathies: Pathobiology and prospects for therapy. J Clin Invest. 2002;110(11):1585–90.
27. Silverman EK, Sandhaus RA. Clinical practice. Alpha-1 antitrypsin deficiency. N Engl J Med. 2009;360(26):2749–57. doi:10.1056/NEJMcp0900449
28. Teckman JH, Qu D, Perlmutter DH. Molecular pathogenesis of liver disease in alpha-1-antitrypsin deficiency. Hepatology. 1996;24(6):1504–16.
29. Perlmutter DH. Alpha-1 antitrypsin deficiency: Importance of proteasomal and autophagic degradative pathways in disposal of liver disease associated protein aggregates. Annu Rev Med. 2011:33345. http://dx.doi.org/10.1146/annurev-med-042409-151920
30. Marciniak SJ, Lomas DA. Alpha-1 antitrypsin deficiency and autophagy. N Engl J Med. 2010;363(19):1863–4. doi:10.1056/NEJMcibr1008007
31. Mayer AS, Stoller JK, Bucher Bartelson B, James Ruttenber A, Sandhaus RA, Newman LS. Occupational exposure risks in individuals with PI*Z alpha-1 antitrypsin deficiency. Am J Respir Crit Care Med. 2000;162(2 Pt 1):553–8.
32. Clark VC, Marek G, Liu C, et al. Clinical and histologic features of adults with alpha-1 antitrypsin deficiency in a non-cirrhotic cohort. J Hepatol. 2018;69(6):1357–64. doi:10.1016/j.jhep.2018.08.005
33. Fromme M, Schneider C V, Pereira V, et al. Hepatobiliary phenotypes of adults with alpha-1 antitrypsin deficiency. Gut. February 2021. doi:10.1136/gutjnl-2020-323729
34. Lowe KE, Hatipoğlu U, Stoller JK. Emphysema in a middle-aged former smoker. Ann Am Thorac Soc. 2020;17(6):762–6. doi:10.1513/AnnalsATS.202001-057CC
35. Elsensohn AN, Curtis JA, Secrest AM, et al. Alpha-1 antitrypsin deficiency panniculitis presenting with severe anasarca, pulmonary embolus and hypogammaglobulinaemia. Br J Dermatol. 2015;173(1):289–91. doi:10.1111/bjd.13611
36. Gross B, Grebe M, Wencker M, Stoller JK, Bjursten LM, Janciauskiene S. New findings in PiZZ alpha-1 antitrypsin deficiency-related panniculitis. Demonstration of skin polymers and high dosing requirements of intravenous augmentation therapy. Dermatology. 2009;218(4):370–5. doi:10.1159/000202982
37. Berden A, Göçeroğlu A, Jayne D, et al. Diagnosis and management of ANCA-associated vasculitis. BMJ. 2012;344(7840). doi:10.1136/bmj.e26
38. Morris H, Morgan MD, Wood AM, et al. ANCA-associated vasculitis is linked to carriage of the Z allele of alpha-1 antitrypsin and its polymers. Ann Rheum Dis. 2011;70(10):1851–6.
39. Deshayes S, Silva NM, Grandhomme F, et al. Clinical effect of alpha-1 antitrypsin deficiency in antineutrophil cytoplasmic antibody-associated vasculitis: Results from a French retrospective monocentric cohort. J Rheumatol. 2019;46(11):1502–8. doi:10.3899/jrheum.180591
40. Deshayes S, Martin Silva N, Khoy K, et al. Prevalence of antineutrophil cytoplasmic antibodies and associated vasculitis in COPD associated with alpha-1 antitrypsin deficiency: An ancillary study to a prospective study on 180 French patients. Chest. 2020;158(5):1919–22. doi:10.1016/j.chest.2020.04.054
41. Ferkingstad E, Oddsson A, Gretarsdottir S, et al. Genome-wide association meta-analysis yields 20 loci associated with gallstone disease. Nat Commun. 2018;9(1):1–11. doi:10.1038/s41467-018-07460-y
42. Schievink WI, Katzmann JA, Piepgras DG, Schaid DJ. Alpha-1 antitrypsin phenotypes among patients with intracranial aneurysms. J Neurosurg. 1996;84(5):781–4.
43. Dako F, Zhao H, Mulvenna A, Gupta S, Simpson S, Kueppers F. Relationship between alpha-1 antitrypsin deficiency and ascending aortic distention. Mayo Clin Proc Innov Qual Outcomes. 2021;5(3):590–595.
44. Tomashefski Jr. JF, Crystal RG, Wiedemann HP, Mascha E, Stoller JK. Alpha 1-Antitrypsin Deficiency Registry Study Group. The bronchopulmonary pathology of alpha-1 antitrypsin (AAT) deficiency: Findings of the Death Review Committee of the national registry for individuals with Severe Deficiency of Alpha-1 Antitrypsin. Hum Pathol. 2004;35(12):1452–61.
45. Parr DG, Stoel BC, Stolk J, Stockley RA. Pattern of emphysema distribution in alpha-1 antitrypsin deficiency influences lung function impairment. Am J Respir Crit Care Med. 2004;170(11):1172–8.
46. Strange C, Stoller JK, Sandhaus RA, Dickson R, Turino G. Results of a survey of patients with alpha-1 antitrypsin deficiency. Respiration. 2006;73(2):185–90.
47. Parr DG, Guest PG, Reynolds JH, Dowson LJ, Stockley RA. Prevalence and impact of bronchiectasis in alpha-1 antitrypsin deficiency. Am J Respir Crit Care Med. 2007;176(12):1215–21.
48. Salahuddin P. Genetic variants of alpha-1 antitrypsin. Curr Protein Pept Sci. 11(2):101–17.
49. Janciauskiene S, Eriksson S, Callea F, et al. Differential detection of PAS-positive inclusions formed by the Z, Siiyama, and Mmalton variants of alpha-1 antitrypsin. Hepatology. 2004;40(5):1203–10.
50. Greulich T, Nell C, Hohmann D, et al. The prevalence of diagnosed alpha-1 antitrypsin deficiency and its comorbidities: Results from a large population-based database. Eur Respir J. 2017;49(1). doi:10.1183/13993003.00154-2016

51. Franciosi AN, Ralph J, O'Farrell NJ, et al. Alpha-1 antitrypsin deficiency–associated panniculitis. J Am Acad Dermatol. 2021. doi:10.1016/j.jaad.2021.01.074
52. Mahr AD, Edberg JC, Stone JH, et al. Alpha-1 antitrypsin deficiency-related alleles Z and S and the risk of Wegener's granulomatosis. Arthritis Rheum. 2010;62(12):3760–7. doi:http://dx.doi.org/10.1002/art.27742
53. Griffith ME, Lovegrove JU, Gaskin G, Whitehouse DB, Pusey CD. C-antineutrophil cytoplasmic antibody positivity in vasculitis patients is associated with the Z allele of alpha-1 antitrypsin, and P-antineutrophil cytoplasmic antibody positivity with the S allele. Nephrol Dial Transplant. 1996;11(3):438–43.
54. Piitulainen E, Mostafavi B, Tanash HA. Health status and lung function in the Swedish alpha-1 antitrypsin deficient cohort, identified by neonatal screening, at the age of 37-40 years. Int J Chron Obstruct Pulmon Dis. 2017;12:495–500. doi:10.2147/COPD.S120241
55. Vreim CE, Wu M, Crystal RG, et al. Survival and FEV1 decline in individuals with severe deficiency of α1-antitrypsin. Am J Respir Crit Care Med. 1998;158(1):49–59. doi:10.1164/ajrccm.158.1.9712017
56. Dawkins PA, Dawkins CL, Wood AM, Nightingale PG, Stockley JA, Stockley RA. Rate of progression of lung function impairment in alpha-1 antitrypsin deficiency. Eur Respir J. 2009;33(6):1338–44.
57. Ejiofor S., Stockley RA. Patterns of exacerbations in alpha-1 antitrypsin deficiency (AATD). Eur Res J. 2015;46:PA3810. doi:10.1183/13993003.congress-2015.pa3810
58. Stoller JK, Tomashefski Jr. J, Crystal RG, et al. Mortality in individuals with severe deficiency of alpha-1antitrypsin: Findings from the National Heart, Lung, and Blood Institute Registry. Chest. 2005;127(4):1196–204.
59. Tanash HA, Nilsson PM, Nilsson J-A, Piitulainen E. Clinical course and prognosis of never-smokers with severe alpha-1 antitrypsin deficiency (PiZZ). Thorax. 2008;63(12):1091–5. doi:10.1136/thx.2008.095497
60. Stoller JK, Brantly M. The challenge of detecting alpha-1 antitrypsin deficiency. COPD. 2013;10 Suppl 1:26–34. doi:10.3109/15412555.2013.763782
61. Greulich T, Rodríguez-Frias F, Belmonte I, Klemmer A, Vogelmeier CF, Miravitlles M. Real world evaluation of a novel lateral flow assay (AlphaKit® QuickScreen) for the detection of alpha-1 antitrypsin deficiency. Respir Res. 2018;19(1):151. doi:10.1186/s12931-018-0826-8
62. Brantly M, Campos M, Davis AM, et al. Detection of alpha-1 antitrypsin deficiency: The past, present and future. Orphanet J Rare Dis. 2020;15(1):96. doi:10.1186/s13023-020-01352-5
63. Jain A, McCarthy K, Xu M, Stoller JK. Impact of a clinical decision support system in an electronic health record to enhance detection of alpha-1 antitrypsin deficiency. Chest. 2011; 140 (1): 198–204.
64. Rahaghi F, Ortega I, Rahaghi N, et al. Physician alert suggesting alpha-1 antitrypsin deficiency testing in pulmonary function test (PFT) results. COPD. 2009;6(1):26–30. doi:10.1080/15412550802587927
65. Campos Hagenlocker, B., Martinez, N. M. Impact of an electronic medical record clinical reminder to improve detection of COPD and alpha-1 antitrypsin deficiency in the veterans administration (VA) system. Am J Respir Crit Care Med. 2011;183.
66. Lam S, Strange C, Brantly M, Stoller JK. A novel detection method to identify individuals with alpha-1 antitrypsin deficiency: Linking prescription of COPD medications with the patient-facing electronic medical record. JCOPDF 2022; 9(1):26–33.
67. Stoller JK, Gildea TR, Ries AL, Meli YM, Karafa MT. Lung volume reduction surgery in patients with emphysema and alpha-1 antitrypsin deficiency. Ann Thorac Surg. 2007;83 (1):241–251. doi:http://dx.doi.org/10.1016/j.athoracsur.2006.07.080
68. Tutic M, Bloch KE, Lardinois D, Brack T, Russi EW, Weder W. Long-term results after lung volume reduction surgery in patients with alpha-1 antitrypsin deficiency. J Thorac Cardiovasc Surg. 2004;128(3):408–13.
69. Wewers MD, Casolaro MA, Sellers SE, et al. Replacement therapy for alpha-1 antitrypsin deficiency associated with emphysema. N Engl J Med. 1987;316(17):1055–62.
70. Chapman KR, Stockley RA, Dawkins C, Wilkes MM, Navickis RJ. Augmentation therapy for alpha-1 antitrypsin deficiency: A meta-analysis. Copd J Chronic Obstr Pulm Dis. 2009;6(3):177–84.
71. Chapman KR, Burdon JG, Piitulainen E, et al. Intravenous augmentation treatment and lung density in severe alpha-1 antitrypsin deficiency (RAPID): A randomised, double-blind, placebo-controlled trial. Lancet. 2015;386(9991):360–8. doi:10.1016/s0140-6736(15)60860-1
72. Barker AF, Iwata-Morgan I, Oveson L, Roussel R. Pharmacokinetic study of alpha-1 antitrypsin infusion in alpha-1 antitrypsin deficiency. Chest. 1997;112(3):607–13.
73. Wencker M, Banik N, Buhl R, Seidel R, Konietzko N. Long-term treatment of alpha-1 antitrypsin deficiency-related pulmonary emphysema with human alpha-1 antitrypsin. Wissenschaftliche arbeitsgemeinschaft zur therapie von lungenerkrankungen (WATL)-alpha1-AT-study group. Eur Respir J. 1998;11(2):428–33.
74. Stoller JK, Fallat R, Schluchter MD, et al. Augmentation therapy with alpha-1 -antitrypsin: Patterns of use and adverse events. Chest. 2003;123(5):1425–34.
75. Gildea TR, Shermock KM, Singer ME, Stoller JK. Cost-effectiveness analysis of augmentation therapy for severe alpha-1 antitrypsin deficiency. Am J Respir Crit Care Med. 2003;167(10):1387–92. doi:10.1164/rccm.200209-1035OC
76. Sandhaus RA, Turino G, Stocks J, et al. Alpha-1 antitrypsin augmentation therapy for PI*MZ heterozygotes: A cautionary note. Chest. 2008;134(4):831–34.
77. Turino GM, Barker AF, Brantly ML, et al. Clinical features of individuals with PI*SZ phenotype of alpha-1 antitrypsin deficiency. Alpha-1 antitrypsin deficiency registry study group. Am J Respir Crit Care Med. 1996;154(6 Pt 1):1718–25. doi:10.1164/ajrccm.154.6.8970361
78. McElvaney GN, Sandhaus RA, Miravitlles M, et al. Clinical considerations in individuals with α1-antitrypsin PI*SZ genotype. Eur Respir J. 2020;55(6). doi:10.1183/13993003.02410-2019
79. Christie JD, Edwards LB, Kucheryavaya AY, et al. The registry of the International Society for Heart and Lung Transplantation: Twenty-eighth adult lung and heart-lung transplant report–2011. J Heart Lung Transplant. 2011;30(10):1104–22. doi:10.1016/j.healun.2011.08.004
80. Cassivi SD, Meyers BF, Battafarano RJ, et al. Thirteen-year experience in lung transplantation for emphysema. Ann Thorac Surg. 2002;74(5):1663–70.
81. Burton CM, Milman N, Carlsen J, et al. The Copenhagen National Lung Transplant Group: Survival after single lung, double lung, and heart-lung transplantation. J Hear Lung Transplant. 2005;24(11):1834–43.
82. Inci I, Schuurmans M, Ehrsam J, et al. Lung transplantation for emphysema: Impact of age on short- and long-term survival. Eur J Cardio-Thorac Surg. 2015;48(6):906–9. doi:10.1093/ejcts/ezu550
83. de Perrot M, Chaparro C, McRae K, et al. Twenty-year experience of lung transplantation at a single center: Influence of recipient diagnosis on long-term survival. J Thorac Cardiovasc Surg. 2004;127(5):1493–1501.
84. Tanash HA, Riise GC, Ekström MP, Hansson L, Piitulainen E. Survival benefit of lung transplantation for chronic obstructive pulmonary disease in Sweden. Ann Thorac Surg. 2014;98(5):1930–35. doi:10.1016/j.athoracsur.2014.07.030
85. Tanash HA, Riise GC, Hansson L, Nilsson PM, Piitulainen E. Survival benefit of lung transplantation in individuals with severe α1-antitrypsin deficiency (PiZZ) and emphysema. J Heart Lung Transplant. 2011;30(12):1342–47. doi:10.1016/j.healun.2011.07.003
86. Banga A, Gildea T, Rajeswaran J, Rokadia H, Blackstone EH, Stoller JK. The natural history of lung function after lung transplantation for α1-antitrypsin deficiency. Am J Respir Crit Care Med. 2014;190(3):274–81. doi:10.1164/rccm.201401-0031OC
87. Cassina PC, Teschler H, Konietzko N, Theegarten D, Stamatis G. Two-year results after lung volume reduction surgery in alpha1-antitrypsin deficiency versus smoker's emphysema. Eur Respir J. 1998;12(5):1028–32.
88. Gelb AF, McKenna RJ, Brenner M, Fischel R, Zamel N. Lung function after bilateral lower lobe lung volume reduction surgery for alpha-1 antitrypsin emphysema. Eur Respir J. 1999;14(4):928–33.

89. Dauriat G, Mal H, Jebrak G, et al. Functional results of unilateral lung volume reduction surgery in alpha-1 antitrypsin deficient patients. Int J COPD. 2006;1(2):201–6.
90. Tuohy MM, Remund KF, Hilfiker R, Murphy DT, Murray JG, Egan JJ. Endobronchial valve deployment in severe alpha-1 antitrypsin deficiency emphysema: A case series. Clin Respir J. 2013;7(1): 45–52. doi:10.1111/j.1752-699X.2012.00280.x
91. Hillerdal G, Mindus S. One-to four-year follow-up of endobronchial lung volume reduction in alpha-1 antitrypsin deficiency patients: A case series. Respiration. 2014;88(4):320–8. doi:10.1159/000365662
92. Vogelmeier C, Kirlath I, Warrington S, Banik N, Ulbrich E, Du Bois RM. The intrapulmonary half-life and safety of aerosolized alpha-1 protease inhibitor in normal volunteers. Am J Respir Crit Care Med. 1997;155(2):536–41.
93. Hubbard RC, Crystal RG. Strategies for aerosol therapy of alpha-1 antitrypsin deficiency by the aerosol route. Lung. 1990;168 Suppl:565–78.
94. Stolk J, Tov N, Chapman KR, et al. Efficacy and safety of inhaled alpha-1 antitrypsin in patients with severe alpha-1 antitrypsin deficiency and frequent exacerbations of COPD. Eur Respir J. 2019;54(5). doi:10.1183/13993003.00673-2019
95. Brantly ML, Chulay JD, Wang L, et al. Sustained transgene expression despite t lymphocyte responses in a clinical trial of rAAV1-AAT Gene therapy. Proc Natl Acad Sci U S A. 2009;106(38):16363–68.
96. Brigham KL, Lane KB, Meyrick B, et al. Transfection of nasal mucosa with a normal alpha-1 antitrypsin gene in alpha-1 antitrypsin-deficient subjects: Comparison with protein therapy. Hum Gene Ther. 2000;11(7):1023–32.
97. Somers A, Jean JC, Sommer CA, et al. Generation of transgene-free lung disease-specific human induced pluripotent stem cells using a single excisable lentiviral stem cell cassette. Stem Cells. 28(10):1728–40.
98. Parfrey H, Dafforn TR, Belorgey D, Lomas DA, Mahadeva R. Inhibiting polymerization: New therapeutic strategies for z alpha-1 antitrypsin-related emphysema. Am J Respir Cell Mol Biol. 2004;31(2):133–9.
99. Zhou A, Stein PE, Huntington JA, Sivasothy P, Lomas DA, Carrell RW. How small peptides block and reverse serpin polymerisation. J Mol Biol. 2004;342(3):931–41. doi:10.1016/j.jmb.2004.07.078
100. Burrows JA, Willis LK, Perlmutter DH. Chemical chaperones mediate increased secretion of mutant alpha 1-antitrypsin (alpha 1-AT) z: A potential pharmacological strategy for prevention of liver injury and emphysema in alpha 1-AT deficiency. Proc Natl Acad Sci U S A. 2000;97(4):1796–1801.
101. Marcus NY, Perlmutter DH. Glucosidase and mannosidase inhibitors mediate increased secretion of mutant alpha1 antitrypsin z. J Biol Chem. 2000;275(3):1987–92.
102. Cantin AM, Woods DE, Cloutier D, Dufour EK, Leduc R. Polyethylene glycol conjugation at Cys232 prolongs the half-life of alpha1 proteinase inhibitor. Am J Respir Cell Mol Biol. 2002;27(6):659–65.
103. Phase 1 Study to Assess the Safety, PK and PD of INBRX-101 in Adults with Alpha-1 Antitrypsin Deficiency - Full Text View – ClinicalTrials.gov. https://www.clinicaltrials.gov/ct2/show/NCT 03815396?term=INBRX+101&rank=1. Published 2019. Accessed April 19, 2021.
104. Hidvegi T, Ewing M, Hale P, et al. An autophagy-enhancing drug promotes degradation of mutant alpha-1 antitrypsin z and reduces hepatic fibrosis. Science 2010;. 329(5988):229–32.
105. Kaushal S, Annamali M, Blomenkamp K, et al. Rapamycin reduces intrahepatic alpha-1-antitrypsin mutant Z protein polymers and liver injury in a mouse model. Exp Biol Med. 2010;235(6):700–9.
106. Evaluation of the Efficacy and Safety of VX-864 in Subjects with the PiZZ Genotype. https://clinicaltrials.gov/ct2/show/NCT04474197. Published 2020. Accessed April 19, 2021.
107. Kaczor MP, Sanak M, Libura-Twardowska M, Szczeklik A. The prevalence of alpha-1 antitrypsin deficiency in a representative population sample from Poland. Respir Med. 2007;101(12):2520–5. doi:10.1016/j.rmed.2007.06.032
108. Kaczor MP, Sanak M, Szczeklik A. Rapid and inexpensive detection of α1-antitrypsin deficiency-related allels s and z by a real-time polymerase chain reaction suitable for a large-scale population-based screening. J Mol Diagnostics. 2007;9(1):99–104. doi:10.2353/jmoldx.2007.060048
109. Saris NE, Nyman MA, Varpela E, Nevanlinna HR. Serum alpha-1 antitrypsin mass concentrations in a Finnish young male population. Scand J Clin Lab Invest. 1972;29(3):249–52.
110. Sveger T, Mazodier P. Alpha-1 antitrypsin screening of 18-year-old men. Thorax. 1979;34(3):397–400.
111. Dahl M, Tybjaerg-Hansen A, Lange P, Vestbo J, Nordestgaard BG. Change in lung function and morbidity from chronic obstructive pulmonary disease in alpha-1 antitrypsin MZ heterozygotes: A longitudinal study of the general population.[Summary for patients in Ann Intern Med. 2002 Feb 19;136(4):I35; PMID: 11848738]. Ann Intern Med. 2002;136(4):270–9.
112. Hoffmann JJ, van den Broek WG. Distribution of alpha-1 antitrypsin phenotypes in two Dutch population groups. Hum Genet. 1976;32(1):43–8.
113. Dijkman JH, Penders TJ, Kramps JA, Sonderkamp HJ, van den Broek WG, ter Haar BG. Epidemiology of alpha-1 antitrypsin deficiency in the Netherlands. Hum Genet. 1980;53(3):409–13.
114. Kimpen J, Bosmans E, Raus J. Neonatal screening for alpha-1 antitrypsin deficiency. Eur J Pediatr. 1988;148(1):86–8.
115. Cook PJ. The genetics of alpha-1 antitrypsin: A family study in England and Scotland. Ann Hum Genet. 1975;38(3):275–87.
116. Webb DR, Hyde RW, Schwartz RH, Hall WJ, Condemi JJ, Townes PL. Serum alpha-1 antitrypsin variants. Prevalence and clinical spirometry. Am Rev Respir Dis. 1973;108(5):918–25.
117. Lieberman J, Gaidulis L, Roberts L. Racial distribution of alpha-1 antitrypsin variants among junior high school students. Am Rev Respir Dis. 1976;114(6):1194–8.
118. Evans HE, Bognacki NS, Perrott LM, Glass L. Prevalence of of alpha-1 antitrypsin Pi types among newborn infants of different ethnic backgrounds. J Pediatr. 1977;90(4):621–4.
119. Morse JO, Lebowitz MD, Knudson RJ, Burrows B. Relation of protease inhibitor phenotypes to obstructive lung diseases in a community. N Engl J Med. 1977;296(21):1190–4. doi:10.1056/nejm197705262962102
120. O'Brien ML, Buist NR, Murphey WH. Neonatal screening for alpha-1 antitrypsin deficiency. J Pediatr. 1978;92(6):1006–10.
121. Dykes DD, Miller SA, Polesky HF. Distribution of alpha-1 antitrypsin variants in a US white population. Hum Hered. 1984;34(5):308–10.
122. Silverman EK, Miletich JP, Pierce JA, et al. Alpha-1 antitrypsin deficiency. High prevalence in the St. Louis area determined by direct population screening. Am Rev Respir Dis. 1989;140(4):961–6.
123. Spence WC, Morris JE, Pass K, Murphy PD. Molecular confirmation of alpha-1 antitrypsin genotypes in newborn dried blood specimens. Biochem Med Metab Biol. 1993;50(2):233–40.
124. Klasen EC, D'Andrea F, Bernini LF. Phenotype and gene distribution of alpha-1 antitrypsin in a North Italian population. Hum Hered. 1978;28(6):474–8.
125. Corda L, Medicina D, La Piana GE, et al. Population genetic screening for alpha-1 antitrypsin deficiency in a high-prevalence area. Respiration. 2011;82(5):418–25. doi:10.1159/000325067
126. Goedde HW, Hirth L, Benkmann HG, et al. Population genetic studies of serum protein polymorphisms in four Spanish populations. II. Hum Hered. 1973;23(2):135–46.
127. Spinola C, Bruges-Armas J, Pereira C, Brehm A, Spinola H. Alpha-1-antitrypsin deficiency in Madeira (Portugal): The highest prevalence in the world. Respir Med. 2009;103(10):1498–502. doi:10.1016/j.rmed.2009.04.012
128. Spinola C, Brehm A, Spinola H. Alpha-1 antitrypsin deficiency in the Cape Verde Islands (Northwest Africa): High prevalence in a Sub-Saharan population. Respir Med. 2010;104(7):1069–72. doi:10.1016/j.rmed.2010.02.012
129. Vandeville D, Martin JP, Ropartz C. Alpha-1 antitrypsin polymorphism of a Bantu population: Description of a new allele PiL. Humangenetik. 1974;21(1):33–8.
130. Massi G, Vecchio FM. Alpha-1-antitrypsin phenotypes in a group of newborn infants in Somalia. Hum Genet. 1977;38(3):265–9.
131. Aljarallah B, Ali A, Dowaidar M, Settin A. Prevalence of alpha-1 antitrypsin gene mutations in Saudi Arabia. Saudi J Gastroenterol. 2011;17(4):256–60. doi:10.4103/1319-3767.82580

132. Harada S, Miyake K, Suzuki H, Oda T. New phenotypes of serum alpha-1 antitrypsin in Japanese detected by gel slab isoelectric focusing. Hum Genet. 1977;38(3):333–6.
133. Aboussouan LS, Stoller JK. Detection of alpha-1 antitrypsin deficiency: A review. Respir Med. 2009;103(3):335–41. doi:10.1016/j.rmed.2008.10.006
134. Alvelestat (MPH966) for the Treatment of ALpha-1 ANTitrypsin Deficiency (ATALANTa). https://clinicaltrials.gov/ct2/show/NCT03679598. Published 2018. Accessed April 19, 2021.
135. Lomas DA, Irving JA, Arico-Muendel C, et al. Development of a small molecule that corrects misfolding and increases secretion of Z α_1-antitrypsin. EMBO Mol Med. 2021;13(3):e13167. doi:10.15252/emmm.202013167
136. Turino GM, Ma S, Lin YY, Cantor JO. The therapeutic potential of hyaluronan in COPD. Chest. 2018;153(4):792–8. doi:10.1016/j.chest.2017.12.016
137. Teckman JH. Lack of effect of oral 4-phenylbutyrate on serum alpha-1 antitrypsin in patients with alpha-1-antitrypsin deficiency: A preliminary study. J Pediatr Gastroenterol Nutr. 2004;39(1):34–7.
138. Wooddell CI, Blomenkamp K, Peterson RM, et al. Development of an RNAi therapeutic for alpha-1 antitrypsin liver disease. JCI Insight. 2020;5(12). doi:10.1172/jci.insight.135348
139. Somers A, Jean J-C, Sommer CA, et al. Generation of transgene-free lung disease-specific human induced pluripotent stem cells using a single excisable lentiviral stem cell cassette. Stem Cells. 2010;28(10):1728–40.
140. Shen S, Sanchez ME, Blomenkamp K, et al. Amelioration of alpha-1 antitrypsin deficiency diseases with genome editing in transgenic mice. Hum Gene Ther. 2018;29(8):861–73. doi:10.1089/hum.2017.227

PART B
Rare Airway Disorders

5

BENIGN CENTRAL AIRWAY DISORDERS

Prince Ntiamoah and Laura K. Frye

Contents

Introduction	33
Idiopathic subglottic stenosis	33
Granulomatosis with polyangiitis	35
Tracheobronchomalacia	37
Relapsing polychondritis	37
Miscellaneous causes of central airway obstruction	38
Conclusion	39
References	39

KEY POINTS

- "Benign" central airway obstruction can be due to a multitude of causes and is associated with significant morbidity.
- Airway stents should be approached with caution and with a plan for long-term management.
- Multidisciplinary management is required for airway manifestations of rheumatologic diseases.

Introduction

Benign central airway obstruction is defined as a nonmalignant process that results in narrowing of the trachea and mainstem bronchi. This term is used to describe multiple etiologies of airway obstruction unrelated to active malignancy and is associated with significant morbidity and mortality. This chapter will review several processes that are associated with benign central airway obstruction, the typical presentation, and management options.

Idiopathic subglottic stenosis

Introduction

Subglottic stenosis (SGS) is obstruction of the airway in the region bounded superiorly by a plane below the glottis and inferiorly by the first two tracheal rings. When no cause is evident after a comprehensive evaluation, this disease process is referred to as idiopathic subglottic stenosis (iSGS) (1). iSGS is a relatively new entity, the first cases being described by Brandenburg in 1972 (2). In addition to a thorough history and physical examination, the initial evaluation should include serologic testing for antineutrophil cytoplasmic antibodies (ANCA), angiotensin-converting enzyme levels (ACE), pulmonary function tests, computerized tomography (CT), and endoscopic examination.

The estimated incidence is 1 in 400,000 and almost exclusively affects women between the third and fifth decades of life. Patients are mainly Caucasian women (3–6).

Etiology

Several etiologies have been proposed for SGS, the most common being trauma secondary to prolonged intubation, excessive endotracheal tube cuff pressure, and tracheostomy. Less frequent causes include infection, gastroesophageal reflux disorder (GERD), systemic diseases, radiation therapy, inhalational injury, occupational exposures, inflammatory bowel disease (IBD), primary and secondary tracheal malignancies, and congenital conditions. It is essential to consider these possibilities in order to identify mimics of iSGS (7–10).

Pathophysiology and risk factors

Most lesions begin at the cricoid cartilage, with the point of maximal stenosis located between its upper edge and the first tracheal ring (5). The stenosis is usually circumferential but may be eccentric. The average length of the stenosed segment is 1 to 3 cm (5, 11). Histopathology of these lesions reveals dense fibrosis of the keloidal type with interspersed fibroblasts. Inflammation tends to be sparse (12). The pathogenesis of iSGS is unclear. The vast majority of patients are women, prompting the theory that estrogen influences the development of stenosis (5, 13). Interestingly, there is no evidence of overexpression of estrogen or progesterone receptors in the cells involved in the disease process (5, 7).

Another hypothesis postulates that trauma from repeated cough may lead to "telescoping" of the first tracheal ring into the ring of the cricoid cartilage, resulting in mechanical injury, ischemia, and anomalous wound repair, possibly potentiated by an abnormal response to estrogen (14). The role of GERD resulting in irritation and subsequent stenosis is a hypothesis supported by multiple observational studies reporting a higher incidence of GERD among this patient population (7).

Clinical Features

The most common symptoms are exertional dyspnea, stridor, chronic cough, and wheezing, with a mean duration before diagnosis ranging from 19 months to 4 years (4, 5). The majority of these symptoms are reported late in the course of the disease when the stenosis reaches more than 50% of the airway diameter (11, 15). In a significant proportion of patients who have central

DOI: 10.1201/9781003089384-5

airway stenosis but no risk factors, the diagnosis is overlooked (15). As many as one-third of patients are misdiagnosed with either asthma or COPD (3–5).

Diagnosis

Pulmonary function tests (PFTs): The flow-volume loop reveals fixed upper airway obstruction associated with a reduction in maximal voluntary ventilation despite preserved muscle strength and patient effort (16).

Imaging: Chest x-ray is of limited value. Chest and neck CT with 3D reconstruction or virtual bronchoscopy (VB) provides invaluable information in the diagnosis (5, 17) and helps define the characteristics and type of stenosis (concentric, complex, hourglass, etc.). The sensitivity of VB for tracheal stenosis is 94–97%, and the specificity is 100% when compared with intraoperative findings (18). Dynamic expiratory CT may allow the identification of airway collapse due to tracheomalacia, which is occasionally associated with iSGS (17).

Bronchoscopy: Endoscopic evaluation is the gold standard in the diagnosis. Flexible endoscopic examination determines fundamental characteristics of iSGS, such as location, extent, and complexity. A concentric web-like stricture measuring less than 1 cm in length without the involvement of the cartilage is referred to as a "simple" stricture while a stricture associated with structural defects is considered "complex" (Figure 5.1).

In cases of severe stenosis, the flexible endoscopic examination can further obstruct the airway and add to respiratory distress. Among patients with preexisting respiratory distress, proceeding directly to rigid endoscopy may be advisable (5, 19, 20). Radial probe endobronchial ultrasound with a balloon can determine the thickness of the lamina propria of the tracheal mucosa, the extent, complexity of the stenosis, and the structure of cartilaginous rings. The latter is helpful in differentiating iSGS from conditions such as relapsing polychondritis (21).

Treatment

Optimal management requires the collaboration and availability of a multidisciplinary team. There is a lack of data to support medical therapy alone for symptomatic iSGS except in GERD.

Therapeutic endoscopy (laryngoscopy or bronchoscopy): Endoscopy has the advantage of being a less invasive procedure that can be performed in the outpatient setting. It is likely to have fewer complications than a surgical approach. However, it has the disadvantage of high recurrence rate, requiring repeated interventions (6, 12, 22, 23). Historically, the treatment of iSGS has

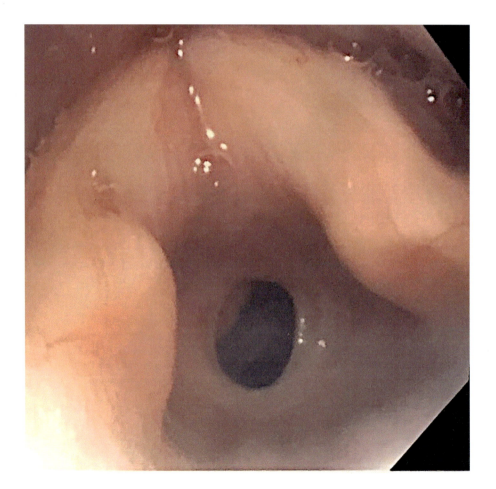

FIGURE 5.1 Bronchoscopy showing simple web-like stenosis.

included dilatation of the involved segment using either bougies or barrels of rigid scopes of increasing diameter. This approach may cause trauma to the treatment site, leading to recurrence. The most common modern-day endoscopic procedure performed for simple iSGS is the "mucosal sparing technique," which is a less invasive approach, involving radial incisions and gentle dilatation (13, 24, 25). Radial incisions are made on the scar, followed by a gentle dilatation using a balloon (13, 26). Complete mucosal ablation of the stenosis promotes recurrent scarring and poor long-term patency (24). Mucosal sparing techniques allow organized tracheal mucosal restructuring and may serve as a platform for fostering normal re-epithelialization and airway repair. Studies have evaluated long-term outcomes after endoscopic management and report initial success. However, this was followed by a recurrence rate of 30% at 6 months and 87% in 5 years (4). In carefully selected patients with a stenosis length of less than 1 cm, endoscopic techniques, usually yield good results (13, 25). In a meta-analysis published by Yamamoto et al. in patients with a stenosis length of less than 1 cm without framework destruction, the success rate of an endoscopic approach was 79%. However, in those with a mean stenosis length of greater than 1 cm, the success rate was only 47% (27). The use of endoscopic procedures should be considered in individuals with complex stenosis to stabilize their airways before surgery or to palliate patients not suitable for surgery (28).

Mitomycin C, a cytotoxic agent isolated from *Streptomyces caespitosus*, inhibits DNA and RNA synthesis. At lower doses, it acts as an inhibitor of fibroblast proliferation (29, 30). It has been used with some success as an adjuvant treatment following mucosal sparing procedures, prolonging the interval to relapse (31–33). A review found that the usual application dose range between 0.1 and 10 mg/mL for 2–5 minutes (34). However, its use is still debatable due to the controversial evidence (35–39). Further studies are required to make an appropriate recommendation (29, 30, 40).

Intralesional injection of steroids is used to decrease scar formation. It acts by delaying collagen synthesis in the early phases of the disease process and by increasing collagen lysis in the later phases of the scar formation (41, 42).

Stents are used to maintain airway patency. Noncovered and partially covered metallic stents are contraindicated in the management of iSGS due to the risk of excessive granulation tissue formation leading to worsening of airway obstruction (13). Several investigators have used straight silicone stents with varying success. Silicone stents usually are placed either temporarily or on a permanent basis when endoscopic treatment has failed, and the patient is not a candidate for surgical management (24, 43, 44). High risks of migration, malposition, infection, and mucus plugging are limitations of this modality (13, 43).

Approximately 20% of patients with iSGS undergo an open surgical approach (6). The most definitive treatment is resection of laryngotracheal stenosis with primary anastomotic reconstruction with a T-tube. This approach has a high rate of success with a decannulation rate of over 95% (5, 27, 45). Age is correlated with unsuccessful airway patency. Another technique with a high decannulation rate is laryngotracheal reconstruction without stenting, but this approach is associated with an increased rate of follow-up surgery and temporary tracheotomy. Laryngoplasty with or without graft has an overall success rate of 76% (27). This procedure may potentially result in voice impairment to a lower pitch, which could be an issue of significant concern, especially to women (27, 45). These complex procedures are best performed in centers of excellence with a high volume of patients (6).

Granulomatosis with polyangiitis

Introduction

Granulomatosis with polyangiitis (GPA) is a multisystem disease of unknown etiology, characterized by necrotizing vasculitis and granuloma formation that affects primarily the upper and lower respiratory tracts and the kidneys. Initially described by Klinger in 1931 as a variant of polyarteritis nodosa, and then in greater detail as a separate entity by Wegener in 1936 and 1939 (46–48). Central airway involvement typically occurs in conjunction with involvement of other organs, but in some instances, it is the sole presenting feature (49). Disease activity in the airway poorly correlates with proteinase-3 (PR3) antineutrophil cytoplasm antibody (ANCA) (50–52). The evaluation and diagnosis of a patient with suspected tracheobronchial GPA requires a combination of clinical assessment, serologic testing, sinus and chest imaging, pulmonary function tests, bronchoscopy, and tissue biopsy. Early recognition and treatment of airway involvement can prevent untoward effects of improper therapy.

The incidence of GPA in the adult population ranges from 3 to 14 cases/million/year, with an increase in annual incidence (53–56). It remains rare in childhood, with peak incidence in the 65- to 70-year-old age group (54). There is no gender-specific incidence, but it is more common in Caucasians (54, 57). Airway involvement occurs in 15–55% of patients with GPA (58).

Risk factors

The initiating event of GPA is a combination of environmental (i.e., infectious agents and/or toxins) and individual risk factors. The pathogen *Staphylococcus aureus* (*S. aureus*) specifically has been associated with ANCA-associated vasculitis (AAV). In GPA, chronic nasal carriage of *S. aureus* is a risk factor for relapse, and prophylactic treatment with co-trimoxazole reduces relapses of GPA by 60% (59, 60). High intensity exposure to silica, propylthiouracil, and levamisole-contaminated cocaine has also been shown to be associated with onset (61–63).

Clinical presentation

Most patients with active GPA present with nasal crusting (69%), chronic rhinosinusitis symptoms (61%), nasal obstruction (58%), and serosanguinous nasal discharge (52%) (64). Cough, dyspnea, wheezing, hoarseness, hemoptysis, and epistaxis are usual symptoms. Stridor is usually a sign of severe laryngeal or tracheal obstruction, signaling more than 70% airway lumen narrowing (65). Airway involvement includes mucosal inflammation, ulceration, hemorrhage, SGS, localized or complex tracheobronchial stenosis, inflammatory pseudotumors, and tracheobronchomalacia (10). Subglottic stenosis occurs in an estimated 8.5–23% of patients with GPA, and GPA accounts for 45% of patients who present with SGS (66, 67). Patients are more likely to present with grade 1 SGS, and higher grades are seen in non-GPA patients.

Diagnosis

Imaging: A majority of patients with GPA will have an abnormal chest radiograph which may show cavitary lung nodules, lobar or segmental atelectasis, infiltrates, pleural opacities, and/or lymphadenopathy. CT is the preferred imaging modality and is usually performed without contrast due to underlying renal insufficiency.

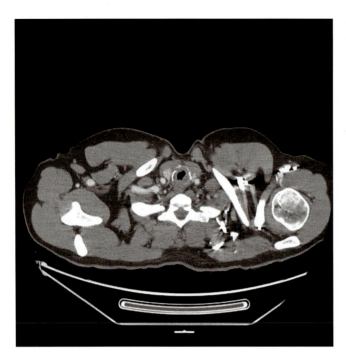

FIGURE 5.2 CT scan demonstrating thickening of tracheal mucosa.

Sinus CT scans disclose mucosal thickening in the nasal cavity and paranasal sinuses in 61 and 75%, respectively. Large airway involvement may consist of focal or elongated segments of stenosis. Other findings include calcifications and thickening of the tracheal rings (68) (Figure 5.2). Bronchial abnormalities, including bronchiectasis and peribronchial thickening, have been reported in 40% of cases (69). Magnetic resonance imaging (MRI) of the trachea and upper airways has also been used in assessing the degree of airway involvement and may demonstrate diffuse thickening of tracheobronchial submucosal tissues and luminal narrowing.

Pulmonary function tests: Pulmonary function tests and flow volume tracings are not uniformly abnormal in all patients and their severity depends on the extent of compromise of the airway lumen. The most frequent abnormality is airflow obstruction with reduced lung volumes and diffusing capacity for carbon monoxide (DLCO). The DLCO may be markedly increased in the presence of active alveolar hemorrhage.

Bronchoscopy: Tracheobronchial manifestations may appear for the first time after remission has been achieved with appropriate immunosuppressive therapy, and it does not necessarily indicate treatment failure. Therefore, bronchoscopy with visualization of airways remains the major diagnostic procedure in the diagnosis, evaluation, and management of airway disease. Endobronchial biopsy can confirm inflammation in 50% of cases, revealing either vasculitis, necrosis, microabscesses, or giant cells (70). However, nondiagnostic biopsies are not unusual even when obtained from abnormal-appearing areas.

Subglottic stenosis occurs independently of systemic GPA activity. It is the most frequent airway manifestation of GPA and may be the initial presenting feature in 1–6% of patients (71). Subglottic inflammation is a common feature in active disease. Erythematous, edematous, and friable mucosa and ulcerations may be seen with lesions typically circumferential. Similar inflammatory processes that occur in the subglottic region can occur at any level in the tracheobronchial tree.

Bronchial inflammation and stenosis are less frequent than subglottic disease and are almost always associated with disease activity elsewhere. Isolated bronchial stenosis has been described. Tracheal or bronchial mass lesions or inflammatory pseudotumors may develop (Figure 5.3). These lesions mimic malignancy and therefore should be biopsied to establish GPA as the etiology. Of note, these lesions may ulcerate and cause hemoptysis (65). Inflammatory pseudotumors are generally a reflection of active disease. Other airway abnormalities of GPA include tracheobronchomalacia, acquired tracheoesophageal fistula, right middle lobe syndrome, and destruction of cartilage.

Pathology

Histologically, the classic description is that of a necrotizing vasculitis with granulomatous inflammation consisting of multinucleated giant cells and palisading histiocytes. A positive lung biopsy precludes the need for a kidney biopsy in many cases

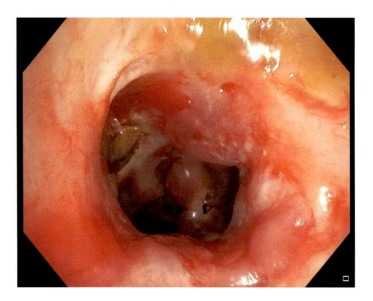

FIGURE 5.3 Bronchoscopy showing ulceration and airway pseudotumors.

(72, 73). All specimens should also be cultured to rule out infectious causes of granulomatous inflammation (e.g., fungal, TB). Cultures for *S. aureus* should also be obtained because chronic nasal carriage is a potential risk factor for relapse.

Treatment

Treatment: Goals of treatment are to improve survival and quality of life while preventing organ failure. This is done through the induction of remission followed by maintenance therapy and often requires a collaborative effort coordinated by a rheumatologist. Untreated GPA is rapidly fatal with median survival of less than 5 months (72). With glucocorticoids alone, death occurs within 1 year from either infection and/or uncontrolled disease (74, 75). Methotrexate, cyclophosphamide, and rituximab followed by azathioprine have been used successfully (76, 77). Predictors of relapse include female gender, African American ethnicity, presentation with severe kidney disease, upper respiratory or pulmonary involvement, and persistent serologic positivity.

Fibrotic scarring stenosis found in GPA does not generally respond to immunosuppressive therapy and, therefore, bronchoscopic treatment is a good alternative. Options for treatment of stenosis include intralesional injection of corticosteroids, electrosurgical incisions or resection, serial/balloon dilation, and local mitomycin-C application (32, 78). It is important to be cognizant of a therapeutic plan that uses a combination of modalities and the potential need for future therapies.

Tracheobronchomalacia

Introduction

Tracheobronchomalacia (TBM) refers to the excessive collapsibility of trachea and bronchi due to structural damage and weakness of the airway cartilage in a diffuse or segmental distribution. TBM produces symptoms due to expiratory flow limitation. Given its diverse symptom profile and heterogenous population, it is frequently mislabeled as difficult to treat asthma, chronic bronchitis, and other respiratory conditions. The flaccidity of the airway is usually most apparent during coughing or forced expiration.

TBM is reported to occur in 12% of patients with respiratory diseases (79). Approximately 23% of patients with COPD on bronchoscopy and 69% of patients with cystic fibrosis on CT chest are reported to have TBM (80). In a retrospective study of dynamic CT scans in 1071 patients with emphysema, approximately 10% men and 17% women had more than 50% reduction in cross-sectional tracheal luminal area at end-expiration (81). There is a clear association between TBM and chronic respiratory diseases (82). If 50% or greater narrowing of the airway lumen is used as a cut off to define TBM, as many as 55–78% of healthy volunteers were found to have TBM (83). Therefore, many experts consider 90% obstruction as a more appropriate cut off point to define patients who warrant treatment (81).

Etiology

In TBM, there is a decrease in the ratio of cartilage to soft tissue. In normal individuals, this ratio is 5:1, while in TBM it is 2:1. In excessive dynamic airway collapse, there is atrophy and decrease in the number of longitudinal elastic fibers of the posterior membrane (84, 85). The underlying causes of TBM can be divided into primary and secondary. Primary TBM is associated with a congenital deficiency of the cartilage. Acquired TBM is caused by trauma, COPD, chronic cough, infection, or connective tissue diseases.

Clinical features

Many patients are asymptomatic, and some studies have shown a poor correlation between the collapsibility and expiratory flow limitation (86). The symptoms include "barking" cough, dyspnea, wheezing, stridor, recurrent chest infections, and respiratory failure (85, 87). Conditions such as congestive heart failure, bronchiectasis, cystic fibrosis, obesity hypoventilation syndrome, vocal cord dysfunction, and chronic gastroesophageal reflux can mimic or coexist with TBM.

Diagnosis

Dynamic airway CT may be used to make a diagnosis of TBM. The radiologist should be alerted of the clinical suspicion for TBM so that they perform inspiratory and expiratory imaging.

Bronchoscopy is the gold standard for diagnosis (88, 89). During bronchoscopy, bowing of the cartilage wall as well as excessive invagination of the posterior wall of the trachea and bronchi is encountered. It is important to evaluate the proximal, mid, and distal trachea as well as the right and left mainstem bronchi and distal airways for obstruction. This will facilitate and guide planned interventions, including stent trial and tracheoplasty.

Management

Therapy is based on the degree of symptoms. Asymptomatic patients do not require treatment or further diagnostic workup. Symptomatic patients should undergo evaluation and management of other comorbid conditions.

If symptoms persist despite optimal medical treatment, patients with diffuse or localized TBM may undergo a stent trial. The stent is used as a temporary measure to evaluate symptomatic changes before considering surgical repair. Patients should be made aware that regardless of the clinical benefit, the stent is a temporizing measure. If patients have significant symptomatic relief after a 1–2-week stent trial, it is removed with consideration of tracheoplasty.

The use of stents for this purpose has been validated by prospective observational trials. In one prospective study, silicone stents were used for moderate to severe diffuse TBM. Following stent placement, 77% of patients reported symptomatic improvement; however, complications were frequent (90).

The ultimate long-term treatment is tracheobronchoplasty with airway stabilization. This surgical procedure has been shown to provide symptomatic benefit (91). In those with a prohibitive surgical risk, definitive stent placement can be explored. However, a proactive approach to the maintenance of stent patency is required. Other surgical alternatives include anterior external splinting, circumferential external splinting, and suture plication of the posterior membrane although experience with these techniques is limited (92–94). More recently, the use of endobronchial laser to cause contraction scarring of the posterior wall and 3D printing and modeling of airway stents are being explored (95–97).

Relapsing polychondritis

Introduction

Relapsing polychondritis (RP) is a rare systemic disease of unknown etiology characterized by recurrent inflammation and destruction of the cartilaginous structures. Pearson et al. suggested the name "relapsing polychondritis" in 1960 to describe the episodic and progressive nature of the cartilaginous destruction (98). Tracheobronchial chondritis is a dreaded complication of RP. Patients present with auricular chondritis, inflammatory arthritis, and nasal chondritis.

Respiratory tract involvement is an uncommon presenting feature, but its incidence increases as the disease progresses. Females develop airway complications more frequently (99–101). Patients who present with respiratory tract involvement have a worse prognosis than those with other organ involvement and have a poorer response to corticosteroids (99, 100, 102).

Clinical presentation
Patients with RP have tracheal collapsibility similar to TBM and as such present with cough, wheezing, and dyspnea.

Management
The mainstay of therapy consists of nonsteroidal anti-inflammatory drugs, high dose corticosteroids, and immunosuppressants (99, 100, 103). There are few therapeutic options available for patients who develop airway complications. During acute exacerbations of respiratory RP, racemic epinephrine may be beneficial in relieving symptoms (104). Surgical interventions may not be beneficial in extensive airway involvement but may be useful for localized disease (102). The surgical options available include tracheostomies and Montgomery T-tubes. Most case reports of surgical resection or tracheoplasties have shown poor outcomes (100, 103, 105). There is a case report of the use of nasal continuous positive airway pressure. It effectively acted as a "pneumatic" splint for the affected airway and prevents tracheobronchial collapse (106).

Miscellaneous causes of central airway obstruction

Involvement of central airways is reported in up to two-thirds of patients with sarcoidosis (107). Granulomas have a predilection for the submucosa of the entire respiratory tract (Figure 5.4). Sarcoidosis of the lower respiratory tract (SLRT) may be subdivided into airway luminal (intrinsic) involvement or extraluminal (extrinsic) compression (Figure 5.5). It is important to distinguish active granulomatous inflammation from fibrotic sequalae of sarcoidosis when formulating a treatment strategy.

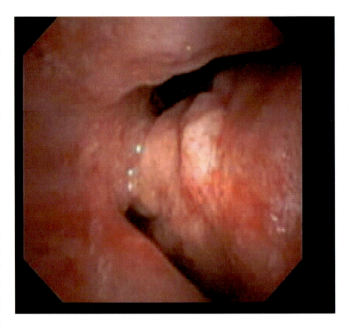

FIGURE 5.4 Bronchoscopy demonstrating mucosal involvement.

The central airways are the most common site of respiratory involvement in IBD (108, 109). The sites of involvement include the vocal cords, subglottic region, and tracheobronchial tree (110, 111). Several patients have developed airway complications for the first time after undergoing colectomy for IBD (108, 112, 113). It is suggested that a reduction in immunomodulating drugs after colectomy for IBD may unmask an underlying airway disease in these patients (112).

Endobronchial tuberculosis (EBTB) is the most important infectious disease of central airways (114). Submucosal granuloma, hyperplastic changes, ulceration, and necrosis of mucosal walls are hallmarks of active disease. Healing occurs with concentric scarring that leads to residual stenosis and atelectasis (115–117). The presence of caseating granulomas or acid-fast bacilli is diagnostic for EBTB. It is apparent that steroids do not

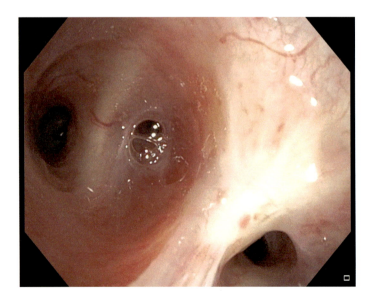

FIGURE 5.5 Bronchoscopy demonstrating lobar and segmental stenosis.

affect the regression of fibrostenotic lesions, but ameliorates inflammation and edema in the early phase of EBTB.

Conclusion

While this review could not provide a review of all etiologies of nonmalignant CAO, it reviews the more common etiologies as well as their presentation, evaluation, and management. While these entities are "benign," they can have significant morbidity and mortality.

References

1. Aravena C, Almeida FA, Mukhopadhyay S, et al. Idiopathic subglottic stenosis: A review. J Thorac Dis. 2020;12(3):1100–1111.
2. Brandenburg JH. Idiopathic subglottic stenosis. Trans Am Acad Ophthalmol Otolaryngol. 1972;76(5):1402–6.
3. Maldonado F, Loisselle A, Depew Z, et al. Idiopathic subglottic stenosis: An evolving therapeutic algorithm. Laryngoscope. 2014;124(2):498–503.
4. Perotin JM, Jeanfaivre T, Thibout Y, et al. Endoscopic management of idiopathic tracheal stenosis. Ann Thorac Surg. 2011;92(1):297–301.
5. Ashiku S, Mathieson D. Idiopathic laryngotracheal stenosis. Chest Surg Clin N Am. 2003;13(2):257–69.
6. Gelbard A, Donovan DR, Ongkasuwan J, et al. Disease homogeneity and treatment heterogeneity in idiopathic subglottic stenosis. Laryngoscope. 2016;126(6):1390–6.
7. Blumin JH, Johnston N. Evidence of extraesophageal reflux in idiopathic subglottic stenosis. Laryngoscope. 2011;121(6):1266–73.
8. Langford CA, Sneller MC, Hallahan CW, et al. Clinical features and therapeutic management of subglottic stenosis in patients with Wegener's granulomatosis. Arthritis Rheum. 1996;39(10):1754–60.
9. Lebovics RS, Hoffman GS, Leavitt RY, et al. The management of subglottic stenosis in patients with Wegener's granulomatosis. Laryngoscope. 1992;102(12):1341–5.
10. Daum TE, Specks U, Colby T V., et al. Tracheobronchial involvement in Wegener's granulomatosis. Am J Respir Crit Care Med. 1995;151(2 I):522–6.
11. Costantino CL, Mathisen DJ. Idiopathic laryngotracheal stenosis. J Thorac Dis. 2016;8(2):S204–9.
12. Grillo HC, Mak EJ, Mathisen DJ, Wain JC. Idiopathic laryngotracheal stenosis and its management. Ann Thorac Surg. 1993;56(1):80–7.
13. Valdez TA, Shapshay SM. Idiopathic subglottic stenosis revisited. Ann Otol Rhinol Laryngol. 2002;111(8):690–5.
14. Damrose EJ. On the development of idiopathic subglottic stenosis. Med Hypotheses. 2008;71(1):122–5.
15. Orphan lung diseases. Orphan Lung Dis. 2011;54.
16. Elizur A, Goldberg MR, Disin, Katz Y. A 14-year-old female with fixed airflow obstruction. Am J Respir Crit Care Med. 2013;188(11):1365.
17. Puchalski J, Musani Ali. Tracheobronchial stenosis: Causes and advances in management. Clin Chest Med. 2013;34(3):557–67.
18. Morshed K, Trojanowska A, Szymanski M, et al. Evaluation of tracheal stenosis: Comparison between computed tomography virtual tracheobronchoscopy with multiplanar reformatting, flexible tracheofiberoscopy and intra-operative findings. Eur Arch Otorhinolaryngol. 2011;268(4):591–7.
19. McCaffrey TV. Classification of laryngotracheal stenosis. Laryngoscope. 1992;102(12 Pt 1):1335–40.
20. Myer C, O'Connor DM, Cotton RT. Proposed grading system for subglottic stenosis based on endotracheal tube sizes. Ann Otol Rhinol Laryngol. 1994;103(4 Pt 1):319–23.
21. Colt C, Murgu S. (2012) Bronchoscopy and Central Airway Disorders. (Edition 1). Philadelphia, PA: Elsevier
22. Smith ME, Roy N, Stoddard K, Barton M. How does cricotracheal resection affect the female voice? Ann Otol Rhinol Laryngol. 2008;117(2):85–9.
23. Nouraei SA, Sandhu GS. Outcome of a multimodality approach to the management of idiopathic subglottic stenosis. Laryngoscope. 2013;123(10):2474–84.
24. Mehta AC, Harris RJ, DeBoer GE. Endoscopic management of benign airway stenosis. Clin Chest Med. 1995; 16(3): 401–13.
25. Mehta AC, Lee FY, Cordasco EM, Kirby T, Eliachar I, DeBoer G. Concentric tracheal and subglottic stenosis. Management using the Nd-YAG laser for mucosal sparing followed by gentle dilatation. Chest. 1993;104(3):673–7.
26. Tremblay A, Marquette CH. Endobronchial electrocautery and argon plasma coagulation: A practical approach. Can Respir J. 2004; 11(4): 305–10.
27. Yamamoto K, Kojima F, Tomiyama K, Nakamua T, Hayashino Y. Meta-analysis of therapeutic procedures for acquired subglottic stenosis in adults. Ann Thorac Surg. 2011;91(6):1747–53.
28. D'Andrilli A, Venuta F, Rendina EA. Subglottic tracheal stenosis. J Thorac Dis. 2016;8(2):S140–7.
29. Eliashar R, Eliachar I, Esclamado R, Gramlich T, Strome M. Can topical mitomycin prevent laryngotracheal stenosis? Laryngoscope. 1999;109(10):1594–600.
30. Penafiel A, Lee P, Hsu A, Eng P. Topical mitomycin-c for obstructing endobronchial granuloma. Ann Thorac Surg. 2006;82(3):E22-3.
31. Smith ME, Elstad M. Mitomycin c and the endoscopic treatment of laryngotracheal stenosis: Are two applications better than one? Laryngoscope. 2009;119(2):272–83.
32. Perepelitsyn I, Shapshay SM. Endoscopic treatment of laryngeal and tracheal stenosis-has mitomycin c improved the outcome? Otolaryngol Head Neck Surg. 2004;131(1):16–20.
33. Roedinger FC, Orloff LA, Courey MS. Adult subglottic stenosis: Management with laser incisions and mitomycin-C. Laryngoscope. 2008;118(9):1542–6.
34. Whited CW, Dailey SH. Is mitomycin C useful as an adjuvant therapy in endoscopic treatment of laryngotracheal stenosis? Laryngoscope. 2015;125(10):2243–4.
35. Rea F, Callegaro D, Loy M, et al. Benign tracheal and laryngotracheal stenosis: Surgical treatment and results. Eur J Cardiothorac Surg. 2002;22(3):352–6.
36. Roh JL, Kim DH, Rha KS, et al. Benefits and risks of mitomycin use in the traumatized tracheal mucosa. Otolaryngol Head Neck Surg. 2007;136(3):459–63.
37. Agrawal N, Morrison GA. Laryngeal cancer after topical mitomycin c application. J Laryngol Otol. 2006;120(12):1075–6.
38. Eliashar R, Gross M, Maly B, Sichel JY. Mitomycin does not prevent laryngotracheal repeat stenosis after endoscopic dilation surgery: An animal study. Laryngoscope. 2004;114(4):743–6.
39. Hartnick CJ, Hartley BE, Lacy PD, et al. Topical mitomycin application after laryngotracheal reconstruction: A randomized, double-blind, placebo-controlled trial. Arch Otolaryngol Head Neck Surg. 2001;127(10):1260–4.
40. Feinstein AJ, Goel A, Raghavan G, et al. Endoscopic management of subglottic stenosis. JAMA Otolaryngol Head Neck Surg. 2017;143(5):500–5.
41. Hirshoren N, Eliashar R. Wound-healing modulation in upper airway stenosis-myths and facts. Head Neck. 2009;31(1):111–26.
42. Wierzbicka M, Tokarski M, Puszczewicz M, Szyfter W. The efficacy of submucosal corticosteroid injection and dilatation in subglottic stenosis of different aetiology. J Laryngol Otol. 2016;130(7):674–9.
43. Martinez-Ballarin JI, Diaz-Jimenez JP, Castro M, Moya JA. Invited commentary. Ann Thorac Surg. 2015;99:453–4.
44. Dumon JF. A dedicated tracheobronchial stent. Chest. 1990;97(2): 328–32.
45. Lorenz RR. Adult laryngotracheal stenosis: Etiology and surgical management. Curr Opin Otolaryngol Head Neck Surg. 2003;11(6):467–472.
46. Garlapati P, Qurie A. Granulomatosis with Polyangiitis. StatPearls Publishing; 2021. http://www.ncbi.nlm.nih.gov/pubmed/32491759
47. Falk RJ, Gross WL, Guillevin L, et al. granulomatosis with polyangiitis (Wegener's): An alternative name for Wegener's granulomatosis. Arthritis Rheum. 2011;63(4):863–4.
48. Mercado U. Wegener's granulomatosis: the man behind the eponym. www.ccjm.org

49. Daum TE, Specks U, Colby TV, et al. Tracheobronchial involvement in Wegener's granulomatosis. Am J Respir Crit Care Med. 1995;151(2 Pt 1):522–6.
50. Hagen EC, Daha MR, Hermans J, et al. Diagnostic value of standardized assays for anti-neutrophil cytoplasmic antibodies in idiopathic systemic vasculitis. EC/BCR project for ANCA assay standardization. Kidney Int. 1998;53(3):743–53.
51. Fidler LM, Kandel S, Fisher JH, Mittoo S, Shapera S. Utility of anti-neutrophil cytoplasmic antibody screening in idiopathic interstitial lung disease. Sarcoidosis Vasc Diffus Lung Dis. 2021;38(2): E2021015.
52. Finkelman JD, Lee AS, Hummel AM, et al. ANCA are detectable in nearly all patients with active severe Wegener's granulomatosis. Am J Med. 2007;120(7).
53. Watts RA, Scott DG, Lane SE. Epidemiology of Wegener's granulomatosis, microscopic polyangiitis, and Churg-Strauss syndrome. Cleve Clin J Med. 2002;69 Suppl 2: SII84-6, E2021015.
54. Lane SE, Watts RA, Scott DG. Epidemiology of systemic vasculitis. Curr Rheumatol Rep. 2005;7(4):270–5.
55. Grisaru S, Yuen GW, Miettunen PM, Hamiwka LA. Incidence of Wegener's granulomatosis in children. J Rheumatol. 2010;37(2): 440–2.
56. Watts RA, Al-Taiar A, Scott DG, AJ MacGregor AJ. Prevalence and incidence of Wegener's granulomatosis in the UK general practice research database. Arthritis Rheum. 2009;61(10):1412–6.
57. Gibelin A, Maldini C, Mahr A. Epidemiology and etiology of Wegener granulomatosis, microscopic polyangiitis, Churg-Strauss syndrome and Goodpasture syndrome: Vasculitides with frequent lung involvement. Semin Respir Crit Care Med. 2011;32(3):264–73.
58. Polychronopoulos VS, Prakash UB, Golbin JM, Edell ES, Specks U. Airway involvement in Wegener's granulomatosis. Rheum Dis Clin North Am. 2007;33(4):755–75.
59. Stegeman CA, Tervaert JW, Sluiter WJ, et al. Association of chronic nasal carriage of *Staphylococcus aureus* and higher relapse rates in Wegener granulomatosis. Ann Intern Med. 1994;120(1):12–7.
60. Kallenberg CGM. Pathogenesis of PR3-ANCA associated vasculitis. J Autoimmun. 2008;30(1-2):29–36.
61. Hogan SL, Cooper GS, Savitz DA, et al. Association of silica exposure with anti-neutrophil cytoplasmic autoantibody small-vessel vasculitis: A population-based, case-control study. Clin J Am Soc Nephrol. 2007;2(2):290–9.
62. Zhang AH, Chen M, Gao Y, Zhao MH, Wang HY. Inhibition of oxidation activity of myeloperoxidase (MPO) by propylthiouracil (PTU) and anti-MPO antibodies from patients with PTU-induced vasculitis. Clin Immunol. 2007;122(2):187–93.
63. Gross RL, Brucker J, Bahce-Altuntas A, et al. A novel cutaneous vasculitis syndrome induced by levamisole-contaminated cocaine. Clin Rheumatol. 2011;30(10):1385–92.
64. Hseu AF, Benninger MS, Haffey TM, Lorenz R. Subglottic stenosis: A ten-year review of treatment outcomes. Laryngoscope. 2014;124(3):736–41.
65. Murgu S, Colt HG. Morphometric bronchoscopy in adults with central airway obstruction: Case illustrations and review of the literature. Laryngoscope. 2009;119(7):1318–24.
66. Lebovics RS, Hoffman GS, Leavitt RY, et al. The management of subglottic stenosis in patients with Wegener's granulomatosis. Laryngoscope. 1992;102(12 Pt 1):1341–45.
67. Cannady SB, Batra PS, Koening C, et al. Sinonasal Wegener granulomatosis: A single-institution experience with 120 cases. Laryngoscope. 2009;119(4):757–61.
68. Sheehan RE, Flint JD, Muller NL. Computed tomography features of the thoracic manifestations of Wegener granulomatosis. J Thorac Imaging. 2003;18(1):34–41.
69. Papiris SA, Manoussakis MN, Drosos AA, Kontogiannis D, Constantopoulos SH, Moutsopoulos HM. Imaging of thoracic Wegener's granulomatosis: The computed tomographic appearance. Am J Med. 1992;93(5):529–36.
70. Arunsurat I, Reechaipichitkul W, So-Ngern A, et al. Multiple pulmonary nodules in granulomatous polyangiitis: A case series. Respir Med Case Reports. 2020;30:101043.
71. Hernandez-Rodriguez J, Hoffman GS, Koening CL. Surgical interventions and local therapy for Wegener's granulomatosis. Curr Opin Rheumatol. 2010;22(1):29–36.
72. Walton EW. Giant-cell granuloma of the respiratory tract (Wegener's granulomatosis). Br Med J. 1958;2(5091):265.
73. Slot MC, Tervaert JW, Boomsma MM, Stegeman CA. Positive classic antineutrophil cytoplasmic antibody (c-ANCA) titer at switch to azathioprine therapy associated with relapse in proteinase 3-related vasculitis. Arthritis Rheum. 2004;51(2):269–73.
74. Hollander D, Manning RT. The use of alkylating agents in the treatment of Wegener's granulomatosis. Ann Intern Med. 1967;67(2):393–8.
75. Hoffman GS. Wegener's granulomatosis. Curr Opin Rheumatol. 1993;5(1):11–7.
76. De Groot K, N Rasmussen N, Bacon PA, et al. Randomized trial of cyclophosphamide versus methotrexate for induction of remission in early systemic antineutrophil cytoplasmic antibody-associated vasculitis. Arthritis Rheum. 2005;52(8):2461–9.
77. Stone JH, Merkel PA, Spiera R, et al. Rituximab versus cyclophosphamide for ANCA-associated vasculitis. 2010;17(4):168.
78. Simpson GT, Strong MS, Healy GB, et al. Predictive factors of success or failure in the endoscopic management of laryngeal and tracheal stenosis. Ann Otol Rhinol Laryngol. 1982;91(4 Pt 1):384–8.
79. Ikeda S, Hanawa T, Konishi T, et al. Diagnosis, incidence, clinicopathology and surgical treatment of acquired tracheobronchomalacia. Nihon Kyobu Shikkan Gakkai Zasshi. 1992;30(6):1028–1035.
80. McDermott S, Barry SC, Judge EE, et al. Tracheomalacia in adults with cystic fibrosis: Determination of prevalence and severity with dynamic cine CT. Radiology. 2009;252(2):577–86.
81. Barros Casas D, Fernández-Bussy S, Folch E, Flandes Aldeyturriaga J, Majid A. Non-malignant central airway obstruction. Arch Bronconeumol (English Ed.) 2014;50(8):345–54.
82. Ochs RA, Petkovska I, Kim HJ, Abtin F, Brown MS, Goldin J. Prevalence of tracheal collapse in an emphysema cohort as measured with end-expiration CT. Acad Radiol. 2009;16(1):46–53.
83. Boiselle PM, O'Donnell CR, Bankier AA, et al. Tracheal collapsibility in healthy volunteers during forced expiration: Assessment with multidetector CT. Radiology. 2009;252(1):255–62.
84. Lima E, Genta PR, Athanazio RA, et al. What is the optimal large airway size reduction value to determine malacia: Exploratory bronchoscopic analysis in patients in mounier-kuhn syndrome. J Thorac Dis. 2021;13(1):425–9.
85. Nuutinen J. Acquired tracheobronchomalacia. Eur J Respir Dis. 1982;63(5):380–387.
86. Loring SH, O'Donnell CR, Feller-Kopman DJ, Ernst A. Central Airway mechanics and flow limitation in acquired tracheobronchomalacia. Chest. 2007;131(4):1118–1124.
87. Gangadharan SP. Tracheobronchomalacia in adults. Semin Thorac Cardiovasc Surg. 2010;22(2):165–73.
88. Carden KA, Boiselle PM, Waltz DA, Ernst A. Tracheomalacia And tracheobronchomalacia in children and adults: An in-depth review. Chest. 2005;127(3):984–1005.
89. Murgu SD, Colt HG Description of a multidimensional classification system for patients with expiratory central airway collapse. Respirology. 2007;12(4):543–50.
90. Ernst A, Majid A, Feller-Kopman D, et al. Airway stabilization with silicone stents for treating adult tracheobronchomalacia: A prospective observational study. Chest. 2007;132(2):609–16.
91. Majid A, Guerrero J, Gangadharan S, et al. Tracheobronchoplasty for severe tracheobronchomalacia: A prospective outcome analysis. Chest. 2008;134(4):801–7.
92. Cho JH, Kim H, Kim J. External tracheal stabilization technique for acquired tracheomalacia using a tailored silicone tube. Ann Thorac Surg. 2012;94(4):1356–8.
93. Ley S, Loukanov T, Ley-Zaporozhan J, et al. Long-term outcome after external tracheal stabilization due to congenital tracheal instability. Ann Thorac Surg. 2010;89(3):918–25.
94. Masaoka A, Yamakawa Y, Niwa H, et al. Pediatric and adult tracheobronchomalacia. Eur J Cardiothorac Surg. 1996;10(2):87–92.
95. Dutau H, Maldonado F, Breen DP, Colchen A. Endoscopic successful management of tracheobronchomalacia with laser: Apropos of a Mounier-Kuhn syndrome. Eur J Cardiothorac Surg. 2011;39(6): 186–8.
96. Morrison RJ, Hollister SJ, Niedner MF, et al. Mitigation of tracheobronchomalacia with 3D-printed personalized medical devices in pediatric patients. Sci Transl Med. 2015;7: 285.

97. Cheng GZ, Folch E, Ochoa S, et al. Creating Personalized Airway Stents via 3D Printing. B103. Fixing a Hole: Advances in Diagnostic and Therapeutic Bronchoscopy. https://www.atsjournals.org/doi/abs/10.1164/ajrccm-conference.2015.191.1_MeetingAbstracts.A3717
98. Pearson CM, Kline HM, Newcomer VD. Relapsing polychondritis. N Engl J Med. 1960;263:5158.
99. McAdam LP, O'Hanlan MA, Bluestone R, Pearson CM. Relapsing polychondritis: Prospective study of 23 patients and a review of the literature. Medicine (Baltimore). 1976;55(3):193–215.
100. Eng J, Sabanathan S. Airway complications in relapsing polychondritis. Ann Thorac Surg. 1991;51(4):686–92.
101. Dunne JA, Sabanathan S. Use of metallic stents in relapsing polychondritis. Chest. 1994;105(3):864–7.
102. Neilly JB, Winter JH, Stevenson RD. Progressive tracheobronchial polychondritis: Need for early diagnosis. Thorax. 1985;40(1):78–9.
103. Irani BS, Martin-Hirsch DP, Clark D, Hand DW, Vize CE, Black J. Relapsing polychondritis—A study of four cases. J Laryngol Otol. 1992;106(10):911–4.
104. Gaffney RJ, Harrison M, Blayney AW. Nebulized racemic ephedrine in the treatment of acute exacerbations of laryngeal relapsing polychondritis. J Laryngol Otol. 1992;106(1):63–4.
105. Goddard P, Cook P, Laszlo G, Glover SC. Relapsing polychondritis: Report of an unusual case and a review of the literature. Br J Radiol. 2014;64(767):1064–7. http://dx.doi.org/101259/0007-1285-64-767-1064.
106. Adliff M, Ngato D, Keshavjee S, Brenaman S, Granton JT. Treatment of diffuse tracheomalacia secondary to relapsing polychondritis with continuous positive airway pressure. Chest. 1997;112(6):1701–4.
107. Polychronopoulos VS, Prakash UB. Airway involvement in sarcoidosis. Chest. 2009;136(5):1371–80.
108. Camus P, Piard F, Ashcroft T, Gal AA, Colby TV. The lung in inflammatory bowel disease. Medicine (Baltimore). 1993;72(3):151–83.
109. Mahadeva R, Walsh G, Flower CD, Shneerson JM. Clinical and radiological characteristics of lung disease in inflammatory bowel disease. Eur Respir J. 2000;15(1):41–8.
110. Kelly JH, Montgomery WW, Goodman ML, Mulvaney TJ. Upper airway obstruction associated with regional enteritis. Ann Otol Rhinol Laryngol. 1979;88(1 Pt 1):95–9.
111. Ulnick KM, Perkins J. Extraintestinal Crohn's disease: Case report and review of the literature. Ear Nose Throat J. 2001;80(2):97–100.
112. Kelly MG, Frizelle FA, Thornley PT, Beckert L, Epton M, Lynch AC. Inflammatory bowel disease and the lung: Is there a link between surgery and bronchiectasis? Int J Colorectal Dis. 2006;21(8):754–7.
113. Eaton TE, Lambie N, Wells AU. Bronchiectasis following colectomy for Crohn's disease. Thorax. 1998;53(6):529–31.
114. Shim YS. Endobronchial tuberculosis. Respirology. 1996;1(2):95–106.
115. Smith LS, Schillaci RF, Sarlin RF. Endobronchial tuberculosis. Serial fiberoptic bronchoscopy and natural history. Chest. 1987;91(5):644–7.
116. Medlar EM. The behavior of pulmonary tuberculous lesions; A pathological study. Am Rev Tuberc. 1955;71(3, Part 2):1–244. Accessed September 22, 2021. https://pubmed.ncbi.nlm.nih.gov/14350209/
117. Chung HS, Lee JH. Bronchoscopic assessment of the evolution of endobronchial tuberculosis. Chest. 2000;117(2):385–92. http://dx.doi.org/10.1378/CHEST.117.2.385

6

BRONCHIOLITIS

Bilal F. Samhouri and Jay H. Ryu

Contents

Background, definition, and classification 42
Specific forms of bronchiolitis 44
Conclusion 47
References 48

Abbreviations

BMT	bone marrow transplant
BOS	bronchiolitis obliterans syndrome
COP	cryptogenic organizing pneumonia
CT	computed tomography
CTD	connective tissue disease
CVID	common variable immunodeficiency
DAB	diffuse aspiration bronchiolitis
DIPNECH	diffuse idiopathic pulmonary neuroendocrine cell hyperplasia
DLCO	diffusing capacity of the lungs for carbon monoxide
DPB	diffuse panbronchiolitis
ECP	extracorporeal photopheresis
FB	follicular bronchiolitis
FEV_1	forced expiratory volume in 1st second
GERD	gastroesophageal reflux disease
GGO	ground-glass opacities
GVHD	graft versus host disease
HIV	human immunodeficiency virus
HSCT	hematopoietic stem cell transplant
IBD	inflammatory bowel disease
MDAD	mineral dust airway disease
mTOR	mechanistic target of rapamycin
PFT	pulmonary function test
PNEC	pulmonary neuroendocrine cell
RA	rheumatoid arthritis
RB	respiratory bronchiolitis
RB-ILD	respiratory bronchiolitis interstitial lung disease
RSV	respiratory syncytial virus
SJS	Stevens–Johnson syndrome
SSA	somatostatin analogs

KEY POINTS

- Bronchiolitis denotes the presence of inflammation and/or fibrosis within the bronchioles.
- Bronchiolitis can be the main pathologic process (i.e., primary bronchiolar disorders) or a minor component in the context of another respiratory disorder predominantly involving the proximal large airways or distal lung parenchyma.
- Bronchiolitis can manifest in various histopathologic patterns, each of which is relatively nonspecific and can be encountered in a myriad of clinical contexts.
- Patients with bronchiolitis may be asymptomatic or may manifest nonspecific respiratory symptoms of variable chronicity. Chest radiography and pulmonary function tests are often normal.
- High-resolution chest CT with expiratory imaging is the gold-standard imaging modality for bronchiolitis and can be sufficiently diagnostic for bronchiolitis in many cases, obviating the need for more invasive diagnostic approaches, namely surgical lung biopsy.
- Once a diagnosis of bronchiolitis is established, potential causes and/or medical comorbidities should be aggressively sought and accordingly managed.
- All patients with bronchiolitis should receive supportive therapy (smoking cessation, control of acid reflux and microbial colonization, in addition to providing supplemental oxygen and referral to lung transplantation when indicated). Certain bronchiolitis subtypes have disease-specific therapies.
- The clinical course of bronchiolitis depends on the underlying etiology, but the prognosis is generally favorable.

Background, definition, and classification

Bronchioles are the smallest constituents in the air-conducting apparatus of the lungs, with an internal diameter of ≤2 mm. Membranous and terminal bronchioles are purely conductive, whereas respiratory bronchioles participate in gas exchange. Respiratory bronchioles along with alveolar ducts and alveolar sacs comprise the pulmonary acinus where gas exchange takes place. Bronchioles harbor smooth muscle cells in their walls but lack cartilage, cilia, and mucus-producing cells (1). Bronchioles also house pulmonary neuroendocrine cells (PNECs) and a large

DOI: 10.1201/9781003089384-6

number of club cells. Club cells serve many functions, such as detoxification of inhaled air, modulation of inflammatory responses, regeneration of bronchiolar epithelium, among others (2). In non-diseased states, bronchioles have a substantial total cross-sectional area and contribute modestly (about 10%) toward total airway resistance (3).

Bronchiolitis is a broad term that denotes the presence of inflammation and/or fibrosis within the bronchioles and is often encountered in radiology and pathology reports. Bronchiolitis can be the main pathologic process in some disorders (primary bronchiolitis, or primary bronchiolar disorder), or can be a minor component in the context of another respiratory disorder. The latter disorders include those primarily centered in larger airways (e.g., chronic bronchitis, bronchiectasis), or the pulmonary parenchyma (e.g., hypersensitivity pneumonitis, cryptogenic organizing pneumonia) (4, 5). Primary bronchiolitides (i.e., disorders in which bronchioles are the dominant sites of the disease process) will be the focus of this chapter.

Several classification schemes for primary bronchiolar disorders have been proposed. These schemes are based on the clinical context, histologic subtype, imaging (high-resolution computed tomography [HRCT]) findings, or a combination thereof (6). Considerable overlap exists amongst these schemes, and universal acceptance and adoption of one scheme over others has not been reached. The authors favor the histology-based classification and will outline this chapter accordingly.

The histopathologic patterns of bronchiolitis can be broadly divided into (1) cellular bronchiolitis, where different types of inflammatory processes are seen within and around the bronchioles, and (2) constrictive bronchiolitis (also referred to as obliterative bronchiolitis or bronchiolitis obliterans), wherein peribronchiolar and/or submucosal fibrosis are the dominant histopathologic features with associated narrowing and/or obliteration of bronchiolar lumen. Forms of cellular bronchiolitis include acute bronchiolitis, respiratory bronchiolitis (RB), follicular bronchiolitis (FB), diffuse panbronchiolitis (DPB), diffuse aspiration bronchiolitis (DAB), and other rare forms (4, 7–9).

The histopathologic subtypes reflect recognizable patterns of bronchiolar injury with associated radiologic manifestations. Apart from RB that is mostly related to smoking, all other patterns can be encountered in a multitude of clinical circumstances. This lack of specificity underscores the necessity of integrating the clinical, laboratory, pulmonary function, and radiological data in determining the cause and clinical relevance of bronchiolitis. Such determination is best accomplished through a multidisciplinary discussion involving clinicians, radiologists, pathologists, and sometimes other specialists such as rheumatologists.

Clinical presentation

Different forms of bronchiolitis have divergent tendencies pertaining to the gender and age group they typically impact. These tendencies mirror those exhibited by the causative disease/exposure and are addressed later as we discuss specific disease variants.

Most patients with bronchiolitis present for evaluation of respiratory symptoms, but some are asymptomatic and present for evaluation of incidentally found radiologic abnormalities or histopathologic findings. Respiratory symptoms, when present, are nonspecific and typically consist of dyspnea, cough, or both.

Depending on the etiology, symptoms can be acute, subacute, or chronic; acute bronchiolitis presents acutely (days), whereas RB, FB, constrictive bronchiolitis, DPB, and DAB present over weeks, months, or even years (7, 8, 10–12).

Lung auscultation may be normal in some patients with bronchiolitis (especially, constrictive bronchiolitis), but may reveal crackles and/or wheezing in others. Pulmonary function test (PFT) results are normal in a sizable subset of patients, particularly in earlier stages of the disease process. When abnormal, any PFT pattern can be observed depending on the subtype of bronchiolitis, and response to bronchodilators is usually absent. Additionally, residual volume may be elevated (especially, constrictive bronchiolitis) reflecting expiratory air trapping, and the diffusing capacity of the lungs for carbon monoxide (DLCO) may be reduced indicating gas-exchange impairment (11–15).

Chest imaging

In bronchiolitis, chest radiography may be normal, but nonspecific findings such as hyperinflation, oligemia, and/or hazy nodular infiltrates are occasionally present (4, 9). Conversely, HRCT of the chest is nearly always abnormal and, as a result, is the imaging modality of choice whenever bronchiolitis is suspected and will provide clues to the subtype of underlying bronchiolitis.

Normal bronchioles cannot be visualized on thin-section CT. When bronchiolitis is present, however, CT scans can depict direct and indirect signs of bronchiolar disease. Direct signs include: (1) bronchiolar wall thickening due to inflammation and/or fibrosis; (2) bronchiolectasis (i.e., dilatation of the bronchioles); (9) and (3) centrilobular micronodules (i.e., opacities ≤3 mm in diameter) (16) that appear secondary to bronchiolar luminal impaction with secretions, inflammatory cells, and/or fibrotic material (Figures 6.1A and 6.1B). When centrilobular nodules are branching and share a stalk, they are termed "tree-in-bud" opacities (17, 18).

Indirect signs of bronchiolitis on CT are mosaic attenuation (i.e., "patchwork regions of differing attenuation") (16) and subsegmental atelectasis (4). Mosaic attenuation on inspiratory images can be an effect of air trapping (Figure 6.1a), as is the case in constrictive bronchiolitis, patchy involvement with infiltrative parenchymal lung disease, or pulmonary vascular disease. To distinguish between these possibilities, expiratory imaging is essential. During expiration, hypo-attenuated regions in air trapping retain their size and hypo-attenuation, in contrast to infiltrative parenchymal lung disease and pulmonary vascular disease (19).

Diagnosis

In view of the often-patchy nature of bronchiolitis and the small amount of tissue obtained, transbronchial and transthoracic (i.e., CT-guided) needle biopsies may not be diagnostic in this context. Thus, securing a histopathological diagnosis of bronchiolitis often requires a surgical lung biopsy.

However, obtaining a histopathological diagnosis is unnecessary in many cases in light of two factors: (1) in the appropriate clinical setting, a compatible chest CT is sufficiently diagnostic; and (2) because of their low specificity, identifying the histologic subtype often has little influence on management decisions (4, 6, 7). For example, mosaic attenuation due to patchy air trapping encountered in a patient with rheumatoid arthritis (RA) is highly likely to be due to RA-related constrictive bronchiolitis and generally does not necessitate histopathologic confirmation. Similarly, centrilobular ground-glass nodules seen predominantly

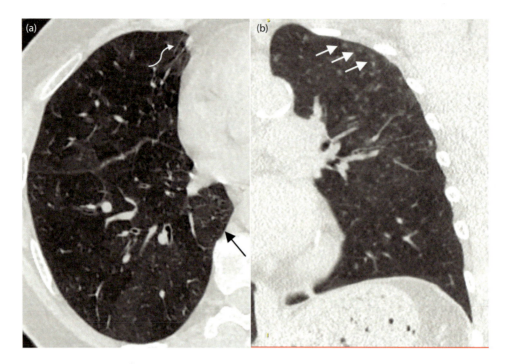

FIGURE 6.1 Chest CT findings in bronchiolitis. (a) An axial CT image that belongs to a patient with DIPNECH, and shows mosaic attenuation, thickened and dilated bronchioles, i.e., bronchiolectasis (black arrow), and subsegmental atelectasis (curved white arrow). (b) A coronal CT image obtained from a patient with respiratory bronchiolitis and displays ground-glass centrilobular nodules (white arrows) that are upper-lung predominant.

in the upper lungs of a smoker likely represents RB and usually does not require a biopsy.

Thus, the diagnosis of bronchiolitis type and cause can be determined in many cases by analyzing the clinical context, imaging findings, selected laboratory tests. When uncertain, lung biopsy may be needed. Whether bronchoscopic or surgical lung biopsy is pursued depends on the imaging findings, type, and extent, as well as consideration of risks along with patient preferences and available local expertise. These issues are explored further for specific forms of bronchiolitis in the following sections.

Management

The general approach to managing bronchiolitis has three pillars: (1) identifying and managing the underlying disease and/or exposure; (2) adequate control of potentially exacerbating conditions (e.g., infection/colonization, gastroesophageal reflux); and (3) providing the optimal supportive care (e.g., smoking cessation, oxygen supplementation when indicated, pulmonary rehabilitation, vaccinations). If respiratory failure ensues despite these interventions, a lung-transplant evaluation becomes warranted (8).

Notably, macrolide antibiotics are beneficial in several forms of bronchiolitis, and this benefit appears to be mediated through the immunomodulatory, rather than the antimicrobial properties that macrolides possess (7). Macrolides can alleviate inflammation via several mechanisms; they inhibit neutrophils' chemotaxis and function, and lower the concentration of many pro-inflammatory mediators including interleukins 1β,4,5,6,8, and others (20).

Specific forms of bronchiolitis

Respiratory bronchiolitis

Histologic RB occurs almost exclusively in smokers, affecting most (if not all) current smokers, and persists in a significant proportion of ex-smokers. Considering the widespread use of cigarettes in the United States (21) and worldwide (22), it is likely that RB is the most prevalent form of bronchiolitis (5, 23, 24). RB is defined by the presence of tan-pigmented macrophages (also called "smokers' macrophages") in the bronchioles and peribronchiolar alveolar spaces (Figure 6.2) (23–25). This finding is commonly associated with mild inflammation in the bronchiolar walls and peribronchiolar interstitium (26).

RB is often not associated with symptoms (4, 5, 27). It is commonly identified as a bystander of uncertain significance on lung tissue specimens obtained for other indications, many of which are smoking-related (e.g., lung cancer and pulmonary Langerhans cell histiocytosis) (23, 24, 28, 29). Because of the growing utilization of chest CT in lung cancer screening among heavy smokers, RB, which manifests as centrilobular ground-glass nodules, has been increasingly encountered as an incidental radiologic abnormality (5). Smoking history, together with centrilobular ground-glass nodules on CT are sufficient to diagnose RB, and invasive tests are not indicated in most cases (5).

RB produces symptoms in only a minority of affected individuals. These symptoms usually include cough, dyspnea, and wheezing, and appear over the course of weeks to months. However, this history may not always be easily discernible since similar symptoms are common among smokers, and subtle changes brought on by RB may go unnoticed by patients and clinicians.

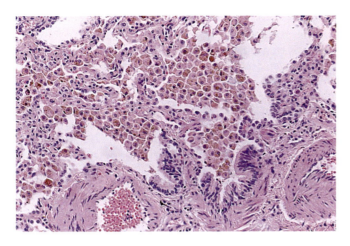

FIGURE 6.2 Histopathologic features of respiratory bronchiolitis. Accumulation of brown pigmented macrophages ("smokers' macrophages") are seen within the respiratory bronchioles and adjacent alveolar airspaces.

When histologic RB is associated with respiratory symptoms, pulmonary function impairment, prominent interstitial abnormalities on CT (e.g., ground-glass opacities, reticular abnormalities), or any combination thereof, the syndrome should be referred to as "RB-ILD" (4, 5, 26, 27, 30, 31). CT abnormalities in RB and RB-ILD are often upper-lung predominant (Figure 6.1b) (30).

Smoking cessation is the cornerstone of therapy, but evidence of RB may persist for years. In one study, 58%, 67%, and 83% of former smokers no longer exhibited tan-pigmented macrophages on lung biopsies obtained at 3, 5, and 20 years after smoking cessation, respectively. In patients with RB, the total amount of cigarette smoke exposure correlates with the presence of peribronchiolar fibrosis (23). As such, patients with RB who continue to smoke may go on to develop RB-ILD (5), a condition that may require therapies beyond smoking cessation, including immunosuppressants (most commonly, glucocorticoids) (32).

Acute bronchiolitis

Histologically, acute bronchiolitis is characterized by infiltration of the bronchiolar walls, submucosa, and adventitia with various inflammatory cells causing airway edema and respiratory epithelial necrosis and sloughing. Consequently, narrowing/occlusion of small airway lumens occurs, and distal air trapping and atelectasis ensue (5, 33).

Acute bronchiolitis is most commonly seen in children, particularly those <2 years of age, who manifest tachypnea and wheezing, classically following an upper respiratory tract infection. The organism most commonly responsible is respiratory syncytial virus (RSV), but other viral (e.g., rhinovirus, influenza, parainfluenza) and nonviral (e.g., mycoplasma, chlamydia, mycobacteria) pathogens have also been implicated. Of children with acute bronchiolitis, 2–3% require hospitalization, and <1% succumb to the disease. Although most affected children recover without long-lasting consequences, an elevated risk of bronchial asthma has been observed, and postinfectious constrictive bronchiolitis (Swyer-James syndrome) can rarely develop leading to chronic airflow limitation (33–35).

In adults, however, acute bronchiolitis is uncommon and comprises approximately 1% of hospital admissions for lower respiratory tract infections. It presents in a similar fashion to community-acquired pneumonia, with acute-onset cough, dyspnea, and fever. Infectious agents are responsible for most cases of acute bronchiolitis in adults, with *Mycoplasma pneumoniae*, influenza virus, and *Haemophilus influenzae* being the organisms most commonly isolated (36). Noninfectious etiologies of acute bronchiolitis include toxic inhalations, Stevens–Johnson syndrome, and others (4). In contrast to pneumonia, acute bronchiolitis displays centrilobular nodules and tree-in-bud opacities without ground-glass or consolidative opacities on CT (5, 37).

In adults, the management consists of supportive therapy, in conjunction with therapies targeted at the underlying cause, if one is identified (5). Acute bronchiolitis is self-limiting with excellent prognosis. In a study of 20 adult patients hospitalized with acute bronchiolitis, all patients recovered and were discharged, including the one patient who needed mechanical ventilation (36).

Constrictive bronchiolitis

Constrictive bronchiolitis (also called obliterative bronchiolitis or bronchiolitis obliterans) is characterized by the presence of peribronchiolar and submucosal fibrosis (4, 12). It is imperative to not confuse constrictive bronchiolitis with another fundamentally different disease, that is, "bronchiolitis obliterans organizing pneumonia" (BOOP). BOOP is an old term that refers to a parenchymal lung disease that belongs in the spectrum of idiopathic interstitial pneumonias when there is no identifiable cause (25). To avoid such confusing terminology, the term "BOOP" has been officially abandoned and replaced with the term "organizing pneumonia" when referring to the histopathologic pattern of lung injury, and "cryptogenic organizing pneumonia" when this pattern of lung injury is of unknown cause (4, 8).

Constrictive bronchiolitis can be found in association with a plethora of heterogeneous conditions and exposures. Constrictive bronchiolitis may also arise as a sequela of other forms of bronchiolitis (e.g., following a bout of acute infectious bronchiolitis) (4, 38). Accordingly, it has been suggested that constrictive bronchiolitis represents the outcome of an ineffective healing process instituted in response to various bronchiolar insults (12), where excessive deposition of fibrotic tissue, rather than tissue regeneration, dominates. Depletion of club cells has been linked to this dysregulated healing process (39–41).

"Bronchiolitis obliterans syndrome" (BOS) is a clinical, rather than a histopathological diagnosis. This term is exclusively used in lung transplant and hematopoietic stem cell transplant (HSCT) recipients, and refers to persistent decline in FEV_1 that cannot be explained by an alternative etiology (42, 43). Amongst lung transplant recipients, BOS is rather common and is the major cause of lung allograft loss and mortality. Constrictive bronchiolitis is the histopathologic abnormality underlying this disorder. Non-immune (e.g., gastroesophageal reflux, airway ischemia) and immune mechanisms, namely chronic cellular and antibody-mediated rejection, play key roles in the pathobiology of BOS (42). In allogeneic HSCT recipients, BOS is a manifestation of graft-versus-host disease (GVHD), particularly chronic GVHD (12, 43).

Constrictive bronchiolitis can occur in association with autoimmune diseases (e.g., RA, inflammatory bowel disease), and cancer (e.g., paraneoplastic autoimmune multi-organ syndrome). In some cases of connective tissue diseases (CTDs), constrictive bronchiolitis may be the presenting manifestation (44).

Certain medications utilized in the management of those conditions (e.g., rituximab, penicillamine, gold, mesalamine, immune checkpoint inhibitors, 5-flourouracil) have also been thought to play a causal role in the development of constrictive bronchiolitis (4, 5).

Constrictive bronchiolitis may also accompany diffuse idiopathic pulmonary neuroendocrine cell hyperplasia (DIPNECH). DIPNECH is a rare entity that mainly affects middle-aged and elderly women. The hallmark pathologic feature of DIPNECH is diffuse and excessive proliferation of PNECs. As a result, the adjacent bronchioles are exposed to supraphysiologic amounts of the bioactive substances normally secreted by PNECs, some of which are pro-fibrotic (e.g., bombesin, 5-hydroxytryptamine) and are thought to underlie the genesis of constrictive bronchiolitis in this context (45).

Several clusters of constrictive bronchiolitis have been reported, and were mostly caused by toxic inhalations occurring in war (e.g., in soldiers returning from Iraq and Afghanistan), and industrial/occupational settings (e.g., workers in the food industry) (5, 7, 12, 40). At times, however, constrictive bronchiolitis is identified without any recognizable association, and is then termed "cryptogenic constrictive bronchiolitis." Cryptogenic constrictive bronchiolitis is usually seen in middle-aged and elderly women (46, 47).

The clinical behavior and prognosis of constrictive bronchiolitis rely on the context within which it occurs. BOS (whether related to lung transplant or HSCT) is slowly progressive in the majority of cases, frequently resulting in respiratory failure and death (42, 48). In toxic inhalation–related constrictive bronchiolitis, progressive respiratory decline is expected unless the causative exposure is discontinued (12). Paraneoplastic, CTD-related, post-infectious, and cryptogenic constrictive bronchiolitis ordinarily follow a more indolent disease course, but some affected individuals may progress to respiratory failure necessitating lung transplantation or causing death (46, 49).

Treatment of constrictive bronchiolitis varies with the clinical setting in which it is identified. In lung transplant recipients, azithromycin has shown some efficacy in preventing and treating BOS. In those with no response to azithromycin, extracorporeal photopheresis (ECP) has shown promising results, with disease stabilization/improvement occurring in >50% of cases (50). Furthermore, immunosuppressive regimens prioritizing tacrolimus over cyclosporine (51), and—based on less robust evidence—mycophenolate over azathioprine (52), were associated with reduced incidence of BOS. Other therapies that deserve further study include montelukast, alemtuzumab, and total lymphoid irradiation, among others (8, 53, 54).

In HSCT recipients with BOS, it is prudent to treat the underlying process, that is chronic GVHD, with immunosuppressive therapies. Additively, a short burst of systemic steroids followed by instituting FAM therapy (i.e., a combination of high-dose inhaled corticosteroids such as fluticasone, azithromycin and montelukast) can preclude disease progression (55). Second-line therapies include ECP and etanercept (43). Importantly, despite recent advances, BOS continues to portend a poor prognosis in both, lung transplant and HSCT recipients. A carefully selected group of patients with BOS unresponsive to other therapies may be considered for (repeat) lung transplantation.

In patients with inhalation-related constrictive bronchiolitis, discontinuing the exposure is the cornerstone of therapy. For DIPNECH-associated constrictive bronchiolitis, highly effective therapies are yet-to-be discovered; however, a potential role for somatostatin analogs and mechanistic target of rapamycin (mTOR) inhibitors (e.g., sirolimus) is supported by limited data (56, 57). In CTD-associated constrictive bronchiolitis, controlling the underlying CTD is the mainstay of therapy. For cryptogenic constrictive bronchiolitis, no proven therapy exists (46, 58).

Follicular bronchiolitis

Infectious and inflammatory stimuli can trigger the genesis of bronchus-associated lymphoid tissue, and if these stimuli persist, continued proliferation of lymphoid tissues results. The abnormal presence of hyperplastic lymphoid follicles and germinal centers within bronchiolar walls defines FB (14). The incidence and prevalence of FB are unknown, but FB appears to be uncommon. Over a period of nearly 9 years, only 12 cases of biopsy-proven FB were identified in a referral center in the United States (15) and 6 cases in a center in China (11).

FB can be encountered in a variety of clinical settings: (1) CTDs, such as RA, Sjögren syndrome, and undifferentiated CTD; (2) congenital and acquired immunodeficiency syndromes, such as common variable immunodeficiency (CVID) and human immunodeficiency virus (HIV) infection; and (3) as a component of various respiratory disorders, including large airway and parenchymal lung diseases (e.g., bronchiectasis, cryptogenic organizing pneumonia). Other associations include autoimmune conditions, infections, and occupational exposures (e.g., nylon and polyethylene) (4, 8, 9, 11, 14, 15). When FB develops in the absence of any recognizable cause, it is then termed "idiopathic FB."

FB can be encountered in both genders, and individuals of all ages. Idiopathic FB preferentially affects middle-aged and elderly women (15). Since many CTDs predominantly affect women (59), and FB tends to appear later in the disease course, CTD-associated FB affects the same demographic as idiopathic FB (14). In contrast, CVID- and HIV-associated FB are commonly diagnosed in young individuals, and while CVID affects both genders equally, HIV is more prevalent among males (60, 61).

In FB, an obstructive pattern is uncommon, and the most commonly encountered PFT abnormality is reduction in DLCO (11, 15). On chest radiography, nonspecific abnormalities, namely bilateral interstitial changes, are recognized in most patients with FB. On CT, direct (most commonly, small nodules) and indirect signs of bronchiolitis can be seen in conjunction with other findings including ground-glass opacities, reticular changes, intrathoracic lymphadenopathy, and cysts (11, 15).

The treatment of FB hinges on controlling the underlying disease when one is identifiable. CTD-associated FB is best treated with immunosuppressive therapies aimed at the underlying CTD (14). Furthermore, HIV-associated FB improves with instituting antiretroviral therapy (62). Although intravenous immunoglobulin may seem promising in patients with CVID-associated FB, its success appears limited (63). In granulomatous-lymphocytic ILD, another CVID-related lung disease, a combination of rituximab and azathioprine has been successfully used (64); however, this regimen should not be routinely implemented in CVID-associated FB until more data concerning its safety and efficacy becomes available.

It has been hypothesized that idiopathic FB develops as a result of a hypersensitivity reaction, or an undiagnosed CTD (14), which prompted clinicians to employ steroids in its management (15, 65). Although steroids have proven beneficial in several cases, relapses were common when steroids were stopped or tapered, warranting the use of a steroid-sparing agent (e.g., mycophenolate, azathioprine). In this setting, azithromycin was also used as a steroid-sparing agent with anecdotal success (15).

Overall, the prognosis of FB is fairly good, and progression to respiratory failure is rare (15, 65). Nonetheless, CVID-associated FB appears to be the most aggressive variant, is progressive, and may sometimes lead to respiratory failure and death (63).

Diffuse panbronchiolitis

DPB is a rare sinobronchial inflammatory disease that has been most reported in young and middle-aged Japanese adults and tends to affect females slightly more than males. Cases outside of Japan have also been reported (8, 66). While its pathogenesis remains elusive, DPB likely has a strong genetic component (67, 68).

Histologically, DPB is characterized by the presence of foamy histiocytes, lymphocytes, and plasma cells, in addition to intraluminal neutrophils. "Pan" in the name indicates that the entire thickness of the bronchiole is involved by the inflammatory process. Early in its course, DPB preferentially affects the respiratory bronchioles, but more proximal airways (i.e., membranous bronchioles, and bronchi) can become involved in advanced disease resulting in bronchiectasis (66).

Like other bronchiolitides, cough and dyspnea are commonly present in DPB. Chronic sinusitis and large-volume sputum production (>50–100 mL per day) are reported by the majority of patients, and their presence is characteristic of DPB (8, 66). Besides the direct (diffuse small nodules and tree-in-bud opacities) and indirect signs of bronchiolar disease on CT, advanced DPB exhibits bronchiectasis that is predominantly peripheral and basilar (4, 8, 66). Importantly, none of the aforementioned clinical, histologic or radiologic features is pathognomonic (4, 66, 69, 70); thus, a summation of the above findings is necessary in order to diagnose DPB (4, 66, 71).

Left untreated, DPB portends a dismal prognosis, with a 5-year survival rate of 51%, that diminishes to 8% in those with *Pseudomonas aeruginosa* superinfection. However, macrolide therapy has dramatically improved outcomes, increasing the 5-year survival rate to 91%. Of macrolides, erythromycin is the agent of choice, but clarithromycin, roxithromycin, and azithromycin are acceptable substitutes. Clinical response is typically noticeable within 2–3 months after the commencement of therapy. Depending on disease severity and response to therapy, macrolides should be prescribed for at least 6 months, and the course may be extended to 2 years or longer (71).

Diffuse aspiration bronchiolitis

DAB is a rare aspiration-related pulmonary syndrome (72, 73). In one autopsy series, DAB was identified in 31/4,880 cases (0.6%). The initial report of DAB was mainly comprised of elderly individuals with obvious aspiration risk (e.g., dementia, debility, dysphagia) (72). However, subsequent reports have demonstrated that DAB can affect younger adults (74, 75), and that the factors predisposing to aspiration may be subtle. In one study that included 20 patients with DAB, esophagogastroduodenoscopy was necessary to diagnose GERD in 4 (20%) individuals who reported no reflux symptoms (75).

On histology, foreign bodies representing food particles can be seen within the bronchioles, often in association with a foreign-body like reaction (5). Lymphoplasmacytic infiltration of bronchiolar cells, with occasional identification of foamy macrophages is another histologic feature of DAB (75).

Most patients with DAB present with chronic respiratory symptoms, most commonly productive cough, whereas a minority present with recurrent pneumonia. Chest radiography typically depicts bilateral nodular and interstitial infiltrates (72, 75), and CT portrays centrilobular nodules and tree-in-bud opacities (75). Treatment of DAB is supportive, and mitigation of the underlying aspiration risk is prudent (5).

Miscellaneous forms of bronchiolitis

Mineral dust airway disease (MDAD) is characterized by fibrosis and pigmentation of the bronchioles, and is related to occupational exposure to different types of mineral dust (e.g., asbestos, silica, etc.) (4). While one study has linked MDAD to airflow abnormalities among dust-exposed workers (76), others have not reached a similar conclusion (4, 77). Therefore, the clinical significance of MDAD remains uncertain, and requires further clarification.

A novel form of bronchiolitis was recently described in five machine-manufacturing workers, all of whom were men and never-smokers. Biopsy showed lymphocytic bronchiolitis, alveolar ductitis, and centrilobular emphysema (BADE). All patients reported chronic dyspnea, which was progressive in three men, necessitating lung transplantation in one man. The causative exposure remains unknown (78).

Conclusion

Bronchiolitis can be classified into several subtypes and can be associated with a host of underlying diseases and exposures. Because of its nonspecific symptoms along with a broad spectrum of PFT and imaging abnormalities, bronchiolitis is a challenging disease to diagnose and manage. Bronchiolitis should be suspected in those reporting respiratory symptoms or manifesting imaging abnormalities in association with a condition/exposure known to cause bronchiolar disease, as well as those presenting with unexplained obstructive lung disease (Table 6.1). In the appropriate clinical context, a chest CT compatible with bronchiolitis can be diagnostic without the need for lung biopsy. In addition to supportive care, identifying and treating the underlying etiology are critical in the management of bronchiolitis (Table 6.2). Prognosis varies depending on the specific type of bronchiolitis, severity, and clinical context.

TABLE 6.1: Clinical Scenarios in Which Bronchiolitis Should Be Suspected

Obstructive lung disease in the absence of another recognizable etiology (e.g., asthma, COPD, bronchiectasis)

Unexplained respiratory symptoms and/or PFT abnormalities in patients with:
- Exposure known to cause bronchiolitis, especially occupational exposures
- Medical condition known to cause bronchiolitis, especially connective tissue diseases
- Lung transplant recipients
- HSCT recipients (particularly allogeneic)

Direct and/or indirect signs of bronchiolar disease on chest CT imaging

Abbreviations: COPD: chronic obstructive pulmonary disease; PFT: pulmonary function test; HSCT: hematopoietic stem cell transplantation.

TABLE 6.2: Summary of the Major Primary Bronchiolitis Subtypes

	Associations	Clinical Features	CT Features	Histology	Management
Respiratory bronchiolitis	Current or previous cigarette smoking; some occupational exposures	Asymptomatic; usually incidental finding on pathology or chest CT scans	Diffuse ground-glass centrilobular nodules, often upper-lung predominant	Tan pigmented macrophages	Elimination of smoking or other inhalational exposures
Acute bronchiolitis	Infections (e.g., mycoplasma, influenza, RSV, H. influenzae); toxic inhalations; SJS	Acute pneumonia-like illness	Centrilobular nodules, tree-in-bud opacities, without GGOs or consolidations	Intense bronchiolar inflammation, with respiratory epithelial necrosis and sloughing	Supportive, treat underlying infection if identified
Constrictive bronchiolitis	BMT and lung transplant recipients (BOS); CTD/IBD; medication-induced; toxic inhalations; post-infectious (Swyer-James syndrome); DIPNECH; idiopathic	Subacute-chronic cough, dyspnea	Mosaic attenuation (inspiratory images), with air trapping on expiratory imaging; bronchial wall thickening; bronchiectasis	Peribronchiolar and submucosal fibrosis; fibrous tissue narrows or obliterates the bronchiolar lumen	• *BMT:* 1st line: FAM* therapy; 2nd line: ECP, etanercept • *Lung transplant:* azithromycin; adjust immunosuppressive regiment; ECP • *Medication- and toxin-induced:* withdraw causative exposure • *CTD/IBD-associated:* treat underlying CTD • *DIPNECH:* (potentially) SSAs, mTOR inhibitors • Idiopathic: no clear evidence or guidelines
Follicular bronchiolitis	CTD; immunodeficiency syndromes; bronchiectasis; COP; occupational exposures; infections; idiopathic	Subacute-chronic cough, dyspnea	Centrilobular nodules, mosaic attenuation, tree-in-bud opacities, subsegmental atelectasis; sometimes GGOs, reticular changes, intrathoracic lymphadenopathy, cysts	Hyperplastic lymphoid follicles and germinal centers involving bronchus-associated lymphoid tissue (BALT)	• *CTD*-associated: treat underlying disease • Exposure-related: discontinue exposure • *Idiopathic:* steroids; may need steroid sparing agent (e.g., mycophenolate); azithromycin
DPB	Mostly Asians, particularly Japanese	Subacute-chronic cough, dyspnea, large-volume sputum, and chronic sinusitis	Centrilobular nodules, tree-in-bud opacities, mosaic attenuation, subsegmental atelectasis; peripheral and basilar predominant bronchiectasis in advanced disease	Foamy macrophages, with lymphoplasmacytic infiltration of bronchioles	Macrolides; erythromycin (1st line); roxithromycin, clarithromycin and azithromycin are alternatives
DAB	Risk factors for aspiration (e.g., GERD, dysphagia, debility, drug use)	Subacute-chronic productive cough, dyspnea; occasionally, recurrent pneumonia	Centrilobular nodules, tree-in-bud opacities; bronchiectasis may also be present	Foreign body (food particles) within bronchioles; foreign body reaction; lymphoplasmacytic infiltration	Mitigate aspiration risk

Abbreviations: BMT: bone marrow transplant; BOS: bronchiolitis obliterans syndrome; COP: cryptogenic organizing pneumonia; CT: computed tomography; CTD: connective tissue disease; DAB: diffuse aspiration bronchiolitis; DIPNECH: diffuse idiopathic pulmonary neuroendocrine cell hyperplasia; DPB: diffuse panbronchiolitis; ECP: extracorporeal photopheresis; GERD: gastroesophageal reflux disease; GGO: ground-glass opacities; IBD: inflammatory bowel disease; mTOR: mammalian target of rapamycin; RSV: respiratory syncytial virus; SJS: Stevens–Johnson syndrome; SSA: somatostatin analogs.

* FAM is a combination therapy that includes: (1) inhaled corticosteroid; (2) azithromycin; and (3) montelukast.

References

1. Brown K, Lynch DT. Histology, Lung. Treasure Island (FL): StatPearls Publishing; 2022 Jan.
2. Rokicki W, Rokicki M, Wojtacha J, Dzeljijli A. The role and importance of club cells (Clara cells) in the pathogenesis of some respiratory diseases. Kardiochirurgia i Torakochirurgia Pol. 2016;13(1):26–30. doi:10.5114/kitp.2016.58961
3. Macklem PT. The physiology of small airways. Am J Respir Crit Care Med. 1998;157(5 II SUPPL.):181–3. doi:10.1164/ajrccm.157.5.rsaa-2
4. Ryu JH, Myers JL, Swensen SJ. Bronchiolar disorders. Am J Respir Crit Care Med. 2003;168(11):1277–92. doi:10.1164/rccm.200301-053SO
5. Ryu JH, Azadeh N, Samhouri B, Yi E. Recent advances in the understanding of bronchiolitis in adults. F1000Research. 2020;9. doi:10.12688/f1000research.21778.1

6. Poletti V, Costabel U. Bronchiolar disorders: Classification and diagnostic approach. Semin Respir Crit Care Med. 2003;24(5):457–63. doi:10.1055/s-2004-815597
7. Ryu JH. Classification and approach to bronchiolar diseases. Curr Opin Pulm Med. 2006;12(2):145–51. doi:10.1097/01.mcp.0000208455.80725.2a
8. Swaminathan AC, Carney JM, Tailor TD, Palmer SM. Overview and challenges of bronchiolar disorders. Ann Am Thorac Soc. 2020;17(3):253–63. doi:10.1513/AnnalsATS.201907-569CME
9. Winningham PJ, Martínez-Jiménez S, Rosado-de-Christenson ML, Betancourt SL, Restrepo CS, Eraso A. Bronchiolitis: A practical approach for the general radiologist. Radiographics. 2017;37(3):777–94. doi:10.1148/rg.2017160131
10. King MS, Eisenberg R, Newman JH, et al. Constrictive bronchiolitis in soldiers returning from Iraq and Afghanistan. N Engl J Med. 2011;365(3):222–30. doi:10.1056/nejmoa1101388
11. Lu J, Ma M, Zhao Q, et al. The clinical characteristics and outcomes of follicular bronchiolitis in Chinese adult patients. Sci Rep. 2018;8(1):1–10. doi:10.1038/s41598-018-25670-8
12. Barker AF, Bergeron A, Rom WN, Hertz MI. Obliterative bronchiolitis. N Engl J Med. 2014;370(19):1820–8. doi:10.1056/NEJMra1204664
13. Hu X, Yi ES, Ryu JH. Bronquiolite aspirativa difusa: Análise de 20 pacientes consecutivos. J Bras Pneumol. 2015;41(2):161–6. doi:10.1590/S1806-37132015000004516
14. Tashtoush B, Okafor NC, Ramirez JF, Smolley L. Follicular bronchiolitis: A literature review. J Clin Diagnostic Res. 2015;9(9):OE01–5. doi:10.7860/JCDR/2015/13873.6496
15. Aerni MR, Vassallo R, Myers JL, Lindell RM, Ryu JH. Follicular bronchiolitis in surgical lung biopsies: Clinical implications in 12 patients. Respir Med. 2008;102(2):307–12. doi:10.1016/j.rmed.2007.07.032
16. Hansell DM, Bankier AA, MacMahon H, McLoud TC, Müller NL, Remy J. Fleischner Society: Glossary of terms for thoracic imaging. Radiology. 2008;246(3):697–722. doi:10.1148/radiol.2462070712
17. Bhalla N, Chang CF, Lee C. Special considerations for tree-in-bud nodules. Ann Am Thorac Soc. 2019; 16:636–8. doi:10.1513/AnnalsATS.201810-727CC
18. Rossi SE, Franquet T, Volpacchio M, Giménez A, Aguilar G. Tree-in-bud pattern at thin-section CT of the lungs: Radiologic-pathologic overview. Radiographics. 2005;25(3):789–801. doi:10.1148/rg.253045115
19. Kligerman SJ, Henry T, Lin CT, Franks TJ, Galvin JR. Mosaic attenuation: Etiology, methods of differentiation, and pitfalls. Radiographics. 2015;35(5):1360–80. doi:10.1148/rg.2015140308
20. Zimmermann P, Ziesenitz VC, Curtis N, Ritz N. The immunomodulatory effects of macrolides-a systematic review of the underlying mechanisms. Front Immunol. 2018;9(MAR). doi:10.3389/fimmu.2018.00302
21. Fast Facts | Fact Sheets | Smoking & Tobacco Use | CDC. Accessed January 31, 2021. https://www.cdc.gov/tobacco/data_statistics/fact_sheets/fast_facts/index.htm
22. Tobacco. Accessed January 31, 2021. https://www.who.int/news-room/fact-sheets/detail/tobacco
23. Fraig M, Shreesha U, Savici D, Katzenstein ALA. Respiratory bronchiolitis: A clinicopathologic study in current smokers, ex-smokers, and never-smokers. Am J Surg Pathol. 2002;26(5):647–53. doi:10.1097/00000478-200205000-00011
24. Cottin V, Streichenberger N, Gamondès JP, Thévenet F, Loire R, Cordier JF. Respiratory bronchiolitis in smokers with spontaneous pneumothorax. Eur Respir J. 1998;12(3):702–4. doi:10.1183/09031936.98.12030702
25. Travis WD, Costabel U, Hansell DM, et al. An official American Thoracic Society/European Respiratory Society statement: Update of the international multidisciplinary classification of the idiopathic interstitial pneumonias. Am J Respir Crit Care Med. 2013;188(6):733–48. doi:10.1164/rccm.201308-1483ST
26. Sieminska A, Kuziemski K. Respiratory bronchiolitis-interstitial lung disease. Orphanet J Rare Dis. 2014;9(1):106. doi:10.1186/s13023-014-0106-8
27. Allan PF, Perkins P. A review of respiratory bronchiolitis and respiratory bronchiolitis-associated interstitial lung disease. Clin Pulm Med. 2004;11(4):219–27. doi:10.1097/01.cpm.0000132889.48916.bb
28. Miller ER, Putman RK, Vivero M, et al. Histopathology of interstitial lung abnormalities in the context of lung nodule resections. Am J Respir Crit Care Med. 2018;197(7):955–8. doi:10.1164/rccm.201708-1679LE
29. Scheidl SJ, Kusej M, Flick H, et al. Clinical manifestations of respiratory bronchiolitis as an incidental finding in surgical lung biopsies: A retrospective analysis of a large Austrian Registry. Respiration. 2016;91(1):26–33. doi:10.1159/000442053
30. Sverzellati N, Lynch DA, Hansell DM, Johkoh T, King TE, Travis WD. American Thoracic Society–European Respiratory Society classification of the idiopathic interstitial pneumonias: Advances in knowledge since 2002. Radiographics. 2015;35(7):1849–71. doi:10.1148/rg.2015140334
31. Attili AK, Kazerooni EA, Gross BH, Flaherty KR, Myers JL, Martinez FJ. Smoking-related interstitial lung disease: Radiologic-clinical-pathologic correlation. Radiographics. 2008;28(5):1383–96. doi:10.1148/rg.285075223
32. Portnoy J, Veraldi KL, Schwarz MI, et al. Respiratory bronchiolitis-interstitial lung disease: Long-term outcome. Chest. 2007;131(3):664–71. doi:10.1378/chest.06-1885
33. Øymar K, Skjerven HO, Mikalsen IB. Acute bronchiolitis in infants, a review. Scand J Trauma Resusc Emerg Med. 2014;22(1):23. doi:10.1186/1757-7241-22-23
34. Justice NA, Le JK. Bronchiolitis. Treasure Island (FL): StatPearls Publishing; 2022 Jan.
35. Ravaglia C, Poletti V. Recent advances in the management of acute bronchiolitis. F1000Prime Rep. 2014;6. doi:10.12703/P6-103
36. Ryu K, Takayanagi N, Ishiguro T, et al. Etiology and outcome of diffuse acute infectious bronchiolitis in adults. Ann Am Thorac Soc. 2015;12(12):1781–1787. doi:10.1513/AnnalsATS.201507-473OC
37. Miller WT, Mickus TJ, Barbosa E, Mullin C, Van Deerlin VM, Shiley KT. CT of viral lower respiratory tract infections in adults: Comparison among viral organisms and between viral and bacterial infections. Am J Roentgenol. 2011;197(5):1088–1095. doi:10.2214/AJR.11.6501
38. Epler GR. Diagnosis and treatment of constrictive bronchiolitis. F1000 Med Rep. 2010;2(1):32. doi:10.3410/M2-32
39. Liu Z, Liao F, Scozzi D, et al. An obligatory role for club cells in preventing obliterative bronchiolitis in lung transplants. JCI Insight. 2019;4(9). doi:10.1172/jci.insight.124732
40. Palmer SM, Flake GP, Kelly FL, et al. Severe airway epithelial injury, aberrant repair and bronchiolitis obliterans develops after diacetyl instillation in rats. PLoS One. 2011;6(3). doi:10.1371/journal.pone.0017644
41. Kelly FL, Kennedy VE, Jain R, et al. Epithelial Clara cell injury occurs in bronchiolitis obliterans syndrome after human lung transplantation. Am J Transplant. 2012;12(11):3076–84. doi:10.1111/j.1600-6143.2012.04201.x
42. Meyer KC, Raghu G, Verleden GM, et al. An international ISHLT/ATS/ERS clinical practice guideline: Diagnosis and management of bronchiolitis obliterans syndrome. Eur Respir J. 2014;44(6):1479–1503. doi:10.1183/09031936.00107514
43. Williams KM. How i treat bronchiolitis obliterans syndrome after hematopoietic stem cell transplantation. Blood. 2017;129(4):448–55. doi:10.1182/blood-2016-08-693507
44. Arcadu A, Ryu JH. Constrictive (obliterative) bronchiolitis as presenting manifestation of connective tissue diseases. J Clin Rheumatol. 2020;26(5):176–80. doi:10.1097/RHU.0000000000001387
45. Samhouri BF, Azadeh N, Halfdanarson TR, Yi ES, Ryu JH. Constrictive bronchiolitis in diffuse idiopathic pulmonary neuroendocrine cell hyperplasia. ERJ Open Res. 2020;6(4):00527–02020. doi:10.1183/23120541.00527-2020
46. Callahan SJ, Vranic A, Flors L, Hanley M, Stoler MH, Mehrad B. Sporadic obliterative bronchiolitis: Case series and systematic review of the literature. Mayo Clin Proc Innov Qual Outcomes. 2019;3(1):86–93. doi:10.1016/j.mayocpiqo.2018.10.003

47. Kraft M, Mortenson RL, Colby T V., Newman L, Waldron JA, King TE. Cryptogenic constrictive bronchiolitis: A clinicopathologic study. Am Rev Respir Dis. 1993;148(4):1093–101. doi:10.1164/ajrccm/148.4_Pt_1.1093
48. Soubani AO, Uberti JP. Bronchiolitis obliterans following haematopoietic stem cell transplantation. Eur Respir J. 2007;29(5):1007–19. doi:10.1183/09031936.00052806
49. Fernández Pérez ER, Krishnamoorthy M, Brown KK, et al. FEV1 over time in patients with connective tissue disease-related bronchiolitis. Respir Med. 2013;107(6):883–9. doi:10.1016/j.rmed.2013.02.019
50. Greer M, Dierich M, De Wall C, et al. Phenotyping established chronic lung allograft dysfunction predicts extracorporeal photopheresis response in lung transplant patients. Am J Transplant. 2013;13(4):911–8. doi:10.1111/ajt.12155
51. Treede H, Glanville AR, Klepetko W, et al. Tacrolimus and cyclosporine have differential effects on the risk of development of bronchiolitis obliterans syndrome: Results of a prospective, randomized international trial in lung transplantation. J Hear Lung Transplant. 2012;31(8):797–804. doi:10.1016/j.healun.2012.03.008
52. Mycophenolate mofetil versus azathioprine immunosuppressive regimens after lung transplantation: preliminary experience - PubMed. Accessed January 31, 2021. https://pubmed.ncbi.nlm.nih.gov/9730425/
53. Benden C, Haughton M, Leonard S, Huber LC. Therapy options for chronic lung allograft dysfunction–bronchiolitis obliterans syndrome following first-line immunosuppressive strategies: A systematic review. J Hear Lung Transplant. 2017;36(9):921–33. doi:10.1016/j.healun.2017.05.030
54. Verleden SE, Sacreas A, Vos R, Vanaudenaerde BM, Verleden GM. Advances in understanding bronchiolitis obliterans after lung transplantation. Chest. 2016;150(1):219–25. doi:10.1016/j.chest.2016.04.014
55. Williams KM, Cheng GS, Pusic I, et al. Fluticasone, azithromycin, and montelukast treatment for new-onset bronchiolitis obliterans syndrome after hematopoietic cell transplantation. Biol Blood Marrow Transplant. 2016;22(4):710–6. doi:10.1016/j.bbmt.2015.10.009
56. Russier M, Plantier L, Derot G, De Muret A, Marchand-Adam S. Diffuse idiopathic pulmonary neuroendocrine cell hyperplasia syndrome treated with sirolimus. Ann Intern Med. 2018;169(3):197–8. doi:10.7326/L17-0634
57. Al-Toubah T, Strosberg J, Halfdanarson TR, et al. Somatostatin analogs improve respiratory symptoms in patients with diffuse idiopathic neuroendocrine cell hyperplasia. Chest. Published online February 2020. doi:10.1016/j.chest.2020.01.031
58. Parambil JG, Yi ES, Ryu JH. Obstructive bronchiolar disease identified by CT in the non-transplant population: Analysis of 29 consecutive cases. Respirology. 2009;14(3):443–8. doi:10.1111/j.1440-1843.2008.01445.x
59. van Vollenhoven RF. Sex differences in rheumatoid arthritis: More than meets the eye... BMC Med. 2009;7:12. doi:10.1186/1741-7015-7-12
60. Pescador Ruschel MA, Vaqar S. Common Variable Immunodeficiency. Treasure Island (FL): StatPearls Publishing; 2020.
61. U.S. Statistics | HIV.gov. Accessed January 13, 2021. https://www.hiv.gov/hiv-basics/overview/data-and-trends/statistics
62. Shipe R, Lawrence J, Green J, Enfield K. HIV-associated follicular bronchiolitis. Am J Respir Crit Care Med. 2013;188(4):510–1. doi:10.1164/rccm.201206-1096IM
63. Costa-Carvalho BT, Wandalsen GF, Pulici G, Aranda CS, Solé D. Pulmonary complications in patients with antibody deficiency. Allergol Immunopathol (Madr). 2011;39(3):128–32. doi:10.1016/j.aller.2010.12.003
64. Chase NM, Verbsky JW, Hintermeyer MK, et al. Use of combination chemotherapy for treatment of granulomatous and lymphocytic interstitial lung disease (GLILD) in patients with common variable immunodeficiency (CVID). J Clin Immunol. 2013;33(1):30–9. doi:10.1007/s10875-012-9755-3
65. Romero S, Barroso E, Gil J, Aranda I, Alonso S, Garcia-Pachon E. Follicular bronchiolitis: Clinical and pathologic findings in six patients. Lung. 2003;181(6):309–19. doi:10.1007/s00408-003-1031-0
66. Poletti V, Casoni G, Chilosi M, Zompatori M. Diffuse panbronchiolitis. Eur Respir J. 2006;28(4):862–71. doi:10.1183/09031936.06.00131805
67. Park MH, Kim YW, Yoon H Il, et al. Association of HLA class I antigens with diffuse panbronchiolitis in Korean patients. Am J Respir Crit Care Med. 1999;159(2):526–9. doi:10.1164/ajrccm.159.2.9805047
68. Sugiyama Y, Kudoh S, Maeda H, Suzaki H, Takaku F. Analysis of HLA antigens in patients with diffuse panbronchiolitis. Am Rev Respir Dis. 1990;141(6):1459–62. doi:10.1164/ajrccm/141.6.1459
69. Iwata M, Colby TV, Kitaichi M. Diffuse panbronchiolitis: Diagnosis and distinction from various pulmonary diseases with centrilobular interstitial foam cell accumulations. Hum Pathol. 1994;25(4):357–63. doi:10.1016/0046-8177(94)90143-0
70. Poletti V, Chilosi M, Trisolini R, et al. Idiopathic bronchiolitis mimicking diffuse panbronchiolitis. Sarcoidosis Vasc Diffus Lung Dis. 2003;20(1):62–8.
71. Kudoh S, Keicho N. Diffuse panbronchiolitis. Clin Chest Med. 2012;33(2):297–305. doi:10.1016/j.ccm.2012.02.005
72. Matsuse T, Oka T, Kida K, Fukuchi Y. Importance of diffuse aspiration bronchiolitis caused by chronic occult aspiration in the elderly. Chest. 1996;110(5):1289–93. doi:10.1378/chest.110.5.1289
73. Hu X, Lee JS, Pianosi PT, Ryu JH. Aspiration-related pulmonary syndromes. Chest. 2015;147(3):815–23. doi:10.1378/chest.14-1049
74. Matsuse T, Teramoto S, Matsui H, Ouchi Y, Fukuchi Y. Widespread occurrence of diffuse aspiration bronchiolitis in patients with dysphagia, irrespective of age. Chest. 1998;114(1):350–51. doi:10.1378/chest.114.1.350-a
75. Hu X, Yi S, Ryu JH. Diffuse aspiration bronchiolitis: analysis of 20 consecutive patients (Bronquiolite aspirativa difusa: análise de 20 pacientes consecutivos). J. Bras Pneumol. doi:10.1590/S1806-37132015000004516
76. Churg A, Wright JL, Wiggs B, Paré PD, Lazar N. Small airways disease and mineral dust exposure. Prevalence, structure, and function. Am Rev Respir Dis. 1985;131(1):139–43. doi:10.1164/arrd.1985.131.1.139
77. Wood C, Yates D. Respiratory surveillance in mineral dust-exposed workers. Breathe. 2020;16(1). doi:10.1183/20734735.0362-2019
78. Cummings KJ, Stanton ML, Nett RJ, et al. Severe lung disease characterized by lymphocytic bronchiolitis, alveolar ductitis, and emphysema (BADE) in industrial machine-manufacturing workers. Am J Ind Med. 2019;62(11):927–37. doi:10.1002/ajim.23038

7

ALLERGIC BRONCHOPULMONARY ASPERGILLOSIS (ABPA)

Sunjay R. Devarajan and Nicola A. Hanania

Contents

Introduction	51
Impact of ABPA in patients with airway diseases	51
Clinical features of ABPA	52
Diagnosis of ABPA	52
Management of ABPA	54
References	55

KEY POINTS

- ABPA is an inflammatory lung disease caused by a dysregulated immune response to inhaled antigen of Aspergillus species, most commonly *Aspergillus fumigatus*.
- Asthma and cystic fibrosis are the two diseases most closely associated with ABPA, which can lead to pulmonary exacerbations and resultant lung function decline.
- Multiple diagnostic criteria exist with the most common findings being elevated serum IgE, sensitization to *Aspergillus fumigatus*, and development of pulmonary infiltrates and bronchiectasis.
- Corticosteroids and antifungal therapies are the mainstays of treatment, but biologic agents are of increasing interest.
- Disease relapse is common, so close follow-up of these patients is required.

Introduction

Aspergillus fumigatus is a ubiquitous saprophytic mold whose spores are inhaled daily by human beings, though related illnesses generally occur in only those with immunological dysregulation or underlying lung disease (1). Several disease manifestations have been ascribed to *A. fumigatus*, namely allergic bronchopulmonary aspergillosis (ABPA), invasive pulmonary aspergillosis (IPA), and chronic pulmonary aspergillosis (CPA), and these may exist on a continuum. In this chapter, we focus the attention on the diagnosis and clinical management of ABPA.

ABPA describes an allergic sensitization (AS,) characterized by immediate cutaneous hypersensitivity or elevated IgE to *A. fumigatus* antigen. The immune response is characterized by both Type 1 and Type 3 hypersensitivity responses (2, 3). It is surmised that *A. fumigatus* spores are first inhaled and then trapped in the mucus of large segmental bronchi (4, 5). Under normal circumstances, inhalation of fungal conidia does not lead to immunologic response; however, idiosyncrasies in innate and/or adaptive immunity result in formation and proliferation *of A. fumigatus* hyphae, which then trigger a pro-inflammatory immune response driven by TH2 CD4+ T-lymphocytes and airway macrophages acting through toll-like receptors (1, 2). Activation of CD4+ T cells also results in a humoral immune response, leading to IgE, IgA, and IgG production by B-lymphocytes and plasma cells which are specifically directed against *A. fumigatus* antigen (6). As a result, *A. fumigatus*-specific IgG antibodies, often referred to as "precipitins antibodies," can be isolated during disease exacerbation (7). Models for direct cellular damage by *A. fumigatus* proteases have also been described (8).

A familial susceptibility to ABPA has been elucidated in certain individuals, such as with genetic expression of HLA molecules DR2, DR4, DR5, and DR7 (9, 10). On the other hand, presence of HLA-DQ2 appears to be protective against development of ABPA (11). As is the case in other disease processes, pathogenesis of ABPA involves both host and environmental factors that blossom into allergic fungal disease like ABPA. It is important to note that only a minority of those with exposure to Aspergillus fumigatus develop overt ABPA, but initial sensitization is viewed as the opening salvo to developing clinically relevant disease. ABPA-associated airways disease is most closely associated with the development of bronchiectasis, which is a final common pathway of many diseases (see Table 7.1).

Impact of ABPA in patients with airway diseases

The prevalence of ABPA in the general population is not well-established (12); however, there are certain high-risk patient populations that deserve special mention. People with asthma and cystic fibrosis (CF) have an outsized risk of ABPA development, which will be expanded upon further. Disease entities known as severe asthma with fungal sensitization (SAFS) and allergic bronchopulmonary mycosis (ABPM), in which some patients with severe asthma are immunologically sensitized to one or more alternate fungi, have been well-described (13, 14), but are outside the scope of this chapter.

Asthma

In general, patients with asthma appear to be at greater risk of ABPA development with estimated prevalence rates of 1–3.5% (2, 12). Studies from higher volume specialty clinics have quoted higher rates, although these may have been subject to referral bias (15). Development of ABPA can have a significant impact on the control of asthma and accelerated loss of lung function, so the presence of this comorbidity should be considered in those patients with difficult-to-control asthma (14, 16).

DOI: 10.1201/9781003089384-7

TABLE 7.1: The Differential Diagnosis of Bronchiectasis

Post-Infectious Complications	Heritable Disease	Immune Dysfunction	Inflammatory Disease
Mycobacterium tuberculosis	Cystic fibrosis	Hypogammaglobulinemia	Rheumatoid arthritis
Non-tuberculous mycobacteria	Alpha-1-antrypsin deficiency	Neutrophil dysfunction	Inflammatory bowel disease
Necrotizing pneumonia	Primary ciliary dyskinesia	HIV/AIDS	Sjögren syndrome
Childhood lower respiratory infection	Marfan syndrome	Other	Sarcoidosis
Acute respiratory distress syndrome	Williams–Campbell syndrome		Other
Other	Mounier–Kuhn syndrome		
	Hyper-IgE syndrome		
	Obstruction & Inhalation	**Other Causes**	
	Recurrent aspiration	Radiation injury	
	Foreign body	Pulmonary fibrosis	
	Endobronchial tumor	Yellow nail syndrome	
	ABPA	Bronchiolitis obliterans	
	Swyer–James syndrome	Other	

Abbreviations: HIV/AIDS: human immunodeficiency virus/acquired immunodeficiency syndrome.

Cystic fibrosis

High prevalence of Aspergillus sp. in respiratory isolates in CF is commonplace (17, 18), depending on fungal culture media used. Estimates of the prevalence of AS in CF, however, range from 20% to 65% (4, 19), and there is a wide range of reported prevalence of overt ABPA in CF. Several diagnostic criteria (discussed in more detail below) for ABPA exist and are variably utilized across studies (19), which, in turn, creates the heterogeneity noted in published prevalence rates. In a European registry study involving 12,447 people with CF across nine countries, the prevalence of ABPA was 7.8%, although though prevalence in this study varied significantly between countries and individual centers (4). Importantly, in this CF population, a diagnosis of ABPA was associated with increased risk for massive hemoptysis and pneumothorax, which are two life-threatening complications seen in this population. Using CF Foundation (CFF) diagnostic criteria, a descriptive Irish study placed the prevalence of ABPA in those presenting with CF-associated pulmonary exacerbations at 12% (20) while a similarly conducted French study in children placed the rate at 9% (21). In stark comparison, a multicenter observational study from the United States reported a lower prevalence of CF-related ABPA of 2%, perhaps attributable to the fact that the study only obtained information on medical conditions that were present within 6 months of study enrollment. ABPA prevalence in this population does not appear to vary by sex although it does rise with age (17).

While patients with CF are at higher risk of ABPA than the general population, more granular risk factors have been identified, such as low body mass index (less than the 3rd percentile) (21), adolescent age, atopy, severity of lung disease, and presence of *Pseudomonas aeruginosa* in sputum isolates (7). Atopic sensitization to common aeroallergens also appears to be a risk factor (22). Aspergillus sputum culture positivity does not appear to impact the risk of ABPA (17).

Specific ABPA diagnostic criteria in CF were established by consensus in 2003 and are also recognized by the CFF: high total serum IgE levels >500 IU/mL, immediate skin hypersensitivity to *A. fumigatus* antigen (prick skin test wheal of ≥3 mm in diameter with surrounding erythema, while the patient is not being treated with systemic antihistamines), elevated precipitating antibody or IgE to Aspergillus antigen, and any typical radiographic findings like central bronchiectasis, mucus plugging, or pulmonary infiltrates (23).

People with CF developing ABPA experience more substantial lung function decline over time relative to control groups, even after taking into account chronic airways infection with *Pseudomonas aeruginosa* (24, 25), which is a well-established source of disproportionate lung function decline in the CF population. Given this, annual screening of serum IgE level is recommended by CFF care guidelines.

Clinical features of ABPA

ABPA typically presents as difficult-to-control, often steroid-dependent asthma accompanied by AS. Other clinical features of ABPA include, but are not limited to, productive cough of mucoid thick sputum, wheezing, fever, hemoptysis, weight loss, malaise, and fatigue. The downstream effects of ABPA include the triggering of asthma exacerbations and airway remodeling with or without bronchiectasis (26), which is classically central (6). Digital clubbing is an uncommon finding, but may be seen in the presence of long-standing bronchiectasis (2, 27). Expectoration of brown mucus plugs, a clinical manifestation previously thought to be pathognomonic for ABPA, can be seen in up to half of patients (27).

Pulmonary function testing (PFT) results vary based on disease control, but are nonspecific because most patients already have underlying airway disease (28). The most common abnormality that is noted during disease exacerbation is airway obstruction, and if disease progresses into a fibrotic stage, this can reduce lung volume and diffusion capacity measurements (29), leading to a mixed pattern of obstruction and restriction.

Diagnosis of ABPA

The Rosenberg/Patterson criteria for diagnosis of ABPA were introduced in 1977 and include seven primary and three secondary components (30, 31). Subsequently, the Greenberger/Patterson criteria followed this diagnostic backbone but included *A. fumigatus* specific IgE and IgG to the criteria. Patterson et al. devised a five-stage classification system that ultimately divided ABPA into two groups: seropositive ABPA without central bronchiectasis (ABPA-S) and ABPA with central bronchiectasis (ABPA-CB) (32). This classification scheme was an attempt to differentiate treatment strategies, and while it was prophetic, it has fallen out of favor (27, 32). Importantly, while patients with ABPA-S may have lower rates of disease exacerbation, this distinction does not appear to correlate with disease severity or serologic findings (28, 33, 34).

Allergic Bronchopulmonary Aspergillosis (ABPA)

More recently, an expert panel from the International Society for Human and Animal Mycology (ISHAM) convened in 2013 to produce a new diagnostic set of criteria for ABPA, which has not been widely adopted. Separate diagnostic criteria exist for people with CF. These diagnostic schemes are summarized in Table 7.2.

Laboratory findings

Peripheral eosinophilia

Peripheral eosinophilia is characterized as mild, moderate, and severe with total counts of 500–1,500/μL, 1,500–5,000/μL, and >5,000/μL, respectively (35). In one retrospective analysis, approximately 75% of patients with ABPA presented with abnormally high levels of peripheral blood eosinophils, and only 40% presented with levels higher than 1,000/μL (36), suggesting that peripheral eosinophilia is a sensitive but nonspecific disease marker. In this group, no association was found between the severity of peripheral eosinophilia and the severity of disease as measured by spirometry.

Serum IgE

An elevation in total serum IgE (typically >1,000 IU/mL in asthma; >500 IU/mL in CF) is a hallmark of ABPA diagnostic criteria, as is elevated specific anti-*A. fumigatus* IgE (28). These serologic studies should be pursued if ABPA is suspected. One analysis found that only a minority of patients with asthma and total serum IgE >1,000 IU/mL met the clinical criteria for ABPA (37), so there is no indication for routine screening for IgE in patients with asthma. CFF patient care guidelines, on the other hand, advocate for yearly screening of serum IgE given the aforementioned higher prevalence in this population.

Skin testing

A. fumigatus skin testing can be performed by skin-prick or intradermal injection with the latter deemed more sensitive but having a requirement of more antigen quantity (29). Both tests are characterized by exposure of skin to diluted Aspergillus antigen. An immediate cutaneous hypersensitivity reaction is marked by development of a wheal and erythema within 1 minute, reaching a maximum size after 10–20 minutes, and followed by resolution within 1 hour (38). There is substantial international variation in the component Aspergillus extract used, which may impact test reliability (29).

Bronchoscopy

Neither bronchoscopy nor histology is required to diagnose ABPA; however, these may have a role when a diagnosis is evasive. Bronchoalveolar lavage studies often reveal the presence of eosinophilia in fluid cell count analysis and an elevation in *A. fumigatus*-specific IgE and IgA (39), while the bronchoscopy itself can reveal airway mucus plugging containing eosinophils and fungal hyphae (7), pathognomonic findings of ABPA. Fungal culture of *A. fumigatus* is an unreliable indicator of disease (28) and could reflect colonization alone.

Imaging

Chest radiography is not a sensitive diagnostic test for ABPA. Obtained early in the disease course, chest radiographs may suggest upper-lobe predominant bronchial wall thickening and hyperinflation, and, advanced disease may be characterized by atelectasis, tubular opacities and "fleeting infiltrates" (29, 40, 41). Chest radiograph findings in people with CF may be indistinguishable from those seen during acute pulmonary exacerbations.

High-resolution computed tomography (HRCT) has replaced bronchography as the test of choice to evaluate for the presence of bronchiectasis with a sensitivity and specificity greater than 90% (41). In ABPA, the most common radiographic abnormality is the presence of bronchiectasis, which is defined by a broncho-arterial ratio (internal diameter of the dilated bronchus divided by the external diameter of the accompanying artery) greater than 1 (41–43). This leads to the classic HRCT finding in ABPA known as the "signet ring sign." If an area of central bronchiectasis

TABLE 7.2: Comparing ABPA Diagnostic Criteria

	Major Criteria	Minor Criteria	Interpretation
Rosenberg/Patterson Criteria (1977)	Presence of asthma	Positive sputum culture for *Aspergillus* sp.	If 6/7 major criteria met, diagnosis is "likely"
	Peripheral eosinophilia	Expectoration of brown mucous plugs	If 7/7 major criteria met, diagnosis is "certain"
	Immediate skin reactivity to Aspergillus antigen	Delayed skin reactivity to Aspergillus antigen	
	Precipitating antibodies to Aspergillus antigen		
	Elevated serum IgE		
	History of pulmonary infiltrates		
	Central bronchiectasis		
International Society for Human and Animal Mycology (ISHAM) (2013)	Detectable IgE against *A. fumigatus*	Precipitating antibodies to *A. fumigatus* or elevated *A. fumigatus* IgG	At least 2 major and 2 minor criteria must be met
	Aspergillus skin test positivity	Radiographic pulmonary opacities	* Patients must have asthma or CF
	Elevated IgE (usually >1,000 IU/mL)	Peripheral eosinophil count >500 cells/uL	
Cystic Fibrosis Foundation ABPA Clinical Care Guidelines (2003)	Acute or subacute clinical deterioration	Precipitating antibodies to *A. fumigatus* or elevated *A. fumigatus* IgG	All 3 major criteria and 2 minor criteria
	Elevated serum IgE >500 IU/mL	New or recent pulmonary opacities not responsive to standard therapy	
	Immediate skin reactivity to Aspergillus		

Source: From (2, 23, 31).

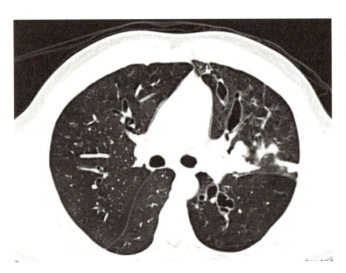

FIGURE 7.1 Cystic bronchiectasis in a person with CF with mucus impaction, known as the "finger-in-glove sign," a characteristic finding of ABPA when using HRCT.

is impacted sufficiently with thick mucus, the so-called "finger-in-glove" sign can be visualized on HRCT (see Figure 7.1). While bronchial mucus plugging in ABPA is generally hypodense, the presence of airway high attenuation mucus (HAM), defined as mucus that is more dense than the chest wall or skeletal muscle, predicts an increased risk of ABPA disease relapse and can be accompanied by higher levels of peripheral blood eosinophils, Aspergillus-specific IgE, and total IgE (27, 44–46). Other HRCT findings include, but are not limited to, centrilobular nodules, pleuroparenchymal fibrosis, tree-in-bud opacities, and mosaic attenuation (44).

Management of ABPA

Systemic corticosteroids
Goals in the treatment of ABPA are to reduce airway inflammation, mucus production and reverse bronchospasm. The cornerstone of treatment is systemic corticosteroids, starting with a dose of 0.5–0.75 mg/kg of prednisone tapered over several months (16, 28). A low maintenance dose may be required to sustain disease remission. Systemic corticosteroids are associated with decreased wheezing, reduction in total serum IgE levels and blood eosinophilia, as well as improvement in opacities on chest imaging (28); however, a host of corticosteroid-related adverse effects may limit both dose and duration of treatment.

Inhaled corticosteroids
Inhaled steroid monotherapy is not recognized as a mainstay of ABPA therapy, and they do not appear to reduce the risk of disease progression (42) in patients with S-ABPA. While robust data are limited, there may be a role for high dose inhaled steroid in reducing the dose of systemic steroids required to achieve disease remission (47).

Antifungal therapies
Several case reports and multiple clinical trials have assessed the efficacy of the triazole antifungal agent, itraconazole, versus placebo and demonstrated effectiveness of antifungal therapy in ABPA (12, 26, 48–51). Stevens et al. conducted a small randomized, double-blinded trial comparing 200 mg of itraconazole twice daily versus placebo over 16 weeks in patients with corticosteroid-dependent ABPA. Favorable overall clinical response was noted in 13 of 28 patients in the itraconazole group compared to only 5 of 27 patients in the placebo group (46% vs. 19%, $p = 0.04$) (48). An open-label phase that followed elicited improvements in the control group without relapses in the treatment group. One randomized, double-blind, placebo-controlled trial compared a treatment regimen of 400 mg of itraconazole versus placebo in 29 patients, stratified on the basis of the presence or absence of bronchiectasis, with stable ABPA over 16 weeks. This study resulted in the treatment arm patients experiencing fewer disease exacerbations that required treatment with systemic corticosteroids, as well as reductions in sputum eosinophil and serum IgE counts (26). While supportive data are not as robust, there may be a role for both voriconazole and posaconazole as alternative antifungal agents in the treatment of ABPA (52, 53).

Data on the utility of inhaled antifungal therapies as a primary treatment strategy are limited. A small randomized control trial demonstrated relative benefit in the use of nebulized Amphotericin B plus inhaled corticosteroid versus inhaled corticosteroid alone, which certainly produces an impetus for larger, blinded, and placebo-controlled studies (54). Unfortunately, nebulized Amphotericin B may not be well-tolerated due to bronchospasm (55).

Systemic steroids versus antifungals
A clinical trial by Agarwal et al. compared itraconazole monotherapy to prednisolone monotherapy in 131 treatments naïve ABPA patients for a period of 4 months. Subjects responded to therapy at the primary endpoint of 6 weeks more frequently in the corticosteroid group compared to the antifungal group (100% and 88%, $p = 0.007$), though there was no statistically significant difference in the time to first exacerbation (56). While prednisolone recipients universally experienced clinical response, patients in the itraconazole arm also experienced positive clinical effects, all while utilizing a medication with a more favorable adverse effect profile. Outside of clinical trials, itraconazole is frequently used in combination with systemic corticosteroids, but caution should be advised in such situations, as corticosteroid effects can be potentiated by itraconazole owing to its potent inhibition of hepatic CYP3A4 activity (57, 58). Specific to CF, retrospective analyses appear to show that addition of itraconazole to systemic corticosteroid therapy appears to reduce the risk of pulmonary exacerbations attributable to ABPA (22).

Targeted biologics
Anti-inflammatory biologics commonly used in severe asthma may have an important role in the management of ABPA. The most well-studied agent is omalizumab, a humanized monoclonal IgG1 antibody that binds free serum IgE and downregulates its production, leading to a significant reduction in relapse, inflammatory markers, total systemic corticosteroid requirement, and serum IgE (59, 60). In a synthesis review of case reports and series, omalizumab resulted in a ~60% decline in serum IgE, improved Asthma Control Test scores, and improved lung function (60) without major adverse effects. Unfortunately, an exploratory study launched specifically to assess the efficacy of omalizumab in CF-related ABPA was terminated early due to adverse effects (61).

In one case report, a female patient with severe asthma and ABPA refractory to treatment, including IgE and anti-IL5 monoclonal antibodies, achieved a complete response when treated with dupilumab, a monoclonal antibody directed against IL-4 (62). Our clinical experience supports these observations, and a randomized control trial is currently underway to study dupilumab and its efficacy in treatment of ABPA in patients with asthma (ClinicalTrials.gov Identifier: NCT04442269).

Mepolizumab and benralizumab, which are monoclonal antibodies directed against the interleukin 5 and its receptor (IL-5), respectively, and result in attenuation of eosinophil activation, have a promising role in the treatment of ABPA, but data to support their use are limited to case reports and case series (63–65).

References

1. Kanj A, Abdallah N, Soubani AO. The spectrum of pulmonary aspergillosis. Respir Med. 2018 Aug;141:121–31.
2. Agarwal R, Chakrabarti A, Shah A, Gupta D, Meis JF, Guleria R, Moss R, Denning DW; ABPA complicating asthma ISHAM working group. Allergic bronchopulmonary aspergillosis: review of literature and proposal of new diagnostic and classification criteria. Clin Exp Allergy. 2013 Aug;43(8):850–73.
3. Murray and Nadel's Textbook of Respiratory Medicine. Murray and Nadel's Textbook of Respiratory Medicine. V. Courtney Broaddus, Robert J. Mason, Joel D. Ernst, Talmadge E. King Jr, Stephen C. Lazarus, John F. Murray, Jay A. Nadel, Arthur Slutsky, Co-Editors. Thoracic Imaging Editor: Michael Gotway. Philadelphia: Elsevier Saunders, 2016.
4. Mastella G, Rainisio M, Harms HK, Hodson ME, Koch C, Navarro J, Strandvik B, McKenzie SG. Allergic bronchopulmonary aspergillosis in cystic fibrosis. A European epidemiological study. Epidemiologic Registry of Cystic Fibrosis. Eur Respir J. 2000 Sep;16(3):464–71.
5. Greenberger PA. Allergic bronchopulmonary aspergillosis. J Allergy Clin Immunol. 2002 Nov;110(5):685–92.
6. Janahi IA, Rehman A, Al-Naimi AR. Allergic bronchopulmonary aspergillosis in patients with cystic fibrosis. Ann Thorac Med. 2017 Apr-Jun;12(2):74–82.
7. Grippi M.A., & Elias J.A., & Fishman J.A., & Kotloff R.M., & Pack A.I., & Senior R.M., & Siegel M.D.(Eds.), (2015). Fishman's Pulmonary Diseases and Disorders, *Fifth Edition*. McGraw Hill
8. Tomee JF, Wierenga AT, Hiemstra PS, Kauffman HK. Proteases from *Aspergillus fumigatus* induce release of proinflammatory cytokines and cell detachment in airway epithelial cell lines. J Infect Dis. 1997 Jul;176(1):300–3.
9. Aron Y, Bienvenu T, Hubert D, Dusser D, Dall'Ava J, Polla BS. HLA-DR polymorphism in allergic bronchopulmonary aspergillosis. J Allergy Clin Immunol. 1999 Oct;104(4 Pt 1):891–2
10. Chauhan B, Santiago L, Hutcheson PS, Schwartz HJ, Spitznagel E, Castro M, Slavin RG, Bellone CJ. Evidence for the involvement of two different MHC class II regions in susceptibility or protection in allergic bronchopulmonary aspergillosis. J Allergy Clin Immunol. 2000 Oct;106(4):723–9.
11. Chauhan B, Hutcheson PS, Slavin RG, Bellone CJ. MHC restriction in allergic bronchopulmonary aspergillosis. Front Biosci. 2003 Jan 1;8:s140–8
12. Denning DW, Pleuvry A, Cole DC. Global burden of allergic bronchopulmonary aspergillosis with asthma and its complication chronic pulmonary aspergillosis in adults. Med Mycol. 2013 May;51(4):361–70.
13. Denning DW, O'Driscoll BR, Powell G, Chew F, Atherton GT, Vyas A, Miles J, Morris J, Niven RM. Randomized controlled trial of oral antifungal treatment for severe asthma with fungal sensitization: The Fungal Asthma Sensitization Trial (FAST) study. Am J Respir Crit Care Med. 2009 Jan 1;179(1):11–18.
14. Greenberger PA, Bush RK, Demain JG, Luong A, Slavin RG, Knutsen AP. Allergic bronchopulmonary aspergillosis. J Allergy Clin Immunol Pract. 2014 Nov-Dec;2(6):703–8
15. Nath A, Khan A, Hashim Z, Patra JK. Prevalence of *Aspergillus* hypersensitivity and allergic bronchopulmonary aspergillosis in patients with bronchial asthma at a tertiary care center in North India. Lung India. 2017 Mar-Apr;34(2):150–4
16. Porsbjerg C, Menzies-Gow A. Co-morbidities in severe asthma: Clinical impact and management. Respirology. 2017 May;22(4):651–61.
17. Milla CE, Wielinski CL, Regelmann WE. Clinical significance of the recovery of Aspergillus species from the respiratory secretions of cystic fibrosis patients. Pediatr Pulmonol. 1996 Jan;21(1):6–10.
18. Bakare N, Rickerts V, Bargon J, Just-Nübling G. Prevalence of Aspergillus fumigatus and other fungal species in the sputum of adult patients with cystic fibrosis. Mycoses. 2003 Feb;46(1-2):19–23
19. Maturu VN, Agarwal R. Prevalence of Aspergillus sensitization and allergic bronchopulmonary aspergillosis in cystic fibrosis: systematic review and meta-analysis. Clin Exp Allergy. 2015 Dec;45(12):1765–78.
20. Chotirmall SH, Branagan P, Gunaratnam C, McElvaney NG. Aspergillus/allergic bronchopulmonary aspergillosis in an Irish cystic fibrosis population: a diagnostically challenging entity. Respir Care. 2008 Aug;53(8):1035–41
21. Jubin V, Ranque S, Stremler Le Bel N, Sarles J, Dubus JC. Risk factors for Aspergillus colonization and allergic bronchopulmonary aspergillosis in children with cystic fibrosis. Pediatr Pulmonol. 2010 Aug;45(8):764–71.
22. Nepomuceno IB, Esrig S, Moss RB. Allergic bronchopulmonary aspergillosis in cystic fibrosis: role of atopy and response to itraconazole. Chest. 1999 Feb;115(2):364–70.
23. Stevens DA, Moss RB, Kurup VP, Knutsen AP, Greenberger P, Judson MA, Denning DW, Crameri R, Brody AS, Light M, Skov M, Maish W, Mastella G; Participants in the Cystic Fibrosis Foundation Consensus Conference. Allergic bronchopulmonary aspergillosis in cystic fibrosis–state of the art: Cystic Fibrosis Foundation Consensus Conference. Clin Infect Dis. 2003 Oct 1;37 Suppl 3:S225–64
24. Kraemer R, Deloséa N, Ballinari P, Gallati S, Crameri R. Effect of allergic bronchopulmonary aspergillosis on lung function in children with cystic fibrosis. Am J Respir Crit Care Med. 2006 Dec 1;174(11):1211–20.
25. Fillaux J, Brémont F, Murris M, Cassaing S, Rittié JL, Tétu L, Segonds C, Abbal M, Bieth E, Berry A, Pipy B, Magnaval JF. Assessment of Aspergillus sensitization or persistent carriage as a factor in lung function impairment in cystic fibrosis patients. Scand J Infect Dis. 2012 Nov;44(11):842–7.
26. Wark PA, Hensley MJ, Saltos N, Boyle MJ, Toneguzzi RC, Epid GD, Simpson JL, McElduff P, Gibson PG. Anti-inflammatory effect of itraconazole in stable allergic bronchopulmonary aspergillosis: a randomized controlled trial. J Allergy Clin Immunol. 2003 May;111(5):952–7.
27. Agarwal R, Gupta D, Aggarwal AN, Saxena AK, Chakrabarti A, Jindal SK. Clinical significance of hyperattenuating mucoid impaction in allergic bronchopulmonary aspergillosis: an analysis of 155 patients. Chest. 2007 Oct;132(4):1183–90.
28. Patterson K, Strek ME. Allergic bronchopulmonary aspergillosis. Proc Am Thorac Soc. 2010 May;7(3):237–44.
29. Shah A, Panjabi C. Allergic aspergillosis of the respiratory tract. Eur Respir Rev. 2014 Mar 1;23(131):8–29.
30. Patterson R, Greenberger PA, Radin RC, Roberts M. Allergic bronchopulmonary aspergillosis: staging as an aid to management. Ann Intern Med. 1982 Mar;96(3):286–91.
31. Rosenberg M, Patterson R, Mintzer R, Cooper BJ, Roberts M, Harris KE. Clinical and immunologic criteria for the diagnosis of allergic bronchopulmonary aspergillosis. Ann Intern Med. 1977 Apr;86(4):405–14.
32. Patterson R, Greenberger PA, Halwig JM, Liotta JL, Roberts M. Allergic bronchopulmonary aspergillosis. Natural history and classification of early disease by serologic and roentgenographic studies. Arch Intern Med. 1986 May;146(5):916–8.
33. Kumar R, Chopra D. Evaluation of allergic bronchopulmonary aspergillosis in patients with and without central bronchiectasis. J Asthma. 2002 Sep;39(6):473–7.
34. Agarwal R, Gupta D, Aggarwal AN, Behera D, Jindal SK. Allergic bronchopulmonary aspergillosis: lessons from 126 patients attending a chest clinic in north India. Chest. 2006 Aug;130(2):442–8.
35. Larsen RL, Savage NM. How I investigate Eosinophilia. Int J Lab Hematol. 2019 Apr;41(2):153–61.
36. Agarwal R, Khan A, Aggarwal AN, Varma N, Garg M, Saikia B, Gupta D, Chakrabarti A. Clinical relevance of peripheral blood eosinophil count in allergic bronchopulmonary aspergillosis. J Infect Public Health. 2011 Nov;4(5-6):235–43.

37. Tay TR, Bosco J, Gillman A, Aumann H, Stirling R, O'Hehir R, Hew M. Coexisting atopic conditions influence the likelihood of allergic bronchopulmonary aspergillosis in asthma. Ann Allergy Asthma Immunol. 2016 Jul;117(1):29–32.e1.
38. Agarwal R, Maskey D, Aggarwal AN, Saikia B, Garg M, Gupta D, Chakrabarti A. Diagnostic performance of various tests and criteria employed in allergic bronchopulmonary aspergillosis: a latent class analysis. PLoS One. 2013 Apr 12;8(4):e61105.
39. Greenberger PA, Smith LJ, Hsu CC, Roberts M, Liotta JL. Analysis of bronchoalveolar lavage in allergic bronchopulmonary aspergillosis: divergent responses of antigen-specific antibodies and total IgE. J Allergy Clin Immunol. 1988 Aug;82(2):164–70.
40. Panse P, Smith M, Cummings K, Jensen E, Gotway M, Jokerst C. The many faces of pulmonary aspergillosis: Imaging findings with pathologic correlation. Radiology of Infectious Diseases. 2016 Dec 1;3(4):192–200.
41. Agarwal R, Khan A, Garg M, Aggarwal AN, Gupta D. Pictorial essay: Allergic bronchopulmonary aspergillosis. Indian J Radiol Imaging. 2011 Oct;21(4):242–52.
42. Agarwal R, Khan A, Aggarwal AN, Saikia B, Gupta D, Chakrabarti A. Role of inhaled corticosteroids in the management of serological allergic bronchopulmonary aspergillosis (ABPA). Intern Med. 2011;50(8):855–60.
43. Kimmig L, Bueno J. Dilated Bronchi: How Can I Tell? Ann Am Thorac Soc. 2017 May;14(5):807–9.
44. Lu HW, Mao B, Wei P, Jiang S, Wang H, Li CW, Ji XB, Gu SY, Yang JW, Liang S, Cheng KB, Bai JW, Cao WJ, Jia XM, Xu JF. The clinical characteristics and prognosis of ABPA are closely related to the mucus plugs in central bronchiectasis. Clin Respir J. 2020 Feb;14(2):140–7.
45. Agarwal R, Sehgal IS, Dhooria S, Aggarwal A. Radiologic Criteria for the Diagnosis of High-Attenuation Mucus in Allergic Bronchopulmonary Aspergillosis. Chest. 2016 Apr;149(4):1109–10.
46. Goyal R, White CS, Templeton PA, Britt EJ, Rubin LJ. High attenuation mucous plugs in allergic bronchopulmonary aspergillosis: CT appearance. J Comput Assist Tomogr. 1992 Jul-Aug;16(4):649–50.
47. Imbeault B, Cormier Y. Usefulness of inhaled high-dose corticosteroids in allergic bronchopulmonary aspergillosis. Chest. 1993 May;103(5):1614–7.
48. Stevens DA, Schwartz HJ, Lee JY, Moskovitz BL, Jerome DC, Catanzaro A, Bamberger DM, Weinmann AJ, Tuazon CU, Judson MA, Platts-Mills TA, DeGraff AC Jr. A randomized trial of itraconazole in allergic bronchopulmonary aspergillosis. N Engl J Med. 2000 Mar 16;342(11):756–62.
49. Denning DW, Van Wye JE, Lewiston NJ, Stevens DA. Adjunctive therapy of allergic bronchopulmonary aspergillosis with itraconazole. Chest. 1991 Sep;100(3):813–9.
50. Salez F, Brichet A, Desurmont S, Grosbois JM, Wallaert B, Tonnel AB. Effects of itraconazole therapy in allergic bronchopulmonary aspergillosis. Chest. 1999 Dec;116(6):1665–8.
51. Germaud P, Tuchais E. Allergic bronchopulmonary aspergillosis treated with itraconazole. Chest. 1995 Mar;107(3):883.
52. Chishimba L, Niven RM, Cooley J, Denning DW. Voriconazole and posaconazole improve asthma severity in allergic bronchopulmonary aspergillosis and severe asthma with fungal sensitization. J Asthma. 2012 May;49(4):423–33.
53. Agarwal R, Dhooria S, Sehgal IS, Aggarwal AN, Garg M, Saikia B, Chakrabarti A. A randomised trial of voriconazole and prednisolone monotherapy in acute-stage allergic bronchopulmonary aspergillosis complicating asthma. Eur Respir J. 2018 Sep 18;52(3):1801159.
54. Ram B, Aggarwal AN, Dhooria S, Sehgal IS, Garg M, Behera D, Chakrabarti A, Agarwal R. A pilot randomized trial of nebulized amphotericin in patients with allergic bronchopulmonary aspergillosis. J Asthma. 2016 Jun;53(5):517–24.
55. Chishimba L, Langridge P, Powell G, Niven RM, Denning DW. Efficacy and safety of nebulised amphotericin B (NAB) in severe asthma with fungal sensitisation (SAFS) and allergic bronchopulmonary aspergillosis (ABPA). J Asthma. 2015 Apr;52(3):289–95
56. Agarwal R, Dhooria S, Singh Sehgal I, Aggarwal AN, Garg M, Saikia B, Behera D, Chakrabarti A. A Randomized Trial of Itraconazole vs Prednisolone in Acute-Stage Allergic Bronchopulmonary Aspergillosis Complicating Asthma. Chest. 2018 Mar;153(3):656–64.
57. Lebrun-Vignes B, Archer VC, Diquet B, Levron JC, Chosidow O, Puech AJ, Warot D. Effect of itraconazole on the pharmacokinetics of prednisolone and methylprednisolone and cortisol secretion in healthy subjects. Br J Clin Pharmacol. 2001 May;51(5):443–50
58. Parmar JS, Howell T, Kelly J, Bilton D. Profound adrenal suppression secondary to treatment with low dose inhaled steroids and itraconazole in allergic bronchopulmonary aspergillosis in cystic fibrosis. Thorax. 2002 Aug;57(8):749–50.
59. Voskamp AL, Gillman A, Symons K, Sandrini A, Rolland JM, O'Hehir RE, Douglass JA. Clinical efficacy and immunologic effects of omalizumab in allergic bronchopulmonary aspergillosis. J Allergy Clin Immunol Pract. 2015 Mar-Apr;3(2):192–9.
60. Li JX, Fan LC, Li MH, Cao WJ, Xu JF. Beneficial effects of Omalizumab therapy in allergic bronchopulmonary aspergillosis: A synthesis review of published literature. Respir Med. 2017 Jan;122:33–42.
61. EUCTR2007-006648-23-IT. An exploratory, randomized, double-blind, placebo controlled study to assess the efficacy of multiple doses of omalizumab (Xolair) in cystic fibrosis complicated by allergic bronchopulmonary aspergillosis - ND. http://www.who.int/trialsearch/Trial2.aspx?TrialID=EUCTR2007-006648-23-IT. 2009
62. Mümmler C, Kemmerich B, Behr J, Kneidinger N, Milger K. Differential response to biologics in a patient with severe asthma and ABPA: a role for dupilumab? Allergy Asthma Clin Immunol. 2020 Jun 26;16:55.
63. Eraso IC, Sangiovanni S, Morales EI, Fernández-Trujillo L. Use of monoclonal antibodies for allergic bronchopulmonary aspergillosis in patients with asthma and cystic fibrosis: literature review. Ther Adv Respir Dis. 2020 Jan-Dec;14:1753466620961648.
64. Schleich F, Vaia ES, Pilette C, Vandenplas O, Halloy JL, Michils A, Peche R, Hanon S, Louis R, Michel O. Mepolizumab for allergic bronchopulmonary aspergillosis: Report of 20 cases from the Belgian Severe Asthma Registry and review of the literature. J Allergy Clin Immunol Pract. 2020 Jul-Aug;8(7):2412–2413.e2.
65. Tolebeyan A, Mohammadi O, Vaezi Z, Amini A. Mepolizumab as possible treatment for allergic bronchopulmonary aspergillosis: A review of eight cases. cureus. 2020 Aug 12;12(8):e9684.

PART C
Rare Pulmonary Vascular Diseases

8

PULMONARY ARTERIOVENOUS MALFORMATIONS (PAVMs) AND HEREDITARY HEMORRHAGIC TELANGIECTASIA (HHT)

Minkyung Kwon, Daniil Gekhman, Carlos Rojas, and Augustine Lee

Contents

Introduction	57
Prevalence and risk factors	57
Hereditary hemorrhagic telangiectasia	57
Clinical presentation	58
Diagnostic evaluation	59
Brief overview of monitoring and management	60
Conclusion	61
References	61

KEY POINTS

- Hereditary hemorrhagic telangiectasia (HHT); also called Osler–Weber–Rendu syndrome, is a genetic vascular condition often manifesting with mucocutaneous telangiectasias and arteriovenous malformations of gastrointestinal tract, lungs, and/or cerebral circulation.
- Contrast-enhanced computed tomography (CT) scan of the chest and transthoracic echocardiography are the best noninvasive modalities to detect PAVMs.
- PAVMs can lead to paradoxical embolization and rupture, and can be considered for angiographic embolization.

Introduction

Pulmonary arteriovenous malformation (PAVM) refers to a vascular anomaly, in which there is a low-resistance fistulous communication between the pulmonary artery and vein. Though it can be acquired, it is most commonly associated with hereditary hemorrhagic telangiectasia (HHT). When lining mucosal services, it can be a cause of hemoptysis and hemorrhage, but the most devastating complications come from the right-to-left shunting of venous blood directly to systemic circulation. Depending on the size and number of PAVMs, the result can be hypoxia and/or paradoxical embolisms through these fistulous connections causing stroke and cerebral abscesses. As effective interventions are available, awareness of the clinical-radiographic features and diagnostic strategies are important for its early detection. Additionally, as HHT is genetically based with autosomal dominant transmission, both the patient and the patient's family should have access to genetics counselors, patient advocacy society ("Cure HHT"), and centers of expertise for HHT patients and families (1).

Prevalence and risk factors

The currently reported prevalence of PAVM is 38 in 100,000 (2). Approximately 90% of patients with PAVMs will have underlying HHT (3), although conversely, PAVMs are present in up to 50% of the HHT population (4–6). The prevalence of HHT is estimated to be as much as 1 in 5,000 (7). Rarely, PAVM can be acquired with reports associated with cardiac surgery or cancer (8).

Hereditary hemorrhagic telangiectasia

Hereditary hemorrhagic telangiectasia, also referred to as Osler–Weber–Rendu syndrome, is an autosomal dominant genetic disorder that has been reported in all populations. While the exact pathophysiologic mechanism has not been fully elucidated, it is thought to be due to a combination of abnormal angiogenesis (9), blood vessel repair (10), and vessel maturation (11). The dominant recognized mutations are referred to as HHT1 when the endoglin gene is affected, HHT2 related to mutations in the activin-receptor like kinase 1 gene (ACVRL1), and JP-HHT (juvenile polyposis syndrome) related to Mutations decapentaplegic homoolog-4 gene (SMAD4) (12). In all, 97% of patients with HHT will have a recognizable mutation, with HHT1 and HH2 accounting for approximately 80% (13).

HHT patients are frequently asymptomatic when young and begin to develop symptoms as they get older (14). Epistaxis is most common, frequently accompanied by telangiectasias on the lips, tongue, and nasal/oral mucosa (15). After initial presentation, further investigation often yields AVMs, most commonly in the gastrointestinal tract, and less commonly in the lung or brain (16). PAVMs may not be apparent in HHT patients, but observation and high level of suspicion is needed as they may develop PAVMs later in life.

Diagnostic criteria of HHT was proposed by Shovlin et al. in 2000 (Curaçao diagnostic criteria, Table 8.1 [17]). This consists of epistaxis, telangiectasias, visceral lesions of AVMs, and family history (first-degree relative with HHT) and patients who met three out of four criteria were thought to be definite HHT. The location, size, and number of AVMs affecting other visceral

DOI: 10.1201/9781003089384-8

TABLE 8.1: Curaçao Criteria

The HHT diagnosis is

Definite	If three criteria are present,
Possible or suspected	If two criteria are present, and
Unlikely	If fewer than two criteria are present

Criteria

1.	Epistaxis	Spontaneous, recurrent nose bleeds
2.	Telangiectasias	Multiple, at characteristic sites: lips, oral cavity, fingers, nose
3.	Visceral lesions	Such as gastrointestinal telangiectasia (with or without bleeding), pulmonary AVM, hepatic AVM, cerebral AVMs, spinal AVM
4.	Family history	A first-degree relative with HHT according to these criteria

organs dictate symptoms and complications, some of which could be devastating (Table 8.2).

Genetic testing for HHT can help establish the diagnosis in patients with suspected HHT or even among asymptomatic relatives. Even when the Curaçao criteria is met, it is recommended that genetic testing be performed to identify the specific mutation, given potential management/monitoring implications (17). Based on the specific symptoms or the genetic mutation, additional screening is often required. For example, in JP-HHT, the

TABLE 8.2: Clinical Features of HHT

Mucocutaneous
- Epistaxis
- Telangiectasias (Figure 8.3)

Neurologic
- Headache, Migraine
- Stroke, thrombotic and hemorrhagic
- Cerebral abscess
- Seizure

Gastrointestinal
- Gastrointestinal bleed
- Abdominal pain
- Portal hypertension
- Cholestasis, anicteric
- Colorectal cancer (juvenile polyposis – HHT)

Hematologic
- Iron deficiency anemia
- Polycythemia
- Venous and arterial thromboembolism

Respiratory
- Dyspnea, platypnea, orthodeoxia
- Hypoxemia (shunting)
- Cyanosis
- Digital clubbing
- Hemoptysis
- Pulmonary hemorrhage
- Hemothorax
- Pulmonary embolism

Cardiovascular
- High-output cardiac failure
- Pulmonary arterial hypertension

SMAD4 mutation confers an increased risk for colorectal cancer, and therefore colonoscopy would be considered (12). Screening for hepatic AVMs are largely driven by symptoms, abnormal liver function tests, or by the presence of downstream complications such as heart failure, portal hypertension, or pulmonary hypertension. If a patient with HHT or suspected HHT has any neurologic symptoms including migraines, seizures, or stroke syndrome, magnetic resonance imaging of the brain should be performed. Given the high morbidity of these complications, consensus guidelines recommend imaging in any patient with suspected or confirmed HHT regardless of symptoms. Similarly, as PAVMs are a mechanism for these devastating cerebral complications, and can be treated, screening for PAVMs are also recommended in all patients, including in pregnant women who are at increased risk for complications of PAVMs.

Clinical presentation

The majority of patients with PAVMs are asymptomatic, and they are typically identified only radiographically as an incidental lung finding. In symptomatic patients, dyspnea and hemoptysis are the most common symptoms. Those with HHT may have epistaxis that will serve as a clue to the underlying diagnosis. Patients with isolated PAVMs typically manifest symptoms/signs in the fifth to sixth decades of life, while HHT often manifests before the age of 20.

As noted earlier, complications of PAVMs can include hypoxia, paradoxic embolism with strokes, cerebral abscesses, pulmonary embolism, pulmonary hemorrhage, and hemothorax (18). Consequently, mortality rates between 4% and 22% have been reported when left untreated (19). Although dyspnea is commonly due to anemia or airflow obstruction rather than right to left shunting itself, large or diffuse PAVMs can drive dyspnea and hypoxia. Occasionally, this can present as platypnea and orthodeoxia when a significant PAVM burden is situated at the bases (20). In addition to dyspnea, patients may also present with hemoptysis, chest pain, digital clubbing. Indirect symptoms may include any neurologic syndrome as well as signs of pulmonary hypertension and heart failure.

Neurologic complications of cerebral abscesses and strokes occur as a result of paradoxical embolization from a microthrombi crossing into systemic circulation via a large enough PAVM. Feeding arteries greater than 2–3 mm in diameter increases the risk of such embolization (21). Non-neurologic systemic embolization has also been reported including infectious endocarditis, and abscesses in the soft tissue, muscle, or spleen (4).

PAVMs can frankly rupture with an estimated lifetime risk of 8% (22). Patients will typically present with hemoptysis (23) due to a ruptured parenchymal or endobronchial PAVM, but pulmonary embolism should be considered in the differential as it can occur in 7–30% of patients with PAVMs (4). When the PAVM approximates the pleura, hemothorax can also occur, with reports up to 3% of HHT patients (4). Pregnancy is a risk factor for PAVM rupture, particularly in the third trimester, therefore counseling (ideally done pre-natal, screening and intervention during the second trimester) is recommended (4).

Pulmonary hypertension has been reported in patients with PAVMs in approximately 10% of patients with HHT (24). HHT patients with ALK-1 or endoglin gene mutation may have heritable pulmonary arterial hypertension that is clinically indistinguishable from idiopathic pulmonary arterial hypertension (25). Although most series of pulmonary hypertension in HHT is limited to noninvasive testing such as echocardiography (26), it is

Pulmonary Arteriovenous Malformations and Hereditary Hemorrhagic Telangiectasia

important to fully assess for both pre- and post-capillary causes of pulmonary hypertension (24) Alternative mechanisms for PH include high-output heart failure (due to hepatic AVMs and/or anemia), venous thromboembolic disease, portal hypertension, hypoxia, or a combination of these. PAVMs may, ironically, ameliorate pulmonary pressures by offloading the right ventricle and pulmonary artery, although the shunting may theoretically be aggravated. Progressive pulmonary hypertension increases the risk that the PAVM will rupture (27).

Diagnostic evaluation

A PAVM can be found as an incidental lung nodule, but also should be suspected in a patient with a history of cerebral infarct or abscess, or in unexplained dyspnea (platypnea), hypoxemia (orthodeoxia), hemoptysis, or hemothorax. When suspected, or in a patient with known HHT, screening of PAVM should first be done with transthoracic contrast-enhanced echocardiography (TTE) (28). Agitated saline (10–20 mL) is injected into a peripheral vein while simultaneously imaging the right and left ventricles. The contrast (microbubbles) is normally visualized in the right ventricle and atrium soon after injection and should not be visualized in the left cardiac chambers, as microbubbles are filtered out by the pulmonary capillary network. The appearance of contrast in the left ventricle is consistent with right-to-left shunt, but if it occurs immediately within one cardiac cycle, it is suggestive of an intracardiac shunt.

When TTE is not helpful or equivocal in confirming PAVM, calculating shunt fraction by 100% oxygen method or radionuclide perfusion scanning can be adjunct tests to identify for the presence and severity of any AVMs. A shunt fraction of >5% is considered abnormal and is calculated from the arterial blood gas analysis (assuming normal arteriovenous extraction) after the patient breathes 100% oxygen for 20 minutes (29). However, its sensitivity may be limited (30). The scintigraphy method typically employs a technetium labeled albumin particles ≥ 20 μm. As these particles should be trapped in the pulmonary capillaries, its detection in the brain or kidney can be used to confirm the presence of shunting and calculate the shunt severity by comparing to the relative uptake in the lungs (31).

Chest radiography is usually considered appropriate in the initial workup of patients with clinically suspected PAVMs as a complimentary examination to TTE to exclude an alternative diagnosis (28). However, chest radiography is limited in the detection of PAVMs with a reported low sensitivity of 70% (32). Contrast CT imaging of the chest is most helpful to locate and confirm PAVMs (33). According to the American College of Radiology appropriateness criteria, CT angiogram (CTA) of the chest with intravenous contrast should be considered in the evaluation of patients with clinically suspected PAVMs (28). CTA can detect, characterize, and help determine the need for and the planning of a potential intervention. The nodule will characteristically demonstrate a dilated feeding pulmonary artery and a draining pulmonary vein (Figure 8.1). The feeding vessel or vessels appear as tubular structures larger than nearby adjacent vessels, whose course is often parallel and seamlessly bending into the sac/nodule. The draining vein is often tortuous and also larger than the adjacent veins. Contrast-enhanced pulmonary arterial angiography will show early phase enhancement (8) and further define the anatomy and course of the PAVMs and the feeding/draining vessels-important in the planning of potential embolization. The PAVM may itself be round, oval, tortuous, or lobular, ranging in size from 0.5 to 5 cm in

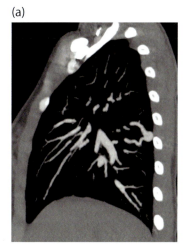

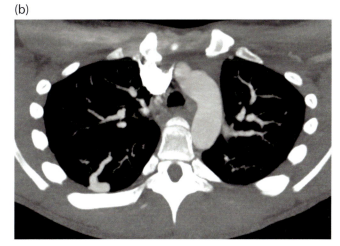

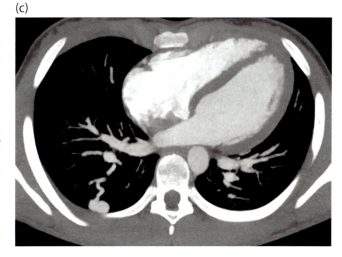

FIGURE 8.1 (a–c) Pulmonary arteriovenous malformation in HHT. A 12-year-old female with HHT. CT chest shows feeding artery, draining vein, and nidus of pulmonary arteriovenous malformation.

diameter (Figure 8.2a, b). Without contrast, it can be mistaken for a solid nodule rather than a vascular lesion, leading to inadvertent biopsy attempt and potential complications thereof.

Magnetic resonance angiography (MRA) is an attractive imaging modality due to the lack of ionizing radiation; however, it has

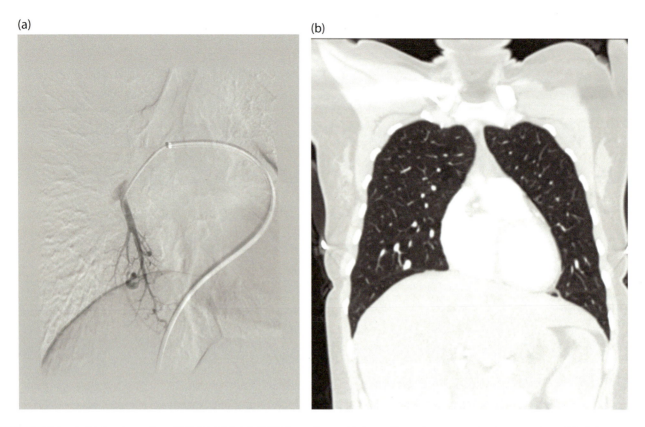

FIGURE 8.2 (a, b) Angiography of PAVM. Multiple PAVMs are located bilaterally, and angiography shows right middle lobe PAVMs.

limited spatial resolution and therefore poor detection of potentially clinically relevant PAVMs of less than 5 mm in size (31).

Brief overview of monitoring and management

Once a PAVM is diagnosed, it is important to determine whether immediate intervention is needed or monitoring would be acceptable. If the PAVM was detected incidentally as part of a lung nodule evaluation in an otherwise asymptomatic patients (i.e., no other significant manifestation of HHT, no stroke, no hypoxia or hemoptysis, etc.), then the radiographic characteristics of the PAVM (size of the feeding vessel and number of lesion) may guide the decision for intervention. Prior recommendation of management planning based on feeding diameter size has been withdrawn, and all PAVMs are considered for treatment when indicated (34).

Pharmacologic agents such as VEGF inhibitors or hormonal therapies (estrogen-progesterone) have been used for epistaxis in HHT, but no data exist for use in isolated PAVMs (35). Management options

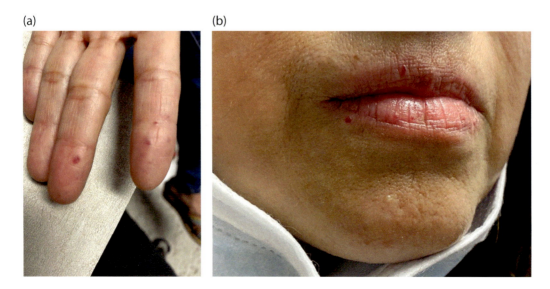

FIGURE 8.3 (a, b) Skin telangiectasias in a patient with hereditary hemorrhagic telangiectasia.

TABLE 8.3: Management of Complications of HHT

Epistaxis	Saline spray or gel, humidification
	Oral tranexamic acid
	Laser, radiofrequency ablation, electrosurgery, sclerotherapy
	Systemic antiangiogenic agents (bevacizumab)
	Septodermoplasty
	Nasal closure
Gastrointestinal bleeding	Esophagogastroduodenoscopy
	Capsule endoscopy
	Colorectal screening for those with SMAD4-HHT
	Obtain hemoglobin level
	Oral or intravenous iron replacement
	Blood transfusions
	Endoscopic argon plasma coagulation
	Oral antifibrinolytics
	Intravenous bevacizumab
Anemia	Iron replacement
	Red blood cell transfusions
	Evaluation for additional causes of anemia
Anticoagulation	Individualized based on the risk of bleeding. Bleeding in HHT is not an absolute contraindication for anticoagulation
	Avoid the use of dual antiplatelet therapy
Liver AVM	Refer to HHT center
	Intravenous bevacizumab for symptomatic high-output cardiac failure
	Liver transplantation for refractory high-output cardiac failure, biliary ischemia, complicated portal hypertension
	Avoid liver biopsy or hepatic artery embolization
Cerebral AVM	Referral to neurovascular expertise
	Transcatheter embolotherapy
	Neurovascular surgery, stereotactic radiosurgery
Pulmonary AVM	Transcatheter embolotherapy
	Antibiotic prophylaxis for procedures with risk of bacteremia
	Avoid intravenous air when placing intravenous access is in place
	Avoidance of SCUBA diving
	Long-term follow-up to detect growth or reperfusion
HHT during pregnancy	Referral to tertiary care center
	Not withholding an epidural anesthesia
	Known, non-high-risk brain AVM can labor and proceed with vaginal delivery

Source: Faughnan ME, Mager JJ, Hetts SW, Palda VA, Lang-Robertson K, Buscarini E, et al. Second international guidelines for the diagnosis and management of hereditary hemorrhagic telangiectasia. Ann Intern Med. 2020;173(12):989–1001.

for various HHT manifestation are enlisted in Table 8.3. Besides possible complications from PAVMs in HHT patients, they are also at risk of high-output heart failure, and gastrointestinal bleeding from extrapulmonary AVMs (1). In addition, cerebral AVMs may cause seizure, migraine, or cerebral hemorrhage from cerebral AVM rupture (36, 37).

Embolization of PAVM is done by angiography using fluoroscopy and injection of contrast material followed by injection of embolizing agent such as balloon, coil, or amplatzer vascular plugs. Success rate has been reported to be greater than 80% and complication rate was reported to be rare, although massive hemoptysis has been reported (38). After embolization, recurrence rate is as high as 70%. PAVM need to be monitored via CT scan 3–6 months postprocedure and every 3–5 years because PAVM may recanalize over time and shunt can recur (31, 39). Although ionizing radiation is increased with CT imaging, TTE unfortunately may not be adequate for follow-up postembolization therapy, since shunting will persist by TTE in approximately 90% (5). For PAVMs causing life-threatening hemorrhage, surgical lung resection may occasionally be indicated. Many patients have lesions distributed not suitable for surgery. For diffuse PAVMs, lung transplantation has been reported as a definitive option. Fukishima et al. described a case of a 7-year-old girl with diffuse PAVMs who underwent successful bilateral lung transplantation with subsequent improvement in hypoxemia and size of cerebral AVMs (40). Lung transplantation is considered only in exceptional cases, and that too only in major HHT/PAVM centers, since even patients who are profoundly hypoxemic have excellent survival relative to lung transplantation.

Pregnancy can increase the risk of PAVM rupture during second and third trimester. If detected after conception, PAVM should be treated starting in the second trimester unless otherwise clinically indicated (34). A patient that does not require immediate intervention needs serial monitoring with TTE during pregnancy. Screening for AVM in HHT is recommended as early as possible, prior to pregnancy planning, as well as generally every 5 to 10 years (36). In patients whose TTE is suggestive of pulmonary AVM(s), low-dose noncontrast chest CT can be used for further confirmation, and guide the need for intervention.

Antibiotic prophylaxis for procedures, particularly dental, are recommended for prevention of bacterial endocarditis and cerebral abscesses in those with both treated and treatment-naïve PAVMs. Extra precautions and care should be taken to avoid air embolism anytime intravenous lines are placed and medications or fluids are injected. Though theoretical, it is recommended to avoid scuba diving due to a perceived elevated risk of decompression complications.

Conclusion

PAVM, as an isolated condition, or as part of HHT, is a rare pulmonary condition that often manifests incidentally. However, these patients may be symptomatic with dyspnea and hemoptysis, and rarely have catastrophic complications such as stroke or cerebral abscesses. Our knowledge of HHT and PAVMs have been evolving with updated guidelines, gearing toward more aggressive screening and judicious selection of candidates for interventions. It is important to care for patients with HHT and PAVMs in a multidisciplinary manner, ideally at a center for excellence.

References

1. Cottin V, Dupuis-Girod S, Lesca G, Cordier JF. Pulmonary vascular manifestations of hereditary hemorrhagic telangiectasia (Rendu-Osler disease). Respiration. 2007;74(4):361–78.
2. Nakayama M, Nawa T, Chonan T, Endo K, Morikawa S, Bando M, et al. Prevalence of pulmonary arteriovenous malformations as estimated by low-dose thoracic CT screening. Intern Med. 2012;51(13):1677–81.
3. van Gent MW, Velthuis S, Post MC, Snijder RJ, Westermann CJ, Letteboer TG, et al. Hereditary hemorrhagic telangiectasia: How accurate are the clinical criteria? Am J Med Genet A. 2013;161A(3):461–6.

4. Cottin V, Chinet T, Lavole A, Corre R, Marchand E, Reynaud-Gaubert M, et al. Pulmonary arteriovenous malformations in hereditary hemorrhagic telangiectasia: A series of 126 patients. Medicine (Baltimore). 2007;86(1):1–17.
5. Begbie ME, Wallace GM, Shovlin CL. Hereditary haemorrhagic telangiectasia (Osler–Weber–Rendu syndrome): A view from the 21st century. Postgrad Med J. 2003;79(927):18–24.
6. Narsinh KH, Ramaswamy R, Kinney TB. Management of pulmonary arteriovenous malformations in hereditary hemorrhagic telangiectasia patients. Semin Intervent Radiol. 2013;30(4):408–12.
7. Geisthoff UW, Nguyen HL, Roth A, Seyfert U. How to manage patients with hereditary haemorrhagic telangiectasia. Br J Haematol. 2015;171(4):443–52.
8. Gill SS, Roddie ME, Shovlin CL, Jackson JE. Pulmonary arteriovenous malformations and their mimics. Clin Radiol. 2015;70(1):96–110.
9. David L, Mallet C, Mazerbourg S, Feige JJ, Bailly S. Identification of BMP9 and BMP10 as functional activators of the orphan activin receptor-like kinase 1 (ALK1) in endothelial cells. Blood. 2007;109(5):1953–61.
10. Dingenouts CK, Goumans MJ, Bakker W. Mononuclear cells and vascular repair in HHT. Front Genet. 2015;6:114.
11. Thalgott J, Dos-Santos-Luis D, Lebrin F. Pericytes as targets in hereditary hemorrhagic telangiectasia. Front Genet. 2015;6:37.
12. Gallione CJ, Repetto GM, Legius E, Rustgi AK, Schelley SL, Tejpar S, et al. A combined syndrome of juvenile polyposis and hereditary haemorrhagic telangiectasia associated with mutations in MADH4 (SMAD4). Lancet. 2004;363(9412):852–9.
13. Vorselaars VM, Velthuis S, Snijder RJ, Vos JA, Mager JJ, Post MC. Pulmonary hypertension in hereditary haemorrhagic telangiectasia. World J Cardiol. 2015;7(5):230–7.
14. Plauchu H, de Chadarevian JP, Bideau A, Robert JM. Age-related clinical profile of hereditary hemorrhagic telangiectasia in an epidemiologically recruited population. Am J Med Genet. 1989;32(3):291–7.
15. Thompson CF, Suh JD, McWilliams J, Duckwiler G, Wang MB. Initial experience of a hereditary hemorrhagic telangiectasia center of excellence. Ear Nose Throat J. 2017;96(6):E33–E6.
16. Bofarid S, Hosman AE, Mager JJ, Snijder RJ, Post MC. Pulmonary vascular complications in hereditary hemorrhagic telangiectasia and the underlying pathophysiology. Int J Mol Sci. 2021;22(7).
17. Shovlin CL, Guttmacher AE, Buscarini E, Faughnan ME, Hyland RH, Westermann CJ, et al. Diagnostic criteria for hereditary hemorrhagic telangiectasia (Rendu–Osler–Weber syndrome). Am J Med Genet. 2000;91(1):66–7.
18. Shovlin CL. Pulmonary arteriovenous malformations. Am J Respir Crit Care Med. 2014;190(11):1217–28.
19. Verkerk MM, Shovlin CL, Lund VJ. Silent threat? A retrospective study of screening practices for pulmonary arteriovenous malformations in patients with hereditary hemorrhagic telangiectasia. Rhinology. 2012;50(3):277–83.
20. Iqbal M, Rossoff LJ, Steinberg HN, Marzouk KA, Siegel DN. Pulmonary arteriovenous malformations: A clinical review. Postgrad Med J. 2000;76(897):390–4.
21. Etievant J, Si-Mohamed S, Vinurel N, Dupuis-Girod S, Decullier E, Gamondes D, et al. Pulmonary arteriovenous malformations in hereditary hemorrhagic telangiectasia: Correlations between computed tomography findings and cerebral complications. Eur Radiol. 2018;28(3):1338–44.
22. Ference BA, Shannon TM, White RI, Jr., Zawin M, Burdge CM. Life-threatening pulmonary hemorrhage with pulmonary arteriovenous malformations and hereditary hemorrhagic telangiectasia. Chest. 1994;106(5):1387–90.
23. Gallitelli M, Pasculli G, Fiore T, Carella A, Sabba C. Emergencies in hereditary haemorrhagic telangiectasia. QJM. 2006;99(1):15–22.
24. Margelidon-Cozzolino V, Cottin V, Dupuis-Girod S, Traclet J, Ahmad K, Mornex JF, et al. Pulmonary hypertension in hereditary haemorrhagic telangiectasia is associated with multiple clinical conditions. ERJ Open Res. 2021 Jan 25;7(1):00078–2020.
25. Trembath RC, Thomson JR, Machado RD, Morgan NV, Atkinson C, Winship I, et al. Clinical and molecular genetic features of pulmonary hypertension in patients with hereditary haemorrhagic telangiectasia. N Engl J Med. 2001;345(5):325–34.
26. Circo S, Gossage JR. Pulmonary vascular complications of hereditary haemorrhagic telangiectasia. Curr Opin Pulm Med. 2014;20(5):421–8.
27. Sperling DC, Cheitlin M, Sullivan RW, Smith A. Pulmonary arteriovenous fistulas with pulmonary hypertension. Chest. 1977;71(6):753–7.
28. Hanley M, Ahmed O, Chandra A, Gage KL, Gerhard-Herman MD, Ginsburg M, et al. ACR appropriateness criteria clinically suspected pulmonary arteriovenous malformation. J Am Coll Radiol. 2016;13(7):796–800.
29. Gossage JR, Kanj G. Pulmonary arteriovenous malformations. A state of the art review. Am J Respir Crit Care Med. 1998;158(2):643–61.
30. Ming DK, Patel MS, Hopkinson NS, Ward S, Polkey MI. The 'anatomic shunt test' in clinical practice; Contemporary description of test and in-service evaluation. Thorax. 2014;69(8):773–5.
31. Trerotola SO, Pyeritz RE. PAVM embolization: An update. AJR Am J Roentgenol. 2010;195(4):837–45.
32. Cottin V, Plauchu H, Bayle JY, Barthelet M, Revel D, Cordier JF. Pulmonary arteriovenous malformations in patients with hereditary hemorrhagic telangiectasia. Am J Respir Crit Care Med. 2004;169(9):994–1000.
33. Dupuis-Girod S, Cottin V, Shovlin CL. The lung in hereditary hemorrhagic telangiectasia. Respiration. 2017;94(4):315–30.
34. Shovlin CL, Jackson JE, Bamford KB, Jenkins IH, Benjamin AR, Ramadan H, et al. Primary determinants of ischaemic stroke/brain abscess risks are independent of severity of pulmonary arteriovenous malformations in hereditary haemorrhagic telangiectasia. Thorax. 2008;63(3):259–66.
35. Garg N, Khunger M, Gupta A, Kumar N. Optimal management of hereditary hemorrhagic telangiectasia. J Blood Med. 2014;5:191–206.
36. Faughnan ME, Mager JJ, Hetts SW, Palda VA, Lang-Robertson K, Buscarini E, et al. Second international guidelines for the diagnosis and management of hereditary hemorrhagic telangiectasia. Ann Intern Med. 2020;173(12):989–1001.
37. Faughnan ME, Palda VA, Garcia-Tsao G, Geisthoff UW, McDonald J, Proctor DD, et al. International guidelines for the diagnosis and management of hereditary haemorrhagic telangiectasia. J Med Genet. 2011;48(2):73–87.
38. Kucukay F, Ozdemir M, Senol E, Okten S, Ereren M, Karan A. Large pulmonary arteriovenous malformations: Long-term results of embolization with AMPLATZER vascular plugs. J Vasc Interv Radiol. 2014;25(9):1327–32.
39. Woodward CS, Pyeritz RE, Chittams JL, Trerotola SO. Treated pulmonary arteriovenous malformations: Patterns of persistence and associated retreatment success. Radiology. 2013;269(3):919–26.
40. Fukushima H, Mitsuhashi T, Oto T, Sano Y, Kusano KF, Goto K, et al. Successful lung transplantation in a case with diffuse pulmonary arteriovenous malformations and hereditary hemorrhagic telangiectasia. Am J Transplant. 2013;13(12):3278–81.

9

DIFFUSE ALVEOLAR HEMORRHAGE (DAH) SYNDROMES

Gaurav Manek and Rendell W. Ashton

Contents

Introduction	63
Pathophysiology	64
Classification	64
Clinical features	64
Diagnostic workup	65
Management	66
Specific types	67
Bibliography	68

Abbreviations

AAV	ANCA-associated vasculitis
ANA	antinuclear antibodies
ANCA	antineutrophil cytoplasmic antibodies
Anti PR3	anti-proteinase 3
APLA	antiphospholipid antibody syndrome
ARDS	acute respiratory distress syndrome
BAL	bronchoalveolar lavage
CD	cluster differentiation
CT	computed tomography
CTD	connective tissue diseases
CXR	plain chest radiography
DAH	diffuse alveolar hemorrhage
EACA	epsilon aminocaproic acid
ECMO	extracorporeal membranous oxygenation
EGPA	eosinophilic granulomatosis with polyangiitis
FVIIa	factor VIIa
GBM	glomerular basement membrane
GGO	ground-glass opacities
GPA	granulomatosis with polyangiitis
Hgb	hemoglobin
IgA	immune globulin A
IPH	idiopathic pulmonary hemosiderosis
MCTD	mixed connective tissue disorder
MPA	microscopic polyangiitis
MPO	myeloperoxidase antibodies
NT-proBNP	N-terminal pro–B-type natriuretic peptide
PEEP	positive end-expiratory pressure
PT-INR	prothrombin time-international normalized ratio
RA	rheumatoid arthritis
RF	rheumatoid factor
SLE	systemic lupus erythematosus
TF	tissue factor
TXA	tranexamic acid

KEY POINTS

- Diffuse alveolar hemorrhage (DAH) is a syndrome characterized by intra-alveolar accumulation of erythrocytes and fibrin through various mechanisms including pulmonary capillaritis, bland alveolar hemorrhage and diffuse alveolar damage.
- Only about a third of patients with DAH have hemoptysis. DAH should be considered in all patients with unexplained opacities on chest imaging and a drop in hemoglobin.
- Bronchoscopy with bronchoalveolar lavage (BAL) with increasingly hemorrhagic return in serial aliquots is diagnostic and it also helps identify or rule out certain underlying etiologies.
- Initial management is supportive, including maintaining oxygenation, using positive end expiratory pressure for tamponade effect, correction of coagulopathy and use of hemostatic agents such as tranexamic acid.
- Corticosteroids, plasmapheresis, immune modulating agents such as rituximab, cyclophosphamide and azathioprine are some of the common therapies used in the treatment of DAH.

Introduction

Diffuse alveolar hemorrhage (DAH) is a clinicopathologic syndrome characterized by loss of integrity of the alveolar-capillary basement membrane leading to intra-alveolar accumulation of erythrocytes and fibrin. Clinically, it can present with hemoptysis, hypoxia, anemia, diffuse infiltrates on chest radiography and even acute respiratory failure. DAH should be distinguished from bronchial circulation bleeding, which is usually due to endobronchial lesions or bronchiectasis. DAH occurs due to damage to the pulmonary microvasculature, caused either by immune or non-immune mechanisms.

DOI: 10.1201/9781003089384-9

Pathophysiology

DAH can be associated with various distinct histopathological patterns representing distinct mechanistic causes of bleeding, including pulmonary capillaritis, bland alveolar hemorrhage and diffuse alveolar damage. Pulmonary capillaritis is a small vessel vasculitis, in which neutrophilic infiltration of the alveolar walls occurs and the walls become fragmented as an apoptotic cycle ensues, releasing cytoplasmic enzymes and oxidative molecules, which cause fibrinoid necrosis and damage to the alveolar-capillary membrane. This leads to accumulation of erythrocytes, fibrin and fragmented neutrophils in the alveolar space, which manifests as the clinical syndrome of DAH. This condition can be seen in systemic vasculitis and connective tissue diseases (CTD). While many of these entities represent systemic diseases involving the pulmonary vasculature, lung allograft rejection and isolated pauci-immune pulmonary capillaritis are lung-limited diseases in which pulmonary capillaritis can also be seen.

Bland alveolar hemorrhage refers to bleeding with no inflammatory infiltrate in the alveolar wall. This histology is seen in settings of structural damage to the alveolar capillary membrane without inflammatory infiltrate, as in antiglomerular basement membrane disease (also called anti-GBM disease or Goodpasture's syndrome), idiopathic pulmonary hemosiderosis (IPH), some drug toxicities, and pulmonary hypertension from left-sided heart disease such as mitral stenosis. Figure 9.1a and b shows representative images of these first two histopathologic patterns, as seen in ANCA-associated vasculitis (AAV), both from the same patient, demonstrating the difficulty with discerning which mechanism is responsible for the bleeding.

Diffuse alveolar damage is a nonspecific histologic pattern associated with complex lung injury in conditions such as acute respiratory distress syndrome, hemopoietic stem cell transplant, and cocaine inhalation. It can cause inflammatory intra-alveolar edema, capillary microthrombi and fibrin deposition, hyaline membrane formation and DAH.

Besides these three common histologic patterns seen in patients with DAH, it can also be associated with diseases such as lymphangioleiomyomatosis, pulmonary veno-occlusive disease, pulmonary capillary hemangiomatosis and various malignancies, each of which causes hemorrhage through some combination of weakening the alveolar basement membrane, disrupting pulmonary capillary integrity and/or increasing intravascular hydrostatic pressure.

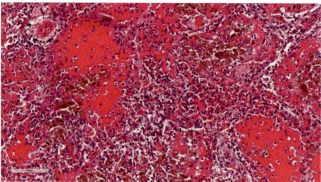

FIGURE 9.1b In addition to blood and hemosiderin-laden macrophages, this image shows capillaritis, characterized by destruction of alveolar septa by an inflammatory infiltrate containing neutrophils and histiocytes. Hematoxylin-eosin, 20× magnification. (Image courtesy of Sanjay Mukhopadhyay, MD.)

Classification

The causes of DAH are many and varied, including autoimmune vasculitis syndromes, CTDs, medication and drug toxicity, coagulopathies, infections, left-sided heart disease, lung transplant rejection, malignancies, and rare pulmonary disorders including lymphangioleiomyomatosis, pulmonary veno-occlusive disease and pulmonary capillary hemangiomatosis. Some diagnoses may cause more than one histologic pattern. Systemic lupus erythematosus (SLE) can cause any of the three main histopathological patterns, and anti-GBM disease can cause pulmonary capillaritis as well as bland pulmonary hemorrhage. Influenza (H1N1), dengue, leptospirosis, malaria and *Staphylococcus aureus* are the main infectious agents that cause DAH while adenovirus, cytomegalovirus, mycoplasma, legionella, strongyloides and invasive aspergillosis are often the culprits in immunocompromised hosts.

Causes of DAH along with their mechanism of injury (immune vs. non-immune) and the corresponding histologic patterns are listed in Table 9.1.

Clinical features

Patients with DAH often present with hemoptysis, although not always. About a third of the patients present without any hemoptysis, and even when present, the hemoptysis is generally intermittent and may be scant. The lungs have a dual blood supply from the pulmonary arterial system and the bronchial arterial system. DAH is generally low-volume bleeding from the pulmonary arterial microcirculation, as opposed to focal bleeding from the bronchial circulation or large pulmonary vessels, which usually presents as massive hemoptysis.

Nonspecific symptoms may include dyspnea, cough, chest pain, fever, and other pulmonary and non-pulmonary symptoms related to the underlying disease, such as joint pain, rash, hematuria or nasal congestion. The symptoms are usually acute

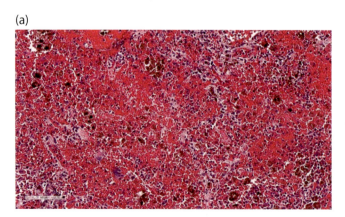

FIGURE 9.1a Intra-alveolar hemorrhage (red blood cells) and hemosiderin in a case of ANCA-associated vasculitis. Although these findings are consistent with hemorrhage, there is no vasculitis or capillaritis in this image. Hematoxylin-eosin, 20× magnification. (Image courtesy of Sanjay Mukhopadhyay, MD.)

Diffuse Alveolar Hemorrhage (DAH) Syndromes

TABLE 9.1: Immune-Mediated and Non-Immune-Mediated Causes of DAH

	Pulmonary Capillaritis	Diffuse Alveolar Damage	Bland Pulmonary Hemorrhage
Immune mediated	AAV, Anti-GBM disease, SLE, APLA, RA, MCTD, scleroderma, Henoch-Schönlein purpura, IgA nephropathy, isolated pauci-immune glomerulonephritis, Behçet syndrome, cryoglobulinemia, drug induced (e.g. propylthiouracil, penicillamine), acute lung transplant rejection, polymyositis, retinoic acid toxicity, myasthenia gravis, ulcerative colitis	SLE, immune-mediated ARDS, hematopoietic stem cell transplantation	SLE, anti-GBM disease
Non-immune mediated		ARDS, crack cocaine inhalation, cytotoxic drugs, radiation pneumonitis	IPH, mitral stenosis, left ventricular dysfunction, atrial tumors, coagulopathies, trimellitic anhydride, drugs (e.g., amiodarone, nitrofurantoin), subacute bacterial endocarditis

Abbreviations: AAV: ANCA-associated vasculitis; APLA: antiphospholipid antibody syndrome; ARDS: Acute respiratory distress syndrome; GBM: glomerular basement membrane; IgA: immune globulin A; IPH: idiopathic pulmonary hemosiderosis; MCTD: mixed connective tissue disorder; RA: rheumatoid arthritis; SLE: systemic lupus erythematosus.

to sub-acute, lasting from hours to several weeks, and can be recurrent.

Patients can be asymptomatic or can present with any level of dyspnea, up to severe respiratory failure, which can be life threatening. Most patients present with dyspnea that is progressive over a few days. A physical exam may reveal crackles or bronchial breath sounds, heart murmurs, S3 or S4. A thorough examination should be done to look for signs of systemic autoimmune disorders.

Other characteristic features include diffuse alveolar opacities on the chest roentgenogram, patchy ground glass opacities on CT imaging, and a decrease in hemoglobin. DAH should be considered in all patients with unexplained opacities on the chest imaging because hemoptysis can be intermittent or absent, and other symptoms can be variable.

Diagnostic workup

Laboratory testing

A complete blood count with differential and coagulation studies should be obtained in all patients. If there is suspicion of a pulmonary-renal syndrome, evaluation of kidney function via urinalysis with microscopy, serum blood urea nitrogen, serum creatinine and possibly kidney biopsy can aid in diagnosing the underlying etiology. Urine toxicology testing should be sent in cases where there may be drug use. If autoimmune diseases are suspected, serological tests including anti-nuclear antibodies (ANA), rheumatoid factor (RF), anti-phospholipid antibodies, lupus anticoagulant, anti-cardiolipin antibodies, anti β-2 glycoprotein 1 antibodies, antiglomerular basement membrane antibodies, antineutrophil cytoplasmic antibodies (ANCA) including c-ANCA and p-ANCA, anti-proteinase 3 (PR3) and myeloperoxidase antibodies (MPO) should be ordered. Infectious evaluation including blood and lower respiratory tract cultures should be sent. Pulmonary function testing may reveal restrictive physiology and often an abnormally high diffusing capacity, due to increased uptake of carbon monoxide. However, testing pulmonary function in acute situations is often not practical. N-terminal pro–B-type natriuretic peptide (NT-proBNP) levels and echocardiography may be obtained if heart failure is suspected.

Imaging

Plain chest radiography (CXR) and computed tomography (CT) are often employed in the diagnostic evaluation. They are useful for screening and localization, but often of limited value in differentiating causes of DAH. In about half of cases, plain chest radiography may be negative. CT scans are superior to CXR in defining the extent and location of pulmonary involvement. Opacities can be unilateral or focal, but diffuse bilateral alveolar opacities or ground glass changes are most commonly seen. Typically, the central and lower lung zones are involved while sparing the apical and peripheral zones (see Figure 9.2). Bilateral consolidation is nonspecific and can be seen in all causes of DAH, but specific clues can be seen on imaging to suggest underlying etiologies. In some cases, where large vessel vasculitis is suspected to be the underlying etiology, CT angiogram or conventional angiogram may be necessary.

Bronchoscopy

Bronchoscopy with bronchoalveolar lavage (BAL) remains an important diagnostic tool to establish and confirm DAH as well as to diagnose or rule out underlying etiologies. When saline is injected into the distal airways and suctioned back, negative pressure disrupts any fragile or inflamed vessels, resulting in increasingly hemorrhagic return with serial aliquots. While this test is very sensitive and characteristic for DAH, false positives can occur in conditions such as tuberculosis. BAL fluid can also be cultured and stained to evaluate for infection.

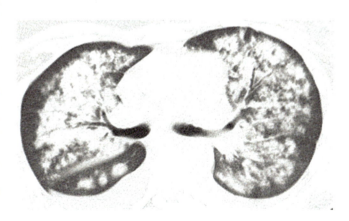

FIGURE 9.2 Chest CT demonstrating diffuse airspace consolidation with striking subpleural sparing in a 44-year-old female with a history of lupus and diffuse alveolar hemorrhage. (Image courtesy of Ruchi Yadav, M.D, Cleveland Clinic)

BAL samples may demonstrate "siderophages" or hemosiderin laden macrophages on microscopic examination. A scoring system has been developed by Golde et al. in which 200–300 macrophages are examined and scored from 0 to 4 depending on intensity of Prussian blue staining. This total is then divided to obtain a mean score for 100 macrophages. A score greater than 100 is suggestive of severe DAH whereas a score of 20–100 is suggestive of mild to moderate DAH. Golde scoring can be time consuming, so another way of establishing the diagnosis of DAH is to note if 20% or more of examined macrophages have positive Prussian blue stain. It can take up to 48 hours after the onset of hemorrhage to detect hemosiderin in the macrophages, and false positive results can occur in diffuse alveolar damage and fluid overload.

Lung biopsy

Biopsy of the lung tissue is infrequently required but may be helpful when the underlying etiology cannot be established based on clinical features, radiographic imaging and serology analysis. Transbronchial biopsies via bronchoscopy generally provide insufficient samples, and surgical lung biopsy may be required to rule out many underlying conditions. Ruling out an underlying autoimmune etiology is important as long-term management depends on the diagnosis. The timing and risks of biopsy should be carefully considered. Biopsies should not be performed in the setting of acute respiratory failure.

Management

Maintaining oxygenation

A prompt, multidisciplinary approach is essential in managing DAH as it can carry a high mortality rate. The most immediate focus should be on reversing hypoxia if possible, via oxygen supplementation devices or, in severe cases, with mechanical ventilation. High levels of positive end-expiratory pressure (PEEP) can have a tamponade effect on the bleeding. Ideal PEEP levels should be individualized to provide adequate oxygenation along with lung-protective ventilation to prevent lung collapse and reduce bleeding. Extracorporeal membranous oxygenation (ECMO) has been successfully used as a supportive strategy in some patients, but the use of ECMO necessitates anticoagulation and the risk of worsening the bleeding must be considered.

Transfusion and correction of coagulopathy

Blood product administration may be required to maintain a hemoglobin level >7 g/dL, platelet count >50,000/μL, prothrombin time-international normalized ratio (PT-INR) <1.5 and fibrinogen levels >100 mg/dL. Correction of coagulopathy can help achieve hemostasis. If bleeding occurs in the setting of anticoagulant medication, specific reversal agents should be used if available.

Specific hemostatic agents

Additional hemostatic agents are available such as tranexamic acid (TXA), factor VIIa, thrombin and epsilon aminocaproic acid (EACA). TXA primarily works by prohibiting conversion of plasminogen into plasmin thereby inhibiting fibrinolysis. TXA has been used intravenously as well as aerosolized/inhaled, and the effect can be dramatic, but may be less useful if the bleeding is profound or recurrent. It also increases the risk of post-operative seizures and has no significant effect of mortality related to bleeding in patients with hematologic malignancies.

EACA works by competitively binding to plasminogen thereby blocking it from binding to fibrin and subsequent fibrinolysis. Thrombin or fibrinogen-thrombin has also been studied and intrapulmonary administration can be considered in DAH refractory to corticosteroids. Thrombin converts fibrinogen to fibrin thereby stabilizing existing clot and providing a meshwork for platelet aggregation and new clot formation, while also promoting vasoconstriction. Recombinant factor VIIa works by activating both the tissue factor (TF) pathway as well as the TF independent pathway of the coagulation cascade, eventually leading to thrombin activation and clot formation. As with other pharmacologic agents, attaining optimal levels of FVIIa in the pulmonary vascular bed requires high systemic doses that in turn can increase thromboembolic complications. FVIIa can also be administered directly into the airway via bronchoscopy in much smaller doses while achieving the same hemostatic effects while decreasing systemic adverse effects. In conditions such as DAH, the alveolar macrophages express TF pathway inhibitors in the airway and locally administered FVIIa can overcome these inhibitors to form the FVIIa-TF complex, which in turn activates the coagulation cascade. It can be used as a final salvage therapy in both immune and non-immune DAH when other measures have failed to control bleeding.

Treating the underlying condition leading to DAH

Treating the underlying condition is vital to controlling DAH, and various therapies including corticosteroids, plasmapheresis, immune modulating agents such as rituximab, cyclophosphamide and azathioprine are available. Corticosteroids remain the mainstay of acute anti-inflammatory therapy and act by reducing alveolar inflammation, edema, thrombotic microangiopathy and inflammatory cell infiltrate. High dose glucocorticoids ("pulse dose," usually 1 g of methylprednisolone or equivalent given daily) is generally recommended for 3–5 days followed by a gradual taper. Corticosteroids can also be used in IPH which is a non-immune cause of DAH but IPH usually does not require further immunomodulatory treatments that would be given for immune-associated DAH conditions. If DAH is due to infection or conditions causing elevated pulmonary pressures (such as mitral valve stenosis or pulmonary veno-occlusive disease), steroids are of little use and may even be counter-productive if they worsen an underlying infection. In immune mediated DAH, high dose steroids are usually helpful while awaiting confirmatory results to guide further therapy. Plasmapheresis can reduce auto antibodies in a rapid fashion and has been used as a treatment modality in DAH due to CTDs, AAV as well as anti-GMB disease. It is usually administered for 2 weeks on alternating days, sometimes as an adjunct to corticosteroids.

Cyclophosphamide, a cell cycle phase alkylating agent and immunosuppressant, is beneficial in some autoimmune DAH. In patients with AAV, the anti-CD20 monoclonal antibody rituximab has been studied, either with or without steroids, as an agent for remission. It has similar efficacy to cyclophosphamide and can be used as an alternative agent in other conditions such as SLE, granulomatosis with polyangiitis (GPA) and pauci-immune pulmonary capillaritis. Prophylactic treatment for *Pneumocystis jirovecii* pneumonia should be included in the treatment regimen of the patients receiving immunosuppressive therapies,

Diffuse Alveolar Hemorrhage (DAH) Syndromes

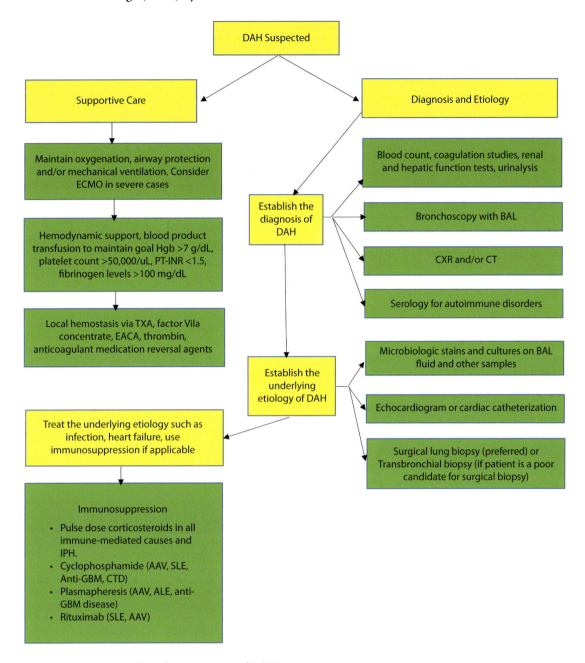

FIGURE 9.3 Diagnostic approach and management of DAH.

including especially with prolonged (more than 1 month) courses of high dose corticosteroids (more than prednisone 20 mg daily or equivalent).

A stepwise approach to management of DAH is outlined in Figure 9.3.

Specific types

ANCA-associated vasculitis

GPA, eosinopohilic granulomatosis with polyangiitis (EGPA) and microscopic polyangiitis (MPA) are the three ANCA-associated vasculitides. GPA is characterized by granulomatous inflammation of the upper and lower respiratory tract and commonly associated with cANCA and anti-proteinase (anti-PR3) antibodies.

EGPA is characterized by eosinophilic granulomatosis. MPA is characterized by absence of granulomatous inflammation and is typically associated with pANCA and antimyeloperoxidase (anti-MPO) antibodies. The three conditions exhibit some clinical overlap with regards to clinical manifestations and seropositivity and are therefore often grouped together as AAV.

Drug-induced AAV is caused by propylthiouracil, antitumor necrosis factor alpha agents, D-penicillamine, minocycline, sulfasalazine and hydralazine, with 50% of these patients exhibiting ANCA seropositivity. Since not all patients will have seropositivity, definitive diagnosis may require a lung and/or kidney biopsy.

On imaging, AAV can demonstrate airspace consolidation with air bronchograms in the early stages. However, diffuse parenchymal lung disease patterns associated with the underlying systemic illness are also seen. Multiple bilateral nodules that can evolve to irregular, thick-walled cavitary lesions, irregular masses with no specific zonal involvement, and bronchial wall thickening are typical; these findings are uncommon in other causes of DAH and suggest GPA. Another clue to GPA is sinus disease detected clinically or on imaging. The involvement of lung apices and/or costophrenic angles suggests other causes. Treatment includes supportive measures and immunosuppression including corticosteroids, cyclophosphamide, azathioprine and rituximab. Plasmapheresis can be of utility if employed early in the disease course.

Anti-GBM disease

This disease is another cause of pulmonary-renal syndrome along with AAV and is characterized by immune complex formation with type 4 collagen and deposition of these complexes in the pulmonary and renal capillary basement membranes. Diagnosis is made through serologic testing for specific antibodies, and if negative, then lung or kidney biopsy demonstrating capillary basement membrane antibody deposition. Patients with anti-GBM disease can also have seropositivity for ANCA antibodies. These patients are regarded as double-positive.

Plain radiographs demonstrate lower lung involvement with coalescing airspace opacities that gradually become reticular while CT scans demonstrate ground-glass opacities (GGO) and septal thickening in a crazy paving pattern; hilar lymphadenopathy may also be seen. Involvement of the apices or pleural effusions should prompt consideration of other diagnoses. Treatment of the underlying disease is via plasmapheresis, corticosteroids and cyclophosphamide. Resolution of the alveolar consolidation occurs in 2–3 days and the complete resolution of residual septal thickening and opacification takes 2–3 weeks.

Systemic lupus erythematosus and other CTDs

While DAH is rare in CTDs, when it is seen, SLE is the most common underlying diagnosis. Patients with SLE can also have secondary antiphospholipid antibody syndrome (APLA). Histopathologically, both capillaritis and bland hemorrhage patterns can be seen. Among CTDs, SLE often presents with pleural effusion, and pulmonary fibrosis is seen in about a third of patients.

Treatment includes corticosteroids and cyclophosphamide. Plasmapheresis can be used to eliminate the auto antibodies that typically occur in SLE and rituximab can be considered in recalcitrant cases. Other CTDs can cause DAH either via capillaritis or immune complex deposition and include rheumatoid arthritis (RA), systemic sclerosis, Sjögren syndrome, myositis and mixed connective tissue disorders.

Isolated pauci-immune pulmonary capillaritis including lung transplant rejection

This is a rare entity characterized by capillaritis on histology with no clinical, serological or radiologic features of any vasculitis or CTD. This can be seen in AAV, RA, APLA, SLE, sarcoidosis and acute lung transplant rejection. The capillaritis can be a *forme fruste* of more complete clinical syndromes, so these patients require long-term follow up to evaluate for subsequent development of the diseases listed. Patients with transplanted lungs require tissue biopsy to differentiate this entity from acute cellular rejection. Treatment is similar to immune-mediated DAH with corticosteroids and cyclophosphamide, with rituximab reserved as a rescue therapy. In lung transplant patients, corticosteroids are the mainstay of treatment with plasmapheresis reserved for severe cases.

Idiopathic pulmonary hemosiderosis

Idiopathic pulmonary hemosiderosis (IPH) is typically a diagnosis of exclusion, when all serologic workup for autoimmune conditions remains negative and biopsy fails to show inflammatory cells or immune complex deposition. The pathogenesis of IPH is poorly understood but genetic and autoimmune mechanisms are thought to play a role. Patients with IPH may have autoantibodies at initial diagnosis or during follow up. There are reports of patients with IPH who later were diagnosed with autoimmune disorders, but also other patients with longstanding IPH whose explant pathology failed to show any capillaritis. Thus, the appearance of antibodies in patients with IPH is thought to reflect immune dysregulation rather than the cause of hemorrhage. There is also an association described between celiac disease and IPH, and consideration should be given to obtaining IgG and IgA tissue transglutaminase antibody, antigliadin antibody and antiendomysial antibody. Isolated diffuse opacities in central and lower lung zones with negative workup for systemic inflammatory diseases are seen in patients with IPH. With time and recurrence, patients with IPH can develop diffuse reticulonodular opacities due to pulmonary fibrosis. Treatment consists of supportive care and corticosteroids.

Hematopoietic stem cell transplant: The pathogenesis of DAH in these patients is poorly understood but diffuse alveolar damage is seen and associated with inflammation and cytokine release. Corticosteroids are employed in treatment of the underlying inflammatory process.

Bibliography

1. Lara AR, Schwarz MI. Diffuse alveolar hemorrhage. Chest. 2010 May;137(5):1164–71.
2. Martínez-Martínez MU, Oostdam DAH, Abud-Mendoza C. Diffuse alveolar hemorrhage in autoimmune diseases. Curr Rheumatol Rep. 2017 May;19(5):27.
3. Colby TV, Fukuoka J, Ewaskow SP, Helmers R, Leslie KO. Pathologic approach to pulmonary hemorrhage. Ann Diagn Pathol. 2001 Oct;5(5):309–19.
4. Thickett DR, Richter AG, Nathani N, Perkins GD, Harper L. Pulmonary manifestations of anti-neutrophil cytoplasmic antibody (ANCA)-positive vasculitis. Rheumatology. 2006 Mar 1;45(3):261–8.
5. Nasser M, Cottin V. Alveolar hemorrhage in vasculitis (primary and secondary). Semin Respir Crit Care Med. 2018 Aug;39(4):482–93.
6. Ioachimescu OC, Stoller JK. Diffuse alveolar hemorrhage: Diagnosing it and finding the cause. Cleve Clin J Med. 2008 Apr;75(4):258, 260, 264–265 passim.
7. Saha BK, Chong WH, Milman NT. Differentiation of idiopathic pulmonary hemosiderosis from rheumatologic and autoimmune diseases causing diffuse alveolar hemorrhage: Establishing a diagnostic approach. Clin Rheumatol. 2022 Feb;41(2):325–36.
8. Krause ML, Cartin-Ceba R, Specks U, Peikert T. Update on diffuse alveolar hemorrhage and pulmonary vasculitis. Immunol Allergy Clin North Am. 2012 Nov;32(4):587–600.
9. von Ranke FM, Zanetti G, Hochhegger B, Marchiori E. Infectious diseases causing diffuse alveolar hemorrhage in immunocompetent patients: A state-of-the-art review. Lung. 2013 Feb;191(1):9–18.
10. Golde DW, Drew WL, Klein HZ, Finley TN, Cline MJ. Occult pulmonary haemorrhage in leukaemia. BMJ. 1975 Apr 26;2(5964):166–8.
11. De Lassence A, Fleury-Feith J, Escudier E, Beaune J, Bernaudin JF, Cordonnier C. Alveolar hemorrhage. Diagnostic criteria and results in 194 immunocompromised hosts. Am J Respir Crit Care Med. 1995 Jan;151(1):157–63.

12. Maldonado F, Parambil JG, Yi ES, Decker PA, Ryu JH. Haemosiderin-laden macrophages in the bronchoalveolar lavage fluid of patients with diffuse alveolar damage. Eur Respir J. 2009 Jun 1;33(6):1361–6.
13. Reisman S, Chung M, Bernheim A. A review of clinical and imaging features of diffuse pulmonary hemorrhage. Am J Roentgenol. 2021 Jun;216(6):1500–9.
14. Abrams D, Agerstrand CL, Biscotti M, Burkart KM, Bacchetta M, Brodie D. Extracorporeal membrane oxygenation in the management of diffuse alveolar hemorrhage. ASAIO J. 2015 Apr;61(2):216–8.
15. de Gracia J, de la Rosa D, Catalán E, Alvarez A, Bravo C, Morell F. Use of endoscopic fibrinogen-thrombin in the treatment of severe hemoptysis. Respir Med. 2003 Jul;97(7):790–5.
16. Heslet L, Nielsen JD, Nepper-Christensen S. Local pulmonary administration of factor VIIa (rFVIIa) in diffuse alveolar hemorrhage (DAH) - a review of a new treatment paradigm. Biologics. 2012;6:37–46.
17. Park JA. Treatment of diffuse alveolar hemorrhage: Controlling inflammation and obtaining rapid and effective hemostasis. IJMS. 2021 Jan 14;22(2):793.
18. Stone JH, Merkel PA, Spiera R, Seo P, Langford CA, Hoffman GS, et al. Rituximab versus cyclophosphamide for ANCA-associated vasculitis. N Engl J Med. 2010 Jul 15;363(3):221–32.
19. Tse JR, Schwab KE, McMahon M, Simon W. Rituximab: An emerging treatment for recurrent diffuse alveolar hemorrhage in systemic lupus erythematosus. Lupus. 2015 Jun;24(7):756–9.
20. Walsh M, Merkel PA, Peh C-A, Szpirt WM, Puéchal X, Fujimoto S, et al. Plasma exchange and glucocorticoids in severe ANCA-associated vasculitis. N Engl J Med. 2020 Feb 13;382(7):622–31.

10

PULMONARY VENO-OCCLUSIVE DISEASE AND PULMONARY CAPILLARY HEMANGIOMATOSIS

Dana Gross, Akhilesh Padhye, Roberto Barrios, and Sandeep Sahay

Contents

Introduction	70
Burden of PVOD/PCH	71
Pathogenesis of PVOD	71
Risk factors for the development of PVOD/PCH	72
Clinical presentation of PVOD/PCH	72
Imaging and diagnostic evaluation	73
Treatment and outcomes	74
Summary and conclusion	74
References	75

KEY POINTS

- Pulmonary veno-occlusive disease (PVOD) and pulmonary capillary hemangiomatosis (PCH) are two rare diseases classified under the subtype of Group 1 Pulmonary Arterial Hypertension (PAH) with a similar hemodynamic profile, but unique pathology, that are very difficult to diagnose and even more difficult to treat.
- Prevalence and incidence of PVOD and PCH is as low as 1–2 cases per million people and 0.1–0.5 cases per million people per year, respectively, although these are likely under-estimated due to difficulties in accurate diagnosis.
- In PVOD and PCH, vascular remodeling begins in the pulmonary venules leading to an initial rise in pressure at the post-capillary side, with progressive increase of pulmonary vascular resistance (PVR) ultimately resulting in right ventricular failure and death.
- There are many potential risk factors for development of PVOD and PCH such as chemotherapy agents, hematopoietic stem cell transplants, exposure to organic solvents or tobacco, autoimmune diseases, or infections such as HIV, but many associations are limited to case reports.
- The EIF2AK4 gene has been found to be responsible for the heritable transmission of both PVOD and PCH.
- PVOD and PCH typically present with nonspecific symptoms like other forms of pulmonary hypertension, however one clue may be development of pulmonary edema when treated with pulmonary vasodilators.
- Although other supporting tests may be useful, transthoracic echo remains the most widely utilized screening test to detect pulmonary hypertension, with right heart catheterization remaining the gold standard for confirmation. Although lung biopsy is ultimately needed for confirmatory diagnosis of PVOD and PCH, it is often not pursued due to prohibitive risk of bleeding.
- Although there are experimental therapies ongoing for PVOD and PCH, targeted therapies for other forms of Group 1 PAH are often ineffective or even harmful. Prognosis is poor, and lung or heart-lung transplantation remains the only definitive treatment option for PVOD/PCH.

Introduction

In the world of evidence-based medicine, accurate diagnosis and effective management of rare diseases remains difficult. Pulmonary veno-occlusive disease (PVOD) and pulmonary capillary hemangiomatosis (PCH) are two such rare diseases, largely considered to be extremely difficult to diagnose and even more difficult to treat. Recently, both diseases have come under considerable attention, which has led to an increased awareness of environmental and genetic risk factors. Despite these advances in knowledge, accurate diagnosis remains a clinical challenge and effective treatments are still almost nonexistent. The prognosis for these patients remains poor and further research is required. It is crucial that more advances be made in early recognition of these entities as well as in treatment options in order to improve the poor prognosis for these patients.

The 6th World Symposium on Pulmonary Hypertension has defined a simplified five-group classification system to categorize pulmonary hypertension (PH) based on etiology (1). Identification of the underlying etiology of pulmonary hypertension is crucial, as the treatment is usually directed specifically at the underlying cause. Under this most recent classification system, PVOD and PCH are rare subtypes of the Group 1 pulmonary arterial hypertension (PAH), as they share hemodynamic and clinical features

Pulmonary Veno-Occlusive Disease and Pulmonary Capillary Hemangiomatosis

with PAH (2). However, the pathology underlying PVOD and PCH is unique, rendering PAH-specific treatments mostly ineffective (2), which translates to poor patient prognosis. In this chapter, we will highlight this unique entity, as well as risk factors, and management considerations for PVOD and PCH. For the purposes of this review, the two diseases present with similar clinical presentations, are evaluated with the same diagnostic tools, and share the same prognosis and treatment considerations, and are therefore largely discussed together.

Burden of PVOD/PCH

The exact incidence of PVOD and PCH is unknown due to a combination of factors. Accurate diagnosis is challenging given that the clinical, hemodynamic, and radiographic presentation often mimics idiopathic PAH leading to misclassification of disease. Surgical or transbronchial biopsy can lead to definitive diagnosis, but is often not pursued due to the high risk for bleeding or other complications (3, 4).

A conservative estimate of prevalence is approximately 1–2 cases per million people and incidence is approximately 0.1–0.5 cases per million people per year (3, 4), which highlights the rarity of these disease entities. However, due to lack of prospective studies and difficulty in obtaining definitive diagnosis, these numbers are still suspected to be an under-estimate of the actual incidence and prevalence (5). Cases are seen to affect both males and females equally (6) and across all age groups from infancy to the seventh decade of life (3, 4). Recent data suggests a bimodal age distribution for PVOD, mostly concentrated in young adults between the ages of 20–30 years and geriatric patients between the ages of 70–80 years (7). The heritable variant has also been described in patients from birth through the fifth decade of life (8).

Pathogenesis of PVOD

To understand PVOD and PCH, it is important to understand the pathology that underlies PAH and how it differs. The hallmark alterations in PAH typically involve excess proliferation of pulmonary artery smooth muscle cells, endothelial cells, fibroblasts, myofibroblasts, and pericytes within the pulmonary arterial wall with loss of *pre-capillary* arteries and perivascular infiltration with inflammatory cells (9). When these cells and proteins accumulate in one place, it forms a lesion that has been referred to as a plexiform lesion (5). These alterations lead to loss and obstructive remodeling of pulmonary arteries and arterioles with subsequent elevation of pulmonary vascular resistance (PVR) (9). However, in PVOD and PCH, the vascular remodeling starts predominantly in the pulmonary venules leading to a rise in pressure at the *post-capillary* side with resultant elevated pressures at the pre-capillary side (4, 10, 11). It is characterized by fibrous intimal thickening, obliteration, and obstruction of the small veins/venules and patchy capillary proliferation (12). Similar to other forms of PH, there is progressive increase of PVR ultimately resulting in right ventricular failure and death (2).

Histologically, PVOD and PCH share many overlapping features with overt features of venous/capillary involvement (13). Typical features of PVOD on lung biopsy include diffuse involvement of venules and septal veins with intimal fibrosis causing luminal narrowing and obliteration (14), along with engorgement of the pulmonary capillaries, which are upstream from the obliterated small veins/venules (15) and dilation of the lymphatics (16) (Figure 10.1). Hemosiderin deposition in the alveoli and thickened interlobular septa are seen in PVOD due to occult pulmonary hemorrhage because of post-capillary obstruction, and interstitial edema most prominent in the interlobular septa progressing into fibrosis, respectively (17) (Figure 10.1, higher magnification). Areas of capillary multiplication within alveolar walls may also be seen in PVOD leading to vessels that resemble arterioles in diameter (18).

The hallmark histologic feature of PCH is abnormal alveolar capillary proliferation, defined as at least two rows of capillaries within the interstitium of alveolar walls. The use of stains such as reticulin and CD-34 can help distinguish it from other mimics of this proliferative process (19, 20). Of note, the plexiform lesion that occurs in small arteries and arterioles in PAH is not seen in either PVOD or PCH (3). PVOD and PCH are often classified

(a)

(b)

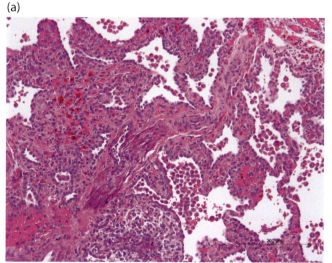
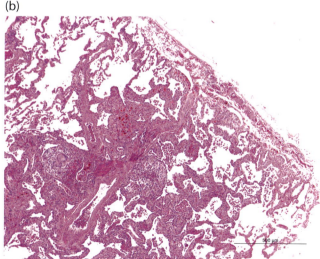

FIGURE 10.1 Sections show an interlobular septum with an occluded vein (200×) (a). At high magnification (500×), ferruginization of elastic fibers can be seen (b). Disruption of the elastic fibers elicits a foreign body reaction with occasional multinucleated giant cells. There are numerous hemosiderin laden macrophages due to repeated episodes of hemorrhage and mild thickening with type 2 proliferation in septa adjacent to the interlobular septa.

together in current literature as variable expression of the same disease. However, it is worth mentioning that there exists an argument for considering them to be two separate entities. One supporting observation for this is the fact that there are cases of PCH that lack pulmonary venous obstruction and alternatively, there are cases of PVOD that do not have the hallmark capillary proliferation characteristic of PCH (18). However, case series of autopsies performed on patients have shown considerable overlap between the two (20).

Risk factors for the development of PVOD/PCH

Many cases of PVOD/PCH are classified as idiopathic, though literature has identified several risk factors and more recently, familial forms of the disease. Understanding these factors is essential for the timely recognition and management of PVOD and PCH. There has been a reported association between various chemotherapeutic agents and development of PVOD, especially with alkylating agents. It is postulated that chemotherapy may damage the pulmonary venule endothelium, though a definitive association between a single agent and PVOD has yet to be established (21). Hematopoietic stem cell transplantation has also been implicated, with several reports of PVOD developing after transplantation (22–31). The mechanism is poorly understood, and data remains scarce.

Occupational exposure to organic solvents (especially trichloroethylene), and tobacco exposure, which may play a synergistic role with organic solvents (7), are also identified risk factors. Autoimmune diseases remain a consistent risk factor for PH and is no exception for patients with PVOD/PCH. Implicated diseases include sarcoidosis, scleroderma, systemic lupus erythematosus and Langerhans cell histiocytosis (6, 32–35). Of special concern is systemic sclerosis, which has more frequent reports associated with PVOD (32). There have been reports of PVOD developing in patients with HIV infections (36, 37). Associations with other infections, prothrombotic states (38), and hormonal factors (39) have been mentioned in literature though the data for this is limited. Overall, the rarity of PVOD and PCH contributes to the lack of data and often the exact mechanistic link between these above exposures and disease is not well established.

Genetic risk factors

A milestone in understanding the development of heritable PVOD/PCH was achieved recently with the discovery of the biallelic mutations of the eukaryotic translation initiation factor 2 alpha kinase 4 (EIF2AK4) gene, which is responsible for the heritable transmission of both PVOD and PCH (18, 40). The presence of this mutation in both PVOD and PCH has provided recent support for the two diseases being variable expressions of the same disease entity. EIF2AK4 mutation is inherited in an autosomal recessive pattern, unlike the autosomal dominant pattern of inheritance seen in familial BMPR2 mutation PAH (16, 41). It also has almost complete penetrance by the age of 50 (40), which differs from the much lower penetrance rate seen in familial BMPR2 PAH (16). The gene encodes a serine-threonine kinase that responds to amino acid deprivation by inducing changes in gene expression, however, the pathophysiologic link between mutation and pathology in the pulmonary vasculature remains unknown (40). In a large population-based study of patients with confirmed or suspected PVOD/PCH, those that were carriers of the mutation were younger on average than those without the mutation and had a 1:1 gender distribution as compared to the male predominance in mutation noncarriers (8). Overall, the discovery of this mutation has led to optimistic advances in our understanding of the molecular and cellular mechanisms underlying these diseases. However, PVOD and PCH still remain orphan lung diseases for which there are no effective therapies and lung transplantation remains the only available option (16).

Clinical presentation of PVOD/PCH

PVOD/PCH typically present with nonspecific symptoms with the most common being exertional dyspnea, fatigue, leg swelling, syncope, or cough (42, 43) (Table 10.1). The nonspecific nature of these symptoms often delays accurate diagnosis until patients have New York Heart Association Functional Class III or IV symptoms (4), which can ultimately delay treatment or early referral to an appropriate PH center. Registries in multiple countries have corroborated this by demonstrating that the mean time from symptom onset to diagnosis of PAH is 2 years (5). Clinically PVOD/PCH is difficult, if not impossible, to distinguish from idiopathic or other forms of PAH. As such, an astute clinician should seek out and recognize identifiable PVOD/PCH-specific risk factors by evaluating for prior oncological treatments, history of connective tissue disease, exposure screening, and family history. Physical examination in PVOD/PCH will largely mimic other forms of PAH. In more mild-moderate pulmonary hypertension, physical examination may be normal, or may reveal splitting of the second heart sound with accentuation of pulmonic valve component. A holosystolic murmur indicative of tricuspid regurgitation may also develop (5). As in other forms of PAH, a physical examination in PVOD/PCH indicating right heart failure include lower extremity edema, ascites, hepatomegaly, and abdominal bloating. A combination of these findings with a history of syncope portends an even worse prognosis (5). Hemoptysis in patients with PH may also be a presenting symptom indicative of pulmonary venous congestion and is more commonly seen in PCH (18, 44). Clubbing and pleural effusions may be a more specific sign of PVOD (16), as these are less commonly seen in other forms of PAH. There are also patients who present with no symptoms at all and are discovered incidentally to have pulmonary hypertension. It is this heterogenous and nonspecific

TABLE 10.1: Common Clinical Symptoms and Physical Examination Findings Commonly Seen in PVOD/PCH

Symptom (Case Series 1, n = 24)	Estimated Percentage at Presentation
Right heart failure (leg swelling, crackles)	54%
Syncope/Near syncope	45%
Clubbing	16%
Raynaud phenomenon	8%
Hemochromatosis	8%
Hemoptysis	4%
Symptom (Case Series 2, n = 11)	
Progressive dyspnea	100%
Nonproductive cough	55%
Viral prodrome	36%
Orthopnea	18%
Paroxysmal nocturnal dyspnea	18%
Atypical chest pain	18%
Near syncope	18%

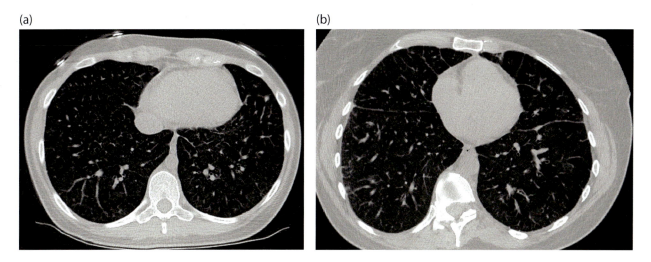

FIGURE 10.2 High-resolution computed tomography of chest showing centrilobular ground glass nodules pathognomic for PVOD (a). Thickening of the interlobular septa bilaterally is shown in a patient with PVOD (b).

presentation that contributes to making this rare subtype of PAH, an already complex disease, so difficult to evaluate.

Imaging and diagnostic evaluation

Transthoracic echocardiography remains the most widely utilized initial test to detect PH (45). Findings on echocardiography indicative of pulmonary hypertension may include tricuspid regurgitation, elevated right ventricular systolic pressure, right ventricular pressure overload with flattening of the interventricular septum, right ventricular dysfunction, or even a right to left shunt via a patent foramen ovale if right-sided pressures are high enough. The presence and greater size of a pericardial effusion portends a poorer prognosis (5). Tricuspid annular plan systolic excursion (TAPSE) has been found to have prognostic indications as well, with lower values associated with higher WHO functional classes in patients with PAH (46). An echocardiogram can also be useful for evaluating for other potential etiologies of PH such as left heart disease or valvular disorders, which are not seen in PVOD/PCH. In addition to an echocardiogram, the initial assessment should also include blood serum testing for etiological causes. In PVOD, special consideration should be given based on individualized risk factors, such as screening for connective tissues disease or HIV. Genetic testing for associated mutations should also be strongly considered in patients with family history of PH.

High-resolution chest computed tomography (CT) is a crucial part of diagnostic evaluation for PVOD/PCH. A triad of enlarged mediastinal lymph nodes, centrilobular ground glass opacities, and smooth thickening of the interlobular septa can be seen (47–50) (Figure 10.2a, b). Presence of two out of three of these findings on CT scan correlates with a sensitivity of 75% and specificity of almost 85% for PVOD/PCH (18). In one study, patients with PCH had larger ground glass opacities than PVOD, though the study population was limited to three patients in each arm (51). CT can also reveal further signs of PH such as central pulmonary vessel enlargement, right ventricular dilation, or pleural effusions. Additional imaging studies such as the ventilation-perfusion scan may show perfusion defects indistinguishable from other conditions like chronic thromboembolic pulmonary hypertension (CTEPH) or PAH (Figure 10.3) (52). Further evaluation

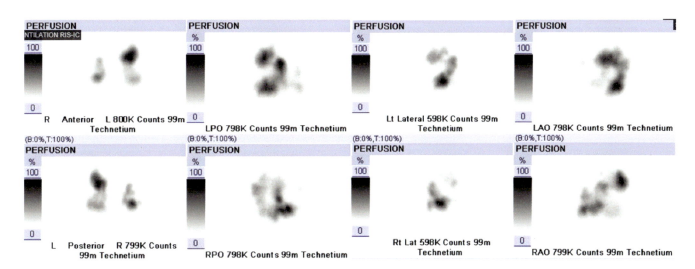

FIGURE 10.3 Ventilation perfusion scan in a patient with PVOD shows bilateral multiple perfusion defects mimicking chronic thromboembolic pulmonary hypertension. A pulmonary arterial angiogram was done to distinguish between the two.

with a pulmonary arterial angiogram may be necessary to confirm (CTEPH). Pulmonary function testing is often indicated in a new diagnosis of PH. Patients with PVOD/PCH will typically have preserved spirometry and lung volumes. However, an out-of-proportion reduction in DLCO to less than 50% predicted is common, which can be a distinguishing feature (43).

Right heart catheterization (RHC) remains the gold standard for confirming a diagnosis of PH (4). The 6th World Health Symposium on Pulmonary Hypertension has proposed defining PH as mean pulmonary artery pressure >20 mmHg, pulmonary vascular resistance ≥3 woods units, and pulmonary artery wedge pressure ≤15 mmHg. Unfortunately, the classic hemodynamic alterations found in PVOD/PCH are similar to PAH despite their differences in post-capillary versus pre-capillary pathology (43). This is because wedging of the balloon during RHC does not reflect post-capillary venule pressures, instead reflecting left atrial pressure, which are normal in both diseases. However, a few small-scale reports have noted potential distinguishing features during RHC in PVOD. First, vasoreactivity testing may lead to development of flash pulmonary edema (42, 53) as dilation of pulmonary arterioles in the setting of obstructed venules can lead to sudden transudative fluid accumulation in the alveoli. For this reason, careful consideration should be taken prior to pursuing vasoreactivity testing if there is a specific suspicion for PVOD/PCH prior to RHC. Second, old literature has theorized that pulmonary artery wedge pressure tracings during flushing may rise disproportionally as the saline flush becomes trapped in the high-pressured, obstructed venules (54). Cardiopulmonary exercise testing (CPET) is another potentially useful as patients with PVOD/PCH often have earlier onset of anaerobic threshold, higher degree of gas exchange impairment, higher ventilatory demand, more dead space, and higher minute ventilation per exhaled carbon dioxide than matched patients with PAH (55). If pursued, bronchoalveolar lavage specimens or sputum cytology can show hemosiderin laden macrophages (17) and may be a supportive of PVOD in the appropriate clinical context. Despite all these above testing modalities, the diagnosis of PVOD and PCH can remain elusive or misdiagnosed as PAH. Histological evaluation via surgical or transbronchial lung biopsy remains the only gold standard for diagnosing PVOD and PCH (4), though these are commonly not pursued due to high risk for uncontrolled bleeding or other complications as previously mentioned. If PVOD/PCH is highly suspected, the onus remains on the astute clinician to utilize clinical history, physical examination, and the above diagnostic testing to establish a diagnosis.

Treatment and outcomes

Prognosis of PVOD/PCH is unfortunately dismal and significantly worse than other forms of PAH, with a mortality rate of 72% in the first year from diagnosis (42) and a mean time of 11.8 months from diagnosis to death or lung transplantation (43). Despite the significant progress in development of several PAH-specific therapies over the past few decades, there remains no medical therapy with proven benefit for PVOD/PCH (4). Therefore, lung transplantation remains the only conclusive treatment.

PAH-specific therapies commonly used to treat Group 1 PAH include phosphodiesterase type 5 inhibitors, endothelin receptor antagonists, prostacyclins, and soluble guanylate cyclase stimulants. Data on the use of these targeted therapies in PVOD/PCH are conflicting. There are some anecdotal reports of patients having functional and hemodynamic improvements, however, there is also an increased risk for PVOD/PCH patients to develop pulmonary edema and worsening respiratory failure on these agents. This is due to PAH-specific therapies having a greater vasodilatory effect on pulmonary arteries rather than veins, which can lead to a sudden increase in hydrostatic pressure and subsequent accumulation of transudative fluid in the alveoli. Despite these possible risks, PAH-specific therapies can still be trialed in PVOD/PCH patients as a bridge to lung transplantation. Literature on its use is very limited, so in general, experienced clinicians may consider a trial of only a *single* agent at a time at the lowest possible dose.

Recent genetic advances in heritable PVOD/PCH have raised questions if such patients respond differently to PAH-targeted treatment. Once again, data on this remain mixed. In case reports on patients with EIF2AK4 mutations, one showed a favorable response to treatment with PAH-targeted therapies (56) while another showed rapid progression with death within 6 months of diagnosis (57). Another population-based study documented satisfactory clinical response in only 4% of all treated PVOD/PCH patients, with development of drug-induced pulmonary edema in 23% of patients with the EIF2AK4 mutation and 21% in those without the heritable mutation. There was no difference in survival in the same study between mutation carriers and noncarriers with 3-year event-free survival rates as low as 32–34% in those that did not receive lung transplant (8), illustrating the paucity of treatment options and poor prognosis in both heritable as well as sporadic forms of PVOD/PCH. There is limited and mixed literature regarding the use of immunosuppressive agents such as glucocorticoids, cyclophosphamides, and azathioprine in PVOD/PCH patients (10). In theory, these medications should be especially useful in PVOD/PCH with autoimmune features, with two case reports showing remission of PVOD/PCH after initiating immunomodulator therapies (58, 59). A more recent case series has expanded upon this and demonstrated improvement in both sporadic and heritable PVOD/PCH after treatment with a combination of glucocorticoid and mycophenolate (60). Ultimately, the data on this treatment approach is limited and the exact drug class, dosage, and timing of immune therapy is not established. In rare occasions, experienced clinicians may trial the lowest possible dose of therapy and titrate based on clinical response. Various other experimental therapies for PVOD/PCH are still undergoing investigation, usually stemming from PAH or hepatic veno-occlusive disease (HVOD) trials. A very recent study on imatinib, a tyrosine kinase inhibitor with anti-angiogenesis properties, had shown some promise with improvement of hemodynamic values, exercise capacity and survival (61).

Lung or heart-lung transplantation remains the only definitive treatment option for PVOD/PCH. At the time of diagnosis, referral for lung transplantation should be made immediately regardless of clinical status, given the lack of effective treatment options and anticipated rapid progression of disease. In fact, the disease is so devastating, that even with early lung transplant referral, PVOD patients remain at increased risk of death while on the transplant waitlist (62). In patients that are able to receive lung transplant, the estimated 5-year survival rate was as high as 73% (8), a remarkable figure that should further encourage early referral.

Summary and conclusion

PVOD and PCH are a set of rare diseases currently classified under Group 1 PAH. However, in comparison to PAH, PVOD/PCH retain their own distinct pathology and therefore respond poorly to currently used PAH targeted therapies. Lung transplantation remains the only definitive treatment necessitating early recognition of these difficult to diagnose diseases. A combination of clinical history, imaging modalities and testing can provide clues, and are important to utilize early. New therapies should ideally target the unique venous pathology found in PVOD/PCH, though the rarity of diseases and challenges in making a definitive diagnosis makes them difficult to study. They therefore remain a diagnostic and therapeutic dilemma for physicians with unfortunate consequence for patients. Recent advances in molecular genetics are promising new developments and may provide us with further avenues for study in the management of these rare diseases.

References

1. Galie N, McLaughlin VV, Rubin LJ, Simonneau G. An overview of the 6th world symposium on pulmonary hypertension. Eur Respir J. 2019;53(1):1802148.
2. Simonneau G, Montani D, Celermajer DS, Denton CP, Gatzoulis MA, Krowka M, et al. Haemodynamic definitions and updated clinical classification of pulmonary hypertension. Eur Respir J. 2019;53(1):1801913.
3. Chaisson NF, Dodson MW, Elliott CG. Pulmonary capillary hemangiomatosis and pulmonary veno-occlusive disease. Clin Chest Med. 2016;37(3):523–34.
4. Montani D, Lau EM, Dorfmuller P, Girerd B, Jais X, Savale L, et al. Pulmonary veno-occlusive disease. Eur Respir J. 2016;47(5):1518–34.
5. Grippi MA. Fishman's pulmonary diseases and disorders. 2015.
6. Hoffstein V, Ranganathan N, Mullen JB. Sarcoidosis simulating pulmonary veno-occlusive disease. Am Rev Respir Dis. 1986;134(4):809–11.
7. Montani D, Lau EM, Descatha A, Jais X, Savale L, Andujar P, et al. Occupational exposure to organic solvents: A risk factor for pulmonary veno-occlusive disease. Eur Respir J. 2015;46(6):1721–31.
8. Montani D, Girerd B, Jais X, Levy M, Amar D, Savale L, et al. Clinical phenotypes and outcomes of heritable and sporadic pulmonary veno-occlusive disease: A population-based study. Lancet Respir Med. 2017;5(2):125–34.
9. Humbert M, Guignabert C, Bonnet S, Dorfmuller P, Klinger JR, Nicolls MR, et al. Pathology and pathobiology of pulmonary hypertension: State of the art and research perspectives. Eur Respir J. 2019;53(1):1801887.
10. Mandel J, Mark EJ, Hales CA. Pulmonary veno-occlusive disease. Am J Respir Crit Care Med. 2000;162(5):1964–73.
11. Montani D, Price LC, Dorfmuller P, Achouh L, Jais X, Yaici A, et al. Pulmonary veno-occlusive disease. Eur Respir J. 2009;33(1):189–200.
12. Pietra GG, Capron F, Stewart S, Leone O, Humbert M, Robbins IM, et al. Pathologic assessment of vasculopathies in pulmonary hypertension. J Am Coll Cardiol. 2004;43(12 Suppl S):25S–32S.
13. Pietra GG, Edwards WD, Kay JM, Rich S, Kernis J, Schloo B, et al. Histopathology of primary pulmonary hypertension. A qualitative and quantitative study of pulmonary blood vessels from 58 patients in the national heart, lung, and blood institute, primary pulmonary hypertension registry. Circulation. 1989;80(5):1198–206.
14. Wagenvoort CA, Wagenvoort N. The pathology of pulmonary veno-occlusive disease. Virchows Arch A Pathol Anat Histol. 1974;364(1):69–79.
15. Schraufnagel DE, Sekosan M, McGee T, Thakkar MB. Human alveolar capillaries undergo angiogenesis in pulmonary veno-occlusive disease. Eur Respir J. 1996;9(2):346–50.
16. Machado RD, Eickelberg O, Elliott CG, Geraci MW, Hanaoka M, Loyd JE, et al. Genetics and genomics of pulmonary arterial hypertension. J Am Coll Cardiol. 2009;54(1 Suppl):S32–S42.
17. Rabiller A, Jais X, Hamid A, Resten A, Parent F, Haque R, et al. Occult alveolar haemorrhage in pulmonary veno-occlusive disease. Eur Respir J. 2006;27(1):108–13.
18. Weatherald J, Dorfmuller P, Perros F, Ghigna MR, Girerd B, Humbert M, et al. Pulmonary capillary haemangiomatosis: A distinct entity? Eur Respir Rev. 2020;29(156):190168.
19. Havlik DM, Massie LW, Williams WL, Crooks LA. Pulmonary capillary hemangiomatosis-like foci. An autopsy study of 8 cases. Am J Clin Pathol. 2000;113(5):655–62.
20. Lantuejoul S, Sheppard MN, Corrin B, Burke MM, Nicholson AG. Pulmonary veno-occlusive disease and pulmonary capillary hemangiomatosis: A clinicopathologic study of 35 cases. Am J Surg Pathol. 2006;30(7):850–7.
21. Ranchoux B, Gunther S, Quarck R, Chaumais MC, Dorfmuller P, Antigny F, et al. Chemotherapy-induced pulmonary hypertension: Role of alkylating agents. Am J Pathol. 2015;185(2):356–71.
22. Bunte MC, Patnaik MM, Pritzker MR, Burns LJ. Pulmonary veno-occlusive disease following hematopoietic stem cell transplantation: A rare model of endothelial dysfunction. Bone Marrow Transplant. 2008;41(8):677–86.
23. Hackman RC, Madtes DK, Petersen FB, Clark JG. Pulmonary venoocclusive disease following bone marrow transplantation. Transplantation. 1989;47(6):989–92.
24. Joselson R, Warnock M. Pulmonary veno-occlusive disease after chemotherapy. Hum Pathol. 1983;14(1):88–91.
25. Knight BK, Rose AG. Pulmonary veno-occlusive disease after chemotherapy. Thorax. 1985;40(11):874–5.
26. Salzman D, Adkins DR, Craig F, Freytes C, LeMaistre CF. Malignancy-associated pulmonary veno-occlusive disease: Report of a case following autologous bone marrow transplantation and review. Bone Marrow Transplant. 1996;18(4):755–60.
27. Seguchi M, Hirabayashi N, Fujii Y, Azuno Y, Fujita N, Takeda K, et al. Pulmonary hypertension associated with pulmonary occlusive vasculopathy after allogeneic bone marrow transplantation. Transplantation. 2000;69(1):177–9.
28. Swift GL, Gibbs A, Campbell IA, Wagenvoort CA, Tuthill D. Pulmonary veno-occlusive disease and Hodgkin's lymphoma. Eur Respir J. 1993;6(4):596–8.
29. Troussard X, Bernaudin JF, Cordonnier C, Fleury J, Payen D, Briere J, et al. Pulmonary veno-occlusive disease after bone marrow transplantation. Thorax. 1984;39(12):956–7.
30. Waldhorn RE, Tsou E, Smith FP, Kerwin DM. Pulmonary veno-occlusive disease associated with microangiopathic hemolytic anemia and chemotherapy of gastric adenocarcinoma. Med Pediatr Oncol. 1984;12(6):394–6.
31. Williams LM, Fussell S, Veith RW, Nelson S, Mason CM. Pulmonary veno-occlusive disease in an adult following bone marrow transplantation. Case report and review of the literature. Chest. 1996;109(5):1388–91.
32. Dorfmuller P, Montani D, Humbert M. Beyond arterial remodelling: Pulmonary venous and cardiac involvement in patients with systemic sclerosis-associated pulmonary arterial hypertension. Eur Respir J. 2010;35(1):6–8.
33. Hamada K, Teramoto S, Narita N, Yamada E, Teramoto K, Kobzik L. Pulmonary veno-occlusive disease in pulmonary Langerhans' cell granulomatosis. Eur Respir J. 2000;15(2):421–3.
34. Johnson SR, Patsios D, Hwang DM, Granton JT. Pulmonary veno-occlusive disease and scleroderma associated pulmonary hypertension. J Rheumatol. 2006;33(11):2347–50.
35. Kishida Y, Kanai Y, Kuramochi S, Hosoda Y. Pulmonary venoocclusive disease in a patient with systemic lupus erythematosus. J Rheumatol. 1993;20(12):2161–2.
36. Escamilla R, Hermant C, Berjaud J, Mazerolles C, Daussy X. Pulmonary veno-occlusive disease in a HIV-infected intravenous drug abuser. Eur Respir J. 1995;8(11):1982–4.
37. Ruchelli ED, Nojadera G, Rutstein RM, Rudy B. Pulmonary veno-occlusive disease. Another vascular disorder associated with human immunodeficiency virus infection? Arch Pathol Lab Med. 1994;118(6):664–6.
38. Tachibana T, Nakayama N, Matsumura A, Nakajima Y, Takahashi H, Miyazaki T, Nakajima H. Pulmonary hypertension associated with pulmonary veno-occlusive disease in patients with polycythemia vera. Intern Med. 2017 Sep 15;56(18):2487–92. doi: 10.2169/internalmedicine.8629-16. Epub 2017 Aug 21. PMID: 28824072; PMCID: PMC5643179.

39. Urisman A, Leard LE, Nathan M, Elicker BM, Hoopes C, Kukreja J, Jones KD. Rapidly progressive pulmonary venoocclusive disease in young women taking oral contraceptives. J Heart Lung Transplant. 2012 Sep;31(9):1031–6. doi: 10.1016/j.healun.2012.05.007. PMID: 22884388.
40. Eyries M, Montani D, Girerd B, Perret C, Leroy A, Lonjou C, et al. EIF2AK4 mutations cause pulmonary veno-occlusive disease, a recessive form of pulmonary hypertension. Nat Genet. 2014;46(1):65–9.
41. Loyd JE, Primm RK, Newman JH. Familial primary pulmonary hypertension: Clinical patterns. Am Rev Respir Dis. 1984;129(1):194–7.
42. Holcomb BW, Jr., Loyd JE, Ely EW, Johnson J, Robbins IM. Pulmonary veno-occlusive disease: A case series and new observations. Chest. 2000;118(6):1671–9.
43. Montani D, Achouh L, Dorfmuller P, Le Pavec J, Sztrymf B, Tcherakian C, et al. Pulmonary veno-occlusive disease: Clinical, functional, radiologic, and hemodynamic characteristics and outcome of 24 cases confirmed by histology. Medicine (Baltimore). 2008;87(4):220–33.
44. Xie WM, Dai HP, Jin ML, Wang Z, Yang YH, Zhai ZG, Wang C. Clinical features and imaging findings in pulmonary capillary hemangiomatosis: Report of two cases and a pooled analysis. Chin Med J (Engl). 2012 Sep;125(17):3069–73. PMID: 22932183.
45. Lau EM, Manes A, Celermajer DS, Galie N. Early detection of pulmonary vascular disease in pulmonary arterial hypertension: Time to move forward. Eur Heart J. 2011;32(20):2489–98.
46. Tello K, Axmann J, Ghofrani HA, Naeije R, Narcin N, Rieth A, et al. Relevance of the TAPSE/PASP ratio in pulmonary arterial hypertension. Int J Cardiol. 2018;266:229–35.
47. Dufour B, Maitre S, Humbert M, Capron F, Simonneau G, Musset D. High-resolution CT of the chest in four patients with pulmonary capillary hemangiomatosis or pulmonary venoocclusive disease. Am J Roentgenol. 1998;171(5):1321–4.
48. Frazier AA, Franks TJ, Mohammed TL, Ozbudak IH, Galvin JR. From the archives of the AFIP: pulmonary veno-occlusive disease and pulmonary capillary hemangiomatosis. Radiographics. 2007;27(3):867–82.
49. Resten A, Maitre S, Humbert M, Rabiller A, Sitbon O, Capron F, et al. Pulmonary hypertension: CT of the chest in pulmonary venoocclusive disease. Am J Roentgenol. 2004;183(1):65–70.
50. Swensen SJ, Tashjian JH, Myers JL, Engeler CE, Patz EF, Edwards WD, et al. Pulmonary venoocclusive disease: CT findings in eight patients. Am J Roentgenol. 1996;167(4):937–40.
51. Miura A, Akagi S, Nakamura K, Ohta-Ogo K, Hashimoto K, Nagase S, et al. Different sizes of centrilobular ground-glass opacities in chest high-resolution computed tomography of patients with pulmonary veno-occlusive disease and patients with pulmonary capillary hemangiomatosis. Cardiovasc Pathol. 2013;22(4):287–93.
52. Seferian A, Helal B, Jais X, Girerd B, Price LC, Gunther S, et al. Ventilation/perfusion lung scan in pulmonary veno-occlusive disease. Eur Respir J. 2012;40(1):75–83.
53. Galie N, Humbert M, Vachiery JL, Gibbs S, Lang I, Torbicki A, et al. 2015 ESC/ERS guidelines for the diagnosis and treatment of pulmonary hypertension: The joint task force for the diagnosis and treatment of pulmonary hypertension of the European Society of Cardiology (ESC) and the European Respiratory Society (ERS): Endorsed by: Association for European Paediatric and Congenital Cardiology (AEPC), International Society for Heart and Lung Transplantation (ISHLT). Eur Heart J. 2016;37(1):67–119.
54. Chawla SK, Kittle CF, Faber LP, Jensik RJ. Pulmonary venoocclusive disease. Ann Thorac Surg. 1976;22(3):249–53.
55. Laveneziana P, Montani D, Dorfmuller P, Girerd B, Sitbon O, Jais X, et al. Mechanisms of exertional dyspnoea in pulmonary veno-occlusive disease with EIF2AK4 mutations. Eur Respir J. 2014;44(4):1069–72.
56. Liang L, Su H, Ma X, Zhang R. Good response to PAH-targeted drugs in a PVOD patient carrying Biallelic EIF_2AK_4 mutation. Respir Res. 2018;19(1):192.
57. Zeng X, Chen F, Rathinasabapathy A, Li T, Adnan Ali Mohammed Mohammed A, Yu Z. Rapid disease progress in a PVOD patient carrying a novel EIF_2AK_4 mutation: A case report. BMC Pulm Med. 2020;20(1):186.
58. Naniwa T, Takeda Y. Long-term remission of pulmonary veno-occlusive disease associated with primary Sjögren's syndrome following immunosuppressive therapy. Mod Rheumatol. 2011;21(6):637–40.
59. Sanderson JE, Spiro SG, Hendry AT, Turner-Warwick M. A case of pulmonary veno-occlusive disease responding to treatment with azathioprine. Thorax. 1977;32(2):140–8.
60. Bergbaum C, Samaranayake CB, Pitcher A, Weingart E, Semple T, Kokosi M, et al. A case series on the use of steroids and mycophenolate mofetil in idiopathic and heritable pulmonary veno-occlusive disease: Is there a role for immunosuppression? Eur Respir J. 2021;57(6):2004354.
61. Ogawa A, Miyaji K, Matsubara H. Efficacy and safety of long-term imatinib therapy for patients with pulmonary veno-occlusive disease and pulmonary capillary hemangiomatosis. Respir Med. 2017;131:215–9.
62. Wille KM, Sharma NS, Kulkarni T, Lammi MR, Barney JB, Bellot SC, et al. Characteristics of patients with pulmonary venoocclusive disease awaiting transplantation. Ann Am Thorac Soc. 2014;11(9):1411–8.

PART D
Rare Diffuse Parenchymal Lung Diseases

11

PLEUROPARENCHYMAL FIBROELASTOSIS (PPFE)

Bhavna Seth and Sonye K. Danoff

Contents

Introduction 77
History 77
Epidemiology 77
Pathogenesis 78
Clinical characteristics 79
Conclusion 82
Acknowledgment 82
References 82

KEY POINTS

- Pleuroparenchymal fibroelastosis (PPFE) is a rare diagnosis of pleural and sub-pleural lung fibrosis, predominantly in the upper lobes of the lung.
- PPFE can be idiopathic or secondary (e.g., post-transplant, short telomere syndrome related, due to infections, autoimmune disease, drug related).
- Pathologically it is characterized by intra-alveolar fibrosis and elastosis (IAFE), i.e. both disordered collagenosis (excess collagen deposition) or elastosis (excess elastin deposition).
- High-resolution computed tomography (HRCT) reveals pleural thickening with associated subpleural fibrosis concentrated in the upper lobes with less marked or no lower lobe involvement.
- No treatment has demonstrated efficacy for PPFE. Treatment approaches are focused on supportive care and transplant evaluation.

Introduction

Pleuroparenchymal fibroelastosis (PPFE) is a rare diagnosis, characterized by a distinct pattern of pleural and sub-pleural lung fibrosis, particularly in the upper lobes of the lung. The unique pathological characteristic is the elastotic fibrosing process associated with intra-alveolar fibrosis and elastosis (IAFE). It may be idiopathic (iPPFE) or due to secondary causes. Secondary causes (Table 11.1) include associations with drugs, autoimmune disease, infections, lung, and bone marrow transplantation. A definitive diagnosis often requires the presence of a multidisciplinary team approach involving a clinician, radiologist, and pathologist (1). The diagnosis is associated with a distinct prognostic and therapeutic approach that is important to recognize. There are currently limited therapeutic options with proven efficacy, which includes lung transplantation.

History

The diagnostic term pleuroparenchymal fibroelastosis was first formally introduced as a unique clinicopathologic entity in 2004 in five cases, by Frankel et al. (2). Prior to this, however, reports of similar cases of what can be ascertained to be PPFE existed. These case reports carried varied titles, such as "chronic idiopathic pneumonia" (3), "idiopathic progressive pleuropulmonary fibrosis" (4), "pulmonary upper-lobe fibrocystic changes" (5), and "pulmonary apical fibrocystic disease" (6). In particular, numerous reports from Japan described a clinical entity with clinicopathological features of PPFE. The first was a series of 13 patients described by Amitani et al. in 1992, called "idiopathic pulmonary upper-lobe fibrosis (idiopathic PULF)" (7). Amitani and colleagues described autopsy and histological examination of lung tissue; however, radiological imaging was limited to chest x-rays. The authors reported idiopathic PULF as a slowly progressive fatal condition after 10–20 years in patients with slender statures and flattened thoracic cages (7, 8). Idiopathic PULF came to be called Amitani disease, a year prior to the description by Frankel et al., who coined the term PPFE (9). In 2013, PPFE was listed as a rare idiopathic interstitial pneumonia, in the revised multidisciplinary consensus classification of Idiopathic Interstitial Pneumonias (10).

Epidemiology

The prevalence and incidence of PPFE is not known, owing to the limited literature, a lack of a standardized case definition, and frequent misdiagnosis. Numerous reports, however, suggest that it may not in fact be as rare as previously considered and is an underreported entity (11). PPFE can be broadly divided into primary or idiopathic (no apparent trigger) or secondary (associated with an underlying disorder) (Table 11.1).

Co-existing interstitial lung disease (ILD) may be common; a few studies have reported ILDs to co-exist with PPFE in as high as 43–75% of cases (12, 13). Similarly, in a 5-year retrospective review of patients listed for lung transplant, one-quarter of 118 patients with fibrotic ILD were found to have radiological features consistent with PPFE (14). Over a 10-year follow up of a referral clinic for interstitial pneumonias, 7.7% of consecutive cases had iPPFE (15). Post-transplant-related PPFE is the most

TABLE 11.1: Causes of Secondary Pleuroparenchymal Pulmonary Fibroelastosis Reported with Notable Features

Condition	Distinguishing Features (if any)	References
Transplant related	May appreciate concomitant bronchiolitis obliterans on histopathology	(13, 24–36, 38–39)
• Form of restrictive allograft syndrome (RAS), complicating lung transplant, and hematopoietic stem cell transplant (pulmonary complication of graft vs. host disease [GVHD])		(16, 29–31)
Interstitial lung disease		(34, 40)
• Usual interstitial pneumonia		
• Hypersensitivity pneumonitis		
Short telomere syndromes	Autosomal dominant, genetic anticipation	(19, 41–43)
Familial history of pulmonary fibrosis	Associated with genetic mutations TERT	
Chronic/Recurrent bronchopulmonary infection	Unclear if colonization or due to opportunistic infection vs. direct pathogenic role	(2, 13, 44, 45)
• Aspergillus		
• Non-tuberculosis mycobacteria		
Autoimmune	Underlining history and physical findings would direct to primary disease process	(5, 46–49)
• Scleroderma		
• Rheumatoid arthritis		
• Psoriasis		
• Chron's disease		
• Systemic lupus erythematosus		
• Giant cell arteritis		
Ankylosis spondylitis		(5)
Amiodarone		(50)
Cytotoxic chemotherapy (e.g. cyclophosphamide, carmustine)		(8)
Radiation	Usually confined to irradiated area	
Malignancy associated		(51, 52)
Occupational lung disease	Calcifications have not been reported within the thickened pleura (8), which helps to separate PPFE from asbestos-induced pleural thickening; a condition that may also affect the apical pleura, although very rarely (28, 53, 54)	(53, 54)
• Asbestos		
• Aluminum		
Amyotrophic lateral sclerosis (ALS)		(55)

common secondary form. However, population level reports after transplantation are sparse. A 9-year single institution registry diagnosed 53 (7.5%) lung and 700 (0.28%) bone marrow transplant recipients with PPFE (16). In a systematic review of more than 20 papers, 76 patients with a rheumatological associated disease also had PPFE with disease progression (17).

The age distribution of cases is bimodal, with two appreciated peaks, the smaller occurring around the third decade of life, and the larger at the sixth decade. A review of 78 cases found a mean age of 49 (range 13–85) (18). There is no clear gender preponderance in published series (8). However, in younger non-transplant patients, a slight female predominance has been noted (12). Female preponderance has also been reported in patients with telomere gene mutation related diseases and PPFE (19). Smoking does not appear to be risk factor associated with PPFE. (8)

Pathogenesis

Pulmonary fibrosis, in general, may occur with collagenosis (excess collagen deposition) or elastosis (excess elastin deposition). Idiopathic pulmonary fibrosis (IPF) is predominantly characterized by coallagenosis, while, PPFE may have both processes (20). The sub-epithelial layer of normal alveolar septa are composed of elastic fibers within the extracellular matrix (ECM). These fibers are composed of elastin, a microfibrillar, highly structured, non-extensible component. These are arranged as mature fibers and contribute to elasticity of the lung. However, when exposed to an inflammatory insult, the ECM may remodel its components, including elastin and collagen, and potentially do so in a disordered fashion (21). Elastosis, or reactivation of elastin synthesis due to upregulation of elastin gene expression is observed in response to injury (22, 23). The disordered proliferation leads to altered pulmonary architecture (20). Histopathology from post-lung transplant patients with PPFE or a restrictive allograft syndrome (RAS) phenotype reveals diffuse alveolar damage that supports the hypothesis of a potential nidus of inflammatory or acute lung injury (24, 25). RAS and PPFE both show IAFE, however have different vascular morphology that may provide further insights into their pathogenesis (26). Histologic evaluation of a reported case 16 years after bone marrow transplant found cellular and fibrotic nonspecific interstitial pneumonia

(NSIP), and bronchiolitis obliterans (BO) concurrently, suggesting a spectrum of disease (27). It remains unclear why injuries leading to PPFE evolve into well-demarcated regions in the upper lobes.

Clinical characteristics

The most common presenting symptoms of PPFE include shortness of breath, and cough (8). Weight loss and lower BMIs are also associated, especially with an intercurrent infection or malignancy. Chest pain may be associated with pneumothorax or pleuritic pain. The diagnosis may be made after a presentation of pneumothorax or asymptomatic incidental imaging. Usually, by the time patients are symptomatic, they have experienced a long duration of asymptomatic disease (28). The clinical course and prognosis after symptoms appear tend to be worse.

On examination, PPFE patients may have a slender, or flattened thoracic cage. The secondary changes from decreased body mass, may produce "platythorax" or a flattened thoracic cage with reduced anterior-posterior diameter of the chest wall. This was frequently reported in cases from Japan, especially in idiopathic PPFE, though it is not clear if this is a congenital association (29). However, a few reports of this feature have also been described in cases with secondary PPFE, such as in two patients after bone marrow transplantation (30). Some authors conjecture that this may be a manifestation of disease progression as a consequence of limited distensibility due to upper lung fibrosis (31). This may also contribute to the appearance of a deeper suprasternal notch, secondary to weight loss, with reduced upper lung volume, and a radiologic appearance of "overlapping" of the posterior tracheal border and spine (28). Clubbed fingers are rare. On auscultation, crackles or crepitations are also unusual.

Pneumothorax is a common presenting feature, after possibly years of an asymptomatic disease course. Unilateral or bilateral pneumothoraces are present in approximately one third of PPFE patients (32). In a series of 120 pneumothorax events across 53 patients with PPFE over approximately 3 years, the cumulative incidence at 1, 2, and 3 years of follow-up was 24.8%, 44.9%, and 53.9%, respectively. Most events were small and asymptomatic, however, 57% of patients had recurrent pneumothorax (33). Among ILD patients registered for lung transplant, PPFE patients have a three times higher history of pneumothorax (14).

Additional clinical features associated with secondary PPFE tend to be related to the underlying condition (Table 11.1). It is important to rule out these potential causes in the evaluation of a patient suspected with PPFE, as management, monitoring, and prognosis for each differ considerably (15).

Diagnosis

Diagnostic evaluation is currently based on clinical history and examination, radiological appearance, and potential surgical biopsy. A multidisciplinary team discussion is often the cornerstone in making the diagnosis and planning a management course. Enomoto et al. developed simple criteria for the diagnosis of iPPFE after ruling out secondary etiologies and appreciation of (1) classic radiological PPFE pattern in the upper lobes and (2) disease progression, in serial radiology follow-up. This was found to successfully discriminate idiopathic interstitial pneumonia (IIP) from iPPFE without the necessity for a surgical lung biopsy, which confers considerable procedural risk, and higher rates of pneumothorax than other ILDs (56).

Radiology

Chest x-ray

Chest radiograph may be of limited utility, especially in early stages, where radiographs are mostly normal. Bilateral irregular thickening in the apices may be appreciated. As the disease course progresses, elevation of the bilateral hilar opacities may be appreciated as well as narrowing of the anterior-posterior chest wall diameter. In more advanced stages, fibrocystic features extending to the lower lungs may also be seen, with reduced lung volume (28).

High-resolution computed tomography

High-resolution computed tomography (HRCT) forms the cornerstone of diagnosis for PPFE. Reddy et al. proposed diagnostic criteria based on radiological evaluation, building off of the histopathology criteria developed by Kusagaya et al. (57), listed in Table 11.2 (58). Key imaging features are demonstrated in Figure 11.1a, b.

Surgical biopsy

The decision on whether a biopsy should be undertaken remains controversial and should be made with a multi-disciplinary team weighing the risks and benefits. Surgical lung biopsies have a high morbidity (13%) and mortality (0–17%) rate in PPFE (59). Additionally, if pursued, specimens should be obtained from at least two sites to facilitate the diagnosis of PPFE and/or a secondary etiology, especially with more diffuse radiological findings. A few recent reports have suggested the potential utility of transbronchial cryo-biopsies and CT-guided needle aspirates to improve sampling and diagnosis (79–100%) with fewer complications. However, these biopsy techniques come with varying degrees of sampling adequacy (52, 60).

Histopathology

A unique feature of PPFE is the presence of (1) homogenous IAFE; (2) juxtaposed to the visceral pleura, with visceral pleural fibrosis; (3) with small fibroblastic foci at the edge of the fibrosis; with (4) mild lymphoblastic infiltrates (45). These features are appreciated with elastin stains such as van Gieson stain. Fibroblastic proliferation may be seen as loose entities at the

TABLE 11.2: Pleuroparenchymal Pulmonary Fibroelastosis Histopathology and Radiological Diagnostic Definitions

Category	Histopathology (57)	HRCT (58)
Definite PPFE	Upper lobe pleural fibrosis with adjacent intra-alveolar fibrosis, with alveolar septal elastosis	Pleural thickening with associated subpleural fibrosis concentrated in the upper lobes with less marked or no lower lobe involvement
Consistent with PPFE	Interalveolar fibrosis present, however, not with significant pleural fibrosis, subpleural, distribution, or absent in an upper lobe biopsy	Upper lobe pleural thickening with associated subpleural fibrosis, but not concentrated in the upper lobes or with coexistent disease elsewhere (present elsewhere)
Inconsistent with PPFE	Absence of features in "definite PPFE" and "consistent with PPFE" categories	Absence of features in "definite PPFE" and "consistent with PPFE" categories

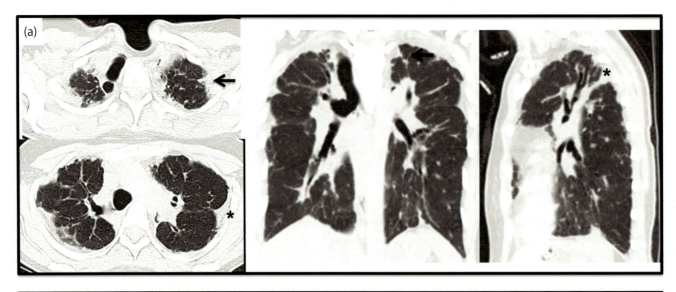
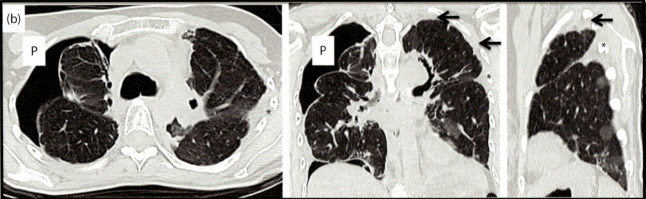

FIGURE 11.1 (a, b) Imaging findings in PPFE include irregular upper lobe pleural thickening (solid arrows) with extension toward the hilum (*) as well as decreased anteroposterior diameter. (a) 32-year-old with a history of intensive chemotherapy for childhood cancer, now with progressive dyspnea on exertion and declining BMI. On exam, she has platythorax and a deep sternal notch. (b) A 56 year old with bone marrow transplant 12 years prior to presentation with progressive dyspnea on exertion and weight loss. The CT demonstrates a spontaneous pneumothorax (P).

juncture of fibrosed and normal lung. Inflammation is generally mild, though may be more prominent surrounding and within pulmonary veins (45).

A usual interstitial pneumonia (UIP) pattern may co-exist in the lower lobes and confers a worse prognosis (35). Key distinguishing features between PPFE and UIP are enumerated in Table 11.3. PPFE associated with post-lung transplant RAS, or post-bone marrow transplant pulmonary GVHD (graft vs. host disease) may have concomitant obliterative bronchiolitis (26). Occasional foci of granulomatous inflammation may be seen in up to 15% of

TABLE 11.3: Distinguishing Features between Histopathological PPFE vs. UIP, and NSIP Patterns

Distribution	UIP Pattern	NSIP Pattern	PPFE Pattern
	Lower lobes initially	Both	Upper lobes
Alveolar structures and fibrosis pattern	Lung parenchyma remodeling. Honeycombing in end-stage fibrosis, effacement of original parenchymal architecture	Diffuse parenchymal involvement not associated with pleural fibrosis (except connective tissue disease related)	Preserved alveolar structure and thickening of the alveoli through elastic fiber deposition. Homogenous intra-alveolar fibrosis
Pleural fibrosis	May be present, with honeycombing	Pleural sparing	Present
Fibroblastic foci	Temporal heterogeneity of fibrosis, interspersed fibroblastic foci near established fibrosis and interspersed normal lung	NSIP, characteristic interstitial process	Homogenous parenchymal distribution, and sparse fibroblastic foci in relation to alveolar walls and the presence of few fibroblastic foci
Elastin van Gieson stain	Sparse, fragmented, and disorganized	Sparse	More marked, especially in relation to the alveolar walls in PPFE. At least double the elastin compared with UIP

Source: Adapted from (31).

TABLE 11.4: **Distinguishing Features between Apical Caps and Pleuroparenchymal Pulmonary Fibroelastosis**

	Apical Caps	PPFE
Age	Older individuals >65 years	Bimodal distribution
Symptoms	Asymptomatic	Progressive
Smoking history	Present	Absent
Pulmonary function	Normal	Restrictive
Extension	Upper <5 cm	May extend beyond
Follow-up radiology	Non-progressive	Progressive
Mass	Localized mass lesion may be associated in apex of upper lobes	Upper lobe pleural thickening with diffuse subpleural fibrosis
Alveolar architecture	Pleural plaques with extensive alveolar collapse	Preservation of alveolar architecture

cases, though it is unclear if this represents a primary or secondary pathology (28).

Intra-alveolar fibrosis (pleural/parenchymal) is not seen in asbestosis, sarcoidosis, or radiation-induced lung disease. However, features unique to these non-PPFE conditions may be present, such as asbestos bodies or sarcoid type granulomas. The distinguishing features between PPFE and a common benign condition of apical caps is reviewed in Table 11.4 (28, 61, 62).

Pulmonary function tests

The pattern of lung function tests in patients with PPFE is unique and has recently been defined with the term "complex restriction" (66). There are key features that help differentiate it from IPF. Due to fibrosis of the upper lobes, the lower lobes may compensate resulting in an increased residual volume/total lung capacity (RV/TLC) ratio, not typically seen in IPF. Forced vital capacity (FVC) and total lung capacity are reduced, consistent with a restrictive pattern, with an increased forced expiratory volume at one second/forced vital capacity (FEV_1/FVC) similar to IPF. Due to the preserved middle and lower lobes, gas transfer tends to be relatively preserved, or mildly reduced even with extensive disease (66).

Over time, the FVC fall in PPFE may become more precipitous compared to the rate of fall for IPF/UIP, with a mean annual FVC loss of 300 mL for patients with PPFE with telomerase mutations vs. 130–210 mL/yr (no mutation) (19). Short telomere syndrome conditions may be associated with an accelerated decline (41).

Biomarkers

Though elevated levels of a few biomarkers (serum and urine) have been identified, their clinical significance, validation and utility are yet to be determined for clinical practice.

- KL-6 is a mucin-like glycoprotein expressed by type II pneumocytes. It is a reliable marker for certain ILDs. It has been found to be normal or near the upper limit of normal in PPFE, with levels that rise with disease progression. While PPFE is an ILD, it is not an interstitial pneumonia like UIP or NSIP. Thus KL-6 levels tend to be higher in UIP/NSIP, as it is associated with inflammatory/fibrosing processes, unlike with PPFE (28).
- Surfactant protein D (SP-D) may also be elevated in PPFE (28).
- LTBP-4 (latent transforming growth factor beta binding protein 4), may help distinguish iPPFE and IPF; levels are higher in iPPFE. Elevation of this marker has been associated with a poorer prognosis (63).
- Depending on whether there is a secondary process, autoantibodies, including rheumatoid factor antineutrophil cytoplasmic antibodies, have also been reported to be associated with PPFE (53, 57, 64).
- Preliminary reports have found urine desmosine to be higher in PPFE vs. IPF, and may be a potentially noninvasive diagnostic tool (65).

Prognosis

The overall prognosis of PPFE is poor. Pneumothorax that fails to resolve despite intervention as well as low BMI are prognostically important for patients with PPFE (67). In an evaluation of PPFE patients on a lung transplant waitlist, a history of pneumothorax and short 6-minute walk test were independently associated with increased mortality (68). Survival across smaller cohorts range between 1.8–14.8 years after diagnosis (28). A larger cohort of 85 patients had a median survival of 11 years, however this was limited by the censoring of 49 patients (8). Patients with iPPFE, were found to have a poorer prognosis than UIP patients for the same gender-age-physiology (GAP) score (69). Enomoto et al. found no difference in survival in PPFE based on the concomitant presence of UIP (36). Post-transplant PPFE, iPPFE, and concomitant UIP also confer a poorer prognosis (25, 37). A survival analysis was performed based on patients with PPFE from four demographic clusters: (1) young male with non-UIP, (2) elderly female non-smoker with low BMI, (3) elderly male smoker with interstitial pneumonia (IP)-like, and (4) younger male smoker with lower lobe lesions (70). Cluster 3 (elderly, men who smoke with IP like features) had the worst outcomes (70). There are no clear guidelines on the best approach to monitor PPFE patients. A proposed follow-up is to check pulmonary function tests every 3–6 months HRCT annually (71). Patients with a family history suggestive of short telomere syndrome should be followed more frequently.

Treatment

No treatment has demonstrated efficacy for PPFE. Empiric low-dose prednisolone has not been formally evaluated, but has a heightened risk of infection, with only one paper reporting benefit (28). Antifibrotic agents have been used on an anecdotal basis, with trial evidence evolving (72, 73). In a trial of 21 patients on nintedanib, nine who received the drug had a significant reduction in their annual relative FVC decline (% predicted), that is, [−13.6 ± 13.4%/year] before nintedanib and [−1.6 ± 6.02%/year] during nintedanib treatment (p = 0.014) (72). An ongoing trial Pirfenidone for Restrictive Chronic Lung Allograft Dysfunction (PIRCLAD), NCT03359863, has demonstrated safety (73, 74).

As for non-pharmacological interventions, in advanced stage, home oxygen therapy is indicated for hypoxemia and pulmonary rehabilitation for functional decline. A follow up of 13 iPPFE patients who participated in a pulmonary rehabilitation demonstrated significant improvement in the 6-minute walk distance as well as quality of life measures (Hospital Anxiety and Depression Scale and and St. George's Respiratory Questionnaire). Recurrent pneumothorax was the most common reason for patients not participating in pulmonary rehabilitation (75). Psychological, nutritional, and palliative support form an ideal part in the care of PPFE.

Lung transplant is currently the only therapeutic option for PPFE. However, extensive pleural thickening may pose technical challenges (32). Additionally, outcomes after transplant are poorer for PPFE patients than with IPF. One year post-transplant, PPFE patients had lower predicted FVCs than patients with IPF (PPFE 48.4% ± 19.5% vs. IPF 68.6% ± 15.5% *P*<0.01) (76). This may be due to extrapulmonary restriction due to platythorax and low BMI. However, in 100 patients (69 IPF, 31 iPPFE), the Kaplan–Meier survival curve did not demonstrate a mortality difference (76). Development of post-transplant PPFE is also a significant risk, with a rate of 7.5% over a 9-year follow-up in a single registry (16).

Conclusion

PPFE is a rare diagnosis, characterized by a distinct pattern of pleural and sub-pleural lung fibrosis, particularly in the upper lobes of the lung. The unique pathology is characterized by an elastotic fibrosing process, associated with IAFE. Treatment approaches are focused on supportive care and transplant evaluation. Novel targeted approaches and evolving interventions are currently under evaluation.

Acknowledgment

Research reported in this publication was supported by the National Heart, Lung, and Blood Institute of the National Institutes of Health under Award Number T32HL007534. The content is solely the responsibility of the authors and does not necessarily represent the official views of the National Institutes of Health.

References

1. Ishii H, Watanabe K, Kushima H, Baba T, Watanabe S, Yamada Y, et al. Pleuroparenchymal fibroelastosis diagnosed by multidisciplinary discussions in Japan. Respir Med. 2018 Aug; 141:190–7.
2. Frankel SK, Cool CD, Lynch DA, Brown KK. Idiopathic pleuroparenchymal fibroelastosis: Description of a novel clinicopathologic entity. Chest. 2004 Dec;126(6):2007–13.
3. Undiagnosable lung disease. Br Med J. 1962 May 19;1(5289):1403–10.
4. Fraisse P, Vandevenne A, Ducolone A, Burghard G. Idiopathic progressive pleuropulmonary fibrosis. Apropos of 2 cases. Rev Pneumol Clin. 1984;40(2):139–43.
5. Kentala E, Repo UK, Lehtipuu AL, Vuornos T. HLA-antigens and pulmonary upper lobe fibrocystic changes with and without ankylosing spondylitis. A report of seven cases. Scand J Respir Dis. 1978 Feb;59(1):8–12.
6. Repo UK, Kentala E, Koistinen J, Lehtipuu AL, Miettinen A, Pyrhönen S, et al. Pulmonary apical fibrocystic disease. A serologic study. Eur J Respir Dis. 1981 Feb;62(1):46–55.
7. Amitani: Idiopathic pulmonary upper lobe fibrosis (IPUF) - Google Scholar [Internet]. [cited 2022 Jan 20]. Available from: https://scholar.google.com/scholar_lookup?journal=Kokyu&title=Idiopathic+pulmonary+upper+lobe+fibrosis&author=R+Amitani&author=A+Niimi&author=F.+Kuse&volume=11&publication_year=1992&pages=693-699&
8. Watanabe K. Pleuroparenchymal fibroelastosis: Its clinical characteristics. Curr Respir Med Rev. 2013 Jun; 9:299–237.
9. Kawabata: Pathology of idiopathic pulmonary upper... Google Scholar [Internet] [cited 2022 Jan 20]. Available from: https://scholar.google.com/scholar_lookup?journal=Nihon+Kyobu+Rinsho.&title=Pathology+of+idiopathic+pulmonary+upper+lobe+fibrosis.&author=Y+Kawabata&author=R+Matsuoka&volume=62&publication_year=0000&pages=S161-S202&
10. Travis WD, Costabel U, Hansell DM, King TE, Lynch DA, Nicholson AG, et al. An official American Thoracic Society/European Respiratory Society Statement: Update of the international multidisciplinary classification of the idiopathic interstitial pneumonias. Am J Respir Crit Care Med. 2013 Sep 15;188(6):733–48.
11. Rosenbaum JN, Butt YM, Johnson KA, Meyer K, Batra K, Kanne JP, et al. Pleuroparenchymal fibroelastosis: A pattern of chronic lung injury. Hum Pathol. 2015 Jan;46(1):137–46.
12. Nakatani T, Arai T, Kitaichi M, Akira M, Tachibana K, Sugimoto C, et al. Pleuroparenchymal fibroelastosis from a consecutive database: A rare disease entity? Eur Respir J. 2015 Apr;45(4):1183–6.
13. Reddy TL, Tominaga M, Hansell DM, von der Thusen J, Rassl D, Parfrey H, et al. Pleuroparenchymal fibroelastosis: A spectrum of histopathological and imaging phenotypes. Eur Respir J. 2012 Aug;40(2):377–85.
14. Tanizawa K, Handa T, Kubo T, Chen-Yoshikawa TF, Aoyama A, Motoyama H, et al. Clinical significance of radiological pleuroparenchymal fibroelastosis pattern in interstitial lung disease patients registered for lung transplantation: A retrospective cohort study. Respir Res. 2018 Aug 30;19(1):162.
15. Shioya M, Otsuka M, Yamada G, Umeda Y, Ikeda K, Nishikiori H, et al. Poorer prognosis of idiopathic pleuroparenchymal fibroelastosis compared with idiopathic pulmonary fibrosis in advanced stage. Can Respir J. 2018; 2018:6043053.
16. Mariani F, Gatti B, Rocca A, Bonifazi F, Cavazza A, Fanti S, et al. Pleuroparenchymal fibroelastosis: The prevalence of secondary forms in hematopoietic stem cell and lung transplantation recipients. Diagn Interv Radiol Ank Turk. 2016 Oct;22(5):400–6.
17. Orlandi M, Landini N, Bruni C, Sambataro G, Nardi C, Bargagli E, et al. Pleuroparenchymal fibroelastosis in rheumatic autoimmune diseases: A systematic literature review. Rheumatol Oxf Engl. 2020 Dec 1;59(12):3645–56.
18. von der Thüsen JH. Pleuroparenchymal fibroelastosis: Its pathological characteristics. Curr Respir Med Rev. 2013 Aug;9(4):238–47.
19. Newton CA, Batra K, Torrealba J, Meyer K, Raghu G, Garcia CK. Pleuroparenchymal fibroelastosis associated with telomerase reverse transcriptase mutations. Eur Respir J. 2017 May;49(5):1700696.
20. Negri EM, Montes GS, Saldiva PH, Capelozzi VL. Architectural remodelling in acute and chronic interstitial lung disease: Fibrosis or fibroelastosis? Histopathology. 2000 Nov;37(5):393–401.
21. Parra ER, Kairalla RA, de Carvalho CRR, Capelozzi VL. Abnormal deposition of collagen/elastic vascular fibres and prognostic significance in idiopathic interstitial pneumonias. Thorax. 2007 May;62(5):428–37.
22. Pierce RA, Albertine KH, Starcher BC, Bohnsack JF, Carlton DP, Bland RD. Chronic lung injury in preterm lambs: Disordered pulmonary elastin deposition. Am J Physiol. 1997 Mar;272(3 Pt 1): L452–60.
23. Raghow R, Kang AH, Pidikiti D. Phenotypic plasticity of extracellular matrix gene expression in cultured hamster lung fibroblasts. Regulation of type I procollagen and fibronectin synthesis. J Biol Chem. 1987 Jun 15;262(17):8409–15.
24. Hirota T, Yoshida Y, Kitasato Y, Yoshimi M, Koga T, Tsuruta N, et al. Histological evolution of pleuroparenchymal fibroelastosis. Histopathology. 2015 Mar;66(4):545–54.
25. Ofek E, Sato M, Saito T, Wagnetz U, Roberts HC, Chaparro C, et al. Restrictive allograft syndrome post lung transplantation is characterized by pleuroparenchymal fibroelastosis. Mod Pathol Off J U S Can Acad Pathol Inc. 2013 Mar;26(3):350–6.
26. Montero MA, Osadolor T, Khiroya R, Salcedo MT, Robertus JL, Rice A, et al. Restrictive allograft syndrome and idiopathic pleuroparenchymal fibroelastosis: Do they really have the Same histology? Histopathology. 2017 Jun;70(7):1107–13.
27. Oo ZP, Bychkov A, Zaizen Y, Yamasue M, Kadota J-I, Fukuoka J. Combination of pleuroparenchymal fibroelastosis with non-specific interstitial pneumonia and bronchiolitis obliterans as a complication of hematopoietic stem cell transplantation - clues to a potential mechanism. Respir Med Case Rep. 2019; 26:244–7.
28. Chua F, Desai SR, Nicholson AG, Devaraj A, Renzoni E, Rice A, et al. Pleuroparenchymal fibroelastosis. A review of clinical, radiological, and pathological characteristics. Ann Am Thorac Soc. 2019 Nov;16(11):1351–9.
29. Kobayashi Y, Sakurai M, Kushiya M, Mizukoshi T, Nishi Y, Choo JH, et al. Idiopathic pulmonary fibrosis of the upper lobe: A case report. Nihon Kokyuki Gakkai Zasshi. 1999 Oct;37(10):812–6.

30. Bondeelle L, Gras J, Michonneau D, Houdouin V, Hermet E, Blin N, et al. Pleuroparenchymal fibroelastosis after allogeneic hematopoietic stem cell transplantation. Bone Marrow Transplant. 2020 May;55(5):982–6.
31. Harada T, Yoshida Y, Kitasato Y, Tsuruta N, Wakamatsu K, Hirota T, et al. The thoracic cage becomes flattened in the progression of pleuroparenchymal fibroelastosis. Eur Respir Rev. 2014 Jun 1;23(132):263–6.
32. Ali MS, Ramalingam VS, Haasler G, Presberg K. Pleuroparenchymal fibroelastosis (PPFE) treated with lung transplantation and review of the literature. BMJ Case Rep. 2019 Apr 20;12(4): e229402.
33. Kono M, Nakamura Y, Enomoto Y, Yasui H, Hozumi H, Karayama M, et al. Pneumothorax in patients with idiopathic pleuroparenchymal fibroelastosis: Incidence, clinical features, and risk factors. Respir Int Rev Thorac Dis. 2021;100(1):19–26.
34. Jacob J, Odink A, Brun AL, Macaluso C, de Lauretis A, Kokosi M, et al. Functional associations of pleuroparenchymal fibroelastosis and emphysema with hypersensitivity pneumonitis. Respir Med. 2018 May; 138:95–101.
35. Oda T, Ogura T, Kitamura H, Hagiwara E, Baba T, Enomoto Y, et al. Distinct characteristics of pleuroparenchymal fibroelastosis with usual interstitial pneumonia compared with idiopathic pulmonary fibrosis. Chest. 2014 Nov;146(5):1248–55.
36. Enomoto Y, Nakamura Y, Satake Y, Sumikawa H, Johkoh T, Colby TV, et al. Clinical diagnosis of idiopathic pleuroparenchymal fibroelastosis: A retrospective multicenter study. Respir Med. 2017 Dec; 133:1–5.
37. von der Thüsen JH, Hansell DM, Tominaga M, Veys PA, Ashworth MT, Owens CM, et al. Pleuroparenchymal fibroelastosis in patients with pulmonary disease secondary to bone marrow transplantation. Mod Pathol Off J U S Can Acad Pathol Inc. 2011 Dec;24(12):1633–9.
38. Konen E, Weisbrod GL, Pakhale S, Chung T, Paul NS, Hutcheon MA. Fibrosis of the upper lobes: A newly identified late-onset complication after lung transplantation? AJR Am J Roentgenol. 2003 Dec;181(6):1539–43.
39. Pakhale SS, Hadjiliadis D, Howell DN, Palmer SM, Gutierrez C, Waddell TK, et al. Upper lobe fibrosis: A novel manifestation of chronic allograft dysfunction in lung transplantation. J Heart Lung Transplant Off Publ Int Soc Heart Transplant. 2005 Sep;24(9):1260–8.
40. Miyamoto A, Uruga H, Morokawa N, Moriguchi S, Takahashi Y, Ogawa K, et al. Various bronchiolar lesions accompanied by idiopathic pleuroparenchymal fibroelastosis with a usual interstitial pneumonia pattern demonstrating acute exacerbation. Intern Med Tokyo Jpn. 2019 May 1;58(9):1321–8.
41. Cecchini MJ, Tarmey T, Ferreira A, Mangaonkar AA, Ferrer A, Patnaik MM, et al. Pathology, radiology, and genetics of interstitial lung disease in patients with shortened telomeres. Am J Surg Pathol. 2021 Jul 1;45(7):871–84.
42. J ER, Robert AH, Bois A. CASE STUDY Familial extensive idiopathic bilateral pleural fibrosis. 1998.
43. Nunes H, Jeny F, Bouvry D, Picard C, Bernaudin J-F, Ménard C, et al. Pleuroparenchymal fibroelastosis associated with telomerase reverse transcriptase mutations. Eur Respir J. 2017 May;49(5):1602022.
44. Piciucchi S, Tomassetti S, Casoni G, Sverzellati N, Carloni A, Dubini A, et al. High-resolution CT and histological findings in idiopathic pleuroparenchymal fibroelastosis: Features and differential diagnosis. Respir Res. 2011 Aug 23; 12:111.
45. Khiroya R, Macaluso C, Montero MA, Wells AU, Chua F, Kokosi M, et al. Pleuroparenchymal fibroelastosis: A review of histopathologic features and the relationship between histologic parameters and survival. Am J Surg Pathol. 2017 Dec;41(12):1683–9.
46. Morales-Ivorra I, Molina-Molina M, Narváez J. Pleuropulmonary fibroelastosis in a patient with systemic lupus erythematosus. Med Clin (Barc). 2019 Jun 21;152(12):513–4.
47. Perruzza M, Fusha E, Cameli P, Capecchi PL, Selvi E, Gentili F, et al. Pleuroparenchymal fibroelastosis (PPFE) associated with giant cell arteritis: A coincidence or a novel phenotype? Respir Med Case Rep. 2019; 27:100843.
48. Enomoto Y, Nakamura Y, Colby TV, Johkoh T, Sumikawa H, Nishimoto K, et al. Radiologic pleuroparenchymal fibroelastosis-like lesion in connective tissue disease-related interstitial lung disease. PloS One. 2017;12(6): e0180283.
49. Bourke S, Campbell J, Henderson AF, Stevenson RD. Apical pulmonary fibrosis in psoriasis. Br J Dis Chest. 1988 Jan; 82:444–6.
50. Oliveira M, Melo N, Mota PC, E Bastos HN, Pereira JM, Carvalho A, et al. Pleuroparenchymal fibroelastosis as another potential lung toxicity pattern induced by amiodarone. Arch Bronconeumol. 2020 Jan;56(1):55–6.
51. Baroke E, Heussel CP, Warth A, Eichinger M, Oltmanns U, Palmowski K, et al. Pleuroparenchymal fibroelastosis in association with carcinomas. Respirol Carlton Vic. 2016 Jan;21(1):191–4.
52. Kronborg-White S, Ravaglia C, Dubini A, Piciucchi S, Tomassetti S, Bendstrup E, et al. Cryobiopsies are diagnostic in pleuroparenchymal and airway-centered fibroelastosis. Respir Res. 2018 Jul 13;19(1):135.
53. Xu L, Rassaei N, Caruso C. Pleuroparenchymal fibroelastosis with long history of asbestos and silicon exposure. Int J Surg Pathol. 2018 Apr;26(2):190–3.
54. Yabuuchi Y, Goto H, Nonaka M, Tachi H, Akiyama T, Arai N, et al. A case of airway aluminosis with likely secondary pleuroparenchymal fibroelastosis. Multidiscip Respir Med. 2019; 14:15.
55. Shintaku M, Takeuchi H, Ando K, Kobayashi Y, Hasegawa H. Amyotrophic lateral sclerosis associated with pleuroparenchymal fibroelastosis. Int J Clin Exp Pathol. 2019;12(10):3956–60.
56. Watanabe K, Ishii H, Kiyomi F, Terasaki Y, Hebisawa A, Kawabata Y, et al. Criteria for the diagnosis of idiopathic pleuroparenchymal fibroelastosis: A proposal. Respir Investig. 2019 Jul;57(4):312–20.
57. Kusagaya H, Nakamura Y, Kono M, Kaida Y, Kuroishi S, Enomoto N, et al. Idiopathic pleuroparenchymal fibroelastosis: Consideration of a clinicopathological entity in a series of Japanese patients. BMC Pulm Med. 2012 Dec 5; 12:72.
58. Reddy TL, Tominaga M, Hansell DM, von der Thusen J, Rassl D, Parfrey H, et al. Pleuroparenchymal fibroelastosis: A spectrum of histopathological and imaging phenotypes. Eur Respir J. 2012 Aug;40(2):377–85.
59. Esteves C, Costa FR, Redondo MT, Moura CS, Guimarães S, Morais A, et al. Pleuroparenchymal fibroelastosis: Role of high-resolution computed tomography (HRCT) and CT-guided transthoracic core lung biopsy. Insights Imaging. 2016 Feb;7(1): 155–62.
60. Hakami A, Zwartkruis E, Radonic T, Nossent EJ, Chua F, Shah PL, et al. Transbronchial cryobiopsy for diagnosis of pleuroparenchymal fibroelastosis. Respir Med Case Rep. 2020; 31:101164.
61. Marinescu D-C, English J, Sedlic T, Kliber A, Ryerson CJ, Wong AW. Pulmonary apical cap as a potential risk factor for pleuroparenchymal fibroelastosis. Chest. 2021 Jun;159(6): e365–70.
62. McLoud TC, Isler RJ, Novelline RA, Putman CE, Simeone J, Stark P. The apical cap. AJR Am J Roentgenol. 1981 Aug;137(2): 299–306.
63. Kinoshita Y, Ikeda T, Kushima H, Fujita M, Nakamura T, Nabeshima K, et al. Serum latent transforming growth factor-β binding protein 4 as a novel biomarker for idiopathic pleuroparenchymal fibroelastosis. Respir Med. 2020 Sep; 171:106077.
64. Yamakawa H, Oda T, Baba T, Ogura T. Pleuroparenchymal fibroelastosis with positive MPO-ANCA diagnosed with a CT-guided percutaneous needle biopsy. BMJ Case Rep. 2018 Feb 24;2018: bcr-2017-223287.
65. Oyama Y, Enomoto N, Suzuki Y, Kono M, Fujisawa T, Inui N, et al. Evaluation of urinary desmosines as a noninvasive diagnostic biomarker in patients with idiopathic pleuroparenchymal fibroelastosis (PPFE). Respir Med. 2017 Feb 1; 123:63–70.
66. Clay RD, Iyer VN, Reddy DR, Siontis B, Scanlon PD. The "Complex restrictive" pulmonary function pattern: Clinical and radiologic analysis of a common but previously undescribed restrictive pattern. Chest. 2017 Dec;152(6):1258–65.
67. Yoshida Y, Nagata N, Tsuruta N, Kitasato Y, Wakamatsu K, Yoshimi M, et al. Heterogeneous clinical features in patients with pulmonary fibrosis showing histology of pleuroparenchymal fibroelastosis. Respir Investig. 2016 May;54(3):162–9.

68. Miyahara S, Waseda R, Tokuishi K, Sato T, Iwasaki A, Shiraishi T. Elucidation of prognostic factors and the effect of anti-fibrotic therapy on waitlist mortality in lung transplant candidates with idiopathic interstitial pneumonias. Respir Investig. 2021 Jul;59(4):428–35.
69. Kato M, Sasaki S, Kurokawa K, Nakamura T, Yamada T, Sasano H, et al. Usual interstitial pneumonia pattern in the lower lung lobes as a prognostic factor in idiopathic pleuroparenchymal fibroelastosis. Respir Int Rev Thorac Dis. 2019;97(4):319–28.
70. Nakamura Y, Mori K, Enomoto Y, Kono M, Sumikawa H, Johkoh T, et al. Prognostic and clinical value of cluster analysis in idiopathic pleuroparenchymal fibroelastosis phenotypes. J Clin Med. 2021 Apr 4;10(7):1498.
71. Cuppens K, Verbeken E, Coolen J, Verschakelen J, Wuyts W. Idiopathic pleuroparenchymatous fibroelastosis: A case report and brief review of the literature. Respir Med Case Rep. 2014; 12:7–9.
72. Nasser M, Si-Mohamed S, Turquier S, Traclet J, Ahmad K, Philit F, et al. Nintedanib in idiopathic and secondary pleuroparenchymal fibroelastosis. Orphanet J Rare Dis. 2021 Oct 9;16(1):419.
73. Sato S, Hanibuchi M, Takahashi M, Fukuda Y, Morizumi S, Toyoda Y, et al. A patient with idiopathic pleuroparenchymal fibroelastosis showing a sustained pulmonary function due to treatment with pirfenidone. Intern Med Tokyo Jpn. 2016;55(5):497–501.
74. Venado A, Dewey K, Montas G, Greenland J, Leard L, Shah R, et al. Safety and tolerability of pirfenidone for restrictive chronic lung allograft dysfunction (PIRCLAD): Interim results. Chest. 2020 Oct 1;158(4): A2389–90.
75. Mori Y, Yamano Y, Kataoka K, Yokoyama T, Matsuda T, Kimura T, et al. Pulmonary rehabilitation for idiopathic pleuroparenchymal fibroelastosis: A retrospective study on its efficacy, feasibility, and safety. Respir Investig. 2021 Nov;59(6):849–58.
76. Shiiya H, Nakajima J, Date H, Chen-Yoshikawa TF, Tanizawa K, Handa T, et al. Outcomes of lung transplantation for idiopathic pleuroparenchymal fibroelastosis. Surg Today. 2021 Aug;51(8):1276–84.

12

IMMUNOGLOBULIN G4-RELATED LUNG DISEASE

Lauren Abplanalp, Hira Iftikhar, and Girish B. Nair

Contents

Introduction 85
Incidence 85
Pathogenesis and risk factors 85
Clinical presentation 86
Imaging patterns of intrathoracic involvement 86
Diagnosis 88
Treatment 89
Conclusion 90
References 90

KEY POINTS

- IgG4-related sclerosing disease is a multi-systemic fibro-inflammatory disease characterized by elevated circulating levels of IgG4, and can affect the pancreas, biliary tract, lung and several other organs of the body.
- IgG4 lung disease may manifest as lung nodules/masses, airway stenosis, pleural nodules/effusion and mediastinal adenopathy/fibrosing mediastinitis.
- Histopathology demonstrates lymphoplasmacytic infiltrate with an increased number of IgG4-positive cells.
- Treatment of IgG4 lung disease typically involves systemic corticosteroids and rarely uses steroid-sparing agents.

Introduction

Immunoglobulin G4-related disease (IgG4-RD) is a rare, systemic fibro-inflammatory disease, characterized by elevated serum IgG4 levels and a histopathology demonstrating lymphoplasmacytic infiltration, fibrosis, and abundant IgG4-positive plasma cells (1). In 2001, Hamano and colleagues noted elevated serum IgG4 levels in patients with sclerosing or autoimmune pancreatitis (2). IgG4-related lesions would subsequently be identified in all organ systems including the biliary system (sclerosing cholangitis), salivary glands (chronic sclerosing sialadenitis or Kuttner tumor), periorbital tissues, liver (inflammatory pseudotumor), kidneys (tubulointerstitial nephritis), lymph nodes, meninges, aorta (inflammatory aneurysm), retroperitoneum (retroperitoneal fibrosis), breast, prostate, thyroid gland, pericardium and skin (3–5). Pulmonary involvement in IgG4-RD was first reported as two case reports of interstitial pneumonia (6, 7). The intrathoracic manifestations of IgG4-RD include interstitial lung disease, lung nodules and masses, bronchial inflammatory changes, mediastinal fibrosis and pleuritis with effusion. Lung involvement may occur in isolation or with other organ involvement and is sometimes difficult to distinguish from malignancy by imaging alone. In this chapter, we describe the characteristic features, diagnosis and treatment options in IgG4-related lung disease.

Incidence

The incidence and prevalence of pulmonary involvement in IgG4-RD remains unknown. Frequency of pulmonary involvement cited in the literature ranges widely from 12.5–51% (5). In a cross-sectional study of 114 patients with IgG4-RD, 16 (14%) were found to have lung or pleural involvement. Age of included patients ranged from 42 to 79, with a median age of 64 years; most studies reported a male predominance of 75–86% for all organ systems with the exception of head and neck involvement (8).

Pathogenesis and risk factors

The pathogenesis of IgG4-RD remains poorly understood. It has been suggested that IgG4 serves as a surrogate marker rather than playing a primary role in pathogenesis (9). T-helper 2 cells (Th2), regulatory T cells and interleukin-10 have been shown to participate in IgG-4 plasma cell infiltration and fibrogenesis; however, the role of Th2 in particular may be overstated and actually be a reflection of atopy alone (8, 10). CD4-positive cytotoxic T lymphocytes (CTLs) have been identified as the major CD4 subset noted in affected tissue and lead to the secretion of pro-fibrotic cytokines including IL-1 β, transforming growth factor-beta 1 (TGF- β1) and interferon-gamma (IFN- γ) (10). Circulating plasmablasts are also increased in patients with active, untreated IgG4-RD and may suggest disease activity due to their reduction with B-cell depletion therapy (10, 11).

The IgG4 isotype is the least abundant subclass, accounting for less than 5% of the total serum IgG4. Its unique properties arise from the fragment antigen-binding (Fab) arm exchange and dissociation of disulfide bonds between its heavy chains. This process results in the antibody's inability to cross-link antigens and form immune complexes. While the physiologic utility remains unknown, another unique property of IgG4 is its ability to bind to the Fc portion of IgG4. This interaction may assist in an anti-inflammatory function (11). A role in the activation of complement by IgG4 has also been implied, but the mechanism remains unknown (12). Genetic susceptibility has been cited with certain human leukocyte antigen (HLA) haplotypes, particularly in Japanese and Korean populations (13).

A higher incidence of pulmonary and extrapulmonary malignancies including lung, colon, prostate, endometrial, renal, gastric and lymphoma have been suggested; however, for unclear reasons. Studies examining patients with lung cancer and cholangiocarcinoma have documented an increase in IgG4 levels and IgG4 plasmacytic infiltrates in and around the tumor. Fujimoto et al. retrospectively analyzed histopathologic specimens in 294 patients with surgically resected lung cancer. In that study, 12% of patients with non-small cell carcinoma had >20 IgG4-positive cells/high power field and 97% of these patients had obliterative phlebitis or arteritis, the distinguishing feature of IgG4-RD. The absence of IgG4-RD pathology in non-neoplastic tissue and absence of systemic IgG4-RD features led the authors to conclude that the IgG4 response was secondary to an unidentified antigen. This increase in IgG4-positive cells was associated with disease-free survival in stage I squamous cell carcinoma and prompted speculation of a protective role in malignancy (5, 14). No environmental or occupational risk factors have been studied (15).

Clinical presentation

Between 53–75% of patients are asymptomatic, with a suspected diagnosis noted on incidental abnormal imaging (15, 16). When symptoms are present, they are largely nonspecific. In a prospective cohort of 248 patients with IgG4-RD, 27 (31%) patients had respiratory symptoms with 23/27 having cough and two cases with dyspnea or chest pain, respectively (16). When compared to patients without intrathoracic disease, IgG4-RD intrathoracic disease had a higher possibility of fever, allergy and more than three extra-thoracic organs involved. Nineteen percent of patients with respiratory symptoms had a history of asthma (1). Similarly, a cross-sectional study demonstrated that 19% of patients with IgG4-RD carried a diagnosis of allergic disorders, including bronchial asthma, sinusitis or allergic rhinitis (8). These diagnoses or asthma-like symptoms may precede the diagnosis of IgG4-RD by months or years (14).

Imaging patterns of intrathoracic involvement

Major pulmonary manifestations are summarized in Table 12.1 and Figures 12.1–12.4.

Parenchymal disease

Lung parenchymal involvement in IgG4-RD can be divided into four major radiographic subtypes: solid nodular type (solid nodular lesions including mass), round shaped ground-glass opacity, alveolar interstitial and bronchovascular type (1, 4, 9). Rounded opacities may appear solid or with ground-glass attenuation and range in size from 0.9 to 5 cm in diameter. Single or multiple rounded nodular opacities may be evident on chest imaging without lobar predilection and along the periphery or involving the hilar bronchus (17). Malignancy, including adenocarcinoma in-situ, is often suspected in the rounded nodular subtype, particularly when presenting as a focal spiculated appearance. As such, some patients have undergone partial resection or lobectomy due to suspicion of malignancy on initial presentation (4).

The alveolar interstitial subtype is radiographically characterized by diffuse ground-glass attenuation in the mid and lower lung zones with accompanying honeycombing (4). Other case reports have cited accompanying bronchiectasis, ill-defined lower lobe predominant consolidation and reticular opacities disease (18, 19). A differential diagnosis of such a presentation will include non-specific interstitial pneumonia, idiopathic interstitial pneumonia and usual interstitial pneumonia.

Radiographic findings of the bronchovascular type involve thickening of the bronchovascular bundles and interlobular septa.

TABLE 12.1: Imaging Patterns of Pulmonary Involvement in IgG4-Related Disease

Parenchymal
    Solitary or multiple nodules
    Solitary or multiple masses
    Nodular or diffuse ground-glass opacities
    Consolidation, often lower lobe predominant
    Reticular opacities
    Thickened bronchovascular bundles
    Thickened interlobular septa
Airway
    Bronchiectasis
    Large central airway stenosis
Pleural Disease
    Nodular lesions along parietal or visceral pleura
    Pleural thickening
    Pleural effusion
Mediastinal Disease
    Mediastinal and/or hilar lymphadenopathy
    Fibrosing mediastinitis

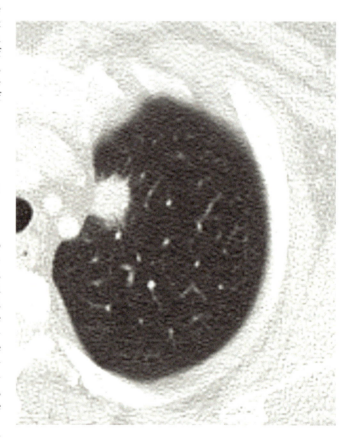

FIGURE 12.1 CT imaging of the left lung in a 39-year-old woman with IgG4-related lung disease presenting as a 1.7 cm spiculated nodule.

Immunoglobulin G4-Related Lung Disease

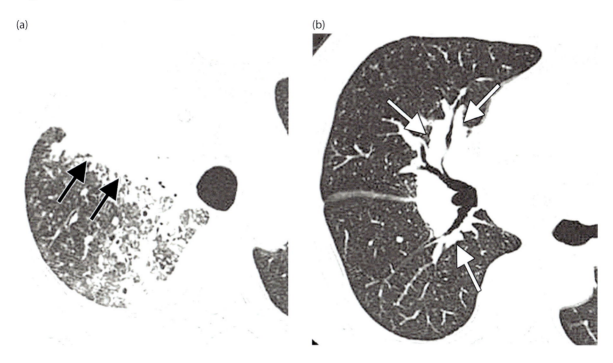

FIGURE 12.2 (a, b) CT imaging of the right lung in a 70-year-old man with IgG4-related lung disease. (a) Arrows outline a mass in the right upper lobe with surrounding ground-glass opacities. (b) Thickening of bronchovascular bundles in the right hilum. (Image republished with permission from RSNA. Inoue D, et al. Immunoglobulin G4-related lung disease: CT findings with pathologic correlations. Radiology. 2009;251[1]:260–70.)

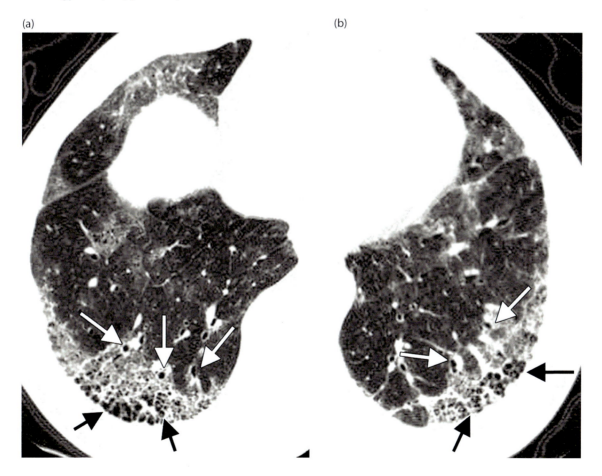

FIGURE 12.3 (a, b) CT imaging of bilateral lower lobes in a 59-year-old man with IgG4-related lung disease showing honeycombing (black arrows) and bronchiectasis (white arrows). Diffuse ground-glass opacities are found in the bilateral middle and lower lobes. (Image republished with permission from RSNA.)

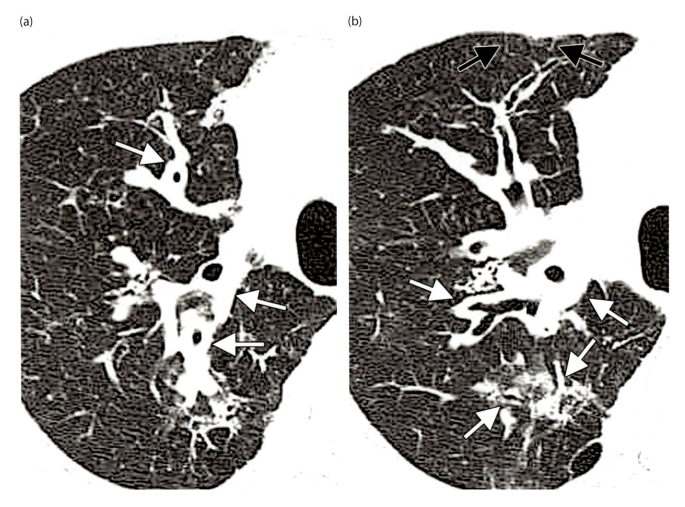

FIGURE 12.4 (a, b) CT imaging of the right lung in a 59-year-old man with IgG4-related disease demonstrated by thickening of the bronchovascular bundles (white arrows). Thickening of interlobular septa noted (black arrows). (Images republished with permission from RSNA. Inoue D, et al. Immunoglobulin G4-related lung disease: CT findings with pathologic correlations. Radiology. 2009;251[1]:260–70.)

Small centrilobular nodules related to hypertrophy of mucosa-associated lymphoid tissue may be present. As above, the differential diagnosis will include lymphoproliferative disorders such as multicentric Castleman disease, sarcoidosis, malignant lymphoma, granulomatosis with polyangiitis, lymphomatoid granulomatosis and lung cancer (lymphangitis carcinoma) with such a presentation (4, 20).

Airway disease
Airway involvement more often occurs in the context of pulmonary parenchymal infiltration. Isolated case reports have documented large central airway stenosis and obstruction as a sequela of mediastinal adenopathy or fibrosis (14).

Pleural disease
Nodular lesions can develop along the visceral or parietal pleural (9). When the parietal pleura is involved, sclerosing inflammation extends into the subpleural fibrous and adipose tissue. Whereas visceral lesions involve the subpleural lung parenchyma cavity (21). Pleural effusion as a presenting finding has been reported in a few case reports, although rare.

Mediastinal disease
The most common intrathoracic finding is mediastinal and/or hilar lymphadenopathy, which has been described in 40–90% of patients.

Multiple lymph nodes are often involved with the most common being mediastinal followed by intra-abdominal and axillary. Lymph nodes are generally less than 2 cm with most lying near the affected organ (9, 21).

Diagnosis

The diagnosis of IgG4-RD relies on clinical, radiological and histopathological findings. The Japanese and Boston criteria are both used for the diagnosis of IgG4-RD (Tables 12.2 and 12.3). The Japanese criteria includes a clinical examination, elevated serum IgG4 concentration (>135 mg/dL), and histopathological examination including marked lymphocyte, plasmacytic infiltration, fibrosis and/or elevated ratio of IgG4+/IgG+ cells >40% (22–24). IgG4-RD is definitively diagnosed in patients who fulfill all three revised comprehensive diagnostic (RCD) criteria. Patients who fulfill criteria points 1) and 3) are diagnosed with probable and possible if criteria points 1) and 2) are fulfilled (25). Organ-specific criteria reinforces the RCD and as such, patients diagnosed with probable or possible, but meet organ-specific criteria for IgG4-RD, are subsequently diagnosed as definite IgG4-RD.

The Boston criteria, although non-organ specific, relies on histological features including lymphoplasmacytic inflammation, fibrosis and obliterative venulitis (17). A tissue biopsy to exclude

TABLE 12.2: The Japanese 2020 Revised Comprehensive Diagnostic (RCD) Criteria for IgG4-RD

1. Clinical and radiological features show diffuse/localized swelling or a mass or nodule in single or multiple organs
2. Serum IgG4 levels >135 mg/dL
3. Histopathological examination shows two of the three following criteria:
   - Dense lymphocyte and plasma cell infiltration with fibrosis
   - Ratio of IgG4-positive plasma cell infiltration with fibrosis
   - Typical tissue fibrosis, particularly storiform fibrosis, or obliterative phlebitis
- Definite: 1 + 2 + 3
- Probable: 1 + 3
- Possible: 1 + 2

TABLE 12.3: The Boston Consensus Criteria

Requires the presence of the following histological feature triad:
1. Lymphoplasmacytic inflammation
2. Fibrosis, usually a storiform pattern
3. Obliterative venulitis

malignancy and other IgG4-mimickers is recommended by the 2012 international consensus (22, 23). Major histopathologic features include dense lymphoplasmacytic infiltrate with IgG4-positive plasma cells, storiform or whorled fibrosis and obliterative phlebitis (Figure 12.5) (14). A tissue IgG4+/IgG+ plasma cell ratio of greater than 40 has a sensitivity of 94.4% and specificity of 85.7% in the diagnosis (24).

IgG4 elevation is encountered in approximately 5% of the normal population and other respiratory conditions including bronchiectasis, asthma, idiopathic pulmonary fibrosis and hypersensitivity pneumonitis (15). An elevated serum IgG4 cutoff of >135 mg/dL has been shown to have a sensitivity of 97% and specificity of 79.6% for the diagnosis of IgG4-RD (24). However, the sensitivity and specificity of the IgG4 level with relation to the diagnosis of intrathoracic disease is unknown (16). This plasma cell concentration is reduced in fibrotic tissue (24).

Bronchoalveolar lavage (BAL) IgG4 level has been suggested as an additional diagnostic tool. The BAL IgG4 level when compared in patients with autoimmune pancreatitis and pulmonary sarcoidosis correlated with the serum IgG4 level (26). The cellular analysis typically reveals a lymphocyte predominant picture. A transbronchial biopsy cannot be used to confirm the diagnosis with rare reporting in case reports.

Pulmonary function testing as a diagnostic tool for IgG4-RD remains unknown. In a clinical review of 16/52 (31%) patients with lung involvement and IgG4-RD, a median diffusion capacity of 41.8% was noted. The severity of the diffusion impairment, which may be dependent on the extent of lymphoplasmacytic infiltration in the alveolar or interlobular septa, can be used as a disease predictor and therapeutic marker (20).

Treatment

Glucocorticoids are recommended as a first-line agent for remission induction. While the optimal dose remains unclear, the international consensus recommends prednisolone 0.6 mg/kg for 2–4 weeks. The dose should then be tapered to 5 mg/day over 3–6 months and then to 2.5–5 mg/day for 3 years (27, 28). Maintenance therapy at 5–10 mg/day was shown to reduce the relapse rate in patients with pancreatic manifestation (3). IgG4-related pulmonary disease has variable response to glucocorticoids. Solitary pulmonary nodules were more refractory to corticosteroid and immunosuppressant therapy when compared to patients with interstitial lung disease, mediastinal mass and bronchial thickening (1). As a subtype, the alveolar consolidative type when treated with corticosteroid therapy alone demonstrated the highest complete response rate with alveolar interstitial type showing the least (29).

Immunosuppressant therapy

Azathioprine, mycophenolate mofetil and rituximab have been used; however, their efficacy has been limited to small

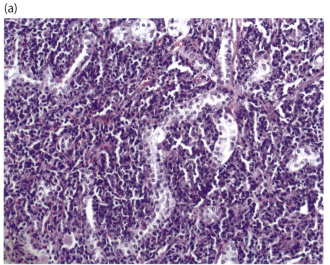
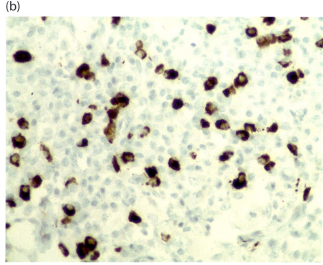

FIGURE 12.5 (a, b) Histologic findings of a 39-year-old woman with IgG-related lung disease presenting as a solitary nodule. (a) There is a marked lymphoplasmacytic inflammatory infiltrate (hematoxylin-eosin stain, original magnification, 20×). (b) IgG4 immunostain showing a large number of IgG4 staining plasma cells (immunohistochemistry staining). (Image courtesy of Dr. Said Hafeez-Khayatta, Department of Pathology, Beaumont Health.)

retrospective case series and reports (22). The protease inhibitor bortezomib has been suggested as a possible therapy due to its benefit in treating multiple myeloma and other B-cell neoplasia. Similar benefits were also seen with cyclophosphamide (30).

Relapse and prognosis

Relapse rates vary across studies, occurring in 25–50% of patients (14). Relapse occurs at a median time of 38 months from glucocorticoid induction. Retreatment with glucocorticoids is indicated in patients with a relapse off treatment and an introduction of a steroid-sparing agent should be considered for continuation of the remission maintenance (22).

The prognosis of IgG4-RD remains ill-defined. IgG4, C3 and C4 have been proposed as prognostic biomarkers (31).

Conclusion

IgG4-RD is a disease known by many names. This heterogenous disease affecting multiple organs by the formation of tumefactive lesions, a dense lymphoplasmacytic infiltrate rich in IgG4 plasma cells and fibrosis. If fibrosis has not set in, immunosuppressants can be helpful. Just like sarcoidosis, it affects many organs but is distinguished by the distinctive histology, which is its hallmark feature despite the organ it involves.

References

1. Fei Y, Shi J, Lin W, Chen Y, Feng R, Wu Q, et al. Intrathoracic involvements of immunoglobulin G4-related sclerosing disease. Medicine (Baltimore). 2015;94(50):e2150.
2. Hamano H, Kawa S, Horiuchi A, Unno H, Furuya N, Akamatsu T, et al. High serum IgG4 concentrations in patients with sclerosing pancreatitis. N Engl J Med. 2001;344(10):732–8.
3. Sekiguchi H, Horie R, Aksamit TR, Yi ES, Ryu JH. Immunoglobulin G4-related disease mimicking asthma. Can Respir J. 2013; 20(2):87–9.
4. Inoue D, Zen Y, Abo H, Gabata T, Demachi H, Kobayashi T, et al. Immunoglobulin G4-related lung disease: CT findings with pathologic correlations. Radiology. 2009;251(1):260–70.
5. Fujimoto M, Yoshizawa A, Sumiyoshi S, Sonobe M, Kobayashi M, Koyanagi I, et al. Stromal plasma cells expressing immunoglobulin G4 subclass in non-small cell lung cancer. Hum Pathol. 2013;44(8):1569–76.
6. Taniguchi T, Ko M, Seko S, Nishida O, Inoue F, Kobayashi H, et al. Interstitial pneumonia associated with autoimmune pancreatitis. Gut. 2004;53(5):770–71
7. Nieminen U, Koivisto T, Kahri A, Farkkila M. Sjögren's syndrome with chronic pancreatitis, sclerosing cholangitis, and pulmonary infiltrations. Am J Gastroenterol. 1997;92(1):139–42.
8. Zen Y, Nakanuma Y. IgG4-related disease: A cross-sectional study of 114 cases. Am J Surg Pathol. 2010;34(12):1812–9.
9. Cheuk W, Chan JK. IgG4-related sclerosing disease: A critical appraisal of an evolving clinicopathologic entity. Adv Anat Pathol. 2010;17(5):303–32.
10. Mattoo H, Stone JH, Pillai S. Clonally expanded cytotoxic CD4(+) T cells and the pathogenesis of IgG4-related disease. Autoimmunity. 2017;50(1):19–24.
11. Wolfson AR, Hamilos DL. Recent advances in understanding and managing IgG4-related disease. F1000Res. 2017;6.
12. Sugimoto M, Watanabe H, Asano T, Sato S, Takagi T, Kobayashi H, et al. Possible participation of IgG4 in the activation of complement in IgG4-related disease with hypocomplementemia. Mod Rheumatol. 2016;26(2):251–8.
13. Stone JH. IgG4-related disease: Nomenclature, clinical features, and treatment. Semin Diagn Pathol. 2012;29(4):177–90.
14. Raj R. IgG4-related lung disease. Am J Respir Crit Care Med. 2013;188(5):527–9.
15. Campbell SN, Rubio E, Loschner AL. Clinical review of pulmonary manifestations of IgG4-related disease. Ann Am Thorac Soc. 2014;11(9):1466–75.
16. Ryu JH, Sekiguchi H, Yi ES. Pulmonary manifestations of immunoglobulin G4-related sclerosing disease. Eur Respir J. 2012;39(1):180–6.
17. Deshpande V, Zen Y, Chan JK, Yi EE, Sato Y, Yoshino T, et al. Consensus statement on the pathology of IgG4-related disease. Mod Pathol. 2012;25(9):1181–92.
18. Kobayashi H, Shimokawaji T, Kanoh S, Motoyoshi K, Aida S. IgG4-positive pulmonary disease. J Thorac Imaging. 2007;22(4):360–2.
19. Yamashita K, Haga H, Kobashi Y, Miyagawa-Hayashino A, Yoshizawa A, Manabe T. Lung involvement in IgG4-related lymphoplasmacytic vasculitis and interstitial fibrosis: Report of 3 cases and review of the literature. Am J Surg Pathol. 2008;32(11):1620–6.
20. Saraya T, Ohkuma K, Fujiwara M, Miyaoka C, Wada S, Watanabe T, et al. Clinical characterization of 52 patients with immunoglobulin G4-related disease in a single tertiary center in Japan: Special reference to lung disease in thoracic high-resolution computed tomography. Respir Med. 2017;132:62–7.
21. Zen Y, Inoue D, Kitao A, Onodera M, Abo H, Miyayama S, et al. IgG4-related lung and pleural disease: A clinicopathologic study of 21 cases. Am J Surg Pathol. 2009;33(12):1886–93.
22. Khosroshahi A, Wallace ZS, Crowe JL, Akamizu T, Azumi A, Carruthers MN, et al. International consensus guidance statement on the management and treatment of IgG4-related disease. Arthritis Rheumatol. 2015;67(7):1688–99.
23. Umehara H, Okazaki K, Masaki Y, Kawano M, Yamamoto M, Saeki T, et al. A novel clinical entity, IgG4-related disease (IgG4RD): General concept and details. Mod Rheumatol. 2012;22(1):1–14.
24. Masaki Y, Kurose N, Yamamoto M, Takahashi H, Saeki T, Azumi A, et al. Cutoff values of serum IgG4 and histopathological IgG4+ plasma cells for diagnosis of patients with IgG4-related disease. Int J Rheumatol. 2012;2012:580814.
25. Umehara H, Okazaki K, Kawa S, Takahashi H, Goto H, Matsui S, et al. The 2020 revised comprehensive diagnostic (RCD) criteria for IgG4-RD. Mod Rheumatol. 2021;31(3):529–33.
26. Tsushima K, Tanabe T, Yamamoto H, Koizumi T, Kawa S, Hamano H, et al. Pulmonary involvement of autoimmune pancreatitis. Eur J Clin Invest. 2009;39(8):714–22.
27. Kamisawa T, Okazaki K, Kawa S, Shimosegawa T, Tanaka M, Research Committee for Intractable Pancreatic D, et al. Japanese consensus guidelines for management of autoimmune pancreatitis: III. Treatment and prognosis of AIP. J Gastroenterol. 2010;45(5):471–7.
28. Kamisawa T, Zen Y, Pillai S, Stone JH. IgG4-related disease. Lancet. 2015;385(9976):1460–71.
29. Kang J, Park S, Chae EJ, Song JS, Hwang HS, Kim SJ, et al. Long-term clinical course and outcomes of immunoglobulin G4-related lung disease. Respir Res. 2020;21(1):273.
30. Khan ML, Colby TV, Viggiano RW, Fonseca R. Treatment with bortezomib of a patient having hyper IgG4 disease. Clin Lymphoma Myeloma Leuk. 2010;10(3):217–9.
31. Tang J, Cai S, Ye C, Dong L. Biomarkers in IgG4-related disease: A systematic review. Semin Arthritis Rheum. 2020;50(2):354–9.

13

EOSINOPHILIC LUNG DISEASES

Nauman A. Khan and Sujith V. Cherian

Contents

Introduction 91
Acute eosinophilic pneumonia 91
Chronic eosinophilic pneumonia 93
Eosinophilic granulomatosis with polyangiitis 95
Parasitic infection causing eosinophilic pneumonia 96
Tropical pulmonary eosinophilia 96
Drug-induced eosinophilic lung disease 96
References 98

KEY POINTS

- Eosinophilic lung diseases are a group of disorders characterized by the presence and presumed pathogenic role of eosinophils, which can be classified phenotypically into (a) predominant airway involvement or (b) predominant parenchymal involvement.
- These are mainly represented by eosinophilic pneumonias, defined by a prominent infiltration of lung parenchyma by eosinophils, which generally heal without significant sequelae.
- Eosinophilic pneumonia may be acute, chronic, or present transiently known as Loeffler syndrome.
- Diagnosis of eosinophilic pneumonia is based on characteristic imaging patterns and the demonstration of eosinophilia in bronchoalveolar lavage during bronchoscopy with >25% eosinophils.
- While peripheral eosinophilia is seen in most of these diseases, it may be absent in idiopathic acute eosinophilic pneumonia initially.
- Loeffler syndrome represents the most common cause of eosinophilic pneumonia worldwide.
- Chronic eosinophilic pneumonia is usually idiopathic while acute eosinophilic pneumonia is often related to drug or tobacco smoke exposure.
- An extensive search for possible etiologies including parasitic and fungal infections, drug exposure and occupational exposures should be performed during evaluation of any patient presenting with eosinophilic lung diseases.

Introduction

Eosinophilic lung diseases are characterized by lung infiltrates accompanied by pulmonary or peripheral eosinophilia (>500 × 10^9 cells/L). The diseases that comprise the group have varying etiologies and can be subtyped into primary and secondary eosinophilic lung diseases (1). Infections, interstitial lung processes, and inflammatory etiologies including autoimmune diseases can be associated with pulmonary eosinophilia, while in some cases no etiology is identified (2) (Table 13.1). Eosinophilic lung diseases can also be classified by phenotype based on anatomy — some forms of eosinophilic lung disease primarily cause airway involvement while others involve the pulmonary parenchyma (3). It is important to subtype eosinophilic lung disorders as treatment and prognosis vary.

Eosinophils are granulocytes and derive from pluripotent CD34+ granulocyte progenitor cells (4). Their primary function is thought to be modulation of innate and adaptive immunity in response to infections, most prominently parasitic infections. They contain granules — primary and secondary that contain numerous mediators that can directly and indirectly lead to inflammation and tissue damage (5). Secondary granules contain mediators such as major basic protein (MBP), cytokines, chemokines, and other factors (6). Eosinophilic lung diseases occur when there is dysregulation of these processes that leads to abnormal airway and parenchymal injury. Primary granules are also known to cause eosinophilic inflammation, because they contain the protein galactin-10, which is responsible for the formation of Charcot-Leyden crystals (7). The chapter's focus is on eosinophilic pneumonias of various types but will not discuss eosinophilic lung diseases with primary airway involvement (Chapter 7).

Acute eosinophilic pneumonia

Acute eosinophilic pneumonia (AEP) was first described in 1989 and is a process that leads to acute respiratory distress syndrome which is typically rapidly progressive (8, 9). AEP is a rare disorder and its incidence is not well-established. Some studies in military personnel report between 9–11 cases per 100,000 person-years, although this is presumed to be predominantly smoking-related AEP (10, 11). It has a strong association with smoking, at times with recent initiation or change in smoking habits (11–14). A recent study noted about one-third of AEP cases to be related to smoking followed by 17% as medication related (15).

AEP can be divided based on etiology into idiopathic and known causes. Known causes include drugs, exposure to inhalants

TABLE 13.1: Eosinophilic Lung Disease Classification by Etiology

Eosinophilic Pneumonia without Known Cause
- Idiopathic acute eosinophilic pneumonia
- Idiopathic chronic eosinophilic pneumonia

Eosinophilic Pneumonia with Known Cause
- Eosinophilic granulomatous polyangiitis
- Drug-induced eosinophilic pneumonia
- Simple pulmonary eosinophilia from parasitic infection

Other Pulmonary Diseases Associated with Eosinophilia
- Organizing pneumonia
- Nonspecific interstitial pneumonia
- Idiopathic pulmonary fibrosis
- Langerhans cell histiocytosis

including cigarette smoking, and infections (10, 12, 15–17). There are several proposed theories for the pathogenesis of AEP, although no explanation is thought to be complete. One likely mechanism is that a Type I hypersensitivity reaction occurs in response to exposure to an external agent (18, 19). Another proposed sequence of events is exposure to a pathogen causing direct injury to various cells including epithelial cells in airways and lung parenchyma that cause production of factors that recruit eosinophils. IL-33 is thought to have an important role in initiating these inflammatory processes (20, 21). Once activated, these eosinophils degranulate and release mediators of inflammation, which causes direct injury to the surrounding lung parenchyma. This can manifest as protein spilling into the alveolar spaces and interstitium as well as induction of surfactant-associated proteins (22–24).

Clinical features

AEP is more common in males, typically between 20–40 years of age with a history of smoking (8–10, 12, 16, 25) (Table 13.2). Onset is usually acute, ranging from days to weeks (16, 25). Nonproductive cough and dyspnea are the most common presenting symptoms (13, 26, 27), and constitutional symptoms including fever can be present (27, 28). Physical examination shows inspiratory crackles and rhonchi. Pleural effusions may be present in some cases (29). In severe disease, acute hypoxemic respiratory failure ensues, and mechanical ventilation may be needed (10, 16). Laboratory studies can show neutrophilic or eosinophilic leukocytosis, which is usually a delayed manifestation (10, 25). Absence of eosinophilia has been reported to be more common in AEP associated with smoking compared with other etiologies (15). Inflammatory markers such as erythrocyte sedimentation rates (ESR) and C-reactive protein (CRP) levels may be elevated. Serum IgE levels may be elevated but its utility may be questionable (26, 30, 31).

Bronchoscopy with broncho-alveolar lavage (BAL) shows a cell count differential of >25% eosinophils often with lymphocytosis and neutrophilia (10, 16, 25). Pleural fluid analysis in the case of associated pleural effusion is exudative and can reveal eosinophilia (>10% eosinophils in pleural fluid cell count) (15). A pulmonary function testing (PFT) (although not able to be performed in most cases) shows a restrictive process with a reduced diffusion capacity of carbon monoxide (DLCO) (31).

TABLE 13.2: Features of Acute Eosinophilic Pneumonia (AEP), Chronic Eosinophilic Pneumonia (CEP), and Eosinophilic Granulomatosis with Polyangiitis (EGPA)

	Acute Eosinophilic Pneumonia	Chronic Eosinophilic Pneumonia	Eosinophilic GPA
Demographic	20–40s, male predominance	40–50s, female predominance	40s and 50s, no gender predilection
Onset	Days–weeks	Weeks–months	Days–months
Association with asthma	No	Yes	Yes, often poorly controlled
Association with smoking	Yes	No	No
Clinical features	Severe cases may develop hypoxemic respiratory failure and ARDS	Respiratory failure less common	Respiratory failure less common
Imaging	Bilateral reticular progressing to alveolar opacities. Diffuse alveolar hemorrhage possible	Peripheral, upper lobe predominant	Migratory, diffuse peripheral ground-glass opacities, bronchial wall thickening may be present
Labs	Peripheral eosinophilia usually absent initially but may develop after a few days	Peripheral eosinophilia frequent	Significant eosinophilia on presentation. MPO-ANCA positivity in some cases. Cardiovascular, neurological, and renal dysfunction possible
BAL	Cell count >25% eosinophils	Cell count >40% eosinophils	Cell counts >40% eosinophils
Histopathology	Clinical condition precludes biopsy in most patients. Diffuse alveolar damage along with interstitial and alveolar eosinophilic infiltration	Alveolar, interstitial inflammation with eosinophilic predominance	Granulomas, perivascular inflammation, fibrinoid necrosis noted
Treatment	Glucocorticoid course for 2 weeks. For severe respiratory failure, high dose and frequency, IV route preferred	Glucocorticoid course for few months, with high rates of recurrence when stopped	Glucocorticoids, cyclophosphamide in severe disease
Alternative treatment	Not studied[a]	Anti-IgE, Anti-IL5 agents under study	Anti-CD-20 therapy or anti-IL-5 therapy, IVIG used in refractory cases
Response/Prognosis	Very good. Relapses may be seen with resumption of cigarette smoking.	Rapid response is usually seen, relapses are frequent requiring prolonged immunosuppression. Progression to fibrosis seen rarely	Response usually good, relapses not very common

[a] Given rapid improvement with corticosteroids and severe hypoxemic respiratory failure at presentation in most patients, studies on alternative therapies are unlikely to occur due to ethical concerns.

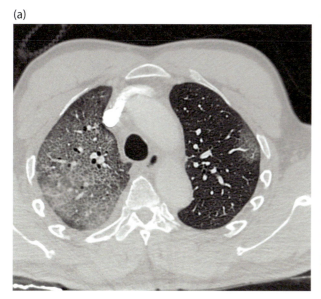 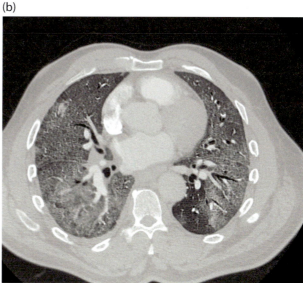

FIGURE 13.1 A 53-year-old man was admitted with acute onset of shortness of breath with a history of crack cocaine abuse. Initially considered to be pulmonary edema, the patient was treated with diuretics without improvement, after which a bronchoscopy was performed, which was consistent with acute eosinophilic pneumonia. Chest CT scans in axial view show bilateral diffuse ground-glass opacities, interlobular septal thickening, and consolidative opacities more over the lower lobes (a) as compared to the upper lobes (b).

Imaging
Chest radiography shows bilateral infiltrates, initially reticular, that progress into alveolar opacities (16, 25, 32). CT chest shows ground-glass opacities (Figure 13.1) and interlobular septal thickening (22, 32, 33). Centrilobular nodules and pleural effusion may be present in AEP from smoking (15, 22, 34).

Histopathology
AEP is characterized on histopathology by significant eosinophils within alveolar spaces, airways, and interstitium to varying degrees. Alveolar involvement can include significant eosinophilic infiltration, hyperplasia of type II pneumocytes, and in advanced disease, fibrinous exudate accumulation and diffuse alveolar damage including hyaline membrane (25, 27, 31). Increased edema within pulmonary interstitium due to eosinophilic and lymphocytic infiltration may be seen (24, 26).

Diagnosis
Diagnosis of AEP currently utilizes the modified Philit criteria including: 1) acute respiratory illness of one month or less duration, 2) pulmonary infiltrates on chest imaging, 3) pulmonary eosinophilia including greater than 25% eosinophils in BAL fluid or eosinophilic pneumonia on lung biopsy, and 4) exclusion of other pulmonary eosinophilic diseases including eosinophilic granulomatosis with polyangiitis (EGPA), allergic bronchopulmonary aspergillosis (ABPA), and hypereosinophilic syndrome (12, 15).

Treatment and prognosis
Treatment in AEP associated with exposures is the elimination of such exposures. In some cases, the disease is self-limited (12, 13, 16, 25, 30, 31). In cases determined to require intervention, mainstay of treatment is systemic glucocorticoid therapy (16, 25, 35). Supportive management in severe cases may include oxygen supplementation and hospitalization at times requiring mechanical ventilation. In case of infection-related AEP, treatment is an antimicrobial agent targeting the isolated microorganism (15).

Glucocorticoid therapy dosage and duration varies on an individual basis. Higher doses, up to intravenous methylprednisolone at 60 mg or greater every 6 hours, are commonly used for severe respiratory failure requiring mechanical ventilation (15). In less severe cases, oral prednisone is used at 40–60 mg daily (12). Glucocorticoid therapy is tapered slowly over 2–4 weeks with monitoring of symptoms, physical exam, and imaging findings (25, 36).

AEP when recognized and treated timely, responds dramatically to glucocorticoid therapy with rapid improvement in respiratory symptoms (12, 37). Radiographic clearance is delayed usually, but complete resolution of chest radiograph can be seen in 1 month (12, 16, 25, 32). Long-term complications are rare when AEP is appropriately diagnosed and treated. Relapses are less common although they have been described. In refractory respiratory failure from AEP, extra-corporeal membranous oxygenation (ECMO) may be required (38).

Chronic eosinophilic pneumonia

Chronic eosinophilic pneumonia (CEP) represents <3% of interstitial lung diseases (2, 39). It occurs more so in females with a stronger association with Caucasian women mostly in their 40s at the time of diagnosis (2, 40–42) (Table 13.2). It has a strong link with prior asthma or other atopic history (2). There is no increased predilection for CEP in smokers (2, 40). An association with radiation therapy has been reported. (43, 44). Lung injury in CEP is caused by degranulation of intracytoplasmic granules releasing proteins, toxins, chemokines, and proinflammatory mediators. IL-5 is thought to be the primary recruiter of eosinophils to the lung (45). IL-25 has also been thought to be associated with chronic eosinophilic inflammation of the lung (46).

Clinical features
CEP has a subacute onset over several weeks to months. Most prominent symptoms include dyspnea, seen in more than 60% of patients and nonproductive cough, which is present in almost all patients with CEP (2). Often, a history of asthma and/or atopy is present. Rhinitis or sinusitis is present in some patients. On physical examination, crackles and wheezing are commonplace, but

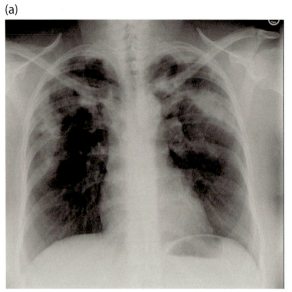
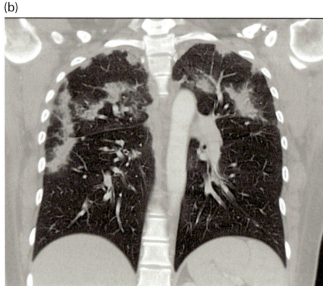

FIGURE 13.2 A 42-year-old woman with a history of bronchial asthma and allergic rhinitis reported worsening shortness of breath of 4 months duration. Chest x-ray shows upper peripheral upper lobe-based consolidative opacities, consistent with photographic negative of pulmonary edema (a), which was confirmed on CT scans in coronal view showing the peripheral consolidative opacities (b). Bronchoscopy with transbronchial biopsies were consistent with chronic eosinophilic pneumonia.

respiratory failure is rare (2, 42, 47, 48). Constitutional symptoms are common such as fatigue, fever, malaise, and night sweats (2). Evaluation for other similar disorders such as EGPA, cryptogenic organizing pneumonia, and idiopathic hypereosinophilic syndrome are important (2, 45). Often, concomitant asthma is present, at times difficult to control despite appropriate escalation of therapy.

Peripheral eosinophilia is often present in CEP with mean eosinophil count of 5–6,000/mm³ (2). Inflammatory markers ESR, CRP, and IgE levels are elevated. PFTs show a mixed obstructive and restrictive defect. DLCO may be reduced (2, 40, 49).

Imaging

The hallmark chest radiograph finding of photographic negative of pulmonary edema is not common in CEP (40, 49–51). CT chest shows ground-glass infiltrates that are bilateral, classically peripheral, and often upper lobe predominant (2, 40). Consolidation with air bronchograms can also be seen. Pleural effusions are not common although pleural-based infiltrates may be seen (52) (Figures 13.2 and 13.3).

Histopathology

Biopsy is often unnecessary for pathologic confirmation if other features are strongly suggestive. Tissue can reveal alveolar and interstitial inflammation with eosinophilic predominance. Alveolar spaces can be filled with fibrinous exudate (40). Accompanying eosinophils, there can also be infiltration of macrophages, lymphocytes, and plasma cells (53) (Figure 13.4).

Diagnosis

Diagnostic criteria include symptoms for longer than 2 weeks duration, eosinophilia on BAL (>40% on cell count differential) and/or peripheral eosinophilia (>1,000 eosinophils/mm³), imaging findings of peripheral, upper lobe predominant infiltrates (3, 54) as well as exclusion of other causes of eosinophilic lung disease. Biopsy though rarely required, may be performed via surgical lung biopsy (SLB) or transbronchial lung biopsy (3, 45, 54); although transbronchial biopsy suffices in most cases in the authors' own experience.

Treatment and prognosis

Treatment is based on immunosuppression, primarily centered around systemic glucocorticoid therapy. Glucocorticoid therapy leads to a rapid improvement in clinical symptoms over several days. Infiltrates on chest imaging also improve with glucocorticoid therapy. There is no established glucocorticoid treatment protocol. Achieving and maintaining a clinical response is the goal of therapy and escalating doses may be initially indicated to achieve this goal (2). Oral prednisone therapy at 0.5–0.6 mg/kg/day has been proposed (40), while another study

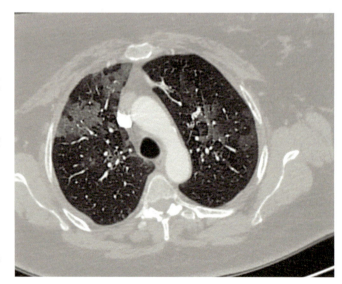

FIGURE 13.3 A 60-year-old woman with a history of bronchial asthma presented with multiple episodes of shortness of breath for which she had been receiving glucocorticoids. CT scans in axial view obtained when she was admitted show bilateral upper lobe ground-glass opacities. Bronchoscopy with broncho-alveolar lavage showed 75% eosinophils, followed by transbronchial biopsies.

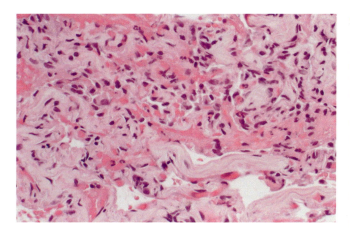

FIGURE 13.4 H: E images in same patient showing significant interstitial and alveolar eosinophil infiltration consistent with chronic eosinophilic pneumonia. (Original magnification 40×). (Images courtesy of Allen Chukwuemekenim Omo-Ogboi, MD, Department of Pathology, UT Health, Houston, Texas.)

suggests prednisolone 30 mg daily (42). There is a significant risk of relapse in as high as half of all patients (2). Hence, the duration of treatment is typically several months with a slow taper. One recent study found the shorter duration of therapy of 3 months may be noninferior to more prolonged courses in preventing relapse (55).

Given the side effects of chronic glucocorticoid therapy (56), steroid-sparing agents should be considered. Studies in steroid-sparing therapy for CEP are still in the early stages. Some targets actively being studied include anti-IgE therapy (57) and anti-IL-5 (58). Targeted therapies for IL-25, IL-33, and IL-4 (59) are being considered in order to limit chronic systemic glucocorticoid therapy (46). Inhaled corticosteroids (ICS) have also been proposed, but may not be particularly effective (60).

Short-term clinical outcomes are generally favorable in CEP. Long-term prognosis may be complicated in cases with frequent relapses (48). Adverse effects such as diabetes mellitus, weight gain, poor bone health, and risk for infections are well established complications of chronic glucocorticoid therapy, and patients should be monitored for them as appropriate (42, 47, 56). Pulmonary function defects may persist from restriction in a significant minority of cases (42).

Eosinophilic granulomatosis with polyangiitis

EGPA is rare with an annual incidence estimated to be fewer than 10 cases per million according to some studies (61–64). There is no gender predilection, although age at diagnosis is usually in the 40 and 50 age groups (61) (Table 13.2). EGPA is classified as a small-vessel vasculitis and characterized by multisystem involvement, which distinguishes it from the other eosinophilic lung diseases discussed here (65).

The primary drivers of pathogenesis of EGPA are eosinophils (66) along with B (67) and T lymphocytes (68), in particular Th-2 lymphocytes. EGPA has an association with certain genomic subtypes (69). Identified environmental exposures include medications, infection, and other allergens (70). Eosinophils release IL-25, which has been shown to lead to activation of Th-2 cells (71). T lymphocytes are present in organs involved with EGPA (72).

Clinical features

The clinical course of EGPA has been divided into three stages: (1) Bronchial asthma and rhinitis, (2) tissue eosinophilia including pulmonary eosinophilia, and (3) extra-pulmonary eosinophilic disease with vasculitis (73). Asthma is often present and uncontrolled, typically preceding the diagnosis of EGPA (74, 75).

The clinical presentation of patients with EGPA have been phenotyped into vasculitic subtype, which is associated with ANCA-positivity and predominantly vasculitic features such as mononeuritis multiplex, glomerulonephritis, and vasculitic skin involvement. The eosinophilic subtype is usually ANCA-negative and characterized by organ damage from eosinophilic infiltration — mainly pulmonary infiltrates but also sinus involvement (66, 73).

Peripheral eosinophilia is usually present and accompanied by increased inflammatory markers. ANCA positivity is noted in one-third to half of all EGPA patients, and usually as myeloperoxidase-ANCA (76–81). In case of renal involvement, an increased serum creatinine and proteinuria may be present (76–81). Most often, PFTs show an obstructive process (82). DLCO can be reduced in cases of pulmonary infiltrates (normal) and may even be increased due to bronchial asthma or, less commonly, from alveolar hemorrhage (82–84).

Imaging

CT scan chest shows diffuse peripheral ground-glass opacities that may be migratory. Bronchial wall thickening and centrilobular nodular infiltrates can be present (85). Occasionally, concomitant pleural effusions are seen (86) (Figure 13.5).

Histopathology

Histopathology of lung tissue with involvement with EGPA shows eosinophil-rich granulomatous inflammation of airways and vasculitis involving small- and medium-sized vessels (87). Fibrinoid necrosis in vessel walls can be seen (88), along with palisading giant cells surrounding an eosinophil-rich necrotic region (87–89). Alveolar hemorrhage may be present (75).

Diagnosis

While diagnostic criteria for EGPA is still undergoing revision, the hallmarks for diagnosis remain the presence of asthma, peripheral eosinophilia, and evidence for organ involvement of vasculitis or eosinophilic infiltration (88, 90). The most commonly utilized criteria are the ACR criteria from 1990 that include clinical findings, with or without tissue biopsy, with four of the following six criteria: Bronchial asthma, peripheral eosinophilia >10%, neuropathy including mononeuropathy or polyneuropathy, pulmonary infiltrates, paranasal sinus abnormalities, or extravascular eosinophilic infiltration on biopsy (88, 90). Lung biopsy is not routinely performed in EGPA, although it may be helpful in lung-limited variants of the disease to confirm the diagnosis (91). Of note, surgical lung biopsies are recommended given the patchy nature of vasculitis and the limited sample size obtained with transbronchial biopsies.

Treatment and prognosis

Treatment recommendations are not well-founded given the limited available data (92). Therapy is centered around systemic glucocorticoids. Dosing depends on the severity of organ involvement and the score on a five-factor score (Table 13.3), which has been shown to predict survival (93, 94). Cyclophosphamide in combination with glucocorticoid pulse therapy have been suggested in severe disease (95). Given a high rate of relapse in EGPA (76–78, 80, 81), steroid-sparing agents are utilized in cases requiring longer-term glucocorticoid therapy, although evidence

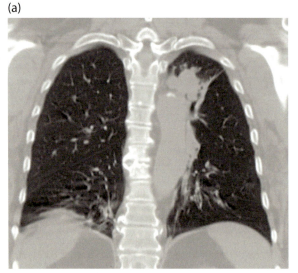 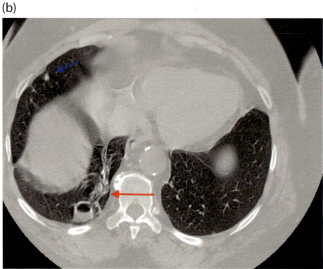

FIGURE 13.5 CT scans in coronal view (a) in a patient with EGPA showing consolidative opacities in left upper lobe and bilateral lower lobe bronchial wall thickening. CT scan in axial view (b) in the same patient shows right lower lobe bronchial thickening and bronchiectasis leading to a cavitary opacity with air-fluid level (red arrow). Also note a nodule in the right middle lobe (blue arrow). (Images courtesy of Daniel Ocazionez-Trujillo, UT Health, Houston, Texas.)

is limited (96). Anti-CD20 therapy with rituximab and anti-IL5 therapy with mepolizumab (97, 98) have been utilized with good results (64, 99). Intravenous immunoglobulin (IVIG) therapy has been shown to benefit in some cases of refractory EGPA for inducing remission (80).

Parasitic infection causing eosinophilic pneumonia

Parasitic infection is the most common cause of eosinophilic pneumonia worldwide. It can manifest as simple pulmonary eosinophilia (SPE) or Loeffler's syndrome, which usually presents as a mild, transient respiratory illness manifesting as cough, wheezing, fever, peripheral eosinophilia, and fleeting pulmonary infiltrates on imaging (100).

It is typically caused by parasites, classically the nematode *Ascaris lumbricoides*, *Strongyloides*, and parasite larvae such as *Toxocara canis*, causing visceral larva migrans (101). In the United States, the most common parasites causing SPE are *Strongyloides*, *Ascaris*, and *Ancylostoma* (102).

Laboratory data show peripheral eosinophilia and BAL may reveal alveolar eosinophilia. Imaging typically reveals transient and migratory areas of consolidation, at times multiple, often peripheral, and upper lobe predominant. Centrilobular nodules with surrounding ground-glass opacities may be seen (85). It usually resolves without intervention in several weeks.

No therapy is indicated for respiratory symptoms, which typically resolve in 4 weeks. Symptom control can be attempted

TABLE 13.3: Five Factor Score in EGPA

a. Age >65 years
b. Cardiovascular insufficiency
c. Gastrointestinal involvement
d. Renal insufficiency (serum creatinine >1.7 mg/dL)
e. Absence of ear, nose, and throat manifestations

Note: Each factor is given 1 point. Score of ≥1 implies a poor prognosis.

with antitussive and antipyretic agents (103). In severe cases, corticosteroid therapy may be beneficial. It is imperative that *Strongyloides* is excluded due to risk of hyperinfection with commencement of steroid therapy. Treatment with antiparasitic agents depends on the individual parasite (104).

Tropical pulmonary eosinophilia

Tropical pulmonary eosinophilia is believed to be a hypersensitivity response to filaria, most commonly *Wuchereria bancrofti* and *Brugia malayi*. It is endemic to South and Southeast Asia, and presents with fatigue, constitutional symptoms, nocturnal cough, and wheezing. Chest radiograph imaging shows diffuse infiltrates (105, 106).

Pathophysiology is thought to be a severe hypersensitivity reaction to filarial antigens, leading to significant eosinophilic infiltration of alveoli. There is a risk of progression to fibrotic disease in the absence of appropriate treatment (105). Diagnosis is based on history of exposure, peripheral eosinophilia, elevated IgE level, diffuse infiltrates, and elevated antifilarial antibody titers (105).

Treatment is diethylcarbamazine at 5 mg/kg/day for 2–4 weeks (105). Relapse rate is high in up to 20% of cases (107). Some cases develop interstitial lung disease with irreversible fibrotic changes (105, 108).

Drug-induced eosinophilic lung disease

Drug-induced eosinophilic lung disease can have a variable presentation and clinical course. Although rarely reported, with a recent review finding only 196 cases reported over almost 30 years, it is likely under-diagnosed and under-reported (109). Respiratory symptoms such as dyspnea, cough, and constitutional symptoms can present acutely, present as AEP, or have a slower and more insidious course as in CEP (109, 110).

Many pharmacologic agents have been found to trigger drug-induced eosinophilic lung disease (Table 13.4). Almost all classes of medications have been described to have an association with

TABLE 13.4: Medications Associated with Drug-Induced Eosinophilic Lung Disease

Antibiotics	Anti-Inflammatory	Chemotherapy	Antimalarial	Antipsychotic	Antihypertensive	Immuno-therapy	Antiarrhythmic	Lipid-Lowering Agents	Other
Daptomycin	Mesalamine	Methotrexate	Dapsone-pyrimethamine	Amitriptyline	Captopril	Ustekinumab	Amiodarone	Simvastatin	Acetaminophen
Minocycline	Sulfasalazine	Gemcitabine	Fansidar	Venlafaxine	Ifenprodil	Interferon-A	Mexiletine		Progesterone
Nitrofurantoin	Ibuprofen	Tegafur uracil UFT	Mefloquine	Risperidone	Hydrochlorothiazide	Infliximab			Diaminodiphenyl sulfone
Azithromycin	Piroxicam		Atovaquone-proguanil	Clozapine		FK-506			Dabigatran
						Abatacept			
Dapsone	Diclofenac	Aminoglutethimide							
Sulfonamide	Balsalazide	Cisplatin		Paroxetine					Ranitidine
Ceftaroline	Benzbromarone			Duloxetine					Sodium cromoglycate
Ethambutol	Nimesulide			Trazadone					Lansoprazole/omeprazole
				Sertraline					
Ampicillin	Bucillamine								Gold
Imipenem	Naproxen								Tryptophan
Isoniazid									Chlorpropamide
Piperacillin-tazobactam									Camostat mesilate
Cefaclor									
Clarithromycin									
Roxithromycin									
Tosufloxacin									
Tetracycline									
Rifampicin/Rifampin									

drug-induced eosinophilic lung disease. The most frequent classes are antibiotics, anti-inflammatory agents, and antiepileptic agents (109, 111–116). The most commonly implicated agents include daptomycin, minocycline, mesalamine, and sulfasalazine (109). In addition, illicit drugs such as cocaine, heroin, and THC products have been shown to trigger the disease as well (117–119). Pathogenesis is not well known and two mechanisms have been proposed — the cytotoxic mechanism and immune-mediated mechanisms, although there is no evidence supporting one over the other and a multifactorial etiology is more likely (109).

The severity of respiratory illness can be significantly higher in acute onset drug-induced eosinophilic lung disease, while chronic presentations were not associated with any severe respiratory illness or cases of mechanical ventilation (109). It is important to note that drug-induced eosinophilic lung disease may not follow the classic gender predilections that are noted in AEP and CEP (109).

Peripheral eosinophilia is commonly noted in both acute and chronic presentations of drug-induced eosinophilic lung disease. BAL can show eosinophilia, and chronic presentation of drug-induced eosinophilic lung disease is typically more frequently associated with eosinophilia on BAL compared to the acute presentation. Lung biopsies are rarely performed (109, 110). There are no diagnostic criteria validated for diagnosis of drug-induced eosinophilic lung disease.

Imaging
CT chest imaging in acute presentations showed diffuse ground-glass opacities and, in chronic presentations, is associated with bilateral peripheral, patchy opacities (109, 110). Migratory opacities have been noted in both acute and chronic presentations of drug-induced eosinophilic lung disease (109).

Treatment
The cornerstone of treatment involves maintaining a high index of suspicion and glucocorticoid therapy. Acute cases are treated with systemic glucocorticoid therapy that usually lead to a rapid response. In chronic presentations of eosinophilic lung disease, treatment may simply be the removal of a triggering agent. In some cases, systemic glucocorticoid therapy may be needed usually with excellent clinical response; there is an association with relapses that can potentially require long-term therapy (109, 110). In chronic presentations, there is a higher recurrence rate. Steroid-sparing agents have been suggested in cases of recurrent disease, although evidence is very limited (109).

References

1. Fernandez Perez ER, Olson AL, Frankel SK. Eosinophilic lung diseases. Med Clin North Am. 2011;95(6):1163–87.
2. Cottin V. Eosinophilic lung diseases. Clin Chest Med. 2016;37(3):535–56.
3. Cottin V, Cordier JF. Eosinophilic lung diseases. Immunol Allergy Clin North Am. 2012;32(4):557–86.
4. Gleich GJ. Historical overview and perspective on the role of the eosinophil in health and disease. Eosinophils in Health and Disease 2013. p. 1–11.
5. Hogan SP, Rosenberg HF, Moqbel R, Phipps S, Foster PS, Lacy P, et al. Eosinophils: Biological properties and role in health and disease. Clin Exp Allergy. 2008;38(5):709–50.
6. Giembycz MA, Lindsay MA. Pharmacology of the eosinophil. Pharmacol Rev. 1999;51(2):213–340.
7. Dvorak AM, Letourneau L, Login GR, Weller PF, Ackerman SJ. Ultrastructural localization of the Charcot-Leyden crystal protein (lysophospholipase) to a distinct crystalloid-free granule population in mature human eosinophils. Blood. 1988;72(1):150–8.
8. Allen JN, Pacht ER, Gadek JE, Davis WB. Acute eosinophilic pneumonia as a reversible cause of noninfectious respiratory failure. N Engl J Med. 1989;321(9):569–74.
9. Badesch DB, King TE, Jr., Schwarz MI. Acute eosinophilic pneumonia: A hypersensitivity phenomenon? Am Rev Respir Dis. 1989;139(1):249–52.
10. Shorr AF, Scoville SL, Cersovsky SB, Shanks GD, Ockenhouse CF, Smoak BL, et al. Acute eosinophilic pneumonia among US military personnel deployed in or near Iraq. JAMA. 2004;292(24):2997–3005.
11. Yoon CG, Kim SJ, Kim K, Lee JE, Jhun BW. Clinical characteristics and factors influencing the occurrence of acute eosinophilic pneumonia in Korean military personnel. J Korean Med Sci. 2016;31(2):247–53.
12. Rhee CK, Min KH, Yim NY, Lee JE, Lee NR, Chung MP, et al. Clinical characteristics and corticosteroid treatment of acute eosinophilic pneumonia. Eur Respir J. 2013;41(2):402–9.
13. Uchiyama H, Suda T, Nakamura Y, Shirai M, Gemma H, Shirai T, et al. Alterations in smoking habits are associated with acute eosinophilic pneumonia. Chest. 2008;133(5):1174–80.
14. Vassallo R. Diffuse lung diseases in cigarette smokers. Semin Respir Crit Care Med. 2012;33(5):533–42.
15. De Giacomi F, Vassallo R, Yi ES, Ryu JH. Acute eosinophilic pneumonia. Causes, diagnosis, and management. Am J Respir Crit Care Med. 2018;197(6):728–36.
16. Philit F, Etienne-Mastroianni B, Parrot A, Guerin C, Robert D, Cordier JF. Idiopathic acute eosinophilic pneumonia: A study of 22 patients. Am J Respir Crit Care Med. 2002;166(9):1235–9.
17. Natarajan A, Shah P, Mirrakhimov AE, Hussain N. Eosinophilic pneumonia associated with concomitant cigarette and marijuana smoking. BMJ Case Rep. 2013;2013.
18. Just N, Carpentier O, Brzezinki C, Steenhouwer F, Staumont-Salle D. Severe hypersensitivity reaction as acute eosinophilic pneumonia and skin eruption induced by proguanil. Eur Respir J. 2011;37(6):1526–8.
19. Liu J, Shen Z, Tian B, Zhang T, Zhang C. Acute eosinophilic pneumonia with sepsis-like symptoms of arthralgia, joint stiffness and lymph node enlargement: A case report. Respir Med Case Rep. 2020;30:101072.
20. Zhao J, Zhao Y. Interleukin-33 and its receptor in pulmonary inflammatory diseases. Crit Rev Immunol. 2015;35(6):451–61.
21. Mato N, Bando M, Kusano A, Hirano T, Nakayama M, Uto T, et al. Clinical significance of interleukin 33 (IL-33) in patients with eosinophilic pneumonia. Allergol Int. 2013;62(1):45–52.
22. Daimon T, Tajima S, Oshikawa K, Bando M, Ohno S, Sugiyama Y. KL-6 and surfactant proteins a and d in serum and bronchoalveolar lavage fluid in patients with acute eosinophilic pneumonia. Intern Med. 2005;44(8):811–7.
23. Nureki S, Miyazaki E, Ando M, Kumamoto T, Tsuda T. CC chemokine receptor 4 ligand production by bronchoalveolar lavage fluid cells in cigarette-smoke-associated acute eosinophilic pneumonia. Clin Immunol. 2005;116(1):83–93.
24. Fujimura M, Yasui M, Shinagawa S, Nomura M, Matsuda T. Bronchoalveolar lavage cell findings in three types of eosinophilic pneumonia: Acute, chronic and drug-induced eosinophilic pneumonia. Respir Med. 1998;92(5):743–9.
25. Pope-Harman AL, Davis WB, Allen ED, Christoforidis AJ, Allen JN. Acute eosinophilic pneumonia. A summary of 15 cases and review of the literature. Medicine (Baltimore). 1996;75(6):334–42.
26. Hayakawa H, Sato A, Toyoshima M, Imokawa S, Taniguchi M. A clinical study of idiopathic eosinophilic pneumonia. Chest. 1994;105(5):1462–6.
27. Tazelaar HD, Linz LJ, Colby TV, Myers JL, Limper AH. Acute eosinophilic pneumonia: Histopathologic findings in nine patients. Am J Respir Crit Care Med. 1997;155(1):296–302.
28. Balbi B, Fabiano F. A young man with fever, dyspnoea and nonproductive cough. Eur Respir J. 1996;9(3):619–21.
29. Cheon JE, Lee KS, Jung GS, Chung MH, Cho YD. Acute eosinophilic pneumonia: Radiographic and CT findings in six patients. AJR Am J Roentgenol. 1996;167(5):1195–9.
30. Umeki S, Soejima R. Acute and chronic eosinophilic pneumonia: Clinical evaluation and the criteria. Intern Med. 1992;31(7):847–56.

31. Ogawa H, Fujimura M, Matsuda T, Nakamura H, Kumabashiri I, Kitagawa S. Transient wheeze. Eosinophilic bronchobronchiolitis in acute eosinophilic pneumonia. Chest. 1993;104(2):493–6.
32. King MA, Pope-Harman AL, Allen JN, Christoforidis GA, Christoforidis AJ. Acute eosinophilic pneumonia: Radiologic and clinical features. Radiology. 1997;203(3):715–9.
33. Johkoh T, Muller NL, Akira M, Ichikado K, Suga M, Ando M, et al. Eosinophilic lung diseases: Diagnostic accuracy of thin-section CT in 111 patients. Radiology. 2000;216(3):773–80.
34. Abe K, Yanagi S, Imadsu Y, Sano A, Iiboshi H, Mukae H, et al. Acute eosinophilic pneumonia with fine nodular shadows. Intern Med. 2003;42(1):88–91.
35. Ajani S, Kennedy CC. Idiopathic acute eosinophilic pneumonia: A retrospective case series and review of the literature. Respir Med Case Rep. 2013;10:43–7.
36. Jantz MA, Sahn SA. Corticosteroids in acute respiratory failure. Am J Respir Crit Care Med. 1999;160(4):1079–100.
37. Jhun BW, Kim SJ, Kim K, Lee JE. Outcomes of rapid corticosteroid tapering in acute eosinophilic pneumonia patients with initial eosinophilia. Respirology. 2015;20(8):1241–7.
38. Sauvaget E, Dellamonica J, Arlaud K, Sanfiorenzo C, Bernardin G, Padovani B, et al. Idiopathic acute eosinophilic pneumonia requiring ECMO in a teenager smoking tobacco and cannabis. Pediatr Pulmonol. 2010;45(12):1246–9.
39. Thomeer MJ, Costabe U, Rizzato G, Poletti V, Demedts M. Comparison of registries of interstitial lung diseases in three European countries. Eur Respir J Suppl. 2001;32:114s–8s.
40. Marchand E, Cordier JF. Idiopathic chronic eosinophilic pneumonia. Orphanet J Rare Dis. 2006;1:11.
41. Allen J, Wert M. Eosinophilic pneumonias. J Allergy Clin Immunol Pract. 2018;6(5):1455–61.
42. Suzuki Y, Suda T. Long-term management and persistent impairment of pulmonary function in chronic eosinophilic pneumonia: A review of the previous literature. Allergol Int. 2018;67(3):334–40.
43. Nakayasu H, Shirai T, Tanaka Y, Saigusa M. Chronic eosinophilic pneumonia after radiation therapy for squamous cell lung cancer. Respir Med Case Rep. 2017;22:147–9.
44. Cottin V, Frognier R, Monnot H, Levy A, DeVuyst P, Cordier JF, et al. Chronic eosinophilic pneumonia after radiation therapy for breast cancer. Eur Respir J. 2004;23(1):9–13.
45. Crowe M, Robinson D, Sagar M, Chen L, Ghamande S. Chronic eosinophilic pneumonia: Clinical perspectives. Ther Clin Risk Manag. 2019;15:397–403.
46. Katoh S, Ikeda M, Matsumoto N, Shimizu H, Abe M, Ohue Y, et al. Possible role of IL-25 in eosinophilic lung inflammation in patients with chronic eosinophilic pneumonia. Lung. 2017;195(6):707–12.
47. Ishiguro T, Takayanagi N, Uozumi R, Tada M, Kagiyama N, Takaku Y, et al. The long-term clinical course of chronic eosinophilic pneumonia. Intern Med. 2016;55(17):2373–7.
48. Naughton M, Fahy J, FitzGerald MX. Chronic eosinophilic pneumonia. A long-term follow-up of 12 patients. Chest. 1993;103(1):162–5.
49. Stoller JK. Eosinophilic Lung Diseases. Murray & Nadel's Textbook of Respiratory Medicine. 6th ed: Elsevier/Saunders; 2016. p. 1221–8.
50. Gaensler EA, Carrington CB. Peripheral opacities in chronic eosinophilic pneumonia: The photographic negative of pulmonary edema. AJR Am J Roentgenol. 1977;128(1):1–13.
51. Zimhony O. Photographic negative shadow of pulmonary oedema. Lancet. 2002;360(9326):33.
52. Suzuki Y, Suda T. Eosinophilic pneumonia: A review of the previous literature, causes, diagnosis, and management. Allergol Int. 2019;68(4):413–9.
53. Saitoh K, Shindo N, Toh Y, Yoshizawa A, Kudo K. Electron microscopic study of chronic eosinophilic pneumonia. Pathol Int. 1996;46(11):855–61.
54. Matsuse H, Shimoda T, Fukushima C, Matsuo N, Sakai H, Takao A, et al. Diagnostic problems in chronic eosinophilic pneumonia. J Int Med Res. 1997;25(4):196–201.
55. Oyama Y, Fujisawa T, Hashimoto D, Enomoto N, Nakamura Y, Inui N, et al. Efficacy of short-term prednisolone treatment in patients with chronic eosinophilic pneumonia. Eur Respir J. 2015;45(6):1624–31.
56. Khan NA, Donatelli CV, Tonelli AR, Wiesen J, Ribeiro Neto ML, Sahoo D, et al. Toxicity risk from glucocorticoids in sarcoidosis patients. Respir Med. 2017;132:9–14.
57. Kaya H, Gumus S, Ucar E, Aydogan M, Musabak U, Tozkoparan E, et al. Omalizumab as a steroid-sparing agent in chronic eosinophilic pneumonia. Chest. 2012;142(2):513–6.
58. Mukherjee M, Sehmi R, Nair P. Anti-IL5 therapy for asthma and beyond. World Allergy Organ J. 2014;7(1):32.
59. Castro M, Corren J, Pavord ID, Maspero J, Wenzel S, Rabe KF, et al. Dupilumab efficacy and safety in moderate-to-severe uncontrolled asthma. N Engl J Med. 2018;378(26):2486–96.
60. Minakuchi M, Niimi A, Matsumoto H, Amitani R, Mishima M. Chronic eosinophilic pneumonia: Treatment with inhaled corticosteroids. Respiration. 2003;70(4):362–6.
61. Mouthon L, Dunogue B, Guillevin L. Diagnosis and classification of eosinophilic granulomatosis with polyangiitis (formerly named Churg-Strauss syndrome). J Autoimmun. 2014;48-49:99–103.
62. Fujimoto S, Watts RA, Kobayashi S, Suzuki K, Jayne DR, Scott DG, et al. Comparison of the epidemiology of anti-neutrophil cytoplasmic antibody-associated vasculitis between Japan and the U.K. Rheumatology (Oxford). 2011;50(10):1916–20.
63. Gonzalez-Gay MA, Garcia-Porrua C, Guerrero J, Rodriguez-Ledo P, Llorca J. The epidemiology of the primary systemic vasculitides in northwest Spain: Implications of the chapel hill consensus conference definitions. Arthritis Rheum. 2003;49(3):388–93.
64. Mohammad AJ, Jacobsson LT, Westman KW, Sturfelt G, Segelmark M. Incidence and survival rates in Wegener's granulomatosis, microscopic polyangiitis, Churg-Strauss syndrome and polyarteritis nodosa. Rheumatology (Oxford). 2009;48(12):1560–5.
65. Jennette JC, Falk RJ, Bacon PA, Basu N, Cid MC, Ferrario F, et al. 2012 Revised International Chapel Hill Consensus conference nomenclature of vasculitides. Arthritis Rheum. 2013;65(1):1–11.
66. Vaglio A, Moosig F, Zwerina J. Churg-Strauss syndrome: Update on pathophysiology and treatment. Curr Opin Rheumatol. 2012;24(1):24–30.
67. Jennette JC, Xiao H, Falk R, Gasim AMH. Experimental models of vasculitis and glomerulonephritis induced by antineutrophil cytoplasmic autoantibodies. Contrib Nephrol. 2011;169:211–20.
68. Guida G, Vallario A, Stella S, Boita M, Circosta P, Mariani S, et al. Clonal CD8+ TCR-vbeta expanded populations with effector memory phenotype in Churg-Strauss syndrome. Clin Immunol. 2008;128(1):94–102.
69. Alberici F, Martorana D, Bonatti F, Gioffredi A, Lyons PA, Vaglio A. Genetics of ANCA-associated vasculitides: HLA and beyond. Clin Exp Rheumatol. 2014;32(3 Suppl 82):S90–7.
70. Furuta S, Jayne DR. Antineutrophil cytoplasm antibody-associated vasculitis: Recent developments. Kidney Int. 2013;84(2):244–9.
71. Terrier B, Bieche I, Maisonobe T, Laurendeau I, Rosenzwajg M, Kahn JE, et al. Interleukin-25: A cytokine linking eosinophils and adaptive immunity in Churg-Strauss syndrome. Blood. 2010;116(22):4523–31.
72. Gioffredi A, Maritati F, Oliva E, Buzio C. Eosinophilic granulomatosis with polyangiitis: An overview. Front Immunol. 2014;5:549.
73. Pagnoux C, Guilpain P, Guillevin L. Churg-Strauss syndrome. Curr Opin Rheumatol. 2007;19(1):25–32.
74. Vaglio A, Buzio C, Zwerina J. Eosinophilic granulomatosis with polyangiitis (Churg-Strauss): State of the art. Allergy. 2013;68(3):261–73.
75. Guillevin L, Cohen P, Gayraud M, Lhote F, Jarrousse B, Casassus P. Churg-Strauss syndrome. Clinical study and long-term follow-up of 96 patients. Medicine (Baltimore). 1999;78(1):26–37.
76. Saku A, Furuta S, Hiraguri M, Ikeda K, Kobayashi Y, Kagami SI, et al. Longterm outcomes of 188 Japanese patients with eosinophilic granulomatosis with polyangiitis. J Rheumatol. 2018;45(8):1159–66.
77. Durel CA, Berthiller J, Caboni S, Jayne D, Ninet J, Hot A. Long-term followup of a multicenter cohort of 101 patients with eosinophilic granulomatosis with polyangiitis (Churg-Strauss). Arthritis Care Res (Hoboken). 2016;68(3):374–87.

78. Comarmond C, Pagnoux C, Khellaf M, Cordier JF, Hamidou M, Viallard JF, et al. Eosinophilic granulomatosis with polyangiitis (Churg-Strauss): Clinical characteristics and long-term followup of the 383 patients enrolled in the French Vasculitis Study Group Cohort. Arthritis Rheum. 2013;65(1):270–81.
79. Sinico RA, Di Toma L, Maggiore U, Bottero P, Radice A, Tosoni C, et al. Prevalence and clinical significance of antineutrophil cytoplasmic antibodies in Churg-Strauss syndrome. Arthritis Rheum. 2005;52(9):2926–35.
80. Tsurikisawa N, Taniguchi M, Saito H, Himeno H, Ishibashi A, Suzuki S, et al. Treatment of Churg-Strauss syndrome with high-dose intravenous immunoglobulin. Ann Allergy Asthma Immunol. 2004;92(1):80–7.
81. Moosig F, Bremer JP, Hellmich B, Holle JU, Holl-Ulrich K, Laudien M, et al. A vasculitis centre based management strategy leads to improved outcome in eosinophilic granulomatosis and polyangiitis (Churg-Strauss, EGPA): Monocentric experiences in 150 patients. Ann Rheum Dis. 2013;72(6):1011–7.
82. Santos YA, Silva BR, Lira PN, Vaz LC, Mafort TT, Bruno LP, et al. Eosinophilic granulomatosis with polyangiitis (formerly known as Churg-Strauss syndrome) as a differential diagnosis of hypereosinophilic syndromes. Respir Med Case Rep. 2017;21:1–6.
83. Saydain G, Beck KC, Decker PA, Cowl CT, Scanlon PD. Clinical significance of elevated diffusing capacity. Chest. 2004;125(2):446–52.
84. Haworth SJ, Savage CO, Carr D, Hughes JM, Rees AJ. Pulmonary haemorrhage complicating Wegener's granulomatosis and microscopic polyarteritis. Br Med J (Clin Res Ed). 1985;290(6484):1775–8.
85. Yeon JJ KKI, Im JS, Chang HL, Ki NL, Ki NK. Eosinophilic lung diseases: A clinical, radiologic, and pathologic overview. Radiographics. 2007. Radiographics. 2007;3(May-June):617–37.
86. Palmucci S, Ini C, Cosentino S, Fanzone L, Di Pietro S, Di Mari A, et al. Pulmonary vasculitides: A radiological review emphasizing parenchymal HRCT features. Diagnostics (Basel). 2021;11(12).
87. Lie JT. Illustrated histopathologic classification criteria for selected vasculitis syndromes. American College of rheumatology subcommittee on classification of vasculitis. Arthritis Rheum. 1990;33(8):1074–87.
88. Masi AT, Hunder GG, Lie JT, Michel BA, Bloch DA, Arend WP, et al. The American college of rheumatology 1990 criteria for the classification of Churg-Strauss syndrome (allergic granulomatosis and angiitis). Arthritis Rheum. 1990;33(8):1094–100.
89. Churg J, Strauss L. Allergic granulomatosis, allergic angiitis, and periarteritis nodosa. Am J Pathol. 1951;27(2):277–301.
90. Lanham JG, Elkon KB, Pusey CD, Hughes GR. Systemic vasculitis with asthma and eosinophilia: A clinical approach to the Churg-Strauss syndrome. Medicine (Baltimore). 1984;63(2):65–81.
91. Nasser M, Thivolet-Bejui F, Seve P, Cottin V. Lung-limited or lung-dominant variant of eosinophilic granulomatosis with polyangiitis. J Allergy Clin Immunol Pract. 2020;8(6):2092–5.
92. Yates M, Watts RA, Bajema IM, Cid MC, Crestani B, Hauser T, et al. EULAR/ERA-EDTA recommendations for the management of ANCA-associated vasculitis. Ann Rheum Dis. 2016;75(9):1583–94.
93. Guillevin L, Lhote F, Gayraud M, Cohen P, Jarrousse B, Lortholary O, et al. Prognostic factors in polyarteritis nodosa and Churg-Strauss syndrome. A prospective study in 342 patients. Medicine (Baltimore). 1996;75(1):17–28.
94. Guillevin L, Pagnoux C, Seror R, Mahr A, Mouthon L, Toumelin PL, et al. The five-factor score revisited: Assessment of prognoses of systemic necrotizing vasculitides based on the French Vasculitis Study Group (FVSG) cohort. Medicine (Baltimore). 2011;90(1):19–27.
95. Ribi C, Cohen P, Pagnoux C, Mahr A, Arene JP, Lauque D, et al. Treatment of Churg-Strauss syndrome without poor-prognosis factors: A multicenter, prospective, randomized, open-label study of seventy-two patients. Arthritis Rheum. 2008;58(2):586–94.
96. Puechal X, Pagnoux C, Baron G, Quemeneur T, Neel A, Agard C, et al. Adding azathioprine to remission-induction glucocorticoids for eosinophilic granulomatosis with polyangiitis (Churg-Strauss), microscopic polyangiitis, or polyarteritis nodosa without poor prognosis factors: A randomized, controlled trial. Arthritis Rheumatol. 2017;69(11):2175–86.
97. Wechsler ME, Akuthota P, Jayne D, Khoury P, Klion A, Langford CA, et al. Mepolizumab or placebo for eosinophilic granulomatosis with polyangiitis. N Engl J Med. 2017;376(20):1921–32.
98. Steinfeld J, Bradford ES, Brown J, Mallett S, Yancey SW, Akuthota P, et al. Evaluation of clinical benefit from treatment with mepolizumab for patients with eosinophilic granulomatosis with polyangiitis. J Allergy Clin Immunol. 2019;143(6):2170–7.
99. Thiel J, Troilo A, Salzer U, Schleyer T, Halmschlag K, Rizzi M, et al. Rituximab as induction therapy in eosinophilic granulomatosis with polyangiitis refractory to conventional immunosuppressive treatment: A 36-month follow-up analysis. J Allergy Clin Immunol Pract. 2017;5(6):1556–63.
100. Allen JN, Davis WB. Eosinophilic lung diseases. Am J Respir Crit Care Med. 1994;150(5 Pt 1):1423–38.
101. Craig JM, Scott AL. Helminths in the lungs. Parasite Immunol. 2014;36(9):463–74.
102. Chitkara RK, Krishna G. Parasitic pulmonary eosinophilia. Semin Respir Crit Care Med. 2006;27(2):171–84.
103. Mann B. Eosinophilic lung disease. Clinical Medicine Circulatory, Respiratory and Pulmonary Medicine. 2008;2:CCRPM.S575.
104. Akuthota P, Weller PF. Eosinophilic pneumonias. Clin Microbiol Rev. 2012;25(4):649–60.
105. Mullerpattan JB, Udwadia ZF, Udwadia FE. Tropical pulmonary eosinophilia–a review. Indian J Med Res. 2013;138(3):295–302.
106. Vijayan VK. Tropical pulmonary eosinophilia: Pathogenesis, diagnosis and management. Curr Opin Pulm Med. 2007;13(5):428–33.
107. Udwadia FE. Tropical eosinophilia: A review. Respir Med. 1993;87(1):17–21.
108. Vijayan VK. Immunopathogenesis and Treatment of Eosinophilic Lung Diseases in the Tropics. Tropical Lung Disease: CRC Press; 2006. p. 46.
109. Bartal C, Sagy I, Barski L. Drug-induced eosinophilic pneumonia: A review of 196 case reports. Medicine (Baltimore). 2018;97(4):e9688.
110. Solomon J, Schwarz M. Drug-, toxin-, and radiation therapy-induced eosinophilic pneumonia. Semin Respir Crit Care Med. 2006;27(2):192–7.
111. Rizos E, Tsigkaropoulou E, Lambrou P, Kanakaki M, Chaniotou A, Alevyzakis E, et al. Risperidone-induced acute eosinophilic pneumonia. In Vivo. 2013;27(5):651–3.
112. Klerkx S, Pat K, Wuyts W. Minocycline induced eosinophilic pneumonia: Case report and review of literature. Acta Clin Belg. 2009;64(4):349–54.
113. Kim JH, Lee JH, Koh ES, Park SW, Jang AS, Kim D, et al. Acute eosinophilic pneumonia related to a mesalazine suppository. Asia Pac Allergy. 2013;3(2):136–9.
114. Anan E, Shirai R, Kai N, Ishii H, Hirata N, Kishi K, et al. [Acute eosinophilic pneumonia caused by several drugs including ibuprofen]. Nihon Kokyuki Gakkai Zasshi. 2009;47(5):443–7.
115. Hirai J, Hagihara M, Haranaga S, Kinjo T, Hashioka H, Kato H, et al. Eosinophilic pneumonia caused by daptomycin: Six cases from two institutions and a review of the literature. J Infect Chemother. 2017;23(4):245–9.
116. Souza CA, Muller NL, Johkoh T, Akira M. Drug-induced eosinophilic pneumonia: High-resolution CT findings in 14 patients. Am J Roentgenol. 2006;186(2):368–73.
117. Reyes F, Vaitkus V, Al-Ajam M. A case of cocaine-induced eosinophilic pneumonia: Case report and review of the literature. Respir Med Case Rep. 2018;23:98–102.
118. Dogan C. Acute eosinophilic pneumonia due to heroin inhalation. Chest. 2020.
119. Antwi-Amoabeng D, Islam R. Vaping is not safe: A case of acute eosinophilic pneumonia following cannabis vapor inhalation. Case Rep Pulmonol. 2020;2020:9496564.

ated giant cells is commonly seen on pathology.
14

HARD METAL LUNG DISEASE AND OTHER RARE OCCUPATIONAL LUNG DISEASES

Matthew Zheng, Robert M. Marron, and Sameep Sehgal

Contents

Introduction 101
Hard metal lung disease 101
Parenchymal lung disease 103
Other metal-related occupational lung diseases 105
Newer occupational lung diseases 106
Conclusion 108
References 108

Abbreviations

BAL	bronchoalveolar lavage
CT	computed tomography
EPMA	electron probe micro-analyzer
GIP	giant cell interstitial pneumonia
HMLD	hard metal lung disease
HRCT	high-resolution computed tomography
HLA	human leukocyte antigen
ICS	inhaled corticosteroids
ILD	interstitial lung disease
PFT	pulmonary function testing
TBLB	transbronchial lung biopsy
WC	tungsten carbide

KEY POINTS

- Hard metal lung disease is caused by exposure to cobalt and tungsten carbide.
- Pulmonary manifestations include occupational asthma, allergic alveolitis, and interstitial lung disease.
- Common occupations associated with exposure include manufacturing of alloys, alloy metal tools, and diamond polishing.
- Giant cell interstitial pneumonitis with multinucleated giant cells is commonly seen on pathology.
- Treatment includes cessation of exposure, corticosteroids, steroid sparing immune suppression, and lung transplantation in refractory disease.
- Siderosis, talcosis, and berylliosis represent other rare occupational lung diseases associated with metals exposure.
- Hypersensitivity pneumonitis develops secondary to continued inhalation of organic antigens such as agricultural dusts, bioaerosols of microorganisms, or reactive chemical species.
- Newer occupational lung diseases described recently include flavor-worker's lung, flock-worker's lung, indium tin oxide lung disease, and bronchiolitis obliterans in military personnel deployed in Afghanistan and Iraq.

Introduction

Occupational lung diseases represent a frequently diagnosed work-related condition. In 2005, the World Health Organization estimated that the most important of these diseases, silicosis, asbestos-related lung diseases, and coal workers' pneumoconiosis, globally, caused 486,000, 376,000, and 366,000 disability-adjusted years of life lost, respectively (1). While these represent pneumoconiosis secondary to inhalation of fibrogenic mineral dust, other rare occupational lung diseases are associated with inhalation of respirable dust from work with metals, noxious fumes or gases, and other organic antigens. These are much rarer as compared to mineral dust pneumoconiosis but represent an important clinical entity, as some of them are not clinically significant but may be associated with unique radiographic appearances. These include siderosis, talcosis, berylliosis, and hard metal lung disease. Hypersensitivity pneumonitis (HP) may be caused secondary to occupational exposure and inhalation of several organic antigens and represents another rare occupational lung disease. Furthermore, several newer occupational lung diseases have been described including flock-worker's lung, flavor-worker's lung, indium tin oxide lung disease, and bronchiolitis obliterans in deployed military personnel in Afghanistan and Iraq. The focus of this chapter will be on hard metal lung diseases, but a brief overview of the other rare occupational lung diseases will also be discussed within.

Hard metal lung disease

Hard metal lung disease (HMLD) refers to an interstitial lung disease (ILD) seen after exposure to metal dusts containing tungsten carbide and cobalt, and is often described in histopathology as a giant cell pneumonitis. The term "hard metal" in industrial use refers to specific composites produced by compacting and heating a powdered mixture of tungsten carbide (~90%) with a small amount of cobalt (~10%) (2). This entity is often confused with other rare ILD associated with another series of elements known as "heavy metals," such as chromium, cadmium, or thallium.

HMLD can present in several manners (Table 14.1), the most common of which is a reactive airway disease without significant parenchymal abnormalities that can resolve quickly with exposure cessation. In more severe presentations, diffuse parenchymal

DOI: 10.1201/9781003089384-14

TABLE 14.1: Characteristics of Hard Metal Lung Disease

	Occupational Asthma	Alveolitis	Interstitial Lung Disease
Clinical presentation	Cough, wheezing, upper respiratory symptoms, dyspnea	Subacute cough, dyspnea, weight loss	Insidious cough, dyspnea, tachypnea, weight loss, finger clubbing
Pulmonary function testing	Normal or obstructive pattern + methacholine with work exposure + cobalt bronchoprovocation testing	Restrictive, or mixed pattern, low DLCO	Restrictive or mixed pattern, low DLCO
Imaging	Mostly normal	Diffuse ground-glass and nodular opacities, mild reticular opacities	Diffuse peripheral-based reticular opacities, occasionally with honeycombing
Pathology	N/A	Lymphocytic predominant alveolitis or bronchiolitis, peribronchiolar inflammation	Giant cell interstitial pneumonia, usual interstitial pneumonia
Establishing diagnosis	Compatible symptoms + history of exposure + obstruction on PFTs/ positive bronchoprovocation test	Compatible symptoms + history of exposure + chest CT with GGO and nodules	Compatible symptoms + history of exposure + chest CT with fibrotic pattern
Treatment	Cessation of exposure, inhaled corticosteroids	Cessation of exposure, glucocorticoids, immunomodulators	Cessation of exposure, glucocorticoids, immunomodulators, lung transplantation

Source: Adapted from Zheng, M., Marron, R.M. & Sehgal, S. Hard Metal Lung Disease: Update in Diagnosis and Management. Curr Pulmonol Rep 9, 37–46 (2020)(https://doi.org/10.1007/s13665-020-00247-x).

disease can range from an allergic alveolitis like HP to an irreversible interstitial fibrotic lung disease (3).

Lung disease in workers exposed to hard metal dust was first described by Jobs and Ballhausen in the 1940s (4). Although the pathologic entity of giant cell interstitial pneumonitis (GIP) had been previously described, the connection between GIP and disease in hard metal workers wasn't established until 1979 by Abraham et al. after analyzing open lung biopsy samples (5, 6). Abraham and colleagues further described 22 cases of GIP with extensive hard metal exposure, which suggested that GIP was pathognomonic for what has become known as HMLD (6). This group also identified the presence of metal content in lung tissue using an electron probe micro-analyzer (EPMA) and found that a group of patients with GIP on pathology had high concentrations of tungsten carbide and cobalt metal alloy (7). These findings were essential in establishing the link between hard metal dust exposure and interstitial lung disease.

Pathophysiology and risk factors

The metal alloys implicated in HMLD are created by a mixture of tungsten carbide and cobalt compacting under high temperatures. This alloy is commonly utilized in in the production of metal sharpening tools due to its durability, which is similar to a diamond's (2). These alloys are also utilized in other industries such as diamond polishing and the production of dental prostheses, which has caused HMLD in workers in those disciplines (8–10).

The production and finishing of these alloys can produce metallic dust particles smaller than 2 μm, which can be inhaled and deposited into alveoli. This induces inflammatory reactions that produce pulmonary disease ranging from reactive airway disease to interstitial fibrosis. Exposure to these particles can lead to development of HMLD (2).

Both components of this alloy, tungsten carbide and cobalt, have been independently implicated in lung disease. Initially tungsten carbide was thought to be the primary driver of the pathology since its insolubility leads to aggregation in lung tissue and was easily detectable (11). Hard metal alloys are primarily composed of tungsten carbide and cobalt forms only a small component of the alloy. Cobalt, however, was found to be pathogenic after a group of diamond polishers using cobalt-containing polishing disks were diagnosed with GIP. Lung pathology of these diamond polishers was compatible with GIP, but a mineralogenic analysis of tissue showed the presence of only cobalt (12–14). The combination of tungsten carbide and cobalt likely has a synergistic effect in the development of lung disease, with cobalt being the main culprit (14). Nonindustrial exposure to cobalt from electronic cigarette use leading to HMLD has also been reported, perhaps due to contamination from cobalt in the heating coil (15).

However, HMLD remains a rare entity, even amongst those with significant exposure. A cross-sectional study from Sprince et al. of workers in tungsten-carbide production reported work-related wheezing in 10.9% and ILD in 0.7% (8).

Pathogenesis

In advanced HMLD, the potential pathways of lung injury could be a combination of maladaptive immunologic responses and oxidative changes. One important difference from pneumoconiosis is that the disease does not seem to be "dose dependent." Total cumulative exposure to tungsten or cobalt does not correlate with severity of parenchymal lung disease.

Bronchoalveolar lavage (BAL) analysis in HMLD shows a pattern similar to hypersensitivity pneumonitis, with predominance of CD8+ cells. It is thus believed that the mechanism could be similar to that of HP due to maladaptive immunological responses (14, 16).

Another theory suggests that the presence of cobalt increases oxidative stress, which creates reactive oxidative species that lead to lung injury. This reaction is enhanced by tungsten carbide, thus adding to the synergistic lung injury. Cobalt chloride exposure in hamsters causes changes seen with oxidative stress. Furthermore, oxygen use has been shown to accelerate HMLD in some patients, giving credence to the oxidative stress theory (2).

Removing exposure

Industries that utilize tools containing titanium carbide and/or cobalt alloys (Table 14.2) should take precautions to educate and protect workers. Workers in these industries should wear respirators during the use of hard metal tools. Per the Occupational Health and Safety Administration, the maximum permissible exposure limit for cobalt is 0.1 mg/m^3 of air as an 8-hour time weighted average (17). Workers should report respiratory

TABLE 14.2: Exposures Associated with Hard Metal Lung Disease

Hard metal production	Manufacturing of alloys
	Sintering and finishing of metal alloy tools
	Finishing/grinding and tool maintenance
Utilization of hard metals or cobalt	Diamond polishing
	Bonded diamond tooling
	Dental prosthesis processing
Miscellaneous	E-cigarette use (vaping)

Source: Adapted from Zheng, M., Marron, R.M. & Sehgal, S. Hard Metal Lung Disease: Update in Diagnosis and Management. Curr Pulmonol Rep 9, 37–46 (2020). (https://doi.org/10.1007/s13665-020-00247-x).

symptoms early and be referred to a specialist evaluation to prevent the progression to severe diseases (18). Cessation of exposure is the most important preventive and treatment tool available.

Reactive airway disease

Workers exposed to cobalt have a 5–10 times higher risk of developing asthma compared to those who are not exposed and 3–4% of exposed workers have a positive cobalt bronchoprovocation test (19). Low molecular weight cobalt dust is an incomplete antigen and can bind to human albumin to induce an IgE-mediated response. This mechanism is like that seen after exposure to platinum, di-isocyanates, and wood dust amongst other agents that cause occupational asthma.

Clinical features

Upper respiratory symptoms, including rhinorrhea, sneezing, congestion, sore throat, and dry cough, are common in occupational asthma and may resolve with cessation of sensitizing-agent exposure. Some patients, however, may have symptoms that progress after extensive exposure over months to years to overt dyspnea, cough, and constitutional symptoms such as malaise, fevers, chills, and weight loss (14, 20).

Patients can present after a wide range of latency periods, varying from months to years, after exposure to cobalt. Symptom onset can be hours after exposure, leading to symptoms developing after leaving the workplace, which makes diagnosis challenging (19).

Establishing diagnosis

Workers exposed to known agents that cause occupational asthma should be screened with a thorough medical history. Symptoms are often nonspecific. Typically, symptoms present after exposure at work with resolution during prolonged periods away from the workplace, such as weekends and vacation. If occupational asthma is suspected, a methacholine challenge should be performed either at work or within 2 hours after the exposure has ended. Lack of bronchoprovocation can help rule out asthma. An alternate method is serial peak expiratory flow rates monitoring. This can be done over 2–3 weeks at work. They should be interpreted with caveats of variations in technique on different attempts and the potential for fabrication (21).

A bronchoprovocation test using cobalt micro-particles can be done in experienced laboratories. This is often considered the gold standard for diagnosing cobalt-related occupational asthma. The concern with this modality is that it can lead to severe bronchospasm in sensitized patients. Rarely, a false negative result may be obtained if the patient has ended exposure for a prolonged period and does not have bronchial hyper-responsiveness to cobalt anymore (21). Some case series have suggested testing for IgE antibodies specific to cobalt-conjugated human serum albumin, which may be helpful (22).

Treatment

The mainstay of management is cessation of exposure. One third of patients report complete resolution of symptoms just with this measure. Persistent symptoms after exposure are commonly seen, especially in those with prolonged or intense exposure. In a small case series, almost 80% of cases had improvement or complete resolution of symptoms on cessation of exposure. Treatment in persistent cases, or when exposure cannot be stopped, is similar to that for asthma, with inhaled corticosteroids being the first-line agent (23–26).

Parenchymal lung disease

Exposure to hard metals can lead to parenchymal damage with varied patterns — hypersensitivity alveolitis and fibrotic diffuse parenchymal lung disease are the two most common. This can often be a spectrum starting as allergic or inflammatory alveolitis and progressing to fibrotic lung disease.

Patients may present with a hypersensitivity pneumonitis-like presentation with episodes characterized by fever, cough, and shortness of breath. Chest CT scans can show diffuse ground-glass opacities and a nodular pattern. These symptoms and radiographic findings may resolve with the removal of exposure. A portion of these patients with repeated alveolitis may progress to irreversible parenchymal changes seen in other fibrotic lung diseases (2).

Clinical features

Through the spectrum of disease, patients can present with a variety of respiratory ailments such as a dry cough and breathlessness. In late fibrotic phases of the disease, tachypnea and hypoxemic respiratory failure, accompanied by fine crackles on lung auscultation and clubbing of fingers, can be observed (14).

Establishing diagnosis

Accurate diagnoses of HMLD can be difficult. The entity can be suggested in the setting of proper exposure history but should be accompanied by supporting evidence in radiographic and pathologic findings compatible with this rare disease. Other etiologies of diffuse parenchymal lung disease, such as connective tissue, sarcoidosis, HP, and other occupational lung disease, should be ruled out (2, 27).

Occupational exposure history

Usually an evaluation of HMLD is preceded by an occupational exposure history consistent with hard metal exposure (Table 14.2). However, the existence of hard metal alloys or cobalt may not be obvious to many clinicians unfamiliar with industrial components. Workers often have occupational health professionals present in their industries and a dialogue between the pulmonologist and those professionals should be initiated. History taking should focus on workplace responsibilities and tools used, making sure to include the trade names of tools and drills used if applicable (2, 14, 27). Unlike some other occupational lung disease, HMLD may be present irrespective of the duration or intensity of the exposure (14).

Radiographic findings

Similar to most interstitial lung diseases, high-resolution computed tomography (HRCT) is required to recognize and characterize HMLD (28). There is a wide heterogeneity in chest CT findings depending on the subtype and severity of disease. In patients with pathologically confirmed HMLD, HRCT findings included diffuse ground-glass opacities (Figure 14.1), centrilobular nodules, multifocal consolidations, and an interstitial fibrosis pattern with traction bronchiectasis as seen in NSIP (Figure 14.2) (29–32). Uncommon findings include peripheral cysts and pneumothoraces (28, 33–35).

Pulmonary function testing

Most patients will demonstrate a restrictive pattern with reduced diffusion capacity on pulmonary function testing. However, in certain cases, an obstructive pattern could be observed if the predominant involvement is in the distal airways (18).

Laboratory findings

Serum and urine measurements of cobalt may help establish cobalt exposure if there is concern of HMLD (36). Bloodwork to rule out other causes of ILD should be done as indicated. Skin-patch testing can be used in many cases to support an allergic hyper-reactivity to cobalt, especially those with dermatitis. However, many workers with HMLD may not have a positive skin test (14).

Bronchoscopy

BAL can assist in the diagnosis of HMLD, but its negative predictive value is low. A low CD4/CD8 cell ratio had been reported in some cases and giant cells present in the BAL fluid, as reported by Kinoshita et al. in their case series, could narrow the diagnosis and preclude necessity for open-lung biopsy. However, giant cells may not be present in most cases and cannot be relied upon as a diagnostic gold standard (37, 38).

Like other ILDs, the transbronchial lung biopsy yield may be too small to reliably support a diagnosis, although it may be diagnostic in some cases (18, 39). The utility of cryobiopsy, which can theoretically produce larger samples, has not been evaluated in HMLD.

Histopathology

Since the earliest descriptions of the disease entity, GIP has been the most common pathological finding. GIP is characterized by airspace filling with alveolar macrophages and numerous multinucleated giant cells along with bronchiolo-centric fibrosis (Figure 14.3). Due to their characteristic engulfment of individually discernable cells (emperipolesis), they are described as "cannibalistic" (5, 14). GIP is not pathognomonic for HMLD. In the absence of heavy metal exposure, it has been seen in ILD due to nitrofurantoin exposure, World Trade Center-associated lung disease, titanium-associated lung disease, and measles (40–44). Given the nonspecific nature of giant cell pneumonitis, an exposure history supporting pathologic evidence is important in the diagnosis of HMLD.

An EPMA can be used to assist in the diagnosis through the detection of tungsten carbide accumulation in lung tissue. In the EPMA analysis performed by Moriyama et al., the tungsten accumulation was mainly found in the giant cells and peribronchiolar fibrosis tissue. Cobalt, however, is not readily identifiable by EPMA due to its solubility (12).

Treatment

Removal of exposure

The primary intervention should be immediate cessation of exposure since specific pharmacologic treatments are based primarily on empiric evidence. Patients should be counselled that most symptoms will subside with cessation exposure, especially in those with reactive airway disease (14, 45). The impact of exposure cessation is lessened in advanced fibrotic disease (46). As in all occupational lung diseases, exposure cessation can be difficult to achieve as it may mean loss of employment for the patient, and the involvement of employer occupational health may be necessary to ensure cessation of exposure without negative financial implications for the patient.

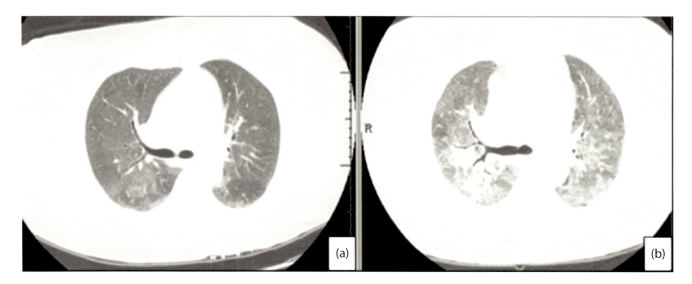

FIGURE 14.1 Giant cell interstitial pneumonia. (a) A cross-sectional axial CT image in a patient with histologically proven GIP demonstrates diffuse ground-glass attenuation. (b) A high-resolution axial CT image of the same patient 4 years later demonstrates progression of diffuse ground-glass attenuation, mosaicism, and peribronchial consolidation. (Reprinted from Respiratory Medicine, volume 129. Adams TN, Butt YM, Batra K, Glazer CS. Cobalt-related interstitial lung disease, pp. 91–97, 2017, with permission from Elsevier.)

Hard Metal Lung Disease and Other Rare Occupational Lung Diseases

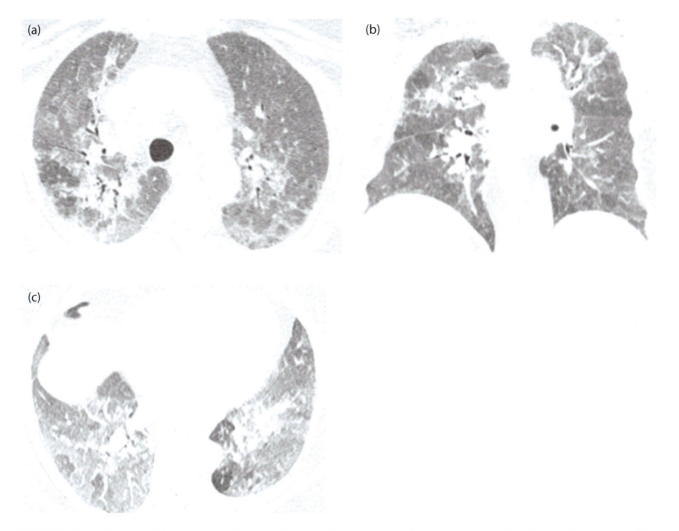

FIGURE 14.2 Hypersensitivity pneumonitis secondary to cobalt exposure. (a) An axial cross-sectional image demonstrates fibrosis with consolidations and traction bronchiectasis as well as surrounding lucent areas. (b) A coronal image in the same patient shows diffuse distribution of the ground-glass opacities, mosaicism, and upper lobe predominant consolidations. (c) This expiratory image demonstrates lobular areas of air trapping. (Reprinted from Respiratory Medicine, volume 129. Adams TN, Butt YM, Batra K, Glazer CS. Cobalt-related interstitial lung disease, pp. 91–97, 2017, with permission from Elsevier.)

Anti-inflammatory agents

The evidence for the efficacy of corticosteroids and immunosuppressive agents are based on only limited cases series. In a review by Chiba et al., of 18 case reports of HMLD treated with corticosteroids, 77.8% of patients showed a favorable response to treatment (47). In their report, corticosteroid responsiveness factors were shorter exposure duration and the finding of GIP on pathology. Patients with a higher burden of fibrotic disease were not as responsive to corticosteroids. Steroid-sparing immunosuppressive agents have been utilized in a few case reports (47). Disease stabilization in a patient with steroid and cyclophosphamide treatment has been reported (48). Azathioprine and cyclosporine have also been used in case reports as adjunct and steroid-sparing agents, but the evidence for their efficacy is not well established (18, 49).

Lung transplantation

Lung transplantation is an option for patients with severe and progressive lung disease. However, there have been reports of recurrence of the disease in single-lung transplant patients, despite cessation of exposure (50).

Other metal-related occupational lung diseases

Siderosis

Siderosis occurs in electric-arc and oxyacetylene welders due to the inhalation of fine divided particles of iron oxide. Usually not associated with clinical impairment, the radiographic appearance is unique with the presence of diffuse high attenuation centrilobular micronodules, which represent accumulation of metal particles within alveolar macrophages. These radiographic opacities are reversible and resolve partially or completely after exposure cessation (32, 51).

Talcosis

Talc is hydrated magnesium silicate used in the leather, ceramic, paper, plastics, rubber, paint, and cosmetic industries. Talc exposure may occur secondary to inhalation or intravenous drug abuse, which can result in non-necrotizing granulomatous inflammation and progressive fibrosis. Radiographically, it is characterized by centrilobular and subpleural nodules with high

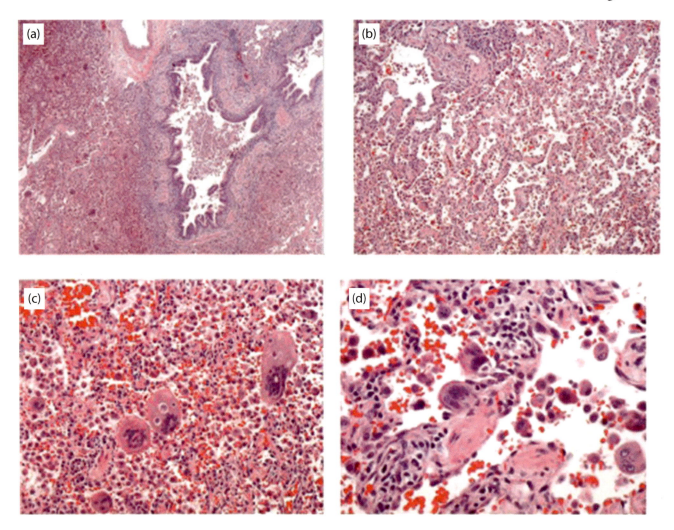

FIGURE 14.3 Giant cell interstitial pneumonia. (a) The hematoxylin and eosin stain shows characteristic intra-alveolar macrophages and multinucleated giant cells in a background of mild interstitial pneumonia, peribronchiolar chronic inflammation, and fibrosis. (b) A higher power shows mild interstitial pneumonia and fibrosis with intra-alveolar macrophages and multinucleated giant cells. (c) A higher power of multinucleated giant cells, several demonstrating emperipolesis. A characteristic halo, thought to be artefactual in nature, can be seen around several of the engulfed inflammatory cells. (d) A high-power view shows multinucleated pneumocytes. (Reprinted from Respiratory Medicine, volume 129. Adams TN, Butt YM, Batra K, glazer CS. Cobalt-related interstitial lung disease, pp. 91–97, 2017, with permission from Elsevier.)

attenuation foci corresponding to talc deposition with relative sparing of lung bases (Figure 14.4 a–c) (51, 52).

Berylliosis

Berylliosis, or chronic beryllium disease, refers to a rare occupational lung disease caused by exposure to beryllium, which is used in aerospace, ceramics, dentistry, nuclear weapons, and nuclear reactors. It is associated with two types of lung injury: 1) An acute chemical pneumonitis and 2) a chronic granulomatous pneumoconiosis very similar to sarcoidosis. Berylliosis may be seen in 5–20% of exposed workers and its incidence and severity is not related to the duration and intensity of exposure. Lung pathology reveals noncaseating granulomas secondary to a delayed hypersensitivity reaction of the beryllium sensitized CD4+ T cells. Indeed, a blood beryllium lymphocyte proliferation test is the initial diagnostic test for suspected berylliosis. A bronchoscopy with BAL and transbronchial biopsy confirms the diagnosis with the demonstration of beryllium-sensitized lymphocytes and noncaseating granulomas, respectively. Radiologically, it is characterized by ground-glass opacities and nodules distributed in a peri-lymphatic distribution, which could then progress to interstitial pulmonary fibrosis, pseudo-plaques, and hilar and mediastinal adenopathy (Figure 14.5 a–c) (53, 54).

Newer occupational lung diseases

Flock-worker's lung

Flock-worker's lung develops from inhalation of respirable flock, an ultra-fine nylon fiber used in the production of fabrics, which is associated with a nongranulomatous ILD with lymphocytic bronchiolitis, and peribronchiolitis with lymphoid hyperplasia (54, 55). Radiologically, it is characterized

Hard Metal Lung Disease and Other Rare Occupational Lung Diseases

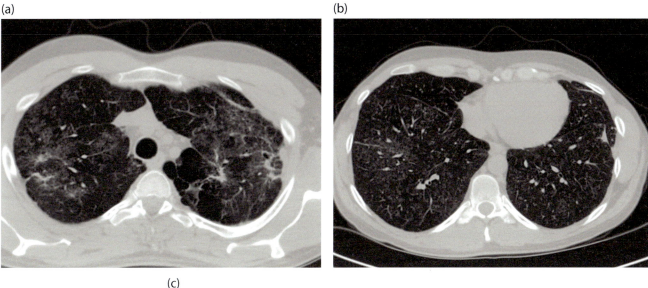

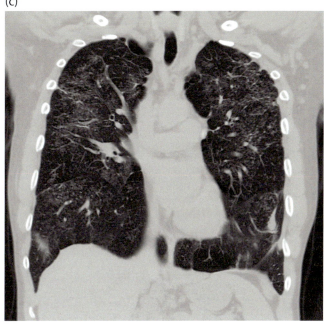

FIGURE 14.4 Talc pneumoconiosis. (a) An axial cross-sectional view of a CT image in a patient with talc pneumoconiosis showing diffuse centrilobular nodules with fibrosis and pleural thickening in the upper lobes. (b) An axial cross-sectional view of CT images showing centrilobular nodules. (c) A coronal view CT images in the same patient showing centrilobular nodules, fibrosis, and pleural thickening, which is more prominent in the upper lobes compared to the lower lobes. (Images courtesy of Daniel Ocazionez-Trujillo MD, UT Health, Houston).

by patchy ground-glass opacities, consolidations, or diffuse micro-nodularity (54).

Flavor-worker's lung
Flavor-worker's lung refers to the development of constrictive bronchiolitis described in patients exposed to the artificial butter flavoring chemical diacetyl (2,3 butanedione). CT imaging shows mosaic attenuation along with expiratory air trapping (54, 56).

Indium tin oxide lung disease
Indium tin oxide, used in the production of transparent conductive films utilized in flat-panel screens, can lead to the development of interstitial lung disease, pulmonary fibrosis, and pulmonary alveolar proteinosis. CT imaging may show subpleural honeycombing, upper lobe pulmonary fibrosis, or ground-glass opacities with a "crazy-paving" appearance (54, 57).

Lung disease in deployed military personnel
Constrictive bronchiolitis was reported in military personnel from Iraq and Afghanistan who were reported to have been exposed to combustion products from the industrial sulfur fires and other noxious gases and fumes. Pulmonary function tests showed a decrease in diffusion capacity and decreased FEV_1 and FVC, although they remained within normal limits in most patients. CT scans showed expiratory air trapping and centrilobular nodules in roughly 25% of patients (54, 58).

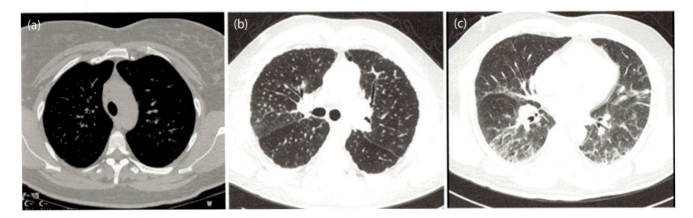

FIGURE 14.5 Chronic beryllium disease or berylliosis transverse CT images from three patients with chronic beryllium disease that highlight the spectrum of imaging abnormalities in chronic beryllium disease, ranging from ground-glass opacification (a), disseminated nodular opacities (b), and ground-glass opacification with septal thickening and fibrosis (c). (Reprinted from CHEST, volume 158. MacMurdo MG, Mroz MM, Culver DA, Dweik RA, Maier LA. Chronic beryllium disease: Update on a moving target, pp. 2458–2466, with permission from Elsevier.)

Conclusion

Occupational lung diseases present a significant and potentially preventable work-related disease. Silicosis, asbestos-related lung disease, and coal workers pneumoconiosis represent the most recognized conditions within this spectrum. Several rare and newer occupational lung diseases exist, each of which requires a high index of suspicion, careful evaluation of occupational exposures, and a good understanding of radiological features to help diagnose them and may obviate the need for lung biopsies in making a confident diagnosis. Pathological patterns are unique in several of these rare occupational lung diseases, which include a granulomatous reaction in berylliosis and giant cell pneumonia in hard metal lung disease. Radiologic patterns described include either fibrosis, expiratory air trapping, centrilobular nodules, or diffuse pulmonary opacities. Cessation of exposure remains a cornerstone of treatment, with the addition of inhaled steroids, systemic steroids, and immunomodulators in the appropriate clinical settings.

References

1. Nelson DI, Concha-Barrientos M, Driscoll T, Steenland K, Fingerhut M, Punnett L, et al. The global burden of selected occupational diseases and injury risks: Methodology and summary. Am J Ind Med. 2005;48(6):400–418.
2. Nemery B, Verbeken EK, Demedts M. Giant cell interstitial pneumonia (hard metal lung disease, cobalt lung). Semin Respir Crit Care Med. 2001;22(4):435–48.
3. Cugell DW, Morgan WK, Perkins DG, Rubin A. The respiratory effects of cobalt. Arch Intern Med. 1990;150(1):177–83.
4. Jobs H. Metalleramiks als staubquelle vom arztlichen und technicheen stnandpunkt. Vertrauensarzt Krankenkasse. 1940;8:142.
5. Liebow AA. Definition and classification of interstitial pneumonias in human pathology. Alveolar Interstitium of the Lung. 8: Karger Publishers; 1975. p. 1–33.
6. Abraham J. Lung pathology in 22 cases of giant cell interstitial pneumonia (GIP) suggests GIP is pathognomonic of cobalt (hard metal) disease. Chest. 1987;91:312.
7. Abraham JL, Burnett BR, Hunt A. Development and use of a pneumoconiosis database of human pulmonary inorganic particulate burden in over 400 lungs. Scanning Microscopy. 1991;5(1):95–104; discussion 5.
8. Sprince NL, Oliver LC, Eisen EA, Greene RE, Chamberlin RI. Cobalt exposure and lung disease in tungsten carbide production. Am Rev Respir Dis. 1988;138:1220–6.
9. Kim Y-H, Chung YK, Kim C, Kim H-J, Joo Y. A case of hypersensitivity pneumonitis with giant cells in a female dental technician. Ann Occup Environ Med. 2013;25(1):1–7.
10. Santhosh L, Venado A, Blanc P, Jones K, Brush D, Ley B. Drilling down on hard metal lung disease: An unusual case of a dental lab technician with rapidly progressive interstitial lung disease. C106 Occupational Lung Epidemiology: American Thoracic Society; 2018. p. A6085–A.
11. Naqvi AH, Hunt A, Burnett BR, Abraham JL. Pathologic spectrum and lung dust burden in giant cell interstitial pneumonia (hard metal disease/cobalt pneumonitis): Review of 100 cases. Arch Environ Occup Health. 2008;63(2):51–70.
12. Moriyama H, Kobayashi M, Takada T, Shimizu T, Terada M, Narita J-I, et al. Two-dimensional analysis of elements and mononuclear cells in hard metal lung disease. Am J Resp Crit Care Med. 2007;176(1):70–7.
13. Demedts M, Gheysens B, Nagels J, Verbeken E, Lauweryns J, Van Den Eeckhout A, et al. Cobalt lung in diamond polishers. Am Rev Resp Dis. 1984;130(1):130–5.
14. Adams TN, Butt YM, Batra K, Glazer CS. Cobalt related interstitial lung disease. Respir Med. 2017;129:91–7.
15. Elliott DRF, Shah R, Hess CA, Elicker B, Henry TS, Rule AM, et al. Giant cell interstitial pneumonia secondary to cobalt exposure from e-cigarette use. Eur Resp J. 2019;54(6).
16. Michetti G, Mosconi G, Zanelli R, Migliori M, Gaffuri G, Villa R, et al. Bronchoalveolar lavage and its role in diagnosing cobalt lung disease. Sci Total Environ. 1994;150(1-3):173–8.
17. Alexandersson R. Blood and urinary concentrations as estimators of cobalt exposure. Arch Environ Health: An International Journal. 1988;43(4):299–303.
18. Takada T, Moriyama H. Hard Metal Lung Disease. A Clinical Guide to Occupational and Environmental Lung Diseases: Springer; 2012. p. 217–30.
19. Cirla AM. Cobalt-related asthma: Clinical and immunological aspects. Sci Total Environ. 1994;150(1-3):85–94.
20. Balmes J. Respiratory effects of hard-metal dust exposure. Occup Med (Philadelphia, Pa). 1987;2(2):327–44.
21. Bernstein JA. Occupational asthma. Allergy and Asthma: Springer; 2016. p. 253–70.
22. Shirakawa T, Kusaka Y, Fujimura N, Goto S, Kato M, Heki S, et al. Occupational asthma from cobalt sensitivity in workers exposed to hard metal dust. Chest. 1989;95(1):29–37.
23. Merget R, Reineke M, Rueckmann A, Bergmann E-M, Schultze-Werninghaus G. Nonspecific and specific bronchial responsiveness in occupational asthma caused by platinum salts after allergen avoidance. Am J Respir Crit Care Med. 1994;150(4):1146–9.
24. Pisati G, Zedda S. Outcome of occupational asthma due to cobalt hypersensitivity. Sci Total Environ. 1994;150(1-3):167–71.

25. Nureki S, Miyazaki E, Nishio S, Ando M, Kumamoto T. Hard Metal lung disease successfully treated with inhaled corticosteroids. Intern Med. 2013;52(17):1957–61.
26. Rachiotis G, Savani R, Brant A, MacNeill SJ, Taylor AN, Cullinan P. Outcome of occupational asthma after cessation of exposure: A systematic review. Thorax. 2007;62(2):147–52.
27. Beckett WS. Occupational respiratory diseases. N Engl J Med. 2000;342(6):406–13.
28. Gotway MB, Golden JA, Warnock M, Koth LL, Webb R, Reddy GP, et al. Hard Metal interstitial lung disease: High-resolution computed tomography appearance. J Thorac Imag. 2002;17(4):314–8.
29. Akira M. Uncommon pneumoconioses: CT and pathologic findings. Radiology. 1995;197(2):403–9.
30. Enriquez LS, Mohammed T-LH, Johnson GL, Lefor MJ, Beasley MB. Hard Metal pneumoconiosis: A case of giant-cell interstitial pneumonitis in A machinist. Respiratory Care. 2007;52(2):196–9.
31. Hahtola PA, Järvenpää RE, Lounatmaa K, Mattila JJ, Rantala I, Uitti JA, et al. Hard Metal alveolitis accompanied by rheumatoid arthritis. Respiration. 2000;67(2):209–12.
32. Kim KI, Kim CW, Lee MK, Lee KS, Park CK, Choi SJ, et al. Imaging of occupational lung disease. Radiographics. 2001;21(6):1371–91.
33. Dunlop P, Müller NL, Wilson J, Flint J, Churg A. Hard Metal lung disease: High-resolution CT and histologic correlation of the initial findings and demonstration of interval improvement. J Thorac Imag. 2005;20(4):301–4.
34. Kaneko Y, Kikuchi N, Ishii Y, Kawabata Y, Moriyama H, Terada M, et al. Upper lobe-dominant pulmonary fibrosis showing deposits of hard metal component in the fibrotic lesions. Intern Med. 2010;49(19):2143–5.
35. Wahbi Z, Arnold A, Taylor AN. Hard Metal lung disease and pneumothorax. Respiratory Medicine. 1997;91(2):103–5.
36. Ichikawa Y, Kusaka Y, Goto S. Biological monitoring of cobalt exposure, based on cobalt concentrations in blood and urine. Int Arch Occup Environ Health. 1985;55(4):269–76.
37. Kinoshita M, Sueyasu Y, Watanabe H, Tanoue S, Okubo Y, Koga T, et al. Giant cell interstitial pneumonia in two hard metal workers: The role of bronchoalveolar lavage in diagnosis. Respirology. 1999;4(3):263–6.
38. Forni A. Bronchoalveolar lavage in the diagnosis of hard metal disease. Sci Total Environ. 1994;150(1-3):69–76.
39. Nakamura Y, Nishizaka Y, Ariyasu R, Okamoto N, Yoshida M, Taki M, et al. Hard metal lung disease diagnosed on a transbronchial lung biopsy following recurrent contact dermatitis. Intern Med. 2014;53(2):139–43.
40. Magee F, Wright J, Chan N, Currie W, Karr G, Hogg J, et al. Two unusual pathological reactions to nitrofurantoin. Histopathology. 1986;10(7):701–6.
41. Hargett CW, Sporn TA, Roggli VL, Hollingsworth JW. Giant cell interstitial pneumonia associated with nitrofurantoin. Lung. 2006;184(3):147–9.
42. Khoor A, Roden AC, Colby TV, Roggli VL, Elrefaei M, Alvarez F, et al. Giant cell interstitial pneumonia in patients without hard metal exposure: Analysis of 3 cases and review of the literature. Human Pathology. 2016;50:176–82.
43. Krajsová B, Tichý T. Giant cell interstitial pneumonia without exposure to hard metals. Ceskoslovenska Patologie. 2013;49(3):141–3.
44. Radoycich GE, Zuppan CW, Weeks DA, Krous HF, Langston C. Patterns of measles pneumonitis. Pediatric Pathology. 1992;12(6):773–86.
45. Zanelli R, Barbic F, Migliori M, Michetti G. Uncommon evolution of fibrosing alveolitis in a hard metal grinder exposed to cobalt dusts. Sci Total Environ. 1994;150(1-3):225–9.
46. Maier LA. Clinical approach to chronic beryllium disease and other nonpneumoconiotic interstitial lung diseases. Journal of Thoracic Imaging. 2002;17(4):273–84.
47. Chiba Y, Kido T, Tahara M, Oda K, Noguchi S, Kawanami T, et al. Hard Metal lung disease with favorable response to corticosteroid treatment: A case report and literature review. The Tohoku J Exp Med. 2019;247(1):51–8.
48. Ratto D, Balmes J, Boylen T, Sharma OP. Pregnancy in a woman with severe pulmonary fibrosis secondary to hard metal disease. Chest. 1988;93(3):663–5.
49. Chiarchiaro J, Tomsic L, Strock S, Veraldi K, Nouraie M, Sellares J, et al. A case series describing common radiographic and pathologic patterns of hard metal pneumoconiosis. Resp Med Case Reports. 2018;25:124–8.
50. Tarabichi Y, Saggar R, Wallace WD, Lynch JP, Saggar R. Primary disease recurrence after single lung transplantation in a patient with prior hard metal exposure. J Heart and Lung Transplant. 2015;34(9):1216–8.
51. Chong S, Lee KS, Chung MJ, Han J, Kwon OJ, Kim TS. Pneumoconiosis: Comparison of imaging and pathologic findings. Radiographics. 2006;26(1):59–77.
52. Akira M, Kozuka T, Yamamoto S, Sakatani M, Morinaga K. Inhalational talc pneumoconiosis: Radiographic and CT findings in 14 patients. AJR Am J Roentgenol. 2007;188(2):326–33.
53. Sharma N, Patel J, Mohammed TL. Chronic beryllium disease: Computed tomographic findings. J Comput Assist Tomogr. 2010;34(6):945–8.
54. Cox CW, Rose CS, Lynch DA. State of the art: Imaging occupational lung disease. Radiology. 2014;270(3):681–96.
55. Kern DG, Crausman RS, Durand KT, Nayer A, Kuhn C, 3rd. Flock worker's lung: Chronic interstitial lung disease in the nylon flocking industry. Ann Intern Med. 1998;129(4):261–72.
56. Kreiss K, Gomaa A, Kullman G, Fedan K, Simoes EJ, Enright PL. Clinical bronchiolitis obliterans in workers at a microwave-popcorn plant. N Engl J Med. 2002;347(5):330–8.
57. Cummings KJ, Nakano M, Omae K, Takeuchi K, Chonan T, Xiao YL, et al. Indium lung disease. Chest. 2012;141(6):1512–21.
58. King MS, Eisenberg R, Newman JH, Tolle JJ, Harrell FE, Jr., Nian H, et al. Constrictive bronchiolitis in soldiers returning from Iraq and Afghanistan. N Engl J Med. 2011;365(3):222–30.

15

ADULT PULMONARY ALVEOLAR PROTEINOSIS

Katherine Richards, Anupam Kumar, and Tisha Wang

Contents

Introduction	110
Pathogenesis and classification	110
Clinical features	110
Radiographic features	111
Diagnosis	111
Treatment	112
References	114

KEY POINTS

- PAP is a rare lung disorder characterized by abnormal surfactant homeostasis resulting in accumulation of lipoproteinaceous material in the lung causing symptoms and abnormal gas exchange.
- Antibodies to GM-CSF, a glycoprotein cytokine critical for lung immunity, alveolar macrophage maturation, and inflammation, is pathogenic for autoimmune PAP (>90% of cases).
- Treatment options for symptomatic PAP include whole lung lavage, supplementation of GM-CSF, and in refractory cases, lung transplantation may be considered.

Introduction

Pulmonary alveolar proteinosis (PAP), first described by Rosen et al. in 1958, is a rare disorder characterized by abnormal pulmonary surfactant homeostasis (1). The accumulation of lipoproteinaceous material in the alveolar spaces causes symptoms and abnormal gas exchange in some patients. It also predisposes patients to secondary infections due to the underlying innate immune deficiency. Patients may have spontaneous resolution of symptoms, or in some instances progress to respiratory failure causing death or need for lung transplantation. Our understanding of the pathogenesis and therapeutic approach to PAP has evolved substantially in the last few decades. This chapter is a brief discussion of the clinical features, pathogenesis, diagnostic approach, and currently available treatment modalities for adult PAP.

Pathogenesis and classification

The fundamental abnormality in PAP is the abnormal surfactant homeostasis of the lung, either due to impaired surfactant clearance or abnormal surfactant production. Pulmonary surfactant is synthesized in the type 2 alveolar epithelial cells and is catabolized by recycling and uptake in the alveolar macrophages. Surfactant proteins (A, B, C, and D), key components for surfactant integrity, also mediate innate immunity of the lung.

Perhaps the most groundbreaking discovery in our understanding of PAP was the identification of the role of granulocyte-macrophage colony-stimulating factor (GM-CSF) in surfactant metabolism and lung immunity (2).

GM-CSF, a 23 kDa dimeric glycoprotein cytokine, is expressed by lung epithelial cells and has a pivotal role in immunity, host defense, and inflammation. Specifically, within the lung, GM-CSF is also critical for terminal differentiation of alveolar macrophages. Nakata and colleagues first reported the presence of GM-CSF-neutralizing antibodies in the serum and bronchoalveolar lavage (BAL) fluid of patients with idiopathic PAP (as it was called then), but noted its absence in secondary PAP or in healthy subjects (2–4). Given the autoimmune basis of pathogenesis, idiopathic PAP is now termed as autoimmune PAP, and constitutes approximately 90% of the patients with PAP. PAP may also be classified as primary PAP (caused by disruption of GM-CSF signaling) and secondary PAP (caused by impaired alveolar macrophage function from another etiology). Genetic defects in the GM-CSF receptor α or β chains (*CSF2RA*, *CSF2RB*) also lead to impaired macrophage maturation in the absence of autoimmunity, and is termed congenital or hereditary PAP. Certain occupational or environmental exposure are known to be directly toxic to alveolar macrophages, such as the original description of acute silicoproteinosis in silica workers (5). Commonly implicated exposures for development of PAP (secondary PAP) are noted in Table 15.1.

Alveolar macrophages are not only crucial for its metabolic functions, but they also play a key role in regulating pulmonary immunity (6). Thus, dysfunctional alveolar macrophages predispose these patients to opportunistic infections. GM-CSF is particularly important for control of *Nocardia* species, and studies have isolated antibodies to GM-CSF as a risk factor for disseminated disease, even in otherwise healthy individuals (7). Secondary infections contribute to approximately 20% of deaths due to PAP and should therefore be considered at every point of the clinical course in a symptomatic patient (8).

Clinical features

PAP has an estimated prevalence of 6.87 per million in the general population (9). The disease was traditionally reported as more common in men with a 2:1 gender predilection, but more recent US-based data suggests no gender predilection (9).

Adult Pulmonary Alveolar Proteinosis

TABLE 15.1: Classification of PAP and Underlying Etiology

Autoimmune PAP	>90% of cases
	Antibodies to GM-CSF causing disruption of GM-CSF signaling
Secondary PAP	5–10% of cases
	Hematologic disorders: Myelodysplasia, leukemia, lymphoma, stem cell or bone marrow transplantation
	Infections: HIV, *Nocardia*, pneumocystis
	Toxic inhalation: Silica, aluminum, titanium, indium
	Drug-induced: Chemotherapy agents, leflunomide, mycophenolate, sirolimus
Congenital or hereditary PAP	<1% of cases
	CSF2RA and CSF2RB mutations, ABCA3 mutation, surfactant production disorders
Unclassified PAP	

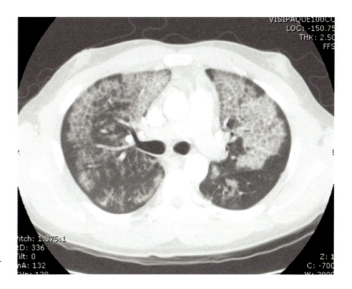

FIGURE 15.1 A CT chest scan demonstrating patchy ground-glass opacities with superimposed interlobular septal thickening in a "crazy paving" pattern.

In addition, no gender predominance was present in sub-analyses of nonsmokers and those without dust exposures (8), which suggests that differential exposures between genders may have accounted for the apparent male predominance rather than the natural history of the disease.

The disease usually presents insidiously in the third to sixth decade of life (8, 10) with variable and nonspecific symptoms. Progressive dyspnea is most reported with an incidence ranging from 50–90% (11, 12). Cough is common and may be productive or nonproductive. Less common symptoms include fatigue, weight loss, chest discomfort, hemoptysis, and arthralgias. Fever is rare and should prompt further workup for an infectious cause. Up to a third of patients may be asymptomatic on presentation (10), likely representing subclinical cases. Physical examination is similarly variable and, in many cases may be nonrevealing. Crackles are present in 15–50% of cases while cyanosis and clubbing are infrequently reported (13).

PAP may present with a combination of characteristic findings on physiologic and laboratory studies. Impairments in gas exchange are frequently evident with reductions in diffusing capacity on pulmonary function testing as well as widening of alveolar to arterial oxygen gradients on arterial blood gas. Pulmonary function testing may also reveal a restrictive ventilatory impairment. A 6-minute walk test can reveal any exertional desaturation and need for oxygen supplementation.

Laboratory testing commonly shows elevations in various serum inflammatory markers including C-reactive protein, erythrocyte sedimentation rate, and lactate dehydrogenase, although none is specific for PAP. In autoimmune PAP, elevated levels of circulating antibodies to GM-CSF are present in both the serum and BAL, although serum titers do not correlate with disease severity (14). In cases of congenital or hereditary PAP, GM-CSF levels may be elevated due to impaired clearance by mutated receptors on alveolar macrophages.

Radiographic features

Chest radiographs show bilateral airspace opacities, classically in a bat-wing appearance with central hilar prominence. High-resolution computed tomography (HRCT) of the chest is the optimal imaging study for further characterization. Patchy ground-glass opacities with superimposed interlobular septal thickening are classically seen in a pattern termed "crazy paving" (Figure 15.1).

The process is usually diffuse, though a lower zone predominance is seen in nearly a quarter of cases (15). Although 83% of patients with PAP are found to have crazy paving on HRCT, it is not pathognomonic for the condition. The pattern has also been described in a variety of other conditions including pulmonary edema, adult respiratory distress syndrome, diffuse alveolar hemorrhage, organizing pneumonia, nonspecific interstitial pneumonia, lipoid pneumonia, sarcoidosis, various malignancies, and infections including pneumocystis pneumonia and COVID-19 pneumonia (16, 17). Significant fibrosis can also be seen in 7% of cases (15), although other findings such as pleural effusions, mediastinal lymph node enlargement, air trapping, and pulmonary nodules are atypical.

Diagnosis

PAP may be strongly suspected on the basis of clinical presentation and HRCT findings, but confirmatory testing and identification of the etiology is essential for the initiation of therapy. BAL in PAP classically has a milky and opaque appearance due to the accumulation of lipoproteinaceous material in the alveoli (Figure 15.2). On microscopic examination, the BAL fluid reveals large foamy macrophages and eosinophilic granules. Extracellular hyaline material stains positive on periodic acid-Schiff staining and lamellar bodies are characteristically seen on electron microscopy (18). BAL can support a diagnosis of PAP when the fluid has this characteristic gross and histologic appearance.

In some cases, the BAL fluid may not have the classic gross appearance, particularly in situations where the lavage is not performed in a heavily involved area of the lung. The addition of transbronchial biopsy can improve diagnostic yield in such cases of uncertainty. Surgical lung biopsy is rarely necessary to establish the diagnosis and adds unnecessary risk, with reports of its use ranging from 8–20% in recent studies (10, 19). Histopathology demonstrates dense acellular eosinophilic material in the airways with mild interstitial inflammation (Figure 15.3). The accumulated material is characteristically periodic acid-Schiff positive.

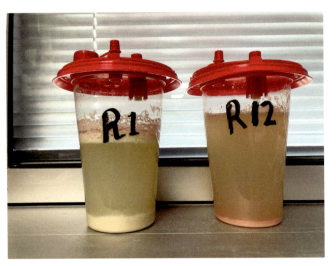

FIGURE 15.2 Bronchoalveolar lavage in PAP classically has a milky and opaque appearance due to the accumulation of lipoproteinaceous material in the alveoli.

Autoimmune PAP, which makes up >90% of PAP cases, can be definitively established by detection of elevated levels of anti-GM-CSF antibodies in the blood. This serum testing has a nearly 100% sensitivity and specificity for the diagnosis of autoimmune PAP, which obviates the need for any invasive procedures. In patients with normal anti-GM-CSF antibody levels, additional history and testing is necessary to discern between secondary PAP, hereditary PAP or unclassifiable PAP. Secondary PAP can usually be identified by normal antibody levels in conjunction with a history of an inhalational exposure, implicated drug exposure, or related disease process. It is noteworthy though that a few patients with PAP due to occupational exposures have also been reported to have anti-GM-CSF antibodies. On the other hand, absence of anti-GM-CSF antibodies, elevated levels of GM-CSF, and the absence of any secondary cause raises suspicion for hereditary PAP, which can be confirmed with genetic testing. An underlying cause is not identified despite extensive workup in a small proportion of cases, which are termed unclassifiable PAP (20).

Treatment

There are currently no international guidelines for the treatment of this rare lung disease. However, expert opinion suggests that treatments should be tailored based upon disease severity as well as the underlying etiology (Figure 15.4). Patients with asymptomatic or minimally symptomatic disease as well as mild physiologic impairments in forced vital capacity (FVC) and diffusing capacity with normal oxygenation are considered to have mild disease. It is reasonable to defer specific PAP therapies for these patients and focus management on the treatment of any secondary causes and avoidance of any implicated exposures. The importance of smoking cessation and preventative vaccines should be emphasized. Patients with mild disease should be monitored closely for progression with follow-up every 3 to 6 months to assess for changes in symptoms, imaging, decline in FVC, diffusing capacity, or oxygenation (20). Symptomatic patients and those with hypoxemia or moderate-to-severe reductions in FVC or diffusing capacity are considered to have moderate-to-severe disease and require more aggressive management.

Whole lung lavage

Whole lung lavage (WLL) has been used as the foundation of therapy for moderate-to-severe PAP since the 1960s (21) and remains the standard of care today. WLL promotes the physical removal of lipoproteinaceous material from the alveoli, which can provide therapeutic benefit in PAP regardless of the cause. Although there have been modifications to the procedure over the years, no standard protocol exists.

WLL is performed under general anesthesia and requires single lung ventilation with a double-lumen endotracheal tube. Extracorporeal membrane oxygenation may be utilized in select cases to support patients who otherwise would not tolerate single-lung ventilation (22). Most centers perform the procedure in two sequential sessions over the course of several days, typically beginning with lavage of the more severely affected lung. During each session, multiple aliquots of warmed saline are systematically infused into and drained from the lung, resulting in gradual clearance of the lavage from milky to clear in appearance.

WLL is largely considered to be a safe procedure when performed at experienced centers. Fever is the most common complication, with a reported incidence of 18%. Hypoxemia is reported in 14% of cases (23). Pneumothorax and pleural effusions related to the procedure are rare. Improvements in both oxygenation and lung function are seen following the procedure (8), but the duration of benefit appears to be limited with many patients experiencing relapse and subsequently requiring additional sessions of WLL. Relapse rates in the literature range from 57–66% (8, 24) with a median duration of benefit of 15 months prior to needing repeat WLL (8). A large survey of PAP patients found that patients require a mean of two-and-a-half WLL procedures within 5 years of their diagnosis (23).

GM-CSF supplementation

Recombinant GM-CSF therapy in humans with autoimmune PAP has been an active area of interest since studies in mice demonstrated a reversal of PAP pathology with GM-CSF replacement therapy (25). Human studies have consistently shown the therapy to be safe and well tolerated, but clinical outcomes have

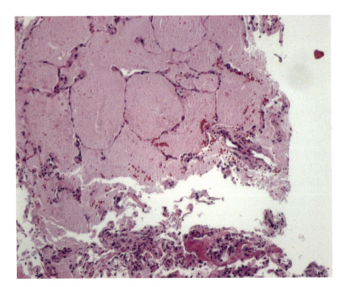

FIGURE 15.3 This histopathology demonstrates dense acellular eosinophilic material in the airways with mild interstitial inflammation.

Adult Pulmonary Alveolar Proteinosis

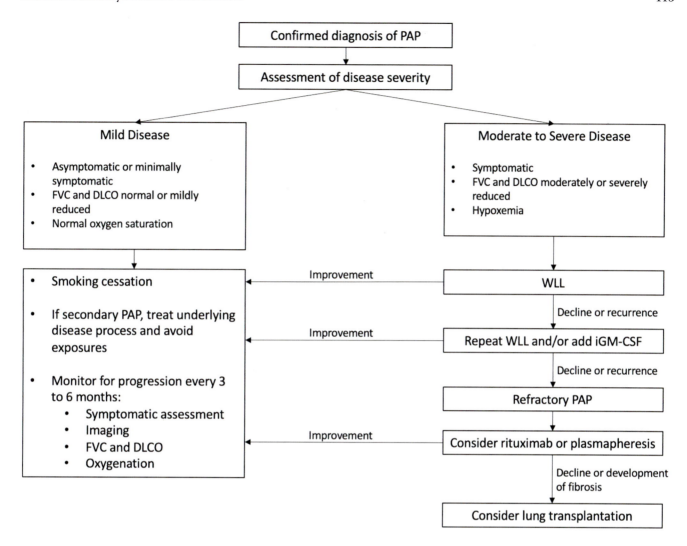

FIGURE 15.4 Treatment algorithm of PAP based on severity and current clinical evidence. *Abbreviations:* FVC: Forced vital capacity, DLCO: Diffusing capacity of lung for carbon monoxide, WLL: Whole lung lavage, iGM-CSF: Inhaled GM-CSF.

been variable. Heterogeneity among the studies in terms of route of administration, dose, frequency of administration, and duration of therapy may contribute to the variability of such results, although the cumulative evidence appears to support clinical benefit.

Recombinant GM-CSF is available in both inhaled and subcutaneous routes of administration for the treatment of autoimmune PAP. Inhaled therapy is associated with higher response rates (26, 27), likely as a result of higher local concentrations and bioavailability in the lungs. Although early studies of inhaled GM-CSF (iGM-CSF) appeared to classify patients into either responders or nonresponders, a later study with longer duration of therapy showed that all patients receiving the treatment were able to reach remission, and many were able to tolerate dose reductions to a lowest-effective dose (28). Two notable randomized-controlled trials have added further insight to this topic. A study of sargramostim in mild-to-moderate autoimmune PAP was associated with a significant improvement in arterial oxygen tension, radiographic lung density, and DLCO, although evidence of symptomatic and functional benefit to patients was less convincing. (29) Another double-blinded, placebo-controlled randomized trial with molgramostim demonstrated statistically significant improvements in both oxygenation and symptom severity, although improvement in walk distance and time to WLL lacked statistical significance (30). Overall, such studies suggest the potential for both physiologic and subjective clinical benefit with iGM-CSF therapy in autoimmune PAP, although the optimal dose, frequency, and duration of treatment have yet to be determined.

With the growing body of evidence for the safety and efficacy of iGM-CSF in autoimmune PAP, some experts advocate that it should no longer be viewed as an "off label" treatment (31). However, it is unclear whether recombinant GM-CSF is noninferior to WLL for use as a single therapy or whether its optimal use would be as an adjunctive therapy to WLL. Unfortunately, randomized controlled trials to answer such questions and obtain regulatory approval remain a challenge to perform due to the rarity of the disease.

Rituximab

Rituximab is a monoclonal antibody that acts to deplete B cells by targeting CD20. Reduction in circulating antibody levels is a downstream effect, making rituximab an appealing therapeutic agent in many autoimmune diseases with pathogenic autoantibodies.

As a result, rituximab has also been considered as a potential treatment of interest for autoimmune PAP. Evidence for its use in the disease has been mixed, with a retrospective analysis showing only 30% of patients with objective improvement following rituximab administration (32), while a small open-label phase II trial demonstrated significant improvement in parameters of oxygenation, imaging, and antibody levels (33). At this time, rituximab is not recommended as a first-line therapy for autoimmune PAP, though it may be considered in refractory cases.

Plasmapheresis

GM-CSF antibody clearance by plasmapheresis has also been proposed as a treatment for autoimmune PAP, although its use has been limited to case reports with variable results. Some reports have shown that plasmapheresis was associated with reduced antibody levels, improvement in arterial oxygenation, and improvement on chest radiography, although others have shown isolated reductions in antibody levels without any significant clinical benefit.

Glucocorticoids

Although glucocorticoids are used in the treatment of many autoimmune disorders, retrospective studies suggest that their use in autoimmune PAP is associated with worsened clinical outcomes (34). Alveolar macrophage function is impaired in PAP and corticosteroids may further suppress their function. This may explain the significant number of new infections seen in patients in the study who had received steroids. Based on the evidence to date, corticosteroids should not be used in the treatment of PAP.

Gene therapy

Gene therapy is a unique and emerging treatment modality in hereditary PAP. Since several specific mutations that result in hereditary PAP have been identified, it is possible that gene-correction therapy with pulmonary macrophage transplantation may provide a novel avenue for treatment. Animal models have shown promising results in terms of both safety and efficacy (35, 36), and application of the therapy in humans is an area of ongoing investigation.

Lung transplantation

Lung transplantation may be considered in rare cases of refractory PAP with persistent clinical decline, particularly in cases with end stage fibrosis. However, it is important to note that cases of recurrent PAP following bilateral lung transplantation have been reported (37, 38). As a result, lung transplantation should be reserved for select cases refractory to WLL and second-line medical therapies. Patients who undergo lung transplantation for PAP should be monitored for signs of recurrence and indications for treatment of PAP following transplantation.

References

1. Rosen SH, Castleman B, Liebow AA. Pulmonary alveolar proteinosis. N Engl J Med. 1958;258(23):1123–1142. doi:10.1056/NEJM195806052582301
2. Tanaka N, Watanabe J, Kitamura T, Yamada Y, Kanegasaki S, Nakata K. Lungs of patients with idiopathic pulmonary alveolar proteinosis express a factor which neutralizes granulocyte-macrophage colony stimulating factor. FEBS Lett. 1999;442(2-3). doi:10.1016/S0014-5793(98)01668-8
3. Kitamura T, Uchida K, Tanaka N, et al. Serological diagnosis of idiopathic pulmonary alveolar proteinosis. Am J Respir Crit Care Med. 2000;162(2 I). doi:10.1164/ajrccm.162.2.9910032
4. Kitamura T, Tanaka N, Watanabe J, et al. Idiopathic pulmonary alveolar proteinosis as an autoimmune disease with neutralizing antibody against granulocyte/macrophage colony-stimulating factor. J Exp Med. 1999;190(6). doi:10.1084/jem.190.6.875
5. Xipell JM, Ham KN, Price CG, Thomas TD. Acute silicoproteinosis. Thorax. 1977;32(1):104–11. doi:10.1136/thx.32.1.104
6. Uchida K, Beck DC, Yamamoto T, et al. GM-CSF autoantibodies and neutrophil dysfunction in pulmonary alveolar proteinosis. N Engl J Med. 2007;356(6). doi:10.1056/nejmoa062505
7. Rosen LB, Pereira NR, Figueiredo C, et al. Nocardia-induced granulocyte macrophage colony-stimulating factor is neutralized by autoantibodies in disseminated/extrapulmonary nocardiosis. Clin Infect Dis. 2015;60(7). doi:10.1093/cid/ciu968
8. Seymour JF, Presneill JJ. Pulmonary alveolar proteinosis: Progress in the first 44 years. Am J Respir Crit Care Med. 2002;166(2). doi:10.1164/rccm.2109105
9. McCarthy C, Avetisyan R, Carey BC, Chalk C, Trapnell BC. Prevalence and healthcare burden of pulmonary alveolar proteinosis. Orphanet J Rare Dis. 2018;13(1). doi:10.1186/s13023-018-0846-y
10. Inoue Y, Trapnell BC, Tazawa R, et al. Characteristics of a large cohort of patients with autoimmune pulmonary alveolar proteinosis in Japan. Am J Respir Crit Care Med. 2008;177(7). doi:10.1164/rccm.200708-1271OC
11. Suzuki T, Trapnell BC. Pulmonary alveolar proteinosis syndrome. Clin Chest Med. 2016;37(3). doi:10.1016/j.ccm.2016.04.006
12. Goldstein LS, Kavuru MS, Curtis-McCarthy P, Christie HA, Farver C, Stoller JK. Pulmonary alveolar proteinosis: Clinical features and outcomes. Chest. 1998;114(5). doi:10.1378/chest.114.5.1357
13. Ioachimescu OC, Kavuru MS. Pulmonary alveolar proteinosis. Chron Respir Dis. 2006;3(3). doi:10.1191/1479972306cd101rs
14. Lin FC, Chang GD, Chern MS, Chen YC, Chang SC. Clinical significance of anti-GM-CSF antibodies in idiopathic pulmonary alveolar proteinosis. Thorax. 2006;61(6). doi:10.1136/thx.2005.054171
15. Holbert JM, Costello P, Li W, Hoffman RM, Rogers RM. CT features of pulmonary alveolar proteinosis. Am J Roentgenol. 2001;176(5). doi:10.2214/ajr.176.5.1761287
16. Rossi SE, Erasmus JJ, Volpacchio M, Franquet T, Castiglioni T, Page McAdams H. "Crazy-paving" pattern at thin-section CT of the lungs: Radiologic-pathologic overview. Radiographics. 2003;23(6). doi:10.1148/rg.236035101
17. Ding X, Xu J, Zhou J, Long Q. Chest CT findings of COVID-19 pneumonia by duration of symptoms. Eur J Radiol. 2020;127. doi:10.1016/j.ejrad.2020.109009
18. Burkhalter A, Silverman JF, Hopkins MB, Geisinger KR. Bronchoalveolar lavage cytology in pulmonary alveolar proteinosis. Am J Clin Pathol. 1996;106(4). doi:10.1093/ajcp/106.4.504
19. Bonella F, Bauer PC, Griese M, Ohshimo S, Guzman J, Costabel U. Pulmonary alveolar proteinosis: New insights from a single-center cohort of 70 patients. Respir Med. 2011;105(12). doi:10.1016/j.rmed.2011.08.018
20. Kumar A, Abdelmalak B, Inoue Y, Culver DA. Pulmonary alveolar proteinosis in adults: Pathophysiology and clinical approach. Lancet Respir Med. 2018;6(7). doi:10.1016/S2213-2600(18)30043-2
21. Ramirez J, Kieffer RF, Ball WC. Bronchopulmonary lavage in man. Ann Intern Med. 1965;63(5). doi:10.7326/0003-4819-63-5-819
22. Hasan N, Bagga S, Monteagudo J, et al. Extracorporeal membrane oxygenation to support whole-lung lavage in pulmonary alveolar proteinosis salvage of the drowned lungs. J Bronchol Interv Pulmonol. 2013;20(1). doi:10.1097/LBR.0b013e31827ccdb5
23. Campo I, Luisetti M, Griese M, et al. Whole lung lavage therapy for pulmonary alveolar proteinosis: A global survey of current practices and procedures. Orphanet J Rare Dis. 2016;11(1). doi:10.1186/s13023-016-0497-9
24. Gay P, Wallaert B, Nowak S, et al. Efficacy of whole-lung lavage in pulmonary alveolar proteinosis: A multicenter international study of GELF. Respiration. 2017;93(3). doi:10.1159/000455179
25. Reed JA, Ikegami M, Cianciolo ER, et al. Aerosolized GM-CSF ameliorates pulmonary alveolar proteinosis in GM-CSF-deficient mice. Am J Physiol — Lung Cell Mol Physiol. 1999;276(4 20-4). doi:10.1152/ajplung.1999.276.4.l556

26. Sheng G, Chen P, Wei Y, Chu J, Cao X, Zhang HL. Better approach for autoimmune pulmonary alveolar proteinosis treatment: Inhaled or subcutaneous granulocyte-macrophage colony-stimulating factor: A meta-analyses. Respir Res. 2018;19(1). doi:10.1186/s12931-018-0862-4
27. Wylam ME, Ten R, Prakash UBS, Nadrous HF, Clawson ML, Anderson PM. Aerosol granulocyte-macrophage colony-stimulating factor for pulmonary alveolar proteinosis. Eur Respir J. 2006;27(3). doi:10.1183/09031936.06.00058305
28. Papiris SA, Tsirigotis P, Kolilekas L, et al. Long-term inhaled granulocyte macrophage-colony-stimulating factor in autoimmune pulmonary alveolar proteinosis: Effectiveness, safety, and lowest effective dose. Clin Drug Investig. 2014;34(8). doi:10.1007/s40261-014-0208-z
29. Tazawa R, Ueda T, Abe M, et al. Inhaled GM-CSF for pulmonary alveolar proteinosis. N Engl J Med. 2019;381(10). doi:10.1056/nejmoa1816216
30. Trapnell BC, Inoue Y, Bonella F, et al. Inhaled GM-CSF (Molgramostim) Therapy Reduces the Need for Whole Lung Lavage in Patients with Autoimmune Pulmonary Alveolar Proteinosis — Long-Term Results from a Randomized, Double-Blind Trial (IMPALA), 2020. doi:10.1164/ajrccm-conference.2020.201.1_meetingabstracts.a2755
31. Papiris SA, Tsirigotis P, Kolilekas L, et al. Pulmonary alveolar proteinosis: Time to shift? Expert Rev Respir Med. 2015;9(3). doi:10.1586/17476348.2015.1035259
32. Soyez B, Borie R, Menard C, et al. Rituximab for auto-immune alveolar proteinosis, a real life cohort study. Respir Res. 2018;19(1). doi:10.1186/s12931-018-0780-5
33. Kavuru MS, Malur A, Marshall I, et al. An open-label trial of rituximab therapy in pulmonary alveolar proteinosis. Eur Respir J. 2011;38(6). doi:10.1183/09031936.00197710
34. Akasaka K, Tanaka T, Kitamura N, et al. Outcome of corticosteroid administration in autoimmune pulmonary alveolar proteinosis: A retrospective cohort study. BMC Pulm Med. 2015;15(1). doi:10.1186/s12890-015-0085-0
35. Arumugam P, Suzuki T, Shima K, et al. Long-term safety and efficacy of Gene-pulmonary macrophage transplantation therapy of PAP in Csf2ra$^{-/-}$ mice. Mol Ther. 2019;27(9). doi:10.1016/j.ymthe.2019.06.010
36. Mucci A, Lopez-Rodriguez E, Hetzel M, et al. iPSC-derived macrophages effectively treat pulmonary alveolar proteinosis in Csf2rb-deficient mice. Stem Cell Rep. 2018;11(3). doi:10.1016/j.stemcr.2018.07.006
37. Divithotawela C, Apte SH, Tan ME, De Silva TA, Chambers DC. Pulmonary alveolar proteinosis after lung transplantation. Respirol Case Rep. 2020;8(5). doi:10.1002/rcr2.566
38. Takaki M, Tanaka T, Komohara Y, et al. Recurrence of pulmonary alveolar proteinosis after bilateral lung transplantation in a patient with a nonsense mutation in CSF2RB. Respir Med Case Rep. 2016;19. doi:10.1016/j.rmcr.2016.06.011

PART E
Rare Diffuse Cystic Lung Diseases

16

LYMPHANGIOLEIOMYOMATOSIS

Rosa M. Estrada-Y-Martin

Contents

Introduction 116
Pathogenesis 116
Pathology 117
Clinical manifestations 118
Diagnosis...118
Other considerations about LAM 123
References...123

KEY POINTS

- Lymphangioleiomyomatosis (LAM) is a rare, low-grade metastasizing neoplasm affecting almost exclusively women.
- It is associated with proliferation of smooth muscle-like cells, called LAM cells spreading via lymphatics with resultant development of lung cysts.
- Diagnosis of LAM should be considered in any young woman presenting with a spontaneous pneumothorax.
- Diagnosis of LAM can be established by characteristic findings on HRCT of the chest with diffuse round bilateral thin-walled cysts of varying sizes along with a lung biopsy with characteristic immunochemical stains or the characteristic HRCT findings along with elevated vascular endothelin growth factor D (VEGF-D), or the presence of angiomyolipomas, lymphangiomas, chylous pleural effusions or ascites and definite or probable tuberous sclerosis.
- mTOR inhibitors are an effective treatment for LAM that should be considered in patients with abnormal lung function, rapid deterioration in lung functions or symptomatic chylous complications.

Introduction

Lymphangioleiomyomatosis (LAM) is a rare, low-grade metastasizing neoplasm that affects almost exclusively women. It is associated with proliferation of smooth muscle-like cells, called "LAM cells." The LAM cells spread via lymphatics and target the lungs. It causes progressive diffuse cystic lung involvement, chylous effusions, renal angiomyolipomas (AMLs) and LAM (1, 2). It was initially reported in the 1930s; however, it was not fully recognized until 1975, when Corrin and Liebow described a disease affecting 28 women of reproductive age that presented with pneumothorax and chylothorax. They also recognized the association with renal AMLs (3). Since their initial review, our understanding and treatment of LAM has improved, nevertheless, the origin of the LAM cells is still unknown. LAM can affect women sporadically (S-LAM) or in persons with tuberous sclerosis (TSC) complex (TSC-LAM). The estimated prevalence of S-LAM is 3.4–7.8 per million women. S-LAM affects only women. LAM occurs in up to 30% of women with TSC, although, more recently, it has been noted that up to 80% of TSC patients have LAM by age 40 (4). Only 5–10% of women with TSC-LAM develop respiratory failure (5). LAM can affect up to 13% of men with TSC (4, 6, 7). Although TSC-LAM has been considered to be less severe; a recent review of the National Heart, Lung, and Blood Institute (NHLBI) LAM registry showed that the rate of decline of forced expiratory volume in 1 second (FEV_1) was similar in S-LAM and TSC-LAM, suggesting lead time bias (1, 8, 9).

Pathogenesis

Variation or mutation of the encoding proteins hamartin and tuberin, TSC1 or TSC2 genes, respectively, cause LAM. TSC-LAM results from one germline mutation and one acquired mutation in either TSC1 or TSC2. S-LAM is not inheritable since it results from two acquired mutations, most commonly in the TSC2 gene (10). These genes are tumor suppression genes that result in the inhibition of the mechanistic target of rapamycin (mTOR) complex 1 signaling (5). The signaling network converges on the rapamycin-sensitive TOR complex (Figure 16.1). A deficiency of encoded proteins, hamartin or tuberin, results in the loss of regulation of the mTOR signaling pathway. TOR proteins are serine/threonine protein kinases, which have a central role in cell growth, proliferation, migration and survival as well as synthesis of proteins and lipids (5, 10). The activation of mTOR kinase and S6 kinase causes increased protein translation with further cellular proliferation, migration and invasion (11). The TSC1-TSC2 cytosolic protein complex acts as a checkpoint that regulates mTOR function in response to upstream changes, inhibiting the GTP binding process Ras homolog enriched in the brain (Rheb). Rheb is a positive regulator of cell growth and mTOR is the catalytic subunit of two complexes, mTORC1 and mTORC2 (10). mTORC1 regulates downstream targets such as ribosomal S6 kinase and the eukaryotic initiation factor 4E-binding protein (4E-BP1) involved in protein translation, cell growth, proliferation, and autophagy. mTORC2 has six

Lymphangioleiomyomatosis

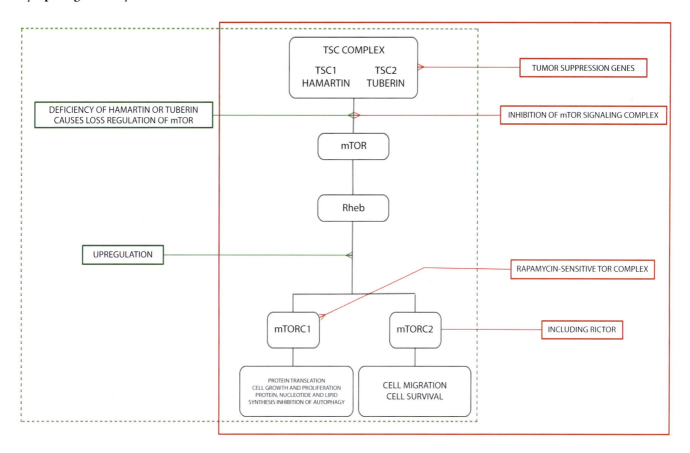

FIGURE 16.1 Simplified mTOR pathway. The TSC complex of TSC1 and TSC2 are tumor suppressors genes. TSC genes encode hamartin or tuberin proteins. The mutation or variation of TSC genes TSC1 or TSC2 result in a loss of regulation of the mTOR signaling pathway, activating Rheb with upregulation of the mTOR signaling complex. TOR proteins have a central role in cell growth, cell proliferation, migration, survival, synthesis of protein and lipid and autophagy. The green dashed box denotes TSC1 or TSC2 variation, upregulation of mTOR1/mTOR2 with subsequently increased protein translation, cell growth proliferation, migration and survival and inhibition of autophagy. The red box denotes normal function. *Abbreviations:* TSC: tuberous sclerosis gene; mTOR: mechanistic target of rapamycin; Rheb: ras homolog enriched in the brain; mTORC: mTOR complex; RICTOR: rapamycin-insensitive companion of mTOR.

subunits including rapamycin-insensitive companion of mTOR (rictor). Upregulation of mTORC2 increases cellular migration and cell survival (10, 12). In essence, mutation of the TSC1/TSC2 tumor suppressive genes results in activation of Rheb, leading to activation of mTORC1 and downstream dysregulation, causing uncontrollable cell growth and proliferation with a reduction of autophagy (10). Of note, elevated mTORC1 (mutations affecting negative regulation of mTORC1) have been associated with multiple neoplasms and diseases such as proteus syndrome, neurofibromatosis type 1, Peutz–Jeghers syndrome, familial adenomatous polyposis and TSC/LAM (13).

The formation of new blood vessels through angiogenesis is necessary for malignant cell to disseminate from the primary tumor to surrounding tissues or to distant organs via lymphatics or blood-stream. Vascular endothelial growth factors are angiogenic mediators. Vascular endothelial factors C (VEGF-C) and D (VEGF-D) are ligands that induce formation of lymphatics and promote the spread of tumor cells to lymph nodes (14). VEGF-D is elevated in patients with LAM (15).

As mentioned previously, LAM can present in patients with TSC (TSC-LAM) or sporadically (S-LAM). TSC is an autosomal dominant disease with high penetrance caused by mutation of one of the TSC genes and characterized by hamartomatous tumors involving the central nervous system, skin, liver, kidneys, heart and eyes. It can manifest early in childhood with seizures and different degrees of cognitive impairment (16, 17). TSC is inherited while S-LAM is not. The majority of TSC cases are the result of *de novo* pathogenic variant. Offsprings have a 50% risk of inheriting the variant. Most individuals affected with TSC and S-LAM have the TSC2 variant (69% TSC and majority of S-LAM) (17). The TSC2 pathogenic variant appears to cause more severe disease than the TSC1 variant in TSC patients (18).

The pathogenesis of cyst formation in LAM is unclear. One of the proposed mechanisms is check-valve obstruction with subsequent distal over-inflation. In LAM, however, the cysts decrease during expiration (as seen in expiratory chest computed tomography [CT] scans), suggesting some degree of distal airway opening (19, 20).

Pathology

LAM is classified as a mesenchymal tumor in the 2015 World Health Organization Classification of Lung Tumors (21). LAM lesions are characterized by proliferation of neoplastic smooth muscle-like cells (LAM cells) in small clusters located on the edges of cysts and along blood vessels, lymphatics and bronchioles

(22). LAM cell infiltration causes obstruction of the bronchioles, vascular wall thickening, lymphatic disruption, venous occlusion and hemorrhage (22). Spindle-shaped and epithelioid LAM cells have antibodies against smooth muscle antigens and stain for å-actin, vimentin and desmin. The epithelioid cells react with human melanin black antibody (HMB-45), a mouse monoclonal antibody that recognized glycoprotein 100. LAM cells are also positive to estrogen, progesterone, ß-catenin, E-catherin and epidermal growth factor receptor (22).

Clinical manifestations

The mean age of diagnosis of S-LAM is 40 years of age in the United States and 39 in the United Kingdom (UK) (23) Dyspnea is the most common symptom of LAM (30–40% in S-LAM and 30–37% in TSC-LAM) (9). Since dyspnea is nonspecific, LAM diagnosis is usually delayed by 3–5 years. Patients are typically misdiagnosed with asthma or chronic obstructive pulmonary disease until an incidental chest CT scan is obtained or the patient suffers a pneumothorax. Other symptoms include fatigue in 70%, cough in 45% and chest pain and wheezes in 40%. Chyloptysis is an uncommon presentation in S-LAM, seen in 20% (23). A high percentage of S-LAM and TSC-LAM suffer a spontaneous pneumothorax during their lifetime (up 73% of S-LAM and 29% TSC-LAM) and is the initial disease presentation in 82% of S-LAM (24, 25). The risk of recurrent pneumothorax is high. Many patients suffer three to four pneumothoraces, (average two) prior to obtaining a diagnosis; as high as 4% of LAM patients have bilateral pneumothoraces (25). The risk of pneumothorax decreases significantly after pleurodesis: from 60 to 66% with conservative management to 27 to 32% with pleurodesis (25).

There are multiple extrapulmonary manifestations of LAM including lymphatic involvement with mediastinal, retroperitoneal or pelvic lymphangiomas; chylous pleural or abdominal effusions; and angiomyolipomas, mainly in the kidneys but also can affect the liver (26, 27) (Figures 16.2 and 16.3). Lymphangiomas have been described to be smaller in size during the morning than later during the day after meals (28, 29) and this may have some diagnostic utility differentiating a mass from a lymphangioma.

There are different clinical phenotypes of LAM with some S-LAM patients presenting mainly after spontaneous pneumothorax and significant pulmonary cysts, while others present with diagnosis of AML without severe lung involvement. Furthermore, others may present mainly with lymphatic involvement with chylous effusions and lymphangiomas.

Diagnosis

LAM should be suspected in every young woman who suffers a spontaneous pneumothorax. Not uncommonly, it is found during screening in a TSC patient or during the workup for dyspnea or, incidentally, after obtaining a chest CT or abdomen CT showing pulmonary cysts in the lower lung fields. LAM should be suspected in patients with a renal AML. Classically, chest CT shows round thin-walled cysts evenly distributed with normal surrounding lung parenchyma. The cysts are bilateral, diffuse, typically 2–5 mm but can be as large as 30 mm (30) (Figures 16.4 and 16.5)

The size of the pulmonary cysts correlates with the risk of pneumothorax. Cysts >0.5 cm have a higher probability of pneumothorax compared to cysts <0.5 cm. Patients with cysts >0.5 cm are also at higher risk of recurrent pneumothorax (31).

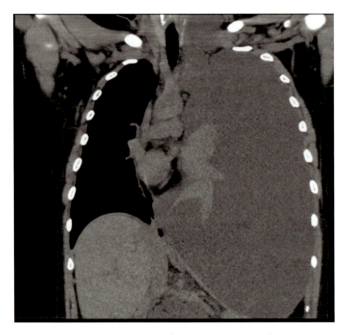

FIGURE 16.2 A 31-year-old woman with massive left pleural effusion with noticed dilated lymphatics in the left neck area. The patient also had abdominal lymphangiomas (not shown). Thoracentesis yielded pleural fluid with chylous appearance. She was diagnosed with S-LAM. Chylothorax and lymphangiomas resolved completely with mTOR inhibitors.

Patients with pneumothorax are usually diagnosed earlier and have faster decline of FEV_1 and DLco. Obviously, this may be related to earlier diagnosis and longer follow up (31). Since the risk of recurrent pneumothorax is high in LAM (69% ipsilateral pneumothorax [32]), pleurodesis should be considered early on with the first spontaneous pneumothorax (25).

AMLs are recognizable in an abdominal CT or MRI by the presence of smooth muscle, blood vessels and macroscopic fat (HU −20) in a renal mass (33). They are highly vascular and can be very large (Figures 16.6a, b).

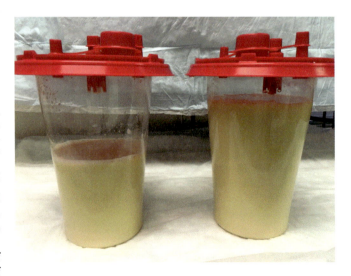

FIGURE 16.3 Pleural fluid obtained from the same patient in Figure 16.2 demonstrating chylothorax.

Lymphangioleiomyomatosis

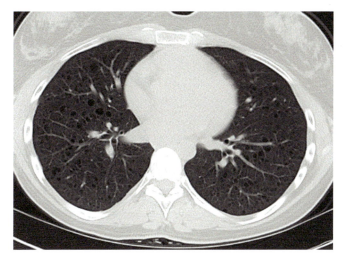

FIGURE 16.4 A 33-year-old woman with a history of dyspnea. Notice diffuse, bilateral cysts up 1 cm in diameter without evidence of pleural effusions, reticulations or GGO.

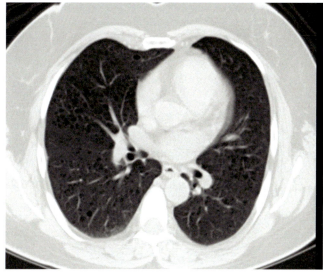

FIGURE 16.5 A 58-year-old woman with dyspnea. Notice bilateral diffuse pulmonary cysts up to 1 cm in diameter without pleural effusions, reticulations or GGO.

TSC patients should be screened for LAM starting at age 18 with a chest CT. Chest CT can be repeated depending on the initial CT findings every 5–10 years in asymptomatic individuals. TSC patients with LAM should be followed like S-LAM patients (17). Some experts have advocated to start screening TSC patients at age 21, considering the potential impact of radiation on breast development and lower probability of severe LAM (34). The evidence of LAM in TSC is age dependent, estimated to be 8% every year or 81% in TSC patients older than 40 (34).

Lung biopsy shows cystic destruction with immunohistochemical workup demonstrating positivity to human melanoma black-45 (HMB-45), å-actin, vimentin, desmin, estrogen and progesterone receptors, as well as ß-catenin, E-catherin and epidermal growth factor receptor (22).

LAM cells have been isolated from blood, bronchoalveolar lavage, urine and other tissues. It is not clinically apparent yet, but supports the theory that LAM is a disseminated neoplasm (35, 36).

The diagnosis of *definite* LAM can be established by characteristic high-resolution computed tomography (HRCT) of chest findings and characteristic lung biopsy with positive immunohistochemical markers, or characteristic HRCT chest and the presence of AML, chylous pleural effusion or ascites, lymphangioma or lymph node involvement. TSC-LAM requires the presence of definite or probable TSC along with the above. *Probable* LAM is suspected by the presence of characteristic HRCT and compatible clinical history or HRCT with AMLs and thoracic or abdominal chylous effusion. *Possible* LAM is suspected with characteristic HRCT (37). Possible LAM diagnosis may require lung biopsy (37–39) (Figure 16.7).

In patients with diffuse cystic lung disease without any evidence of TSC, AML or elevated VEGF-D, lung biopsy is recommended. Transbronchial lung biopsy should be attempted first since the yield is substantial (50%). In patients with more severe cystic lung involvement by chest CT the yield is even higher (up to 79%) without increasing the risk of procedure-related complications (39, 40).

(a)

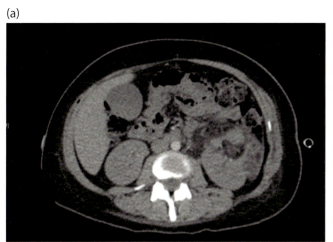

(b)

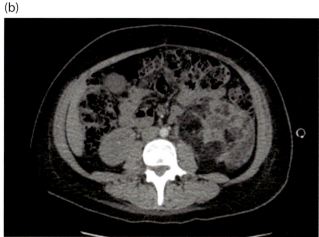

FIGURE 16.6 (a) and (b) Abdominal CT images of a 24-year-old woman with S-LAM showing large left renal mass with low densities consistent with fat in an AML.

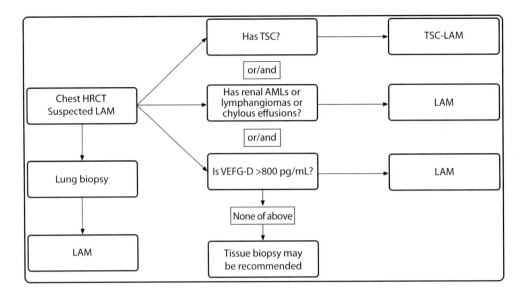

FIGURE 16.7 LAM diagnosis. Diagnosis is dependent on the presence of renal AMLs, lymphangiomas, chylous effusions, VEFG-D >800 pg/mL or TSC. Absence of any presentation may require lung biopsy.

Pulmonary function testing (PFT) demonstrates an obstructive pattern in 61% of patients with LAM, and decreased diffusion capacity in 57%. Thirty percent of S-LAM patients have normal lung function (24, 41). The average FEV_1 declines by 89 mL/yr, which decreases with older age. Menopausal women's FEV_1 declines 74 mL/yr compared to 118 mL/yr in pre-menopausal women (8). Of note, the average FEV_1 decline in the placebo group in the landmark Multicenter International Lymphangioleiomyomatosis Efficacy of Sirolimus (MILES) trial (discussed next) was −12.2 mL per month (−134 ± 182 mL per year) (42). Other studies have confirmed this finding with the average decline of FVC in LAM patients is 50 ± 30 mL per year (1.2% ± 0.6%), FEV_1 by 100 mL ± 30 mL per year and DLco decreased by 1.1 ± 0.1 mL/min per mmHg (4.8% ± 0.9% predicted) per year (43) (Figure 16.8). Dyspnea and fatigue have correlated with the presence of abnormal pulmonary function, obstructive pattern, air trapping and decreased diffusion capacity (23). Twenty-five to thirty percent of LAM patients can respond to bronchodilators (44). Patients with a positive bronchodilator response have a faster decline in pulmonary function (113 mL/year compared to 83 mL/year) (8).

Serum VEGF-D correlates with disease severity and treatment response. In the previously mentioned MILES trial, VEGF-D levels were higher in patients with LAM with hypoxemia requiring oxygen and those who had bronchodilator response. VEGF-D

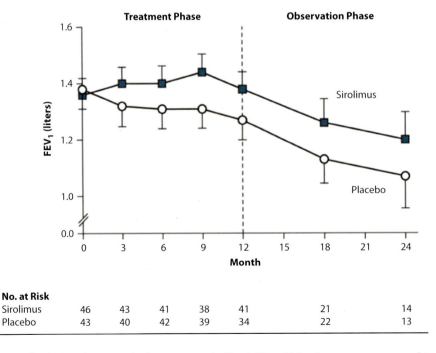

FIGURE 16.8 The FEV_1 of LAM patients on sirolimus group declined 19 ± 124 mL per year compared to −134 ± 182 mL per year in the placebo group. (From Efficacy and Safety of Sirolimus in Lymphangioleiomyomatosis. 364 (17):1602. Copyright [2011] Massachusetts Medical Society. Reprinted with permission from Massachusetts Medical Society.)

Lymphangioleiomyomatosis

levels declined after treatment with sirolimus with higher serum VEFG-D found to correlate with higher improvement in FEV_1 and FVC in patients treated with sirolimus. At the same time, decrease in VEGF-D with treatment was found to be associated with improvement in lung function (45) (Figure 16.9).

VEGF-D (but not VEGF-C) in patients with S-LAM and TSC-LAM has diagnostic implications. Elevated VEGF-D >800 pg/mL with a characteristic HRCT of the chest obviates the need for lung biopsy, however, a VEGF-D <800 pg/mL does not exclude the diagnosis of LAM (37, 46, 47). VEFG-D can also distinguish LAM from other cystic lung diseases (46).

Cancer antigen 125 (CA-125), an ovarian cancer marker, has been found to be elevated in 25% of LAM patients without evidence of ovarian malignancy. Serum CA-125 is associated with lymphatic involvement, disease progression, lower predicted FEV_1 and decreases after treatment with sirolimus (48).

The risk of pneumothorax during air travel is approximately 1–2% per 100 flights, even so, many LAM patients who suffered pneumothorax during air travel had symptoms of dyspnea and chest pain a few days prior to their trip. Pneumothorax is more common in patients that suffered previous pneumothoraces (49, 50).

Pregnancy can accelerate lung function decline. Sixteen LAM patients with before and after pregnancy studies from the UK and US showed FEV_1 decrease from 77 to 64%. DLco decreased from 66 to 57% (51). Pneumothorax was frequent during pregnancy, up to 66% in a survey of 328 LAM patients (52). Some patients suffered bilateral pneumothoraces during their pregnancy. There were no other increased pregnancy complications and newborns were healthy (51, 52). However, CT scores, which correlate with decline in lung function, increased in all patients. CT score is a measurement of the difference in texture between areas adjacent to or remote from the cysts (53).

A complete PFT, 6-minute walk and HRCT of the chest are routinely followed in LAM patients, although the frequency with which these tests should be performed is unclear. PFTs are usually obtained every 6–12 months and HRCT every 1–3 years if clinically stable (11). A new CT protocol has been developed with ultra-low dose chest CT that does not compromise imaging definition and avoids unnecessary and harmful radiation, thus allowing for more frequent chest CTs without significantly increasing the cumulative risk of breast radiation and consequent breast cancer (54).

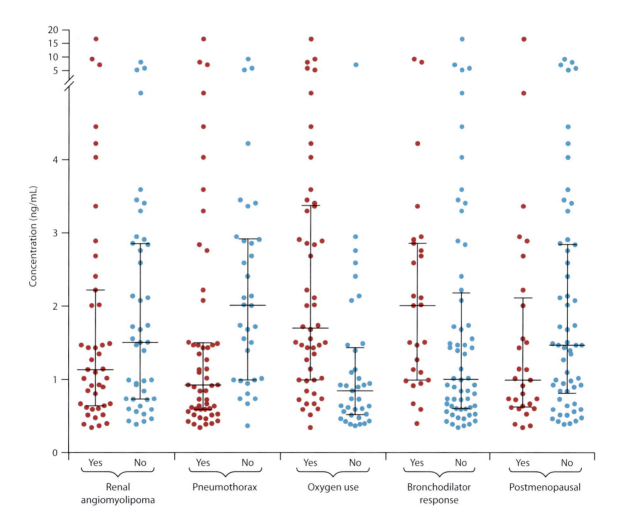

FIGURE 16.9 VEGF-D concentration is higher in LAM patients requiring oxygen, positive bronchodilator response, history of pneumothorax, presence of angiomyolipoma and menopausal status. (Reprinted from Lancet Respiratory Medicine, volume 6, Young L, Lee HS et al., Serum VEGF-D a Concentration as a Biomarker of LAM Severity and Treatment Response: A Prospective Analysis of the Multicenter International Lymphangioleiomyomatosis Efficacy of Sirolimus [MILES] trial, p. 448, copyright (2013), with permission from Elsevier.)

Differential diagnosis

The differential diagnosis of LAM includes any diffuse cystic lung disease including Birt–Hogg–Dubé syndrome, Langerhans cell histiocytosis, lymphocytic interstitial pneumonia and amyloidosis, to name a few (55–57) (Table 16.1).

Prognosis

LAM progresses more rapidly in younger patients, pre-menopausal women, during pregnancy and with the use of estrogens. Patients that present with pneumothorax tend to be younger at presentation (41). Higher VEFG-D correlates with more rapid decline of pulmonary lung function but at the same time also correlates with response to mTOR inhibitors (45). In the NHLBI LAM registry, the progression to death or transplant at 5-, 10-, 15-, and 20-year survival rates were 94%, 85%, 75% and 64% respectively (8). The main predictors of disease progression or death are menopausal status (initial FEV_1) and DLco (8). Following S-LAM diagnosis, the estimated mean transplant-free survival is 23–29 years (23, 58).

LAM can affect men with TSC (10–12%), however, they usually have milder pulmonary disease and are almost never symptomatic (17).

Treatment

With better understanding of the LAM molecular and genetic dysregulation affecting the mTOR signaling pathway, the potential benefit of mTOR inhibitors was considered. Rapamycin is a macrolide antibiotic discovered in the 1970s as a product of *Streptomyces hygrocopicus* in soil samples from Easter Island (Rapa-Nui Island) (59). Rapamycin binds to FK506-binding protein 12 in the cytosol, which directly binds to mTORC1, resulting in the dissociation of raptor and inhibition of mTORC1 (10). Initial studies in patients with TSC and AMLs demonstrated not only that angiomyolipomas regressed with sirolimus (a rapamycin drug) but also that there was an improvement in FEV_1, FVC and air trapping (60).

The MILES study, a randomized controlled trial (RCT) of 89 patients with LAM, showed that sirolimus, an mTOR inhibitor, decreased the decline of lung function, decreased VEGF-D as well as improved symptoms and quality of life. At 12 months, the FEV_1 of LAM patients on sirolimus group declined 19 ± 124 mL per year compared to -134 ± 182 mL per year in the placebo group. In patients with moderate LAM, there was a 10% decrease of FEV_1 per year when sirolimus was stopped. During the follow-up year, the sirolimus and placebo groups had the same decline of lung function, suggesting the mTOR inhibitors should be continued indefinitely (Figure 16.8). The most common adverse events were mucositis, diarrhea, nausea, hypercholesterolemia, acneiform rash and leg edema (42). mTOR inhibitors can also cause pneumonitis (61). Observational studies evaluating comparison of lung functions between pre- and post-treatment with sirolimus in a group with rapidly progressive LAM showed an increase in FVC by 90 ± 20 mL ($3.2\% \pm 0.5\%$ predicted) per year and an

TABLE 16.1: Differential Diagnosis of Cystic Lung Diseases

	Clinical Presentation	Inheritance	Radiographic Findings	Diagnosis	Treatment
LAM	Spontaneous pneumothorax and/or progressive dyspnea	TSC 1 (tuberin) or TSC2 (hamartin) TSC (autosomal dominant) S-LAM is not inherited	Round, diffuse, and small cysts (2–5 mm) without GGO. Pleural effusions or AML or abdominal/pelvic lymphangiomas may be present	Presence of Chylothorax/chylo-ascites or AML or lymphangiomas Presence of TSC Elevated VEGF-D >800 pg/mL Lung biopsy LAM cells that stain positive for HMB-45, estrogen and progesterone receptors, smooth muscle actin, vimentin and desmin	mTOR inhibitors
BHD	Fibrofolliculomas or trichodiscomas Personal or family history of pneumothorax or renal carcinomas	Autosomal dominant Folliculin gene	Round or lentiform, well defined (2–80 mm) Basilar, interlobular septa or sub-pleural predilection and proximal vessels	Genetic testing Skin biopsy can support diagnosis (punch biopsy)	None currently
PLCH	Cigarette smoker Young adults	None	Bizarre cysts and nodules, more in upper and middle lobes, almost complete costophrenic angle sparing	BA: >5% CD1 a- reactive cells Lung biopsy positive CD-1a and S-100	Smoking cessation Selective cases Immunomodulators or BRAF inhibitors
LIP	Commonly associated with Sjögren's disease, SLE, or HIV	None	Cysts are randomly distributed (3–50 mm), may have septae, perivascular in distribution and may have associated GGO and centrilobular nodules	Polyclonal lymphocytic infiltration within alveolar septa, sometimes along bronchi and vessels	Treatment of underlying disease Corticosteroids
Amyloidosis	Hematologic or rheumatologic diseases	None	Cysts are rare, multiple and round and often peri-vascular or sub-pleural. Associated calcified nodules seen in majority of cases	Biopsy demonstrating apple-green birefringence on Congo red stain	Treatment of underlying disease

Abbreviations: LAM: lymphangioleiomyomatosis; TSC: tuberous sclerosis complex; GGO: ground-glass opacity; AML: angiomyolipoma; VEGF-D: vascular endothelial growth factor-D; HMB-45: Human Melanoma Black-45; BHD: Birt–Hogg–Dubé syndrome; PLCH: pulmonary Langerhans cell histiocytosis; BAL: bronchoalveolar lavage; BRAF: B-raf murine sarcoma viral oncogene homolog B; SLE: systemic lupus erythematosus.

increase in FEV_1 by 50 ± 20 mL (1.8% ± 0.5% predicted) over a period of 2.5 years post-treatment with sirolimus. The same group pre-treatment showed a decrease of FVC by 50 ± 30 mL per year (1.2% ± 0.6%), decrease in FEV_1 by 100 mL ± 30 mL per year and decrease in DLco by 1.1 ± 0.1 mL/min per mmHg (4.8% ± 0.9% predicted) per year (43). Thus, based on observational studies and the MILES trial, it is recommended to start sirolimus in LAM patients with FEV_1 <70% (1, 62). Everolimus another mTOR inhibitor, may be as effective as sirolimus with a similar side effect profile in the phase II study (63).

mTOR inhibitor serum levels should be followed during treatment. The ideal serum level for patients with LAM is still to be determined, but probably lower levels compared to renal transplant patients are likely effective. There is an ongoing trial, the MILED trial, that may shed some light on early- and low-dose sirolimus in LAM in the next few years (64).

Sirolimus is also indicated for the treatment of chylous effusion (chylothorax or chylous ascites) and angiomyolipomas in patients with LAM or TSC (43). Patients with lymphatic involvement, including chylous effusions, have a better a response to mTOR inhibitors (61, 65).

Other considerations about LAM

Apart from being used as a diagnostic marker, VEGF-D levels can be used to assess treatment response in patients with LAM (45, 47). AMLs larger than 4 cm are at high risk of bleeding and embolization is recommended (11). Twenty to thirty percent of LAM patients respond to bronchodilators. Bronchodilator responders have faster decline of lung function than non-responders. Bronchodilators may improve quality of life in some LAM patients (44, 66). Pneumothorax in LAM should be treated with chemical or surgical pleurodesis from the initial event due to the risk of recurrence. Pleurodesis may increase perioperative bleeding after lung transplantation, however, it should not exclude a patient for undergoing lung transplantation since it does not affect the length of post-operative stay or outcomes (39, 67). Patients with moderate-to-severe LAM should be counseled about the possibility that pregnancy may accelerate the decline of lung function. Vaccinations are recommended for all LAM patients, but patients taking mTOR inhibitors should avoid live attenuated vaccines.

References

1. McCormack FX, Gupta N, Finlay GR, Young LR, Taveira-DaSilva AM, Glasgow CG, et al. Official American Thoracic Society/Japanese Respiratory Society clinical practice guidelines: Lymphangioleiomyomatosis diagnosis and management. Am J Resp Crit Care Med. 2016;194(6):748–61.
2. Krymskaya VP, McCormack FX. Lymphangioleiomyomatosis: A monogenic model of malignancy. Annu Rev Med. 2017;68:69–83.
3. Corrin B, Liebow AA, Friedman PJ. Pulmonary lymphangiomyomatosis. A review. Am J Pathol. 1975;79(2):348–82.
4. Adriaensen ME, Schaefer-Prokop CM, Duyndam DA, Zonnenberg BA, Prokop M. Radiological evidence of lymphangioleiomyomatosis in female and male patients with tuberous sclerosis complex. Clin Radiol. 2011;66(7):625–8.
5. Henske EP, Jozwiak S, Kingswood JC, Sampson JR, Thiele EA. Tuberous sclerosis complex. Nat Rev Dis Primers. 2016;2:16035.
6. Harknett EC, Chang WY, Byrnes S, Johnson J, Lazor R, Cohen MM, et al. Use of variability in national and regional data to estimate the prevalence of lymphangioleiomyomatosis. QJM. 2011;104(11):971–9.
7. Moss J, Avila NA, Barnes PM, Litzenberger RA, Bechtle J, Brooks PG, et al. Prevalence and clinical characteristics of lymphangioleiomyomatosis (LAM) in patients with tuberous sclerosis complex. Am J Resp Crit Care Med. 2001;164(4):669–71.
8. Gupta N, Lee HS, Ryu JH, Taveira-DaSilva AM, Beck GJ, Lee JC, et al. The NHLBI LAM registry: Prognostic physiologic and radiologic biomarkers emerge from a 15-year prospective longitudinal analysis. Chest. 2019;155(2):288–96.
9. Taveira-DaSilva AM, Jones AM, Julien-Williams P, Yao J, Stylianou M, Moss J. Severity and outcome of cystic lung disease in women with tuberous sclerosis complex. Eur Respir J. 2015;45(1):171–80.
10. Moir LM. Lymphangioleiomyomatosis: Current understanding and potential treatments. Pharmacol Ther. 2016;158:114–24.
11. McCormack FX. Lymphangioleiomyomatosis: A clinical update. Chest. 2008;133(2):507–16.
12. Sarbassov DD, Ali SM, Kim DH, Guertin DA, Latek RR, Erdjument-Bromage H, et al. Rictor, a novel binding partner of mTOR, defines a rapamycin-insensitive and raptor-independent pathway that regulates the cytoskeleton. Curr Biol. 2004;14(14):1296–302.
13. Manning BD. Game of TOR - the target of rapamycin rules four kingdoms. N Engl J Med. 2017;377(13):1297–9.
14. Stacker SA, Caesar C, Baldwin ME, Thornton GE, Williams RA, Prevo R, et al. VEGF-D promotes the metastatic spread of tumor cells via the lymphatics. Nat Med. 2001;7(2):186–91.
15. Seyama K, Kumasaka T, Souma S, Sato T, Kurihara M, Mitani K, et al. Vascular endothelial growth factor-d is increased in serum of patients with lymphangioleiomyomatosis. Lymphat Res Biol. 2006;4(3):143–52.
16. Crino PB, Nathanson KL, Henske EP. The tuberous sclerosis complex. N Engl J Med. 2006;355(13):1345–56.
17. Northrup H, Koenig MK, Pearson DA, Au KS. Tuberous Sclerosis Complex. In: Adam MP, Ardinger HH, Pagon RA, Wallace SE, Bean LJH, Stephens K, et al., editors. GeneReviews (®). Seattle (WA): University of Washington, Seattle.
18. Au KS, Williams AT, Roach ES, Batchelor L, Sparagana SP, Delgado MR, et al. Genotype/phenotype correlation in 325 individuals referred for a diagnosis of tuberous sclerosis complex in the United States. Genet Med. 2007;9(2):88–100.
19. Lee KN, Yoon SK, Choi SJ, Goo JM, Nam KJ. Cystic lung disease: A comparison of cystic size, as seen on expiratory and inspiratory HRCT scans. Korean J Radiol. 2000;1(2):84–90.
20. Seaman DM, Meyer CA, Gilman MD, McCormack FX. Diffuse cystic lung disease at high-resolution CT. AJR. 2011;196(6):1305–11.
21. Travis WD, Brambilla E, Nicholson AG, Yatabe Y, Austin JHM, Beasley MB, et al. The 2015 World Health Organization classification of lung tumors: Impact of genetic, clinical and radiologic advances since the 2004 classification. J Thorac Oncol. 2015;10(9):1243–60.
22. Ferrans VJ, Yu ZX, Nelson WK, Valencia JC, Tatsuguchi A, Avila NA, et al. Lymphangioleiomyomatosis (LAM): A review of clinical and morphological features. J Nippon Med Sch. 2000;67(5):311–29.
23. Cohen MM, Pollock-BarZiv S, Johnson SR. Emerging clinical picture of lymphangioleiomyomatosis. Thorax. 2005;60(10):875–9.
24. Ryu JH, Moss J, Beck GJ, Lee JC, Brown KK, Chapman JT, et al. The NHLBI lymphangioleiomyomatosis registry: Characteristics of 230 patients at enrollment. Am J Resp Crit Care Med. 2006;173(1):105–11.
25. Cooley J, Lee YCG, Gupta N. Spontaneous pneumothorax in diffuse cystic lung diseases. Curr Opin Pulm Med. 2017;23(4):323–33.
26. Derweduwen AM, Verbeken E, Stas M, Verschakelen J, Coolen J, Verleden G, et al. Extrapulmonary lymphangioleiomyomatosis: A wolf in sheep's clothing. Thorax. 2013;68(1):111–3.
27. Matsui K, Tatsuguchi A, Valencia J, Yu Z, Bechtle J, Beasley MB, et al. Extrapulmonary lymphangioleiomyomatosis (LAM): Clinicopathologic features in 22 cases. Hum Pathol. 2000;31(10):1242–8.
28. Taveira-DaSilva AM, Jones AM, Julien-Williams P, Shawker T, Glasgow CG, Stylianou M, et al. Effect of fasting on the size of lymphangioleiomyomas in patients with lymphangioleiomyomatosis. Chest. 2015;148(4):1027–33.
29. Avila NA, Dwyer AJ, Murphy-Johnson DV, Brooks P, Moss J. Sonography of lymphangioleiomyoma in lymphangioleiomyomatosis: Demonstration of diurnal variation in lesion size. AJR. 2005;184(2):459–64.

30. Abbott GF, Rosado-de-Christenson ML, Frazier AA, Franks TJ, Pugatch RD, Galvin JR. From the archives of the AFIP: Lymphangioleiomyomatosis: Radiologic-pathologic correlation. Radiographics. 2005;25(3):803–28.
31. Steagall WK, Glasgow CG, Hathaway OM, Avila NA, Taveira-Dasilva AM, Rabel A, et al. Genetic and morphologic determinants of pneumothorax in lymphangioleiomyomatosis. Am J Physiol Lung Cell Mol Physiol. 2007;293(3):L800–8.
32. Young LR, Almoosa KF, Pollock-Barziv S, Coutinho M, McCormack FX, Sahn SA. Patient perspectives on management of pneumothorax in lymphangioleiomyomatosis. Chest. 2006;129(5):1267–73.
33. Manoukian SB, Kowal DJ. Comprehensive imaging manifestations of tuberous sclerosis. AJR. 2015;204(5):933–43.
34. Cudzilo CJ, Szczesniak RD, Brody AS, Rattan MS, Krueger DA, Bissler JJ, et al. Lymphangioleiomyomatosis screening in women with tuberous sclerosis. Chest. 2013;144(2):578–85.
35. Steagall WK, Pacheco-Rodriguez G, Darling TN, Torre O, Harari S, Moss J. The lymphangioleiomyomatosis lung cell and its human cell models. Am J Respir Cell Mol Biol. 2018;58(6):678–83.
36. Crooks DM, Pacheco-Rodriguez G, DeCastro RM, McCoy JP, Jr., Wang JA, Kumaki F, et al. Molecular and genetic analysis of disseminated neoplastic cells in lymphangioleiomyomatosis. Proc Natl Acad Sci U S A. 2004;101(50):17462–7.
37. Johnson SR, Cordier JF, Lazor R, Cottin V, Costabel U, Harari S, et al. European Respiratory Society guidelines for the diagnosis and management of lymphangioleiomyomatosis. Eur Respir J. 2010;35(1):14–26.
38. Johnson SR, Taveira-DaSilva AM, Moss J. Lymphangioleiomyomatosis. Clin Chest Med. 2016;37(3):389–403.
39. Gupta N, Finlay GA, Kotloff RM, Strange C, Wilson KC, Young LR, et al. Lymphangioleiomyomatosis diagnosis and management: High-resolution chest computed tomography, transbronchial lung biopsy, and pleural disease management. An official American Thoracic Society/Japanese Respiratory Society clinical practice guideline. Am J Respir Crit Care Med. 2017;196(10):1337–48.
40. Okamoto S, Suzuki K, Hayashi T, Muraki K, Nagaoka T, Nishino K, et al. Transbronchial lung biopsy for The diagnosis of lymphangioleiomyomatosis: The severity of cystic lung destruction assessed by The modified goddard scoring system as a predictor for establishing The diagnosis. Orphanet J Rare Dis. 2020;15(1):125.
41. Taveira-DaSilva AM, Moss J. Epidemiology, pathogenesis and diagnosis of lymphangioleiomyomatosis. Expert Opin Orphan Drugs. 2016;4(4):369–78.
42. McCormack FX, Inoue Y, Moss J, Singer LG, Strange C, Nakata K, et al. Efficacy and safety of sirolimus in lymphangioleiomyomatosis. N Engl J Med. 2011;364(17):1595–606.
43. Taveira-DaSilva AM, Hathaway O, Stylianou M, Moss J. Changes in lung function and chylous effusions in patients with lymphangioleiomyomatosis treated with sirolimus. Ann Intern Med. 2011;154(12):797–805, W-292-3.
44. Taveira-DaSilva AM, Steagall WK, Rabel A, Hathaway O, Harari S, Cassandro R, et al. Reversible airflow obstruction in lymphangioleiomyomatosis. Chest. 2009;136(6):1596–603.
45. Young L, Lee HS, Inoue Y, Moss J, Singer LG, Strange C, et al. Serum VEGF-D A concentration as A biomarker of lymphangioleiomyomatosis severity and treatment response: A prospective analysis of the multicenter international lymphangioleiomyomatosis efficacy of sirolimus (MILES) trial. Lancet Respir Med. 2013;1(6):445–52.
46. Young LR, Vandyke R, Gulleman PM, Inoue Y, Brown KK, Schmidt LS, et al. Serum vascular endothelial growth factor-d prospectively distinguishes lymphangioleiomyomatosis from other diseases. Chest. 2010;138(3):674–81.
47. Gupta N, Hagner M, Wu H, Young LR, Palipana A, Szczesniak RD, et al. Serum vascular endothelial growth factor-c as a marker of therapeutic response to sirolimus in lymphangioleiomyomatosis. Ann Am Thorac Soc. 2020.
48. Glasgow CG, Pacheco-Rodriguez G, Steagall WK, Haughey ME, Julien-Williams PA, Stylianou MP, et al. CA-125 in disease progression and treatment of lymphangioleiomyomatosis. Chest. 2018;153(2):339–48.
49. Pollock-BarZiv S, Cohen MM, Downey GP, Johnson SR, Sullivan E, McCormack FX. Air travel in women with lymphangioleiomyomatosis. Thorax. 2007;62(2):176–80.
50. Wajda N, Gupta N. Air travel-related spontaneous pneumothorax in diffuse cystic lung diseases. Curr Pulmonol Rep. 2018;7(2):56–62.
51. Taveira-DaSilva AM, Johnson SR, Julien-Williams P, Johnson J, Stylianou M, Moss J. Pregnancy in lymphangioleiomyomatosis: Clinical and lung function outcomes in two national cohorts. Thorax. 2020;75(10):904–7.
52. Cohen MM, Freyer AM, Johnson SR. Pregnancy experiences among women with lymphangioleiomyomatosis. Respir Med. 2009;103(5):766–72.
53. Yao J, Taveira-DaSilva AM, Colby TV, Moss J. CT grading of lung disease in lymphangioleiomyomatosis. AJR. 2012;199(4):787–93.
54. Hu-Wang E, Schuzer JL, Rollison S, Leifer ES, Steveson C, Gopalakrishnan V, et al. chest CT scan at radiation dose of a posteroanterior and lateral chest radiograph series: A proof of principle in lymphangioleiomyomatosis. Chest. 2019;155(3):528–33.
55. Park S, Lee EJ. Diagnosis and treatment of cystic lung disease. Korean J Intern Med. 2017;32(2):229–38.
56. Gupta N, Vassallo R, Wikenheiser-Brokamp KA, McCormack FX. Diffuse cystic lung disease. Part I. Am J Respir Crit Care Med. 2015;191(12):1354–66.
57. Gupta N, Vassallo R, Wikenheiser-Brokamp KA, McCormack FX. Diffuse cystic lung disease. Part II. Am J Respir Crit Care Med. 2015;192(1):17–29.
58. Oprescu N, McCormack FX, Byrnes S, Kinder BW. Clinical predictors of mortality and cause of death in lymphangioleiomyomatosis: A population-based registry. Lung. 2013;191(1):35–42.
59. Sehgal SN. Sirolimus: Its discovery, biological properties, and mechanism of action. Transplant Proc. 2003;35(3 Suppl):7S–14S.
60. Bissler JJ, McCormack FX, Young LR, Elwing JM, Chuck G, Leonard JM, et al. Sirolimus for angiomyolipoma in tuberous sclerosis complex or lymphangioleiomyomatosis. N Engl J Med. 2008;358(2):140–51.
61. Takada T, Mikami A, Kitamura N, Seyama K, Inoue Y, Nagai K, et al. Efficacy and safety of long-term sirolimus therapy for Asian patients with lymphangioleiomyomatosis. Ann Am Thorac Soc. 2016;13(11):1912–22.
62. Feemster LC, Lyons PG, Chatterjee RS, Kidambi P, McCormack FX, Moss J, et al. Summary for clinicians: Lymphangioleiomyomatosis diagnosis and management clinical practice guideline. Ann Am Thorac Soc. 2017;14(7):1073–5.
63. Goldberg HJ, Harari S, Cottin V, Rosas IO, Peters E, Biswal S, et al. Everolimus for the treatment of lymphangioleiomyomatosis: A phase II study. Eur Respir J. 2015;46(3):783–94.
64. Ando K, Kurihara M, Kataoka H, Ueyama M, Togo S, Sato T, et al. Efficacy and safety of low-dose sirolimus for treatment of lymphangioleiomyomatosis. Respir Investig. 2013;51(3):175–83.
65. Taveira-DaSilva AM, Jones AM, Julien-Williams P, Stylianou M, Moss J. Long-term effect of sirolimus on serum vascular endothelial growth factor d levels in patients with lymphangioleiomyomatosis. Chest. 2018;153(1):124–32.
66. Johnson J, Johnson SR. Cross-sectional study of reversible airway obstruction in LAM: Better evidence is needed for bronchodilator and inhaled steroid use. Thorax. 2019;74(10):999–1002.
67. Almoosa KF, Ryu JH, Mendez J, Huggins JT, Young LR, Sullivan EJ, et al. Management of pneumothorax in lymphangioleiomyomatosis: Effects on recurrence and lung transplantation complications. Chest. 2006;129(5):1274–81.

17

LYMPHOCYTIC INTERSTITIAL PNEUMONIA AND ASSOCIATED CYSTIC LUNG DISEASES

Evelyn Lynn, Liam Jeremiah Chawke, Aurelie Fabre, David J. Murphy, and Cormac McCarthy

Contents

Lymphocytic interstitial pneumonia 125
Epidemiology and clinical features of LIP 125
Radiological features of LIP 126
Histopathological features of LIP 127
Management of LIP 128
Follicular bronchiolitis 129
Pulmonary amyloidosis and light chain deposition disease 129
Conclusion.. 130
References... 130

KEY POINTS

- Lymphocytic interstitial pneumonia (LIP) is a rare diffuse cystic lung disease, it is mostly associated with autoimmune conditions and immunodeficiency, most classically Sjögren's syndrome and HIV.
- Patients usually present with a cough or progressive dyspnea that can precede the diagnosis by many months or years.
- High-resolution CT thorax is required to confirm diagnosis and shows pulmonary cysts, which can be subpleural, parenchymal, parenchymal with nodules, and parenchymal with ground-glass opacification. Surgical biopsy is rarely necessary but if required video-assisted thoracoscopy (VATS) is the preferred method.
- Approximately 5% of patients transform to lymphoma, which is more common in those with serum dysproteinemias.
- Treatment of LIP requires controlling the underlying disease, and in some cases, corticosteroids or immunosuppressive therapies are required.

Lymphocytic interstitial pneumonia

Lymphocytic interstitial pneumonia (LIP) belongs to the idiopathic interstitial pneumoniae that are part of a larger group of diffuse or interstitial lung diseases (12). Initially classified by Liebow and Carrington (1) in 1969 as part of the chronic interstitial pneumonias, the American Thoracic Society (ATS) and European Respiratory Society (ERS) consensus statement further defined the clinical manifestations, pathology, and radiological features of idiopathic interstitial pneumonias (IIPs), with an update issued in 2011 (12, 13). This update, intended to supplement the 2002 statement (14), subdivided IIPs into four groups and assigned LIP to the "rare" group (15). While these disease entities share many features (8), each has a distinct histological pattern and CT findings (8, 14). In LIP, it is the lymphocytic infiltration of the lung parenchyma that distinguishes it from other patterns of interstitial pneumonias (14). Following the initial recognition of LIP as its own disease entity, it was considered a paraneoplastic phenomenon (12) where it was believed a large number of patients progressed to develop lymphoma. More recently with the wide adoption of immunohistochemistry and molecular testing clinically, the few cases that would have previously been misclassified as LIP are now correctly diagnosed as low-grade lymphomas, mostly extranodal marginal zone B-cell lymphomas of mucosa-associated lymphoid tissue (MALT) (15). Another development since the initial 2002 ATS/ERS criteria is the diagnosis of cellular NSIP in those previously thought to have LIP (3, 15).

Epidemiology and clinical features of LIP

LIP is extremely rare (10, 12, 15, 16). While prevalence is uncertain (2), it is twice as likely to occur in women as men (3, 17). The disease typically presents in the fifth decade of life, especially in those with autoimmune disease, most classically Sjögren's syndrome (2, 11). It also occurs in immunodeficiency conditions including HIV infection, particularly in children (1, 8, 9). Indeed, the Centers for Disease Control and Prevention has defined LIP in those with HIV as an AIDS defining illness (15).

The most common presenting symptom is cough, often present for many months or years prior to diagnosis (10). Other symptoms include progressive dyspnea (12, 18). Infrequently, patients present with systemic symptoms including fever, night sweats, arthralgia, and weight loss or evidence of underlying disease such as symptoms of associated autoimmune disorders described (1, 2, 15, 19). On examination, the majority of patients are found to have bibasilar inspiratory crackles (2) and lymphadenopathy though the latter is often more common in those with underlying Sjögren's disease (12). Patients may also exhibit features of underlying disease such as autoimmune or immune-deficiency conditions. Up to 80% of patients have evidence of dysproteinemias (15), and patients found to have monoclonal gammopathy or hypogammaglobulinemia must be investigated for

TABLE 17.1: Clinical Conditions Associated with Lymphoid Interstitial Pneumonia

Idiopathic	
Connective tissue disease	Sjögren's syndrome
	Systemic lupus erythematosus
	Rheumatoid arthritis
Immunodeficiency	Human immunodeficiency virus (HIV)
	Acquired immune-deficiency syndrome (AIDS)
	Common variable immune deficiency (CVID)
	Severe combined immune deficiency (SCID)
Infection	Epstein–Barr virus (EBV)
	Human T-cell lymphotropic virus type-1 (HTLV-1)
	Human herpes virus-6
	Pneumocystis carinii
Other autoimmune disorders	Myasthenia gravis
	Pernicious anemia
	Hashimoto's thyroiditis
	Chronic active hepatitis
Hematological disorders	Dysproteinemia
	Amyloidosis

lympho-proliferative disorders (12) (Table 17.1). Approximately 5% of patients transform to lymphoma, which is more common in those with serum dysproteinemias. Pulmonary function testing usually reveals a restrictive ventilatory defect with a decrease in the forced vital capacity, and forced expiratory volume over 1 second (2, 15). There is also a decrease in the diffusion capacity of the lung for carbon monoxide (DLCO) (16) and those with advanced disease may be hypoxemic.

LIP is an inflammatory pulmonary reaction of the bronchus associated lymphoid tissue. LIP should be considered when there is a high-resolution CT (HRCT) scan demonstrating cysts in the correct clinical context. HRCT is the imaging modality of choice (20). A pulmonary cyst is characterized radiologically as a rounded airspace parenchymal lucency, or a low attenuation area with a well-defined interface with the normal lung (21). In diffuse cystic lung disease, cysts can be subpleural, parenchymal, parenchymal with nodules, and parenchymal with ground-glass opacification. They can vary in their number, distribution, and location (7, 22). Cyst formation in LIP is multifactorial due to potential ischemia caused by vascular obstruction, post-obstructive bronchiolar ectasia, or bronchiolar compression by lymphoid tissues (16).

LIP is a clinicopathological condition that infers a diffuse involvement of the lung parenchyma by reactive lymphoid tissue (19). A polyclonal hypergammaglobulinemia can be seen in about 75% of cases, or rarely a monoclonal increase in IgG or IgM (12, 23, 24). LIP should be considered when there is a clinical history of an autoimmune disorder and investigations such as ANA, anticyclic citrullinated peptide antibodies, anti-SSA/Ro, anti-SSB/LA antibodies, EBV titers, HIV, human T-cell lymphotropic virus, rheumatoid factor, serum and urine electrophoresis, thyroid function tests, and IgG4 should be performed (19) in the setting of a characteristic HRCT. Idiopathic LIP is extremely rare. It is recommended that patients with a diagnosis of LIP are assessed for autoimmune diseases and other associated syndromes (12).

Radiological features of LIP

It is postulated that cysts along with intrathoracic lymphadenopathy are present in around 60–80% (25) of patients and form <10% of the total lung parenchyma (26). The distribution of LIP changes is predominantly in the lower lung fields (27, 28). Typically, cysts are thin-walled, <3 mm in thickness, and are of varying size and morphology, which may be ill-defined (25, 28, 29). The presence of characteristic cysts may be the only evidence of LIP on imaging (25, 27). The diagnosis of LIP should be considered in patients with lung cysts and immunological abnormalities. The appearance of a few scattered cysts in a patient with Sjögren's syndrome is very likely to indicate LIP (25) (Figure 17.1). Other radiological findings consist of poorly defined centrilobular (25) and subpleural micronodules, bilateral diffuse areas of ground-glass opacification (which may resolve over serial imaging when treatment is commenced [25]), bibasilar reticulation, and peribronchovascular interstitial thickening (28, 29), reticular

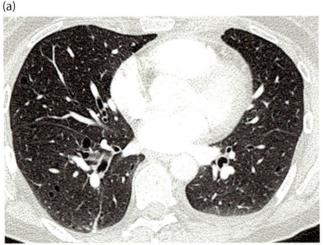
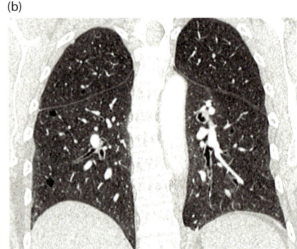

FIGURE 17.1 The axial (a) and coronal (b) images of the chest in a 60-year-old male with Sjögren's syndrome and lymphocytic interstitial pneumonia, demonstrating bilateral cysts that are thin-walled and randomly distributed.

Lymphocytic Interstitial Pneumonia and Associated Cystic Lung Diseases

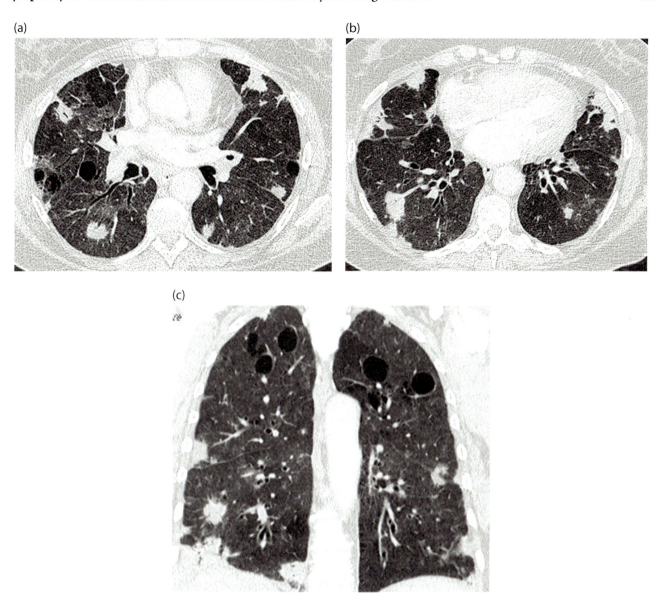

FIGURE 17.2 The axial (a, b) and coronal (c) images from a CT chest scan in a 55-year-old female with a history of mixed connective tissue disease, LIP, and subsequent lymphoma. Thin-walled cysts are visible as well as nodular lymphoma.

abnormalities, intrathoracic lymphadenopathy, and formation of thin-walled cysts, usually in the basal regions (23, 26, 30–32).

HRCT is required not only to confirm the diagnosis of LIP (2), but it is also important to distinguish between LIP and its differentials as treatment, disease progression, and prognosis differ vastly between each (8). The HRCT changes often correlate with the histopathological findings of distribution of pulmonary lymphatics and peribronchiolar distribution of the lymphoid cells. The HRCT imaging must be correlated with clinical presentation and pathological findings (8). Where cysts exist, they are usually deep in the lung parenchyma and the result of peribronchiolar cellular infiltration seen on biopsy samples (15, 30). A fine linear or reticular pattern may be found on HRCT (29), and perivascular honeycombing has also been reported, though it is rare (8, 15). Fifty percent of patients have a reticular pattern on CT, with some patients noted to have lung nodules and consolidation as CT features. Nodules need to be carefully followed as they may transition to lymphoma occasionally and in some cases

associated with amyloid (Figures 17.2 and 17.3). Pleural effusion has been described but is rare (15). Follow-up CT studies show that the ground-glass opacity improves in the majority of cases of lymphoid interstitial pneumonia, although cysts remain, with rare cases developing honeycomb change (33). As with all cystic lung disease, accurate interpretation of imaging combined with clinical findings and appropriate genetic testing can facilitate diagnosis without the requirement for lung biopsy (34).

Histopathological features of LIP

Bronchoscopy and bronchoalveolar lavage (BAL) are useful in excluding an alternative diagnosis, in particular where the differential includes infectious and malignant causes of cystic lung disease (35, 36). Surgical lung biopsy is rarely required but, when necessary, a video-assisted thoracoscopy (VATS) is the biopsy method of choice (37). Transbronchial forceps biopsy can be performed, but the diagnostic yield is lower compared to a VATS

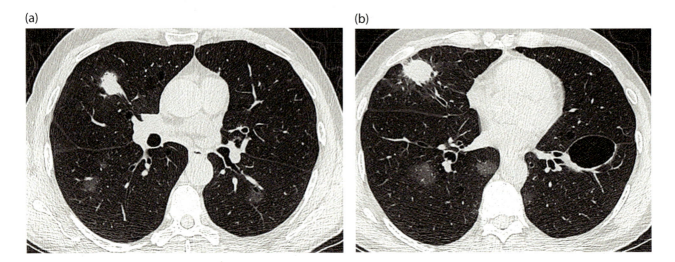

FIGURE 17.3 (a, b) CT chest images of a 50-year-old male with a history of Sjögren's syndrome, LIP, and nodular amyloid. Bilateral thin-walled cysts and nodules associated with amyloidosis are evident.

surgical lung biopsy (17). There has been no recommendation for or against the use of cryoprobe assisted transbronchial lung biopsies in LIP (38). This technique has been used with some success in patients with lymphangioleiomyomatosis (39, 40). A decision to proceed with a biopsy should be made in conjunction with clinicians, radiologists, and pathologists (3, 8, 10), and likewise, when a biopsy is performed, the results should be discussed in tandem with multidisciplinary team discussion.

Cysts likely form as a result of ischemia due to vascular obstruction, post-obstructive alveolar dilatation, or compression of bronchioles by lymphoid tissue leading to a check-valve mechanism (35). On histological examination of LIP, lymphoid tissue is present in the hilar and intrapulmonary nodes, in the lung parenchyma itself, and in the bronchus-associated lymphoid tissue (BALT) (17). Lymphocytes, plasma cells, and histiocytes deposit in the alveolar septa leading to lymphoid cell hyperplasia and alveolar macrophage increase (3, 17), resulting in expansion of the septa (3, 15). The airspaces and vessels may eventually become filled with infiltrates, macrophages, or proteinaceous fluid (15). Though uncommon, nonnecrotizing granulomas may be seen, although they are usually inconspicuous and loosely arranged (41). In those with advanced disease, biopsy may reveal interstitial fibrosis and honeycombing (24). A classic feature of LIP is polyclonal cellular infiltrates (17). Histologically, LIP is characterized by light chains that are inflammatory in nature and either form nodular lymphoid aggregates or may contain germinal centers (3, 14, 15) (Figure 17.4). Those with Sjögren's may have deposits of amyloid (15, 17) (Figure 17.5). The pattern of distribution in LIP differs from lymphoma where the changes are largely distributed along the intralobular septa, bronchoalveolar bundles, and pleura (3, 15). Where lymphoma is suspected, immunohistochemistry is required. Lymphoma typically demonstrates monoclonal B-cell proliferations (41). Additionally, LIP can resemble a cellular subtype of nonspecific interstitial pneumonia type pattern. The overlapping features include lymphohistiocytic infiltration of the interalveolar septa.

Management of LIP

To date, there have been no randomized controlled trials to determine the optimal treatment for LIP, whereas control of the underlying disease in secondary LIP appears to be most important (17, 18). The course trajectory of LIP tends to be variable and unpredictable; on one hand, spontaneous improvement has been reported while on the other hand, patients may develop complications such as superimposed infections, progressive pulmonary disease, and, rarely, lymphoma (42). The 5-year survival rate is approximately 70% (41), whereas the median survival rate is from 5–11.5 years (16). Mortality is generally related due to pulmonary fibrosis or lymphoma (2, 16), hence it is difficult to determine whether treatment alters disease progression (43). Treatment recommendations are largely based on case series and case reports and generally consist of corticosteroids and other immunosuppressive agents as well an antiretroviral therapy in HIV-infected patients (2, 44). Depending on the disease severity, appropriate commencement regimes for corticosteroids are 0.75 mg/kg/day for an initial 3-month period, following by a dose reduction by 0.25 mg/kg/day for every 6–12 weeks (2). The optimum duration of treatment is unclear due to lack of longitudinal data. Nodules and ground-glass opacification appear to respond well to the corticosteroid therapy, but is it unclear what effect therapy has on cyst formation or progression (33).

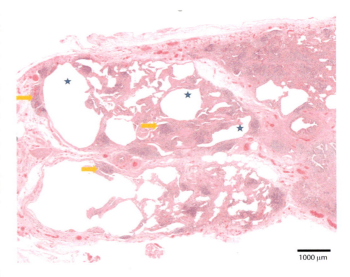

FIGURE 17.4 The histology of lymphoid interstitial pneumonia showing cystic spaces (stars) and lymphoid aggregates within the wall of the cysts (yellow arrows).

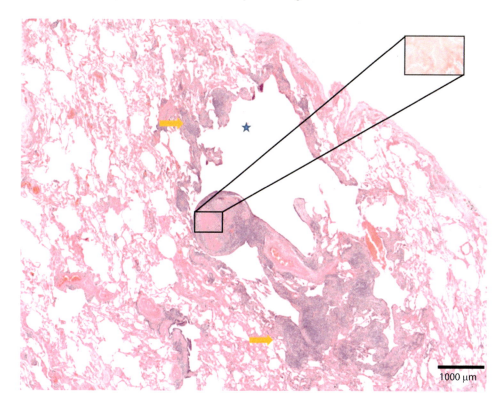

FIGURE 17.5 An amyloid deposition, as evidenced by Congo red stain, in a patient with LIP (insert: Congo red stain). The cystic spaces (stars) and lymphoid aggregates within the wall of the cysts (yellow arrows) are denoted.

Other immunosuppressive agents that have been used with some success include rituximab (4), cyclophosphamide (45), azathioprine, and hydroxychloroquine. Their use has been reported with varying success. Currently there is no indication for use of antifibrotics in LIP. There may be a limited role for intravenous gamma globulin therapy in patients with hypogammaglobulinemia (46).

Approximately two-thirds of patients respond to corticosteroid therapy (2) with the remaining one-third progressing to either fulminant respiratory failure or developing complications from the use of immunosuppressive therapies (2). Up to 50% of patients may die within 5 years of diagnosis (2, 15). Relapses can occur in some cases, and in those refractory to treatment, lung transplantation is an option; however, longitudinal data is limited (16, 32).

Follicular bronchiolitis

An important differential/spectrum of LIP is follicular bronchiolitis (FB), classified as a reactive lymphoid disorder that also affects the lungs (47). It is classified as one of the reactive pulmonary lymphoid disorders as part of the lymphoproliferative pulmonary diseases (48). Like LIP, it is most commonly associated with connective tissue diseases like Sjögren's syndrome, rheumatoid arthritis, HIV, and other immunodeficient states (48–51). Associated respiratory symptoms include cough and dyspnea, although many patients can be asymptomatic, especially in mild disease. A HRCT is required as part of the diagnostic workup. Classical radiological findings in FB, like LIP, are diffuse cystic lung disease (oval in shape, 4 mm–5 cm in size, with a basal predominance) (52) including small centrilobular nodules that are associated with patchy ground glass opacities (53). Other supportive radiological features include evidence of bronchial wall thickening, bronchiolectasis/bronchiectasis, and air trapping as evidenced by mosaicism expiratory phases on a CT (54). Classical CT features suggestive of FB in the clinical context of SS may obviate the need for a lung biopsy, however outside of this, a surgical lung biopsy may be required for formal diagnosis, as well as excluding pulmonary lymphoma or amyloidosis, which is known to complicate cystic lung disease (55). FB is characterized histologically by the presence of prominent hyperplastic lymphoid follicles, as well as well-defined reactive germinal centers distributed along the bronchovascular bundles (56). This ultimately leads to narrowing and obliteration of the bronchioles in contrast to LIP. FB is mainly bronchiolocentric, whereas LIP is better characterized by interstitial involvement. An interstitial inflammatory infiltrate is seen in about 20% of cases in LIP and FB (41). Treatment largely consists of treating the underlying condition in patients infected with HIV, or immunodeficient states (50, 52). In autoimmune conditions such as Sjögren's syndrome or rheumatoid arthritis, treatments consist of corticosteroids, azathioprine, cyclophosphamide, and mycophenolate mofetil. No randomized controlled trials exist comparing various pharmacological therapies in FB.

Pulmonary amyloidosis and light chain deposition disease

There are three forms of pulmonary amyloid, (57) diffuse alveolar-septal amyloidosis, nodular pulmonary amyloidosis, and tracheobronchial amyloidosis. Isolated pulmonary involvement in amyloidosis is relatively rare (58, 59), and features of the associated underlying disease such as Sjögren's syndrome-associated LIP can be present on imaging. Rarely, pulmonary amyloidosis can present as diffuse cystic lung disease (60). In these cases, the cysts are numerous and are small- to moderate-sized, thin-walled, and most often rounded (61). Peribronchovascular and subpleural cysts are common and nodules are often calcified. Biopsy is always required to diagnosis amyloid and clinicians should be cognizant of the risk of bleeding (62). All cases require correct diagnosis and close follow-up as treatment may vary depending on specific amyloid type (57). Underlying chronic conditions such as plasma cell dyscrasia must be ruled out.

Light chain deposition disease (LCDD) is a rare disorder characterized by deposition of extracellular light chains in tissue leading to destruction of the structure and function of that organ. It most often occurs in patients who have underlying plasma cell or lymphoproliferative disease where there is excess production of monoclonal light chains (63). Similar to amyloid, two histological patterns have been described: diffuse and nodular. Nodular disease is more commonly associated with plasma cell disease and thus the distinction may be important when treatment is being considered. Nonfibrillary amorphous deposition of monotypic kappa light chains occurs in the basement membrane of alveolar walls, small airways, and vessels (60, 63). This leads to emphysematous-like changes and small airway dilation. In comparison to amyloidosis, it does not stain positive on Congo red or exhibit apple-green birefringence under polarized light. Renal disease is the most common result of this deposition, where patients can present with rapidly deteriorating renal function (60, 64).

Isolated pulmonary LCDD is very rare and mostly asymptomatic (60). While LCDD itself was first described by Randall et al. in 1976 (63), Colombat et al. (65) documented the first cases of LCDD presenting as cystic pulmonary disease. Patients present with a spectrum of symptoms from shortness of breath to severe end-stage respiratory compromise, while in others the disease is found incidentally. Radiological findings vary from thin-walled cysts, either small sub-2 cm cysts, diffusely distributed cysts similar to those seen in LAM, or larger cystic changes associated with reticulonodular opacities similar to PLCH. Solid and subsolid pulmonary nodules are also common features of LCDD (60, 66). PET-CT displays variable fluorodeoxyglucose (FDG) uptake within nodules (60). In some cases, biopsy may be required, mostly to distinguish between LCDD and amyloid disease. Treatment centers around identifying the underlying lymphoproliferative disease, if present, and managing that. In those with end-stage respiratory failure, lung transplantation may be required.

Conclusion

LIP is a benign lymphoproliferative disorder characterized radiologically as a diffuse cystic lung disease. Several autoimmune diseases have been implicated in LIP, with idiopathic LIP being extremely rare. A thorough diagnostic evaluation is required to exclude other differential diagnoses such an infectious and malignant causes. An HRCT is required for definitive diagnosis, with surgical lung biopsy reserved when there is doubt regarding the diagnosis. Limited data exists for treatment of LIP, whereas treatment of the underlying causes is usually sufficient in most cases. Despite the low risk of transformation to lymphoma, consideration should be given to surveillance imaging periodically, with biopsies performed of any uncharacteristic enlarging nodules/opacites (5, 37). The optimal time for surveillance and frequency requires further studies. Other lymphoproliferative and associated conditions need to be considered in the diagnostic workup.

References

1. Liebow AA. The interstitial pneumonias. Frontiers of Pulmonary Radiology. 1969:102–41.
2. Swigris JJ, Berry GJ, Raffin TA, Kuschner WG. Lymphoid interstitial pneumonia: A narrative review. Chest. 2002;122(6):2150–64.
3. Travis WD, Costabel U, Hansell DM, King TE, Jr., Lynch DA, Nicholson AG, et al. An official American Thoracic Society/European Respiratory Society statement: Update of the international multidisciplinary classification of the idiopathic interstitial pneumonias. Am J Respir Crit Care Med. 2013;188(6):733–48.
4. Flament T, Bigot A, Chaigne B, Henique H, Diot E, Marchand-Adam S. Pulmonary manifestations of Sjögren's syndrome. Eur Respir Rev. 2016;25(140):110–23.
5. Obaidat B, Yazdani D, Wikenheiser-Brokamp KA, Gupta N. Diffuse cystic lung diseases. Respir Care. 2020;65(1):111–26.
6. Sharma A, Ali M, Arya V. Lymphoid interstitial pneumonia in a patient with rheumatoid arthritis. Rheumatology (Oxford, England). 2019;58(5):928.
7. Raoof S, Bondalapati P, Vydyula R, Ryu JH, Gupta N, Raoof S, et al. Cystic lung diseases: Algorithmic approach. Chest. 2016;150(4):945–65.
8. Lynch DA, Travis WD, Muller NL, Galvin JR, Hansell DM, Grenier PA, et al. Idiopathic interstitial pneumonias: CT features. Radiology. 2005;236(1):10–21.
9. Davies CW, Juniper MC, Gray W, Gleeson FV, Chapel HM, Davies RJ. Lymphoid interstitial pneumonitis associated with common variable hypogammaglobulinaemia treated with cyclosporin a. Thorax. 2000;55(1):88–90.
10. Oliveira DS, Araújo Filho JA, Paiva AFL, Ikari ES, Chate RC, Nomura CH. Idiopathic interstitial pneumonias: Review of the latest American Thoracic Society/European Respiratory Society classification. Radiol Bras. 2018;51(5):321–7.
11. Dalvi V, Gonzalez EB, Lovett L. Lymphocytic interstitial pneumonitis (LIP) in Sjögren's syndrome: A case report and A review of the literature. Clin Rheumatol. 2007;26(8):1339–43.
12. Demedts M, Costabel U. ATS/ERS international multidisciplinary consensus classification of the idiopathic interstitial pneumonias. European Respiratory Journal. 2002;19(5):794–6.
13. Raghu G, Collard HR, Egan JJ, Martinez FJ, Behr J, Brown KK, et al. An official ATS/ERS/JRS/ALAT statement: Idiopathic pulmonary fibrosis: Evidence-based guidelines for diagnosis and management. Am J Respir Crit Care Med. 2011;183(6):788–824.
14. Larsen BT, Colby TV. Update for pathologists on idiopathic interstitial pneumonias. Archives of Pathology & Laboratory Medicine. 2012;136(10):1234–41.
15. Tian X, Yi ES, Ryu JH. Lymphocytic interstitial pneumonia and other benign lymphoid disorders. Semin Respir Crit Care Med. 2012;33(05):450–61.
16. Cha SI, Fessler MB, Cool CD, Schwarz MI, Brown KK. Lymphoid interstitial pneumonia: Clinical features, associations and prognosis. Eur Respir J. 2006;28(2):364–9.
17. Arcadu A, Moua T, Yi ES, Ryu JH. lymphoid interstitial pneumonia and other benign lymphoid disorders. Semin Respir Crit Care Med. 2016;37(3):406–20.
18. Tian X, Yi ES, Ryu JH. Lymphocytic interstitial pneumonia and other benign lymphoid disorders. Semin Respir Crit Care Med. 2012;33(5):450–61.
19. Panchabhai TS, Farver C, Highland KB. Lymphocytic interstitial pneumonia. Clin Chest Med. 2016;37(3):463–74.
20. Gupta N, Meraj R, Tanase D, James LE, Seyama K, Lynch DA, et al. Accuracy of chest high-resolution computed tomography in diagnosing diffuse cystic lung diseases. Eur Respir J. 2015;46(4):1196–9.
21. Ryu JH, Swensen SJ. Cystic and cavitary lung diseases: Focal and diffuse. Mayo Clinic Proceedings. 2003;78(6):744–52.
22. Carignan S, Staples CA, Müller NL. Intrathoracic lymphoproliferative disorders in the immunocompromised patient: CT findings. Radiology. 1995;197(1):53–8.
23. DeCoteau WE, Tourville D, Ambrus JL, Montes M, Adler R, Tomasi TB, Jr. Lymphoid interstitial pneumonia and autoerythrocyte sensitization syndrome. A case with deposition of immunoglobulins on the alveolar basement membrane. Arch Intern Med. 1974;134(3):519–22.
24. Guinee DG, Jr. Update on nonneoplastic pulmonary lymphoproliferative disorders and related entities. Arch Pathol Lab Med. 2010;134(5):691–701.

25. Lee KC, Kang EY, Yong HS, Kim C, Lee KY, Hwang SH, et al. A stepwise diagnostic approach to cystic lung diseases for radiologists. Korean J Radiol. 2019;20(9):1368–80.
26. Ichikawa Y, Kinoshita M, Koga T, Oizumi K, Fujimoto K, Hayabuchi N. Lung cyst formation in lymphocytic interstitial pneumonia: CT features. J Comput Assist Tomogr. 1994;18(5):745–8.
27. Escalon JG, Richards JC, Koelsch T, Downey GP, Lynch DA. Isolated cystic lung disease: An algorithmic approach to distinguishing Birt–Hogg–Dube syndrome, lymphangioleiomyomatosis, and lymphocytic interstitial pneumonia. Am J Roentgenol. 2019:1–5.
28. Sverzellati N, Lynch DA, Hansell DM, Johkoh T, King TE, Jr., Travis WD. American Thoracic Society–European Respiratory Society classification of the idiopathic interstitial pneumonias: Advances in knowledge since 2002. Radiographics. 2015;35(7):1849–71.
29. Aquilina G, Caltabiano DC, Galioto F, Cancemi G, Pino F, Vancheri A, et al. Cystic interstitial lung diseases: A pictorial review and a practical guide for the radiologist. Diagnostics (Basel, Switzerland). 2020;10(6):346.
30. Johkoh T, Muller NL, Pickford HA, Hartman TE, Ichikado K, Akira M, et al. Lymphocytic interstitial pneumonia: Thin-section CT findings in 22 patients. Radiology. 1999;212(2):567–72.
31. Vilela VS, Dias MM, Salgado Â A, da Silva BRA, Lopes AJ, Bessa EJC, et al. Pulmonary hypertension in systemic sclerosis: Diagnosis by systematic screening and prognosis after three years follow-up. BMC Pulmon Med. 2021;21(1):251.
32. Silva CI, Flint JD, Levy RD, Müller NL. Diffuse lung cysts in lymphoid interstitial pneumonia: High-resolution CT and pathologic findings. J Thorac Imaging. 2006;21(3):241–4.
33. Johkoh T, Ichikado K, Akira M, Honda O, Tomiyama N, Mihara N, et al. Lymphocytic interstitial pneumonia: Follow-up CT findings in 14 patients. J Thorac Imaging. 2000;15(3):162–7.
34. Trotman-Dickenson B. Cystic lung disease: Achieving a radiologic diagnosis. Eur J Radiol. 2014;83(1):39–46.
35. Baldi BG, Carvalho CRR, Dias OM, Marchiori E, Hochhegger B. Diffuse cystic lung diseases: Differential diagnosis. J Bras Pneumol. 2017;43(2):140–9.
36. Luppi F, Sebastiani M, Silva M, Sverzellati N, Cavazza A, Salvarani C, et al. Interstitial lung disease in Sjögren's syndrome: A clinical review. Clin Exp Rheumatol. 2020;38 Suppl 126 (4):291–300.
37. Gupta N, Vassallo R, Wikenheiser-Brokamp KA, McCormack FX. Diffuse cystic lung disease. Part II. Am J Respir Crit Care Med. 2015;192(1):17–29.
38. American Thoracic Society/European Respiratory Society International Multidisciplinary Consensus Classification of the Idiopathic Interstitial Pneumonias. This joint statement of the American Thoracic Society (ATS), and the European Respiratory Society (ERS) was adopted by the ATS board of directors, June 2001 and by the ERS Executive Committee, June 2001. Am J Respir Crit Care Med. 2002;165(2):277–304.
39. Yoshida M, Awano N, Inomata M, Kuse N, Tone M, Yoshimura H, et al. Diagnostic usefulness of transbronchial lung cryobiopsy in two patients mildly affected with pulmonary lymphangioleiomyomatosis. Respir Investig. 2020;58(4):295–9.
40. Gupta N, Wikenheiser-Brokamp K, Zander D, Balestra R, Selvaraju A, Niehaus K, et al. Successful diagnosis of lymphangioleiomyomatosis with transbronchial lung cryobiopsy. Lymphology. 2017;50(3):154–7.
41. Nicholson AG, Wotherspoon AC, Diss TC, Hansell DM, Du Bois R, Sheppard MN, et al. Reactive pulmonary lymphoid disorders. Histopathology. 1995;26(5):405–12.
42. Banerjee D, Ahmad D. Malignant lymphoma complicating lymphocytic interstitial pneumonia: A monoclonal B-cell neoplasm arising in A polyclonal lymphoproliferative disorder. Hum Pathol. 1982;13(8):780–2.
43. Nicholson AG. Lymphocytic interstitial pneumonia and other lymphoproliferative disorders in the lung. Semin Respir Crit Care Med. 2001;22(4):409–22.
44. Nordgren B, Friden C, Demmelmaier I, Bergstrom G, Lundberg IE, Nessen T, et al. An outsourced health-enhancing physical activity program for people with rheumatoid arthritis: Study of the maintenance phase. J Rheumatol. 2018;45(8):1093–100.
45. Dong X, Gao YL, Lu Y, Zheng Y. Characteristics of primary Sjögren's syndrome related lymphocytic interstitial pneumonia. Clin Rheumatol. 2021;40(2):601–12.
46. Popa V. Lymphocytic interstitial pneumonia of common variable immunodeficiency. Ann Allergy. 1988;60(3):203–6.
47. Poletti V, Ravaglia C, Tomassetti S, Gurioli C, Casoni G, Asioli S, et al. Lymphoproliferative lung disorders: Clinicopathological aspects. Eur Respir Rev. 2013;22(130):427–36.
48. Tashtoush B, Okafor NC, Ramirez JF, Smolley L. Follicular bronchiolitis: A literature review. J Clin Diagn Res. 2015;9(9):Oe01–5.
49. Shipe R, Lawrence J, Green J, Enfield K. HIV-associated follicular bronchiolitis. Am J Respir Crit Care Med. 2013;188(4):510–1.
50. Camarasa Escrig A, Amat Humaran B, Sapia S, León Ramírez JM. Follicular bronchiolitis associated with common variable immunodeficiency. Arch Bronconeumol. 2013;49(4):166–8.
51. Kadura S, Raghu G. Rheumatoid arthritis-interstitial lung disease: Manifestations and current concepts in pathogenesis and management. Eur Respir Rev. 2021;30(160).
52. Fisseler-Eckhoff A, Märker-Hermann E. Interstitial lung disease associated with connective tissue disease. Der Pathologe. 2021;42(1):4–10.
53. Pipavath SJ, Lynch DA, Cool C, Brown KK, Newell JD. Radiologic and pathologic features of bronchiolitis. Am J Roentgenol. 2005;185(2):354–63.
54. Howling SJ, Hansell DM, Wells AU, Nicholson AG, Flint JD, Müller NL. Follicular bronchiolitis: Thin-section CT and histologic findings. Radiology. 1999;212(3):637–42.
55. Borie R, Wislez M, Antoine M, Copie-Bergman C, Thieblemont C, Cadranel J. Pulmonary mucosa-associated lymphoid tissue lymphoma revisited. Eur Respir J. 2016;47(4):1244–60.
56. Tashiro K, Ohshima K, Suzumiya J, Yoneda S, Yahiro M, Sugihara M, et al. Clonality of primary pulmonary lymphoproliferative disorders; Using in situ hybridization and polymerase chain reaction for immunoglobulin. J Leuk Lymphoma. 1999;36(1–2):157–67.
57. Khoor A, Colby TV. Amyloidosis of the lung. Arch Pathol Lab Med. 2017;141(2):247–54.
58. Georgiades CS, Neyman EG, Barish MA, Fishman EK. Amyloidosis: Review and CT manifestations. Radiographics. 2004;24(2):405–16.
59. Lee SH, Ko YC, Jeong JP, Park CW, Seo SH, Kim JT, et al. Single nodular pulmonary amyloidosis: Case report. Tuberc Respir Dis. 2015;78(4):385–9.
60. Baqir M, Moua T, White D, Yi ES, Ryu JH. Pulmonary nodular and cystic light chain deposition disease: A retrospective review of 10 cases. Respir Med. 2020;164:105896.
61. Zamora AC, White DB, Sykes AM, Hoskote SS, Moua T, Yi ES, et al. Amyloid-associated cystic lung disease. Chest. 2016;149(5):1223–33.
62. Milani P, Basset M, Russo F, Foli A, Palladini G, Merlini G. The lung in amyloidosis. Eur Respir Rev. 2017;26(145).
63. Randall RE, Williamson WC, Jr., Mullinax F, Tung MY, Still WJ. Manifestations of systemic light chain deposition. Am J Med. 1976;60(2):293–9.
64. Buxbaum J, Gallo G. Nonamyloidotic monoclonal immunoglobulin deposition disease. Light-chain, heavy-chain, and light- and heavy-chain deposition diseases. Hematol/Oncol Clin North Am. 1999;13(6):1235–48.
65. Colombat M, Stern M, Groussard O, Droz D, Brauner M, Valeyre D, et al. Pulmonary cystic disorder related to light chain deposition disease. Am J Respir Crit Care Med. 2006;173(7):777–80.
66. Sheard S, Nicholson AG, Edmunds L, Wotherspoon AC, Hansell DM. Pulmonary light-chain deposition disease: CT and pathology findings in nine patients. Clin Radiol. 2015;70(5):515–22.

18

BIRT–HOGG–DUBÉ SYNDROME

Stephan A. Reyes and Rosa M. Estrada-Y-Martin

Contents

Introduction	132
Epidemiology and genetics	132
Pathology	133
Clinical presentation	133
Diagnostic evaluation	134
Monitoring and management	135
References	136

KEY POINTS

- Birt–Hogg–Dubé syndrome (BHD) is a rare cause of cystic lung disease with an incidence of two cases per million people and an estimated prevalence of at least 200 families affected worldwide.
- It is an autosomal dominant disorder affecting the folliculin gene located on chromosome 17p11.2 as the most common mutation.
- BHD is associated with manifestations in three organ systems: Cutaneous manifestations with fibrofolliculomas and trichodiscomas, pulmonary findings with multiple cysts, and risk of spontaneous pneumothorax and renal involvement with renal cell cancer (chromophobe and oncocytoma).
- Pulmonary cysts in BHD tend to be large (>2 cm), elliptical in shape, may have internal septation, and are predominantly located in the lower lobes in close proximity to the pleura and subpleural area as well as fissures.
- Early identification and diagnosis of BHD is essential due to risk of development of renal tumors and pneumothorax.
- There is no treatment available currently for BHD.

Introduction

Folliculin disease also known as Birt–Hogg–Dubé syndrome (BHD) or Hornstein–Knickenberg, is a rare genetic disease characterized by skin lesions (fibrofolliculomas and trichodiscomas), pulmonary cysts with recurrent spontaneous pneumothorax, and renal tumors. Cystic lung diseases are a rare spectrum of disorders characterized by the presence of greater than five parenchymal cysts on high-resolution computed tomography (HRCT) of the chest (1). The most common acute presentation is pneumothorax, manifested with acute chest pain, dyspnea, and occasionally, cough (2). Most patients are asymptomatic. Lung cysts are incidentally found when obtaining a CT of the chest or abdomen (visualizing lower lung cuts).

Interestingly, BHD was first described in 1975 by German physicians Hornstein and Knickenberg (3), and later by Canadian physicians Birt, Hogg, and Dubé in 1977 (4). Both groups noted families with small, pale, dome-shaped skin tumors that appeared on the face, neck, and upper torsos leading to the idea of a novel hereditary disease (5). The clinical features were expanded upon in 1999, including the pulmonary cysts and pneumothoraces (6). The mutation of the folliculin gene (FLCN) was recognized in 2002 (7).

Epidemiology and genetics

The prevalence of BHD is estimated at two cases per million (8). There are at least 200 families affected by this rare disorder. This disorder is inherited in an autosomal dominant pattern, and patients with a pathologic mutation express at least one feature of BHD 90–95% of the time, indicating a very high penetrance (9). The expression of the phenotype can vary even between family members (5) (Figure 18.1).

Genetically, the gene that is implicated in BHD is the FLCN gene on chromosome 17p11.2 (9). While the most common variation site appears to be in exon 11 with an insertion or deletion mutation (considered to be a "hot spot"), there have been more than 200 different reported pathological variations throughout all 14 exons of the gene (5). Mutations of multiple varieties have been noted, including frameshift, nonsense, splice-site variants, duplications, and deletions (5, 10). In some way, all the detected variations result in protein truncation and a loss of function of FLCN. As mentioned before, these variations are inherited in an autosomal dominant manner, but there are also *de novo* mutations in individuals without any known family history (11).

The FLCN gene is expressed in a variety of different tissues within the human body, including the skin, nephrons, stromal cells, pneumocytes of the lung, pancreas, parotid gland, breast, prostate, and cerebrum (7). The FLCN gene plays an important role as a tumor suppressor gene. FLCN interacts with two major proteins: Folliculin-interacting protein 1 (FNIP1) and folliculin-interacting protein 2 (FNIP2) (12, 13). FLCN plays a role in regulating the mammalian target of rapamycin (mTOR) pathway, however, it is unclear whether it is in an activating or regulatory role, or both (14). mTOR is an important protein kinase that plays a role in cell proliferation by regulating cell growth, metabolism, and survival (15). It is possible that mutations cause changes in binding patterns leading to variation in the

Birt–Hogg–Dubé Syndrome

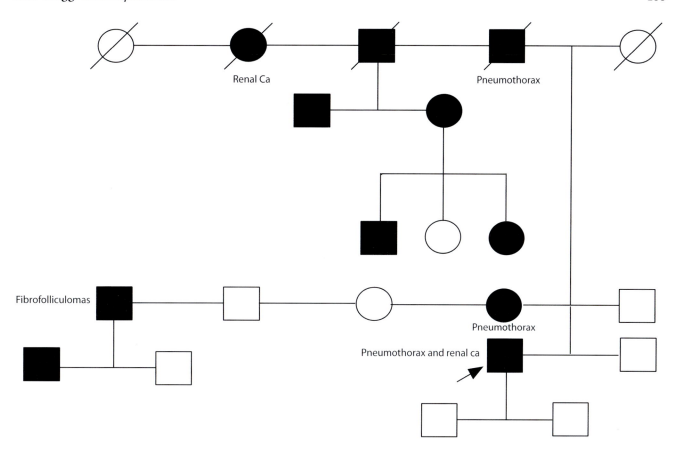

FIGURE 18.1 Pedigree of a 39-year-old man with multiple pneumothoraces and a 1 cm renal mass (arrow). FLCN exon 9 c102del (p/Arg341Glyfs*12). His children are asymptomatic (both younger than 10 years of age). Notice the high penetrance of BHD with multiple generations of family members affected. Square denotes male, circle denotes female. Darkened figure denotes affected individuals, crossed line indicates deceased.

regulatory function of FLCN. In addition to mTOR, other potential targets of FLCN include the autophagy pathway, adenosine monophosphate-activated protein kinase (AMPK) pathway, and cell motility via ciliogenesis (14). The exact mechanisms of action of FLCN and its relevant pathways when it comes to its phenotypic expression, however, remain unclear.

Pathology

Fibrofolliculomas and trichodiscomas are present in the majority of persons with BHD syndrome. Fibrofolliculomas are folliculosebaceous hamartomas that arise from mesodermal and ectodermal components. There are anastomosing strands of infundibular epithelial cells from a normal follicle in the dermis. The epithelial strands are encapsulated by a well-demarcated, loose mucin-rich or thick connective tissue stroma. Trichodiscomas are derived from the pilosebaceous mesenchyme instead of a larger epithelial prominence such as in fibrofolliculomas (16).

Wedge biopsy of unruptured pulmonary cysts demonstrate cystic alveoli and fusion of the epithelium of the cyst to the visceral pleura, partially incorporated into the parenchyma, interlobular septum, and/or bronchovascular bundle and are diagnostic of BHD. The lining cells are often flattened respiratory epithelium without fibrosis or inflammation. Biopsy of a ruptured cyst is not useful in diagnosing BHD and it may be difficult to distinguish from other etiologies due to inflammation, mechanical stress, and remodeling (17).

Clinical presentation

BHD syndrome has three major classical presentations: Cutaneous manifestations with fibrofolliculomas, trichodiscomas and/or acrochordons, pulmonary findings with cysts, and renal findings with renal cell carcinoma. Although the penetrance is high, there is quite a large variability in phenotypic expression as some patients may have just one feature, or multiple findings, or be asymptomatic (10).

The classical cutaneous triad described by Birt, Hogg, and Dubé is fibrofolliculomas, trichodiscomas, and acrochordons (commonly called skin tags) and are seen in up to 80% of BHD patients (4, 18). However, it must be noted that acrochordons are nonspecific to BHD and are seen commonly throughout the general population. The characteristic lesions are the fibrofolliculoma and trichodiscomas, a benign hair follicle tumor, which are small, pale, dome-shaped papules, typically present in the second or third decades of life (18, 19). These lesions appear more commonly on the face, the retro-auricular, the nuchal region, and the upper chest (4, 20, 21) (Figure 18.2).

Pulmonary involvement is also very common in BHD and is seen in greater than 80% of patients with the presence of multiple bilateral pulmonary cysts (19, 22). Interestingly, the pulmonary cysts present later than the cutaneous findings as they are commonly noted in the fourth to fifth decade of life. Radiographically using HRCT of the chest, the pulmonary cysts are variable in size and shape. The cysts are thin-walled, round, or elliptical in shape

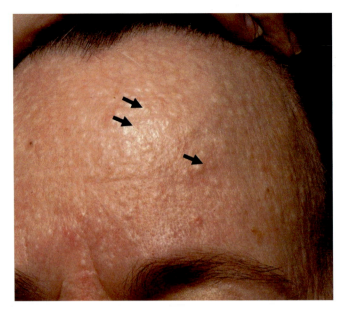

FIGURE 18.2 Frontal fibrofolliculomas. Pale, small, dome-shaped lesions. (Reprinted from Gene, volume 640, Schmidt L S and Linehan W M, FLCN: The Causative Gene for Birt–Hogg–Dubé Syndrome, p. 31, copyright [2018], with permission from Elsevier).

with a predominance for the lower lobes and fissures that usually account for <30% of the total lung field (23, 24). BHD cysts are more irregular with internal septation, tend to be attached to the pleura or subpleural areas, usually greater than 2 cm, have air-cuff sign (cysts encompassing the bronchovascular bundle), and may form concave indentation of mediastinal fat (25) (Figure 18.3). This is different from other cystic pulmonary diseases — the cysts in pulmonary Langerhans cell histiocytosis (PLCH) present with nodules, cavitated nodules and cysts, classically with sparing of the costophrenic areas, while in LAM the cysts are usually uniformly round and thin-walled that do not spare the juxtaphrenic recess (26) (see Table 16.1, Differential Diagnosis of Cystic Lung Diseases, in Chapter 16). Pneumothorax can be the only pulmonary manifestation in up 38% of the BHD patients (27, 28). While pneumothorax may be the only pulmonary presentation the risk of recurrence is up to 75% (27). Interestingly, pulmonary function appears to be stable over time despite these large cysts (29). This is unlike the other major cystic lung diseases, as they often have progressive decline in lung function (1).

Renal involvement is seen in approximately one-third of patients by the fifth decade of life, and it involves either cyst formation and importantly, renal tumors (6, 22). These tumors are often chromophobe renal cell carcinomas, in approximately 34% of patients, or a mass that has features of both chromophobe renal cell carcinoma and renal oncocytoma called a hybrid oncocytoma, seen in approximately 50% of patients (30). These tumors are often bilateral and multicentric with varying sizes (28). In a small number of patients, papillary renal cell carcinoma and clear cell carcinoma have been reported (31) (Figure 18.4). While the genetics of BHD syndrome still are not completely understood, the phenotypic manifestations cutaneous, pulmonary, and renal involvement are better defined (Table 18.1).

Diagnostic evaluation

Given the rarity of the disease, there has not been a validated and accepted set of diagnostic criteria for BHD syndrome. The disease is usually suspected after a recurrent episode of spontaneous pneumothorax. Recurrent pneumothorax has been described in up to 63–75% of cases (32, 33). BHD syndrome should be suspected in a young adult presenting with spontaneous pneumothorax and especially in persons with family history of pneumothorax, cutaneous findings, or renal tumors. Due to phenotypic expression seen in BHD syndrome, the absence of skin or renal findings does not exclude BHD syndrome as a potential diagnosis. In young patients with spontaneous pneumothorax,

(a)

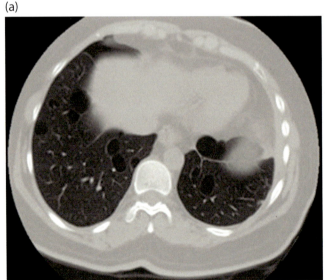

(b)

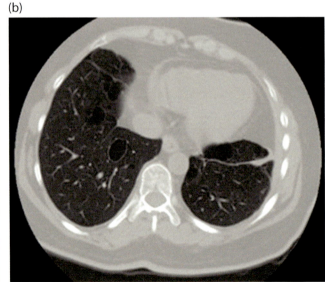

FIGURE 18.3 (a) and (b) CT scans from a 56-year-old woman with genetically proven BHD. She had first spontaneous pneumothorax at age 30. Multiple irregular pulmonary cysts, more evident in the lower lobes, some near fissure and subpleural areas (abutting the mediastinal pleura). Notice left pleural thickening due to previous pneumothorax with chest tube placement and pleurodesis. Two of her four children had spontaneous pneumothoraces before her final diagnosis.

Birt–Hogg–Dubé Syndrome

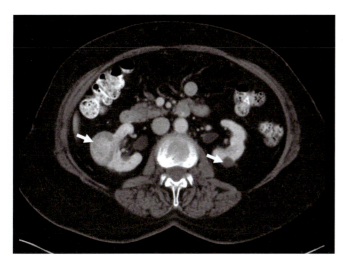

FIGURE 18.4 Abdomen CT scan showing multifocal renal tumors in a patient with BHD. (Reprinted from Gene, volume 640, Schmidt L S and Linehan W M, FLCN: The Causative Gene for Birt–Hogg–Dubé Syndrome, p. 31, copyright [2018], with permission from Elsevier.)

chest CT is a cost-effective screening tool to diagnose diffuse cystic lung diseases, including BHD syndrome (33). The overall characteristics of the cysts seen in BHD are rather unique and make it possible to distinguish them from other diffuse cystic diseases such as LAM and PLCH. Although, less common as a presentation, bilateral and/or multifocal chromphobe renal cell carcinoma or hybrid oncocytic carcinoma presenting before the age of 50 should prompt investigation for BHD syndrome, especially if there is a family history (14).

There have been proposed, but unvalidated, diagnostic criteria to help in the diagnosis of BHD in suspected patients (Table 18.2) (34). A recommended stepwise approach to confirm the diagnosis has also been suggested with the first step being biopsy of a skin lesion followed by genetic testing of the FLCN (35). The testing of the gene almost always confirms the diagnosis and allows for detection of at-risk family members so they may be referred to genetic counseling (28, 35). However, if the genetic test is negative, it does not rule-out BHD syndrome. The genetic mutation detection rate is approximately 85% (18, 19, 36).

TABLE 18.1: Summary of Clinical Findings in BHD Syndrome

Feature	% of Patients with Feature	Comment
Cutaneous	~80%	Characteristic lesions are fibrofolliculoma and trichodiscomas. Begin to appear by second and third decade of life.
Pulmonary cysts	>80%	Commonly noted by fourth and fifth decade of life. No significant loss of lung function.
Spontaneous pneumothorax	Up to 38%	Recurrence in up to 75%.
Renal cell tumors	Up to 50%	Mainly chromphobe and hybrid oncocytic type. Sometimes papillary and clear cell.

TABLE 18.2: BHD Diagnostic Criteria (Diagnosis Made with One Major Criterion or Two Minor Criteria)

Major Criteria	Minor Criteria
Five or more fibrofolliculomas and/or trichodiscomas One must be confirmed histologically	Multiple lung cysts that are bilaterally located with or without pneumothorax No other cause must be diagnosed or suspected
Genetic testing indicating heterozygous pathogenic variant in FLCN	Renal cancer before 50 years of age Multifocal or bilateral renal cancer Renal cancer of hybrid oncocytic histology First-degree relative with BHD syndrome

Monitoring and management

Early identification and diagnosis of the disease is important due to the risk of renal tumors and rate of pneumothorax. A basic evaluation after initial diagnosis is suggested in all patients (Table 18.3) (37). When it comes to pulmonary involvement, there is no specific treatment for the cystic disease and no trials have evaluated the role of mTOR inhibitors for pulmonary disease (10). Within this context, much of the focus falls on managing and preventing pneumothoraces (38). Initially, conservative management of the first episode of pneumothorax was suggested, however, due to the high risk of recurrence, chemical or mechanical pleurodesis is now recommended after the first episode (33, 38). The risk of recurrence of pneumothorax following conservative management of second pneumothorax is up to 93% (32). In patients with LAM, who have similar pneumothorax recurrence rates, the evidence suggests that pleurodesis is effective in decreasing the risk of recurrence with significant reduction in costs and morbidities of future hospitalizations (39). Routine pulmonary function testing and is not generally recommended since pulmonary function does not significant change over time. Patients with abnormal lung function tests at baseline may benefit from periodic measurements of lung function (38). Air travel is considered safe unless they have abnormal lung function with poor reserve or multiple pneumothoraces (38). These cases should be evaluated prior to travelling.

For renal involvement, after the initial screen for renal tumors, it has been recommended that they have screening MRIs every 3 to 4 years lifelong (40). Interestingly, due to the fact the tumors have low malignant potential, surgery can be postponed until reaching a size threshold (3 cm) to maximize nephron-sparing and kidney function (30, 40, 41).

Management of the cutaneous manifestations is cosmetic as the lesions have no malignant risk (10). Topical mTOR inhibitors have proven to be ineffective in treating fibrofolliculomas (42).

TABLE 18.3: Summarizing Initial Evaluations after Diagnosis of BHD Syndrome

System	Evaluation
Integumentary	Detailed dermatologic examinations
Pulmonary	HRCT of chest to screen for pulmonary cysts[a]
Renal	MRI of abdomen/pelvis to screen for renal tumors
Other	Referral to genetic counselor

[a] If a patient presents with pneumothorax before official diagnosis, then the patient should have HRCT of chest.

References

1. Ennis S, Silverstone EJ, Yates DH. Investigating cystic lung disease: A respiratory detective approach. Breathe (Sheff). 2020;16(2):200041.
2. Ferreira Francisco FA, Soares Souza A, Jr., Zanetti G, Marchiori E. Multiple cystic lung disease. Eur Respir Rev. 2015;24(138):552–64.
3. Happle R. Hornstein–Knickenberg syndrome vs. Birt–Hogg–Dubé syndrome: A critical review of an unjustified designation. J Eur Acad Dermatol Venereol. 2020;34(4):885–7.
4. Birt AR, Hogg GR, Dube WJ. Hereditary multiple fibrofolliculomas with trichodiscomas and acrochordons. Arch Dermatol. 1977;113(12):1674–7.
5. Schmidt LS, Linehan WM. Molecular genetics and clinical features of Birt–Hogg–Dube syndrome. Nat Rev Urol. 2015;12(10):558–569.
6. Toro JR, Glenn G, Duray P, et al. Birt–Hogg–Dubé syndrome: A novel marker of kidney neoplasia. Arch Dermatol. 1999;135(10):1195–202.
7. Nickerson ML, Warren MB, Toro JR, et al. Mutations in a novel gene lead to kidney tumors, lung wall defects, and benign tumors of the hair follicle in patients with the Birt–Hogg–Dube syndrome. Cancer Cell. 2002;2(2):157–64.
8. Muller ME, Daccord C, Taffe P, Lazor R. Prevalence of Birt–Hogg–Dube syndrome determined through epidemiological data on spontaneous pneumothorax and bayes theorem. Front Med (Lausanne). 2021;8:631168.
9. Steinlein OK, Ertl-Wagner B, Ruzicka T, Sattler EC. Birt–Hogg–Dubé syndrome: An underdiagnosed genetic tumor syndrome. J Dtsch Dermatol Ges. 2018;16(3):278–83.
10. Daccord C, Good JM, Morren MA, Bonny O, Hohl D, Lazor R. Birt-Hogg-Dubé syndrome. Eur Respir Rev. 2020;29(157).
11. Menko FH, Johannesma PC, van Moorselaar RJ, et al. A de novo FLCN mutation in A patient with spontaneous pneumothorax and renal cancer; A clinical and molecular evaluation. Fam Cancer. 2013;12(3):373–9.
12. Baba M, Hong SB, Sharma N, et al. Folliculin encoded by the BHD gene interacts with a binding protein, FNIP1, and AMPK, and is involved in AMPK and mTOR signaling. Proc Natl Acad Sci U S A. 2006;103(42):15552–7.
13. Hasumi H, Baba M, Hong SB, et al. Identification and characterization of a novel folliculin-interacting protein FNIP2. Gene. 2008;415(1-2):60–7.
14. Schmidt LS, Linehan WM. FLCN: The causative gene for Birt–Hogg–Dube syndrome. Gene. 2018;640:28–42.
15. Zarogoulidis P, Lampaki S, Turner JF, et al. mTOR pathway: A current, up-to-date mini-review (review). Oncol Lett. 2014;8(6):2367–70.
16. Collins GL, Somach S, Morgan MB. Histomorphologic and immunophenotypic analysis of fibrofolliculomas and trichodiscomas in Birt–Hogg–Dube syndrome and sporadic disease. J Cutan Pathol. 2002;29(9):529–33.
17. Furuya M, Nakatani Y. Birt–Hogg–Dube syndrome: Clinicopathological features of the lung. J Clin Pathol. 2013;66(3):178–86.
18. Schmidt LS, Nickerson ML, Warren MB, et al. Germline BHD-mutation spectrum and phenotype analysis of a large cohort of families with Birt–Hogg–Dube syndrome. Am J Hum Genet. 2005;76(6):1023–33.
19. Toro JR, Wei MH, Glenn GM, et al. BHD mutations, clinical and molecular genetic investigations of Birt–Hogg–Dube syndrome: A new series of 50 families and A review of published reports. J Med Genet. 2008;45(6):321–31.
20. Spring P, Fellmann F, Giraud S, Clayton H, Hohl D. Syndrome of Birt–Hogg–Dubé, A histopathological pitfall with similarities to tuberous sclerosis: A report of three cases. Am J Dermatopathol. 2013;35(2):241–5.
21. Tong Y, Schneider JA, Coda AB, Hata TR, Cohen PR. Birt–Hogg–Dubé syndrome: A review of dermatological manifestations and other symptoms. Am J Clin Dermatol. 2018;19(1):87–101.
22. Zbar B, Alvord WG, Glenn G, et al. Risk of renal and colonic neoplasms and spontaneous pneumothorax in the Birt–Hogg–Dube syndrome. Cancer Epidemiol Biomarkers Prev. 2002;11(4):393–400.
23. Lee JE, Cha YK, Kim JS, Choi JH. Birt–Hogg–Dubé syndrome: Characteristic CT findings differentiating it from other diffuse cystic lung diseases. Diagn Interv Radiol. 2017;23(5):354–9.
24. Agarwal PP, Gross BH, Holloway BJ, Seely J, Stark P, Kazerooni EA. Thoracic CT findings in Birt–Hogg–Dubé syndrome. Am J Roentgenol. 2011;196(2):349–52.
25. Park HJ, Chae EJ, Do KH, Lee SM, Song JW. Differentiation between lymphangioleiomyomatosis and Birt–Hogg–Dubé syndrome: Analysis of pulmonary cysts on CT images. Am J Roentgenol. 2019;212(4):766–72.
26. Beddy P, Babar J, Devaraj A. A practical approach to cystic lung disease on HRCT. Insights Imaging. 2011;2(1):1–7.
27. Toro JR, Pautler SE, Stewart L, et al. Lung cysts, spontaneous pneumothorax, and genetic associations in 89 families with Birt–Hogg–Dubé syndrome. Am J Respir Crit Care Med. 2007;175(10):1044–53.
28. Gupta N, Sunwoo BY, Kotloff RM. Birt–Hogg–Dubé syndrome. Clin Chest Med. 2016;37(3):475–86.
29. Daccord C, Cottin V, Prevot G, et al. Lung function in Birt–Hogg–Dubé syndrome: A retrospective analysis of 96 patients. Orphanet J Rare Dis. 2020;15(1):120.
30. Pavlovich CP, Walther MM, Eyler RA, et al. Renal tumors in the Birt–Hogg–Dubé syndrome. Am J Surg Pathol. 2002;26(12):1542–52.
31. Benusiglio PR, Giraud S, Deveaux S, et al. Renal cell tumour characteristics in patients with the Birt–Hogg–Dubé cancer susceptibility syndrome: A retrospective, multicentre study. Orphanet J Rare Dis. 2014;9:163.
32. Cooley J, Lee YCG, Gupta N. Spontaneous pneumothorax in diffuse cystic lung diseases. Curr Opin Pulm Med. 2017;23(4):323–33.
33. Gupta N, Kopras EJ, Henske EP, et al. Spontaneous pneumothoraces in patients with Birt–Hogg–Dubé syndrome. Ann Am Thorac Soc. 2017;14(5):706–13.
34. Menko FH, van Steensel MA, Giraud S, et al. Birt–Hogg–Dubé syndrome: Diagnosis and management. Lancet Oncol. 2009;10(12):1199–1206.
35. Gupta N, Vassallo R, Wikenheiser-Brokamp KA, McCormack FX. Diffuse cystic lung disease. Part II. Am J Respir Crit Care Med. 2015;192(1):17–29.
36. Sattler EC, Reithmair M, Steinlein OK. Kidney cancer characteristics and genotype-phenotype-correlations in Birt–Hogg–Dubé syndrome. PLoS One. 2018;13(12):e0209504.
37. Sattler EC, Steinlein OK. Birt–Hogg–Dubé Syndrome. In: Adam MP, Ardinger HH, Pagon RA, et al., eds. GeneReviews(®). Seattle (WA): University of Washington, Seattle.
38. Gupta N, Seyama K, McCormack FX. Pulmonary manifestations of Birt–Hogg–Dubé syndrome. Fam Cancer. 2013;12(3):387–96.
39. Almoosa KF, Ryu JH, Mendez J, et al. Management of pneumothorax in lymphangioleiomyomatosis: Effects on recurrence and lung transplantation complications. Chest. 2006;129(5):1274–81.
40. Stamatakis L, Metwalli AR, Middelton LA, Marston Linehan w. Diagnosis and management of BHD-associated kidney cancer. Fam Cancer. 2013;12(3):397–402.
41. Herring JC, Enquist EG, Chernoff A, Linehan WM, Choyke PL, Walther MM. Parenchymal sparing surgery in patients with hereditary renal cell carcinoma: 10-year experience. J Urol. 2001;165(3):777–81.
42. Gijezen LM, Vernooij M, Martens H, et al. Topical rapamycin as A treatment for fibrofolliculomas in Birt–Hogg–Dubé syndrome: A double-blind placebo-controlled randomized split-face trial. PLoS One. 2014;9(6):e99071.

19

PULMONARY LANGERHANS CELL HISTIOCYTOSIS AND OTHER HISTIOCYTIC LUNG DISEASES

Maryam Kaous, Bihong Zhao, and Isabel C. Mira-Avendano

Contents

Pulmonary langerhans cell histiocytosis (PLCH)	137
Pathogenesis	137
Pathology	138
Radiology	138
Pulmonary function testing	138
Management	138
Erdheim–Chester disease	138
Introduction	138
Rosai–Dorfman disease	141
Introduction	141
Conclusion	142
References	143

KEY POINTS

- Histiocytic neoplasms are rare neoplasms originating from cells of the myeloid lineage and primarily include Langerhans cell histiocytosis, Erdheim–Chester disease and Rosai–Dorfman disease.
- Pulmonary Langerhans cell histiocytosis is usually associated with cigarette smoking and is characterized by the presence of nodules and bizarre-shaped cysts typically within the upper lobes.
- Erdheim–Chester disease affects the lung in up to 50% of patients and is characterized by diffuse interstitial opacities, ground-glass opacities and pleural effusions.
- Rosai–Dorfman disease affects the lung in 10–20% of patients and is associated with interstitial and septal thickening in the lung bases along with pleural effusions.
- *BRAFV600E* mutations appear in a significant proportion of patients with Langerhans cell histiocytosis and Erdheim–Chester disease.
- Newer therapies targeting the different mutations are being developed with important clinical implications, highlighting the need to diagnose these entities earlier.

PULMONARY LANGERHANS CELL HISTIOCYTOSIS (PLCH)

Pulmonary Langerhans cell histiocytosis (PLCH) is an uncommon cause of diffuse lung disease and represents approximately 3% of all cases referred for evaluation of interstitial lung disease. The disease is seen principally in adults between the ages of 20 and 40 years (1, 2). Men and women are affected in equal proportion (2, 3). PLCH, particularly when isolated to the lung, is a smoking-related lung disease (2–4). At least 90% of adults with isolated PLCH are active or former smokers (2), and cigarette smoking has been reported to precipitate the onset of PLCH in adolescents previously in remission from disease earlier in childhood (5). The role of smoking is less clear when Langerhans cell histiocytosis (LCH) arises in the context of a multisystem disease.

Pathogenesis

PLCH is characterized by the accumulation of Langerhans cells in different organs, which can present with mild isolated compromise or more systemic/fatal disease. The latter is more frequent in children. In adults, the more common presentation is with isolated lung compromise, as PLCH.

Epidermal Langerhans cells are dendritic cells of myeloid origin that populate the skin before birth and are maintained locally under steady-state conditions; however, in reaction to injury or inflammation, these cells have the potential to migrate to the epidermis and differentiate into Langerhans-like cells (6). They then present the antigens and migrate to adjacent lymph nodes, triggering an inflammatory reaction. The *BRAFV600* mutation is found in 60% of the LCH cells. BRAF is a central kinase of the RAS-RAMEK signal transduction pathway that is involved in numerous cells functions.

The initial phenomenon in PLCH is the accumulation of CD1a-expressing myeloid cells in a subepithelial distribution over the peribronchiolar area. Cigarette smoke perhaps activates it through the cytokines such as tumor necrosis factor-α, granulocyte-macrophage colony-stimulating factor (GM-CSF) and transforming growth factor-β from airway epithelial cells (7, 8).

The persistence of activated Langerhans cells and other immune cells results in the formation of nodules and subsequent airway remodeling and cystic changes.

Accumulation of Langerhans cells and other immune cells around respiratory bronchioles is the initial histopathologic finding. Those bronchiolocentric lesions evolve from highly cellular micro- and macro-nodules to a paucicellular and then stellate-shaped fibrotic scars. While most patients who develop the disease are smokers, it is pertinent to note that it develops only in a small minority of smokers; hence a genetic predisposition or environmental trigger are plausible. It is possible that somatic mutations affecting the mitogen-activated protein kinase (MAPK) pathway may be the critical endogenous factor that predisposes smokers to PLCH development (9, 10). Both Braf proto-oncogene (BRAF) and neuroblastoma RAS viral oncogene (NRAS) mutations have been found in PLCH lesions and in circulating myeloid CD1a+ cells (11, 12).

Whether PLCH is a reactive or a clonal neoplastic process has been a subject of debate (13). The low frequency of mitotic figures or cytogenetic abnormalities, reports of spontaneous resolution and the inflammatory nature of the nodules favor the theory of a reactive immune granulomatous reaction. On the other hand, the occasionally aggressive natural course of PLCH in some patients with progressive disease and the efficacy of chemotherapy in certain severe forms of PLCH favor a neoplastic mechanism.

Pathology

In the early stages, PLCH corresponds to an inflammatory bronchiolitis, then nodules of varying sizes (0.5–1.5 cm) may be seen and, in advanced cases, the predominant finding is bullous and cystic destruction of the middle and upper lobes. Also, destruction of distal bronchioles with poorly formed granulomas comprised of Langerhans cells, which stain positive with S-100 and CD1a markers is characteristic (Figure 19.1a–c) (14). Electron microscopic evaluation shows cytoplasmic granules, referred to as "Birbeck granules," which are pathognomonic for Langerhans cells (15).

Radiology

In chest x-rays (CXR), nodular and reticulonodular opacities are seen in early course of the disease, while cystic changes and hyperinflation are seen in advanced cases. The findings in HRCT and CXR, will be different based on the stage of the disease. In cases of recent onset, nodules are common, vary in size from a few millimeters to 2 cm in size, and may show central cavitation (16). In more advanced disease, lung cysts tend to predominate (17). The combination of nodular and cystic changes may result in a highly characteristic radiographic appearance (Figure 19.1d and e). The lung cysts often vary in size, have thin walls and tend to be pleomorphic. Moreover, they tend to spare the lung bases. PLCH lesions are frequently fluorodeoxyglucose avid and positron emission tomography scanning may be helpful to determine the extent of thoracic disease activity, as well as to detect occult extrapulmonary disease, present in approximately 10–15% of patients (18).

Pulmonary function testing

PLCH can affect any area of the lung with consequent changes in lung function tests, which could demonstrate restriction, obstruction or mixed patterns. Up to 20% of patients can have normal pulmonary function tests (PFT) at the initial stage of the disease and one-third can develop obstructive pattern, while restrictive or mixed patterns have a higher prevalence (2, 3).

Diagnosis and clinical manifestations

PLCH should be considered in smokers or former smokers presenting with pulmonary nodules and/or cystic lesions, especially in the upper lobes, and in the setting of a prior history of spontaneous pneumothorax, which could be the presentation in up to 30% of patients (pneumothorax occurs over the course of the disease in 40% of patients). The diagnosis can be delayed for years in some patients with mild clinical and radiologic findings.

Twenty percent of patients do not report symptoms and the diagnosis is suspected because of incidental radiologic findings. More common clinical symptoms are cough and dyspnea. Physical examination is usually unrevealing with unremarkable lung auscultation or may show signs of airway obstruction and limitation with wheezing. Of note, pulmonary arterial hypertension seems to be relatively common in patients with advanced PLCH, with one study reporting echocardiography measurements of pulmonary artery systolic pressures >35 mmHg in 88% of patients (19).

HRCT must be considered in any patient with suspected diagnosis of PLCH, and a provisional diagnosis of PLCH is possible in most cases within the appropriate clinical context. On the other hand, lung biopsy should be considered if the radiologic findings are inconsistent and if treatment is contemplated. Transbronchial biopsy may have a diagnostic yield of up to 50%; however, surgical biopsy is definitive. The identification of >5% CD1a+ bronchoalveolar lavage (BAL) cells has high specificity but low sensitivity and is infrequently used as a sole diagnostic test (20, 21).

Management

Smoking cessation is the most important intervention. In most cases, the disease does not progress following smoking cessation. There is limited evidence supporting the use of systemic corticosteroids, coming only from retrospective data with confounding factors due to the smoking cessation associated with the use of corticosteroids in some of those trials, which makes it difficult to define which intervention explained the results (22–24).

Various chemotherapy agents have been reported to induce disease remission in patients with isolated progressive pulmonary disease or multisystem LCH with lung involvement (25–27). Cladribine, a purine nucleoside commonly used in the treatment of "hairy" cell leukemia, seems to have efficacy in both multisystem and isolated PLCH (26, 28–30). Another treatment option for patients with mutated *BRAFV600E* is the use of the targeted inhibitors of the BRAF/MAPK/MEK pathways, vemurafenib and trametinib (31). Use of these agents should be restricted to patients with confirmed mutation and in progressive disease following smoking cessation. One report suggested that in patients who have BRAF wild type and progressive disease, the use of inhibitors of the downstream MEK pathway such as cobimetinib may also be a potential alternative therapy (32).

ERDHEIM–CHESTER DISEASE

Introduction

In 1930, Jakob Erdheim and William Chester described a rare, non-inherited, non-Langerhans cell histiocytosis (now called Erdheim–Chester disease [ECD]) as "lipoid granulomatose" (33). ECD is a form of systemic histiocytosis characterized by foamy histiocytes or lipid laden macrophages surrounded by fibrosis, which leads to a xanthomatous infiltration of tissues. CD68+ CD1a–histiocytes on biopsy distinguish ECD from Langerhans cell histiocytosis (LCH) in which histiocytes are CD68+ CD1a+, positive for S-100 protein and contain Birbeck granules (34). Recent data also suggest that the *BRAFV600E* gene mutation is associated with development of the disease (35).

Incidence and risk factors

ECD is an exceedingly rare disorder and less than 600 cases have been identified worldwide. Presentation may occur in the fifth decade of life with a slight male predominance (36).

Pulmonary Langerhans Cell Histiocytosis and Other Histiocytic Lung Diseases

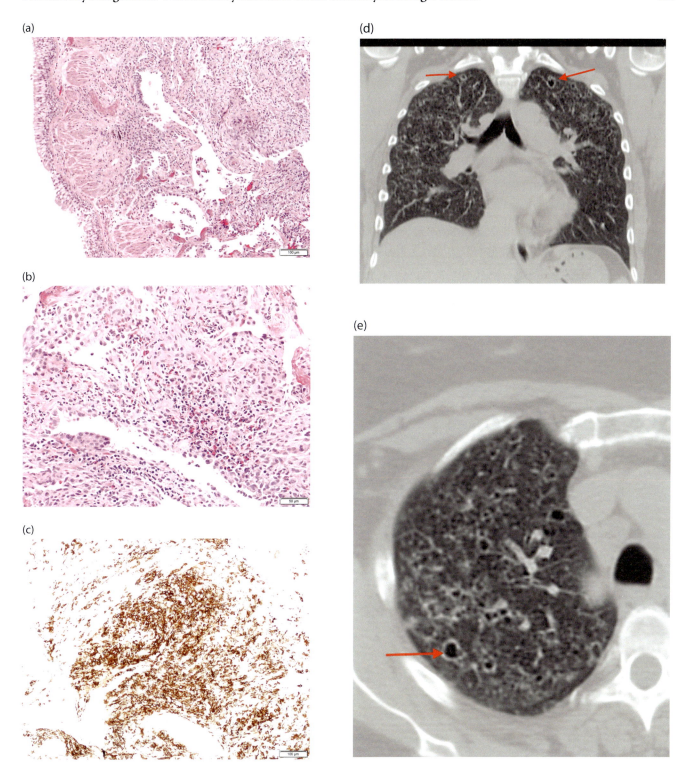

FIGURE 19.1 47-year-old woman with 30 pack-year smoking history who presented with shortness of breath. (a): Transbronchial biopsies were performed given CT findings. Langerhans cell infiltrate shows peribronchial/peribronchiolar pattern, extending to alveolar septum, forming a peribronchial nodule under lower power view. Lightly pigmented macrophages (Smoker's macrophages) are present in and around the infiltrating cells. Cysts are formed by contraction on surrounding alveolar walls. (b): The Langerhans cells have a pale basophilic nucleus with characteristic sharp nuclear infoldings, imparting a "crumpled tissue paper" nuclear contour. Eosinophils in variable numbers occupy the innermost of the infiltration. (c): Immunohistochemical (IHC) stain for CD1a is usually positive in PLCH. In most cases, however, the morphology of the lesions is sufficiently compelling that a definitive diagnosis can be established without the aid of IHC. (d): CT in coronal reconstruction showing bizarre-shaped cysts and nodules (red arrows) that are predominantly located in the upper lobes. (e): Axial section of CT images showing the bizarre-shaped cysts and nodules (red arrow) in the same patient.

Unlike PLCH, smoking association has not been identified in ECD, and no specific risk factors have been identified.

Pathogenesis

ECD pathogenesis is still under investigation. Proposed mechanisms include systemic pro-inflammatory cytokine-chemokine networks, which then recruit and activate histiocytes to form changes in tissues typical of ECD (35). This hypothesis forms the basis for research into therapy targets. Interleukin-6 (IL-6) has been found to be strongly positive on autopsy studies of patients with ECD and found on multiple cell types including macrophages, pneumocytes, endothelial cells and histiocytes. IL-6 plays a major role in osteoclast differentiation, and this could explain the osteosclerosis so commonly seen in ECD (37).

BRAFV600E mutations have also been noted in biopsies as well as in circulating monocytes (38). Histiocytes carrying BRAF mutations have been linked to oncogene mutation and inflammatory cytokine/chemokine activation (35). Molecular analysis in patients with ECD has also shown other coexisting driver mutations, like MAP kinase (MAPK) of myeloid neoplasms. Up to 10% of ECD patients may have a concomitant myeloid malignancy (39).

Diagnosis and clinical manifestations

Clinical presentation of patients can be variable, which also contributes to the longer latency period to diagnosis (on average, about a year). Manifestations can range from limited disease to systemic fatal disease. Fever, weight loss, fatigue, and weakness are common manifestations (39). Patients with ECD will typically manifest with skeletal symptoms, diabetes insipidus (DI), neurological and constitutional symptoms (40). CD68+ and CD1a- histiocytic infiltration on histologic specimens coupled with characteristic skeletal abnormalities are important for diagnosis of ECD.

Laboratory tests should include complete blood count, complete metabolic panel and inflammatory markers, including C-reactive protein (CRP). CRP levels are elevated in >80% of cases (41). Patients may also present with anemia and leukocytosis. Biopsy specimens of involved organs will show foamy histiocytic infiltration of tissues with a xanthogranulomatous pattern that is CD68+ and CD1a- (41).

Skeletal manifestations are the most common symptom in 90% of patients involved, whether silent or symptomatic (36). In up to 50% of patients, this may be the presenting symptom. Assessment of long bones should occur with both radiographs and bone scintigraphy (Figure 19.2a). Uptake of bilateral long bones at bone

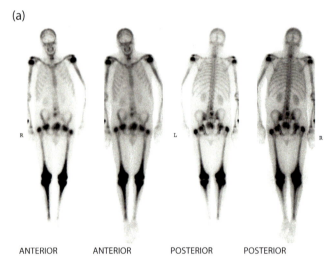

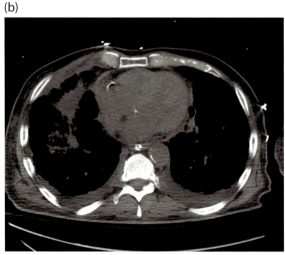

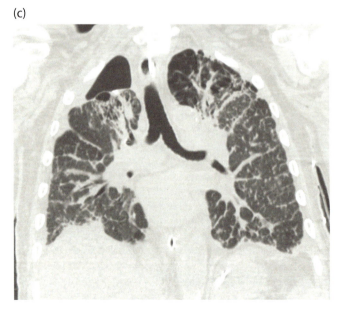

FIGURE 19.2 (a): Technetium-99m bone scintigraphy showing increased uptake and osteosclerosis at the meta-diaphyseal bones predominantly at the knees in a 75-year-old patient with Erdheim–Chester disease. (b): CT scan of the chest in an axial reconstruction in mediastinal windows showing bilateral pleural and pericardial thickening and effusions in the same patient. (c): CT scan of the same patient in lung window showing diffuse interstitial thickening along with pleural thickening. (Images courtesy of Daniel Ocazionez-Trujillo MD, UT Health, Houston.)

scintigraphy is pathognomonic for the disease (36), most prominent in the lower extremities.

Neurologic involvement portends a poor prognosis. About half of the patients have central nervous system (CNS) involvement (35). Magnetic resonance imaging (MRI) and computed tomography (CT) scans are the modality of choice for investigation of CNS disease. Patients may present with headaches, papilledema, exophthalmos, panhypopituitarism and DI. DI is a common presentation in ECD (39). Visual disturbances and blurred vision are seen with exophthalmos from retro-orbital space infiltration (42, 43).

Other manifestations include pulmonary, cutaneous or cardiovascular involvement. Renal involvement in the form of retroperitoneal fibrosis and an appearance of a "hairy" kidney on imaging may be detected in up to 30% of patients. Patients may complain of dysuria, abdominal pain and kidney failure if hydronephrosis is also present (35).

Cardiovascular involvement, in up to 36–62% of patients, includes circumferential periaortic encasement, pericardial effusion, valvular disease, pseudotumoral infiltration on the right side of the heart and consequently heart failure (39).

Skin manifestations have been reported in up to 27% of patients with xanthelasmas being the most common manifestation (44).

Pulmonary disease

Though pulmonary involvement is present in only about 20–30% of patients (45), it portends a poor prognosis. Time to diagnosis of pulmonary disease in ECD can often be long, with an average time span in studies showing around 29 months (45). Patients present with shortness of breath or cough. Depending on level of involvement, spirometry may be normal or show restriction on spirometry with decreased or normal carbon monoxide diffusing lung capacity (DLCO). Patients with ECD may develop interstitial lung disease (46). Lung biopsy samples from patients show histiocytes with foamy cytoplasm, lymphocytes and plasma cells. Histiocytes stain positive for CD68 but negative for CD1a. BAL fluid can be sent for testing of CD68+ and CD1a– histiocytes. Pleural effusions may occur in those with cardiac involvement as well (45, 46).

Chest CT will show diffuse interstitial infiltrates (Figure 19.2b, c), ground-glass opacities or centrilobular opacities (46). Consolidation is rarely seen. Up to half the patients tend to have lung parenchymal involvement and 40% of the patients may have pleural involvement as well (45). Interlobular septal thickening, centrilobular nodules and ground-glass nodules may be the more common manifestations seen on CT. The histiocytic infiltrates seen in ECD tend to follow a lymphangitic distribution, which explains why lesions are seen along septa and the bronchovascular bundles (45–47).

Management

Prognosis of ECD is poor without treatment. Limited data exists for treatment in ECD, and treatment options are largely limited to symptom control. Treatment targeting inhibition of inflammation is the mainstay of therapy and leads to symptom resolution in about 68% of patients (35). Corticosteroids, immunotherapy and chemotherapy have been utilized in treatment plans of ECD patients. Interferon-alpha (IFN) has been studied for therapy in recent years and is currently first-line therapy as it is beneficial in patients with CNS and cardiovascular involvement (35, 48). There are also reports on treatment with interleukin-1 receptor antagonist anakinra, thought to be helpful in targeting the cytokine response in ECD (49).

If first-line treatments with IFN-alpha or anakinra are unsuccessful, BRAF inhibitor vemurafenib has also been utilized as *BRAFV600E* mutation in histiocytes have been seen in 57% of ECD patients (48).

ROSAI–DORFMAN DISEASE

Introduction

Destombes-Rosai–Dorfman disease (RDD) is part of a group of histiocytoses including ECD and LCH, of which LCH is the most common (50). The disease was first described as a "sinus histiocytosis with massive lymphadenopathy" by Dr. Paul Destombes in 1965 and was then recognized as a clinicopathological syndrome by Dr. Rosai and Dr. Dorfman in 1969. RDD is a rare non-Langerhans cell histiocytosis characterized by massive cervical lymphadenopathy and more common in children than adults. Extranodal lymphadenopathy can also be seen (51). Pathology specimens with CD68+, PS100– and CD1a– histiocytes are seen (51). Though no clear cause has been identified for *RDD*, *KRAS* and *MAP2K1* mutations may be implicated, as in other histiocytic disorders (52). These mutations form the basis for therapy targets if needed as most cases are self-limited (53).

Epidemiology

RDD is an extremely rare disease with an estimated prevalence of 1:200,000 (54). The mean age at onset of disease is 20.6 years and is more commonly reported in children and young adults (52). The disease may have a slight male predominance.

Pathogenesis

The exact pathology and etiology of RDD is poorly understood. No clear causative agent for development of RDD has been described. Generally, RDD has been recognized as a non-neoplastic histiocytic disorder characterized by cells that are polyclonal and reactive (54–56). Whole genome sequencing of RDD cases has demonstrated kinase mutations, including *KRAS*, *MAP2K1*, *NRAS*, and *ARAF*. Though *BRAFV600E* mutations may be seen in LCH and ECD, these mutations are generally absent in RDD (54).

Diagnosis and clinical presentation

Patients with RDD typically present with massive painless cervical lymphadenopathy associated with constitutional symptoms such as fever, night sweats and weight loss. Evaluation should include a thorough physical exam and history, as identification of associated disorders with RDD is important. Diagnosis requires histopathological evaluation, characterized by sinus histiocytic proliferation and histiocytic engulfment of intact lymphocytes or plasma cells, a phenomenon known as emperipolesis, and positive staining of S100 protein, CD68+ and CD1a– (52, 56). Immunohistochemical evaluation is necessary to exclude LCH. Up to 40% of cases may be seen with extranodal involvement (52). The disease may be classified based on presentation into sporadic, familial or cutaneous forms. The most common presentation of RDD is the sporadic form, which includes the classic nodal and extranodal forms, as well as neoplasia-associated RDD and immune disease-associated RDD (55).

Laboratory findings may be nonspecific, including anemia, leukocytosis and elevation of inflammatory markers like erythrocyte sedimentation rate (57). Imaging can be targeted for organ systems involved vs. full body PET/CT imaging in specific patients (54). However, expert consensus regarding extent of imaging is lacking.

CNS involvement is very rarely reported with <5% of cases affected, in which intracranial lesions may be seen (52). Otherwise, ophthalmic involvement in the form of a mass in the orbital tissue, conjunctiva or uveitis, or nasal cavity involvement may be seen up to 11% of RDD cases (54). Less common manifestations include intrathoracic and GI manifestations. The clinical course can range from lymphadenopathy alone to exacerbations to remissions lasting several years (52).

Pulmonary

Lung involvement in RDD is relatively rare. Symptoms are often nonspecific. Moyon et al. described their RDD patient cohort with lung involvement as most commonly presenting with chronic dyspnea and dry cough in up to 47% of patients. Fulminant pulmonary failure as a presenting symptom is atypical (51). BAL is nonspecific. Patients may have a lymphocytic predominance in the BAL fluid, however, this is not commonly observed. PFTs most commonly are normal; however, a small percent of patients may have DLCO. Restrictive pattern on PFTs may occasionally be seen (51).

Imaging

In patients with pulmonary clinical signs of involvement, nearly all patients may have abnormalities noted on chest CT (51). However, changes observed on CT are nonspecific. Interlobular septal thickening, nodules, ground-glass opacities, peribronchovascular and perilobular consolidation can be observed in patients with RDD on CT.

Management

As presentation can be variable, therapy depends on the extent of disease. Therapy options for patients should be individualized and determined at a specialty center. Patients presenting with suddenly enlarged nodes that spontaneously regress can be managed with expectant management. Surgery can also be considered, especially in cases where extensive nodal disease may lead to end-organ compromise. However, patients with widespread multimodal disease and systemic symptoms with multiple exacerbations will require systemic treatment (51, 56).

Corticosteroids are helpful in alleviating symptoms and nodal size; however, recurrence can still occur. Other options in widespread disease include radiotherapy, chemotherapy and immunomodulatory therapy (55). Chemotherapeutic agents such as methotrexate, 6-mercaptopurine, alkaloids, and azathioprine have been used with mixed results (54). Cobimetinib (a MEK 1/2 inhibitor) has been utilized in RDD patients for therapy.

Conclusion

Histiocytic neoplasms are rare neoplasms with an annual incidence of <5 cases/million, of which there are several types, but that primarily include LCH, EDD and RDD (Table 19.1). Owing to their rarity and diverse clinical manifestations, they pose a major diagnostic challenge for many clinicians. Misdiagnosis and delayed diagnosis are common, leading to frustration for patients and physicians alike. Maintaining a high index of suspicion is key

TABLE 19.1: Features of LCH, ECD, and RDD Based on Clinical Characteristics and Histopathological Characteristics

Organ Involvement	LCH	EDD	RDD
Respiratory	Pulmonary nodules initially followed by cysts in later stages. Seen in 60% of cases.	Mediastinal infiltration along with pleural and interlobular septal thickening. Affects 50% of patients.	Mainly involves large airways and sinuses. Rarely causes pleural effusion with interstitial and septal thickening in bases. Involvement seen in 10–20% of patients.
Cardiac	Pulmonary arterial hypertension in up to 88% of patients.	Right atrial and atrio-ventricular groove infiltration. Pericardial and myocardial infiltration seen on cardiac MRI. These findings may be seen in 40–70% of patients.	Seen very rarely in <5% of patients. Infiltration of right atrium, right ventricle are rare cardiac manifestations.
Vascular	Very rarely affected.	Peri-aortic infiltration or "coated" aorta seen in 50–80% of patients.	Peri-aortic and carotid sheath infiltration in <5% of cases.
Retroperitoneum	Rarely reported.	Perinephric infiltration ("hairy kidneys") seen in 40–50% of patients.	Affects 5–10% of patients with hilar masses, subcapsular infiltration.
Lymph nodes	Lymphadenopathy reported in 5–10% of patients.	Never reported.	Most common manifestation is isolated or generalized lymphadenopathy in up to 50% of patients.
Bones	Osteolytic lesions seen in 60% of patients.	Long-bone osteosclerosis at metadiaphysis is pathognomonic and seen in 95% of patients.	Osteolytic lesions may be seen in up to 15% of patients.
Endocrine	Diabetes insipidus may be seen in 40–70% of patients. May be the initial presenting feature.	Diabetes insipidus may be seen in 40–70% of patients. May be the initial presenting feature.	Never reported.
Histopath Characteristics			
BRAFV600E	+/−	+/−	−
CD68	+	+	+/−
CD1a	+	−	−
Langerin	+	−	−

Source: Used with permission from Reference (58).

to diagnosis of these neoplasms — for which a good understanding and knowledge of these rare entities is necessary to help in early and correct diagnosis. Moreover, introduction of targeted therapies results in better outcomes once they are diagnosed in a timely manner (58).

References

1. Arico M, Girschikofsky M, Genereau T, Klersy C, McClain K, Grois N, et al. Langerhans cell histiocytosis in adults. Report from the International Registry of the Histiocyte Society. Eur J Cancer. 2003;39(16):2341–8.
2. Vassallo R, Ryu JH, Schroeder DR, Decker PA, Limper AH. Clinical outcomes of pulmonary Langerhans'-cell histiocytosis in adults. N Engl J Med. 2002;346(7):484–90.
3. Travis WD, Borok Z, Roum JH, Zhang J, Feuerstein I, Ferrans VJ, et al. Pulmonary Langerhans cell granulomatosis (histiocytosis X). A clinicopathologic study of 48 cases. Am J Surg Pathol. 1993;17(10):971–86.
4. Mogulkoc N, Veral A, Bishop PW, Bayindir U, Pickering CA, Egan JJ. Pulmonary Langerhans' cell histiocytosis: Radiologic resolution following smoking cessation. Chest. 1999;115(5):1452–5.
5. Bernstrand C, Cederlund K, Ashtrom L, Henter JI. Smoking preceded pulmonary involvement in adults with Langerhans cell histiocytosis diagnosed in childhood. Acta Paediatr. 2000;89(11):1389–92.
6. Allen CE, Merad M, McClain KL. Langerhans-cell histiocytosis. N Engl J Med. 2018;379(9):856–68.
7. Churg A, Tai H, Coulthard T, Wang R, Wright JL. Cigarette smoke drives small airway remodeling by induction of growth factors in the airway wall. Am J Respir Crit Care Med. 2006;174(12):1327–34.
8. Hellermann GR, Nagy SB, Kong X, Lockey RF, Mohapatra SS. Mechanism of cigarette smoke condensate-induced acute inflammatory response in human bronchial epithelial cells. Respir Res. 2002;3:22.
9. Brown NA, Elenitoba-Johnson KSJ. Clinical implications of oncogenic mutations in pulmonary Langerhans cell histiocytosis. Curr Opin Pulm Med. 2018;24(3):281–6.
10. Howarth DM, Gilchrist GS, Mullan BP, Wiseman GA, Edmonson JH, Schomberg PJ. Langerhans cell histiocytosis: Diagnosis, natural history, management, and outcome. Cancer. 1999;85(10):2278–90.
11. Mourah S, How-Kit A, Meignin V, Gossot D, Lorillon G, Bugnet E, et al. Recurrent NRAS mutations in pulmonary Langerhans cell histiocytosis. Eur Respir J. 2016;47(6):1785–96.
12. Roden AC, Hu X, Kip S, Parrilla Castellar ER, Rumilla KM, Vrana JA, et al. BRAF V600E expression in Langerhans cell histiocytosis: Clinical and immunohistochemical study on 25 pulmonary and 54 extrapulmonary cases. Am J Surg Pathol. 2014;38(4):548–51.
13. Yousem SA, Colby TV, Chen YY, Chen WG, Weiss LM. Pulmonary Langerhans' cell histiocytosis: Molecular analysis of clonality. Am J Surg Pathol. 2001;25(5):630–6.
14. Colby TV, Lombard C. Histiocytosis X in the lung. Hum Pathol. 1983;14(10):847–56.
15. Radzikowska E. Pulmonary Langerhans' cell histiocytosis in adults. Adv Respir Med. 2017;85(5):277–89.
16. Hartman TE, Tazelaar HD, Swensen SJ, Muller NL. Cigarette smoking: CT and pathologic findings of associated pulmonary diseases. Radiographics. 1997;17(2):377–90.
17. Brauner MW, Grenier P, Tijani K, Battesti JP, Valeyre D. Pulmonary Langerhans cell histiocytosis: Evolution of lesions on CT scans. Radiology. 1997;204(2):497–502.
18. Krajicek BJ, Ryu JH, Hartman TE, Lowe VJ, Vassallo R. Abnormal fluorodeoxyglucose PET in pulmonary Langerhans cell histiocytosis. Chest. 2009;135(6):1542–9.
19. Chaowalit N, Pellikka PA, Decker PA, Aubry MC, Krowka MJ, Ryu JH, et al. Echocardiographic and clinical characteristics of pulmonary hypertension complicating pulmonary Langerhans cell histiocytosis. Mayo Clin Proc. 2004;79(10):1269–75.
20. Chollet S, Soler P, Dournovo P, Richard MS, Ferrans VJ, Basset F. Diagnosis of pulmonary histiocytosis X by immunodetection of Langerhans cells in bronchoalveolar lavage fluid. Am J Pathol. 1984;115(2):225–32.
21. Xaubet A, Agusti C, Picado C, Guerequiz S, Martos JA, Carrion M, et al. Bronchoalveolar lavage analysis with anti-T6 monoclonal antibody in the evaluation of diffuse lung diseases. Respiration. 1989;56(3–4):161–6.
22. Friedman PJ, Liebow AA, Sokoloff J. Eosinophilic granuloma of lung. Clinical aspects of primary histiocytosis in the adult. Medicine (Baltimore). 1981;60(6):385–96.
23. Callebaut W, Demedts M, Verleden G. Pulmonary Langerhans' cell granulomatosis (histiocytosis X): Clinical analysis of 8 cases. Acta Clin Belg. 1998;53(5):337–43.
24. Benyounes B, Crestani B, Couvelard A, Vissuzaine C, Aubier M. Steroid-responsive pulmonary hypertension in a patient with Langerhans' cell granulomatosis (histiocytosis X). Chest. 1996;110(1):284–6.
25. Saven A, Burian C. Cladribine activity in adult langerhans-cell histiocytosis. Blood. 1999;93(12):4125–30.
26. Dimopoulos MA, Theodorakis M, Kostis E, Papadimitris C, Moulopoulos LA, Anastasiou-Nana M. Treatment of Langerhans cell histiocytosis with 2 chlorodeoxyadenosine. Leuk Lymphoma. 1997;25(1–2):187–9.
27. Tazi A, Lorillon G, Haroche J, Neel A, Dominique S, Aouba A, et al. Vinblastine chemotherapy in adult patients with langerhans cell histiocytosis: A multicenter retrospective study. Orphanet J Rare Dis. 2017;12(1):95.
28. Giona F, Caruso R, Testi AM, Moleti ML, Malagnino F, Martelli M, et al. Langerhans' cell histiocytosis in adults: A clinical and therapeutic analysis of 11 patients from A single institution. Cancer. 1997;80(9):1786–91.
29. Aerni MR, Aubry MC, Myers JL, Vassallo R. Complete remission of nodular pulmonary Langerhans cell histiocytosis lesions induced by 2-chlorodeoxyadenosine in a non-smoker. Respir Med. 2008;102(2):316–9.
30. Pardanani A, Phyliky RL, Li CY, Tefferi A. 2-Chlorodeoxyadenosine therapy for disseminated Langerhans cell histiocytosis. Mayo Clin Proc. 2003;78(3):301–6.
31. Lorillon G, Jouenne F, Baroudjian B, de Margerie-Mellon C, Vercellino L, Meignin V, et al. Response to trametinib of a pulmonary Langerhans cell histiocytosis harboring a MAP2K1 deletion. Am J Respir Crit Care Med. 2018;198(5):675–8.
32. Diamond EL, Durham BH, Ulaner GA, Drill E, Buthorn J, Ki M, et al. Efficacy of MEK inhibition in patients with histiocytic neoplasms. Nature. 2019;567(7749):521–4.
33. Chester W. Über lipoidgranulomatose. Virchows Archiv für pathologische Anatomie und Physiologie und für klinische Medizin. 1930;279(2):561–602.
34. Veyssier-Belot C, Cacoub P, Caparros-Lefebvre D, Wechsler J, Brun B, Remy M, et al. Erdheim–Chester disease. Clinical and radiologic characteristics of 59 cases. Medicine (Baltimore). 1996;75(3):157–69.
35. Campochiaro C, Tomelleri A, Cavalli G, Berti A, Dagna L. Erdheim–Chester disease. Eur J Intern Med. 2015;26(4):223–9.
36. Cavalli G, Guglielmi B, Berti A, Campochiaro C, Sabbadini MG, Dagna L. The multifaceted clinical presentations and manifestations of Erdheim–Chester disease: Comprehensive review of the literature and of 10 new cases. Ann Rheum Dis. 2013;72(10):1691–5.
37. Stoppacciaro A, Ferrarini M, Salmaggi C, Colarossi C, Praderio L, Tresoldi M, et al. Immunohistochemical evidence of a cytokine and chemokine network in three patients with Erdheim–Chester disease: Implications for pathogenesis. Arthritis Rheum. 2006;54(12):4018–22.
38. Cangi MG, Biavasco R, Cavalli G, Grassini G, Dal-Cin E, Campochiaro C, et al. BRAFV600E-mutation is invariably present and associated to oncogene-induced senescence in Erdheim–Chester disease. Ann Rheum Dis. 2015;74(8):1596–602.
39. Starkebaum G, Hendrie P. Erdheim–Chester disease. Best Pract Res Clin Rheumatol. 2020;34(4):101510.
40. Kenn W, Stäbler A, Zachoval R, Zietz C, Raum W, Wittenberg G. Erdheim–Chester disease: A case report and literature overview. Eur Radiol. 1999;9(1):153–8.

41. Haroche J, Arnaud L, Cohen-Aubart F, Hervier B, Charlotte F, Emile JF, et al. Erdheim–Chester disease. Curr Rheumatol Rep. 2014;16(4):412.
42. Dion E, Graef C, Miquel A, Haroche J, Wechsler B, Amoura Z, et al. Bone involvement in Erdheim–Chester disease: Imaging findings including periostitis and partial epiphyseal involvement. Radiology. 2006;238(2):632–9.
43. Della Torre E, Dagna L, Mapelli P, Mellone R, Grazia Sabbadini M. Erdheim–Chester disease: Imaging-guided therapeutic approach. Clin Nucl Med. 2011;36(8):704–6.
44. Cives M, Simone V, Rizzo FM, Dicuonzo F, Cristallo Lacalamita M, Ingravallo G, et al. Erdheim–Chester disease: A systematic review. Crit Rev Oncol Hematol. 2015;95(1):1–11.
45. Arnaud L, Pierre I, Beigelman-Aubry C, Capron F, Brun AL, Rigolet A, et al. Pulmonary involvement in Erdheim–Chester disease: A single-center study of thirty-four patients and A review of the literature. Arthritis Rheum. 2010;62(11):3504–12.
46. Egan AJ, Boardman LA, Tazelaar HD, Swensen SJ, Jett JR, Yousem SA, et al. Erdheim–Chester disease: Clinical, radiologic, and histopathologic findings in five patients with interstitial lung disease. Am J Surg Pathol. 1999;23(1):17–26.
47. Rush WL, Andriko JA, Galateau-Salle F, Brambilla E, Brambilla C, Ziany-bey I, et al. Pulmonary pathology of Erdheim–Chester disease. Mod Pathol. 2000;13(7):747–54.
48. Haroche J, Cohen-Aubart F, Emile JF, Arnaud L, Maksud P, Charlotte F, et al. Dramatic efficacy of vemurafenib in both multisystemic and refractory Erdheim–Chester disease and Langerhans cell histiocytosis harboring the BRAF V600E mutation. Blood. 2013;121(9):1495–500.
49. Dagna L, Corti A, Langheim S, Guglielmi B, De Cobelli F, Doglioni C, et al. Tumor necrosis factor α as a master regulator of inflammation in Erdheim–Chester disease: Rationale for the treatment of patients with infliximab. J Clin Oncol. 2012;30(28):e286–90.
50. Papo M, Cohen-Aubart F, Trefond L, Bauvois A, Amoura Z, Emile JF, et al. Systemic histiocytosis (Langerhans cell histiocytosis, Erdheim–Chester disease, Destombes-Rosai–Dorfman disease): From oncogenic mutations to inflammatory disorders. Curr Oncol Rep. 2019;21(7):62.
51. Moyon Q, Boussouar S, Maksud P, Emile JF, Charlotte F, Aladjidi N, et al. Lung involvement in Destombes-Rosai–Dorfman disease: Clinical and radiological features and response to the MEK inhibitor cobimetinib. Chest. 2020;157(2):323–33.
52. Jacobsen E, Shanmugam V, Jagannathan J. Rosai–Dorfman Disease with activating KRAS mutation - response to Cobimetinib. N Engl J Med. 2017;377(24):2398–9.
53. Garces S, Medeiros LJ, Patel KP, Li S, Pina-Oviedo S, Li J, et al. Mutually exclusive recurrent KRAS and MAP2K1 mutations in Rosai–Dorfman disease. Mod Pathol. 2017;30(10):1367–77.
54. Abla O, Jacobsen E, Picarsic J, Krenova Z, Jaffe R, Emile JF, et al. Consensus recommendations for the diagnosis and clinical management of Rosai–Dorfman-Destombes disease. Blood. 2018;131(26):2877–90.
55. Bruce-Brand C, Schneider JW, Schubert P. Rosai–Dorfman disease: An overview. J Clin Pathol. 2020;73(11):697–705.
56. Haroche J, Abla O. Uncommon histiocytic disorders: Rosai–Dorfman, juvenile xanthogranuloma, and Erdheim–Chester disease. Hematology Am Soc Hematol Educ Program. 2015;2015:571–8.
57. Cai Y, Shi Z, Bai Y. Review of Rosai–Dorfman disease: New insights into the pathogenesis of this rare disorder. Acta Haematol. 2017;138(1):14–23.
58. Goyal G, Young JR, Koster MJ, Tobin WO, Vassallo R, Ryu JH, et al. The Mayo clinic Histiocytosis Working Group consensus statement for the diagnosis and evaluation of adult patients with histiocytic neoplasms: Erdheim–Chester disease, Langerhans cell histiocytosis, and Rosai–Dorfman disease. Mayo Clin Proc. 2019;94(10):2054–71.

PART F
Rare Pulmonary Neoplasms

20

PRIMARY PULMONARY LYMPHOPROLIFERATIVE NEOPLASMS

Bibi Aneesah Jaumally, Khalid Mohamed Ahmed, and Saadia A. Faiz

Contents

Introduction 145
Primary pulmonary lymphoproliferative neoplasms 145
Lymphoproliferative disorders in the immunocompromised patient 149
Conclusion 151
References 151

KEY POINTS

- Primary pulmonary lymphoproliferative neoplasms are rare tumors, comprising 0.4% of all primary lung cancers, <1% of non-Hodgkin's lymphoma and 3–4% of all extranodal non-Hodgkin's lymphoma.
- Although secondary involvement of the lung by lymphoma is much more common, primary pulmonary lymphoproliferative neoplasms represent a distinct entity with favorable prognosis in most cases.
- Primary pulmonary lymphomas are defined as clonal lymphoid proliferation affecting one or both lungs (parenchyma and/or bronchi) with no extrapulmonary involvement at the time of diagnosis or 3 months after diagnosis.
- Mucosa-associated lymphoid tissue type (MALT) lymphomas are the most common type followed by diffuse large B-cell lymphomas. They are more common in patients with chronic immunosuppression such as HIV and collagen vascular diseases.

Introduction

Primary pulmonary lymphoproliferative neoplasms are rare, but awareness of these entities is important for prompt diagnosis and treatment. These neoplasms can occur in both immunocompetent and immunocompromised individuals. Secondary lymphomatous pulmonary involvement commonly occurs with Hodgkin's and non-Hodgkin's lymphoma (NHL). This chapter will focus on primary lymphomatous malignant disease affecting the pulmonary system.

Primary pulmonary lymphoproliferative neoplasms

Primary pulmonary lymphoproliferative neoplasms are defined as clonal lymphoid proliferation affecting one or both lungs (parenchyma and/or bronchi) without any extrathoracic manifestation of lymphoma at diagnosis for the following 3 months (1). These typically manifest with monoclonal lymphoid proliferation, and their behavior may range from indolent, as with pulmonary mucosa-associated lymphoid tissue (MALT) lymphoma, to more aggressive, as seen with diffuse large B-cell lymphoma and lymphomatoid granulomatosis (LyG). Primary pulmonary lymphoma is rare and accounts for 0.4% of all primary pulmonary neoplasms, 3.6% of extranodal lymphomas, and less than 0.5–1.0% of all lymphomas (2). However, clinical and radiographic features may be identical to lung cancer, so histologic confirmation is imperative for definitive diagnosis with important therapeutic and prognostic implications.

Pulmonary mucosa-associated lymphoid tissue lymphoma

Pulmonary MALT lymphoma is a low-grade, B-cell, extranodal lymphoma, and is the most common primary pulmonary lymphoproliferative neoplasm. It was first described in 1983 and has also been referred to as bronchial-associated lymphoid tissue (BALT) lymphoma (3). BALT refers to the specialized lymphoid tissues found around the respiratory mucosa of small bronchi and bronchioles; they are not prominent in the normal human lung but becomes evident after chronic antigen exposure (2). MALT lymphoma arises from monoclonal proliferation of B-cell progenitor cells thought to be driven by chronic antigen stimulation (either autoantigens or a microbial origin) (1).

Epidemiology and clinical features

Pulmonary MALT lymphoma is the most common pulmonary lymphoproliferative neoplasm (70–80%). The disease predominantly affects adults (median age 68 years), but it can develop in younger individuals who are immunosuppressed or human immunodeficiency virus (HIV) positive (4). The tumor is slightly more common in women.

Up to 30% of patients with MALT lymphoma have either an associated autoimmune condition such as Sjögren's disease, Hashimoto's thyroiditis, systemic lupus erythematosus, rheumatoid arthritis, or a persistent infection such as Hepatitis C or HIV. Unlike gastrointestinal MALT lymphoma and *Helicobacter pylori*, an association between a specific pathogen and pulmonary MALT lymphoma has not been reported (5). MALT lymphoma has also been associated with a smoking history, exposure to certain drugs or toxins, as well as with underlying pre-existing pulmonary conditions (6).

Approximately 30% of patients are asymptomatic, whereas others may have nonspecific symptoms such as cough, shortness of breath, chest pain, and, occasionally, hemoptysis. Clinical findings are nonspecific and often confused with a pneumonia-like process not responsive to antibiotics. Fever and weight loss have also been described in more aggressive illness. Monoclonal gammopathy has been reported in 40% of patients, but associated amyloidosis is rare (7, 8).

Radiographic findings

MALT lymphoma can manifest as pulmonary nodules, patchy irregular consolidation, or nonspecific opacities. They may originally be detected on chest radiograph, but computed tomography of the chest is the ideal modality for baseline and longitudinal assessment. Lesions can occur in a unilateral distribution and may be solid, mixed solid and ground-glass, or purely ground-glass in appearance. Single or multiple nodules or areas of consolidation are the most common patterns, and bronchiectasis, bronchiolitis or diffuse interstitial lung disease patterns are less common (9). Hilar and mediastinal lymphadenopathy has been described in about one-third of patients (6). Endobronchial disease may be localized or present as diffuse thickening in the tracheobronchial tree (10, 11).

Positive emission tomography (PET) has been shown to have a high detection rate of MALT lymphoma in up to 80% of patients and has been described as a worthwhile modality to aid both in diagnostic and for surveillance purposes (6, 12). However, fluorodeoxyglucose (FDG) uptake may be lower and therefore not reliable in indolent cases, hence the routine use of PET imaging in the staging of MALT lymphoma remains controversial.

Pathology

Minimally invasive modalities, including bronchoscopy with transbronchial or endobronchial biopsies and percutaneous image-guided biopsies, can yield tissue for diagnosis. If needed, surgical lung biopsies and resection may be considered. Histopathological assessment is the gold standard for diagnosis, and immunohistochemical staining has also been useful for accurate diagnosis (13).

MALT lymphoma is characterized by a proliferation of clonal marginal-zone lymphocytes that invade epithelial structures and form characteristic lymphoepithelial lesions (14). Microscopically, it is defined by a triad of reactive lymphoid follicles, diffuse infiltration by small lymphocytes, and lymphoepithelial lesions (2). Occasionally, there are small germinal centers with effacement of the lymphoid follicle's architecture with infiltration of marginal zone cells (2, 15).

Immunohistochemistry and/or flow cytometry findings include light chain restriction and cells that are strongly positive for CD20, CD79a, IgM, and may express bcl-2 (2). Neoplastic cells are negative for CD5, CD10, CD23, cyclin D1, and bcl-6, and these properties can be particularly useful especially in cases of small biopsy samples as they help differentiate between a reactive and neoplastic process (2). Cytogenetic abnormalities, t (11:18) (q21;q21), may be found in 40–50% of MALT lymphoma (16) (Figures 20.1 and 20.2).

Prognosis and treatment

MALT lymphomas generally portend a good prognosis and tend to have an indolent course with a 5-year survival rate of greater than 80%. No difference in survival is observed between gastrointestinal and nongastrointestinal lymphoma and between

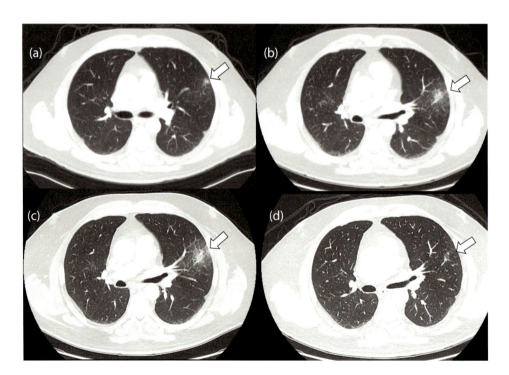

FIGURE 20.1 MALT lymphoma. (a): A middle-aged man incidentally found to have a new 1 cm irregular marginated noncavitated nodule in the left upper lobe with surrounding ground-glass opacity (arrow). (b): After 18 months, the previously noted left upper subpleural nodular opacity had improved, but the adjacent lung parenchyma demonstrated new ill-defined nodular opacities (arrow) and surrounding ground-glass opacities with septal thickening. (c): At 24 months, imaging reveals persistent opacity in the left upper lobe comprised of a central irregular opacity (arrow) surrounded by ground-glass opacities and interlobular septal thickening, which had progressed. Bronchoscopy with transbronchial biopsy confirmed extranodal marginal zone lymphoma of mucosa-associated tissue (MALT lymphoma). Immunohistochemical stains showed the neoplastic cells were positive for CD20 and CD43. (d): He received treatment with four doses of rituximab and 30 months later, imaging revealed resolution of the left upper lobe nodule with minimal residual opacity (arrow).

Primary Pulmonary Lymphoproliferative Neoplasms

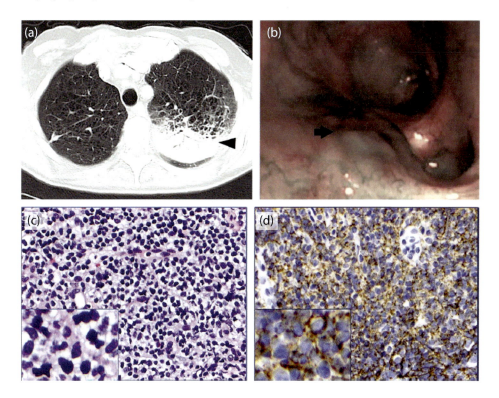

FIGURE 20.2 Parenchymal and endobronchial lymphoma. An elderly woman presented with abdominal mass and pulmonary infiltrate. (a): A CT scan showed left upper lobe consolidative opacities (black arrowhead). (b): Bronchoscopy revealed smooth raised lesions (black arrow) found overlying the left mainstem carina near the left upper lobe. Biopsies of the endobronchial abnormality and left upper lobe were obtained and revealed mucosa-associated lymphoid tissue (MALT) lymphoma. (c): Similar histologic features of both areas were noted with a dense lymphoid infiltrate composed of predominantly small lymphocytes with irregular nuclei, condensed chromatin and small to moderate amounts of pale cytoplasm. Occasional large cells and plasma cells are present. (d): Anti-CD20 immunohistochemistry demonstrates lymphocytes are B cells in endobronchial biopsy. (Reprinted from Clinics in Chest Medicine, Volume 38. Bashoura L, Eapen GA, Faiz SA. Pulmonary Manifestations of Lymphoma and Leukemia, pp. 187–200, with permission from Elsevier.)

localized or disseminated disease (14). However, some cases can rarely transform into high-grade B-cell lymphoma (13).

An individualized approach is usually taken for management considerations. Locally, advanced disease has responded to radiotherapy and surgery with or without chemotherapy, and in some cases, expectant management is preferred with frequent follow up. For patients with more advanced symptoms, anti-CD20 monoclonal antibody (rituximab or obinutuzumab) with or without chemotherapy is considered, and the decision to incorporate chemotherapy depends on goals of therapy and patient risk factors. However, current data suggests improved progression-free survival, but not overall survival (17).

Primary pulmonary diffuse large B-cell lymphoma

Primary pulmonary diffuse large B-cell lymphoma (P-DLBCL) is an extremely rare type of NHL that arises directly from lung tissue and represents about 0.4% of all NHL. It is under-recognized mainly due to its systemic nature as it spreads quickly to lymph nodes and extrathoracic sites. About half the cases arise *de novo* with the remaining half arising from large cell transformation from MALT lymphoma, so overlap of both clinical and radiographic features with MALT lymphoma are present.

Epidemiology and clinical features

P-DLCBL is the second most common type of primary pulmonary lymphoproliferative neoplasms (10–20% of cases). The incidence of P-DLBCL peaks between ages 50 and 70 with a slight preponderance for males. However, given its aggressive nature and tendency to spread, the true incidence may be underestimated. P-DLCBL has also been associated with underlying chronic infections, inflammatory conditions, or immunosuppression such as transplant or HIV patients. In HIV-positive patients, it has been associated with the Epstein–Barr virus (EBV). There is also an association with long-term methotrexate, cyclosporin A, and certain murine monoclonal antibody use (6, 18).

Patients typically present with respiratory symptoms such as cough and dyspnea and "B symptoms" such as fever, sweats, and weight loss. It develops more often in immunocompromised individuals.

Radiographic findings

The most common presentation includes solitary or multiple pulmonary nodules, which are well circumscribed rounded lesions that are more prominent in the lower lobes with a peripheral distribution. About half of the lesions demonstrate central cavitation and necrosis on imaging, especially in HIV-infected patients (15). P-DLBCL may also present as a single peripheral mass that shows a sharp transition from the adjacent lung. Mediastinal lymph node enlargement and pleural effusion may be present. PET imaging is likely to show FDG avidity (6, 18).

Pathology

Bronchial, transbronchial, or transthoracic biopsy samples are usually adequate for diagnosis. Tissue is easily obtained from core needle biopsies since these tumors localize peripherally. Identification of large cells mitoses and necrosis on pathology warrants additional testing to distinguish from other lymphomas, poorly differentiated carcinoma, germ cell tumors, and melanoma (1, 2).

Microscopically, there are sheets of large atypical cells that are at least two times larger than a mature lymphocyte, and features include centroblastic or immunoblastic morphology, coarse nuclear chromatin, prominent nucleoli, and a rim of amphophilic to slightly eosinophilic cytoplasm (2). Areas of necrosis and effacement of the lung and airway architecture, with invasion into bronchial walls, blood vessels and pleura, are characteristics of P-DLCBL and its aggressive behavior. Immunohistochemistry findings are strongly positive cells for CD20 and CD79a and light chain restriction. The Ki67-labeling index is 60–90%, and CD20 maybe useful when extensive necrosis is present as "ghost" tumor cells may still express it (2).

Prognosis and treatment

Median survival times have been reported ranging from 3 to 10 years (2). Conversely, despite P-DLCBL being an aggressive malignancy, complete remission is possible in many cases with systemic treatment.

Surgical resection is an option in localized lesions, however, P-DLCBL is usually widespread by the time of diagnosis and hence combination chemotherapy and radiation are usually the treatment of choice. Patients with underlying HIV infection or immunosuppression from transplant are at higher risk for disease progression or relapse as well as worsening general conditions due to opportunistic infections. In a large case series of 77 cases, >90% of patients with P-DLCBL who were treated with cyclophosphamide, doxorubicin, vincristine, and prednisone (CHOP) therapy achieved complete remission and the relapsed cases also had a favorable response to conventional chemotherapy (19).

Pulmonary lymphomatoid granulomatosis (LyG)

LyG is a rare extranodal neoplastic lymphoproliferative disorder initially described in 1972 by Averill Liebow and associates (20). They described overlapping features of a "lymphoma-like" process and a "limited form of Wegener granulomatosis," so the term LyG emerged; however, granulomas are not typically observed. LyG is associated with EBV and has a propensity for lymphocytic invasion of vascular walls on biopsy. Unlike MALT lymphoma and P-DLBCL, LyG most commonly involves the lungs, has an angiocentric distribution, and is challenging to prove clonality.

Epidemiology and clinical features

LyG generally presents between the ages of 30 and 50 years and peaks between 50 and 60 years, but it can present at any age. Males are more affected by the disease than females. A proportion of patients who develop LyG has an underlying immunodeficiency or a lymphoproliferative disease. Some patients developed LyG while on immunosuppressive medications, with resolution of the disease upon cessation of those medications.

The majority (90%) of patients are symptomatic and may have nonspecific symptoms present for months, including fatigue, cough, and shortness of breath (21). Fever might be present. Due to the rarity of the disease and nonspecific symptoms, diagnosis is usually delayed for several months. It can also affect the skin (50%), brain (30%), kidneys, and the gastrointestinal system (1). Skin manifestations may include erythematous plaques and nodules with predominance on the trunk and extremities (22). Neurologic symptoms vary depending on localization of the disease, but radiographic findings on an MRI must be differentiated from sarcoidosis, lymphoma, or vasculitis. Finally, renal involvement (mass) and ear, nose and throat manifestations often help differentiation from granulomatosis with polyangiitis (23).

Radiographic findings

About 80% will present with bilateral pulmonary nodules with a predilection for lung bases and a peribronchial and vascular distribution (21, 24). Nodules may coalesce and cavitate, and subsequent mass-like lesions with or without cavitation must be differentiated from both infection and other malignancies. Migratory nodules that wax and wane and the reverse halo sign have also been described (15). A pulmonary mass with poorly defined margins is another common presentation (Figure 20.3).

Pathology

Tissue biopsy remains the gold standard for diagnoses, and often surgical lung biopsy may be needed. High-grade LyG shows an

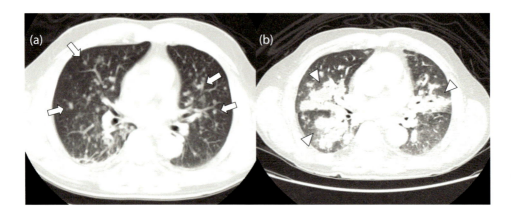

FIGURE 20.3 Lymphomatoid granulomatosis (LyG). A middle-aged man presented with increased dyspnea, productive cough and weight loss. (a): CT of the chest reveals scattered small ill-defined nodules in both lungs (arrows). A CT-guided biopsy and wedge resection of the right middle lobe confirmed lymphomatoid granulomatosis of the lung. (b): Despite systemic therapy, he progressively worsened, and imaging 3 months later showed increased nodular consolidation (arrowheads) throughout all lobes of the lung with predominance centrally with coalescence into larger mass-like formation.

angiocentric polymorphous mononuclear infiltrate composed of numerous small lymphocytes, plasma cells, histiocytes, and large atypical EBV-positive B cells, which resemble immunoblasts (15). LyG arises from proliferation of atypical large B cells and defective cytotoxic T cells. It is thought that EBV-infected B cells release chemokines, which attract reactive T cells, producing vascular damage and an impaired immunological response that then leads to the proliferation of damaged B cells in a malignant process (25). LyG is classified from grade 1 to grade 3 depending on the number of tumoral cells. Fibrinoid necrosis of the vessel wall may also occur. Giant cells or true granulomas are not a histological feature.

Prognosis and treatment

LyG patients have variable outcomes based on the extent of disease. Median survival ranges from 2 to 4 years (2, 26, 27). Respiratory insufficiency, hemoptysis, neurological complications, and infection are common causes of death (1). Poor prognostic factors include age younger than 25 years, neurologic involvement, hepatosplenomegaly, leukopenia, persistent fever, and the number of tumoral cells and degree of necrosis seen on histology. Older asymptomatic patients with unilateral lung involvement have a more favorable prognosis.

Treatment varies according to the grade of LyG, and for localized disease could include surgery or radiation (28). Careful assessment of a patient's medication and medical history is crucial, for in some cases cessation of immunomodulating medications might be an adequate treatment for LyG. Low-grade disease may be followed closely. Treatment with the antiviral, antiproliferative cytokine interferon alfa-2b has shown promising results. High-grade disease and more extensive disease require similar treatment strategies as in those with diffuse large B-cell lymphoma, as LyG can progress to lymphoma.

Lymphoproliferative disorders in the immunocompromised patient

Primary effusion lymphoma

Primary effusion lymphoma (PEL) is a rare form of lymphoma involving the pleura, pericardium, or peritoneum in immunocompromised patients (1). Human herpesvirus 8 (HHV-8) plays a role in the pathogenesis of PEL. PEL was first described in 1995, and the World Health Organization (WHO) classification intentionally separates it from solid lymphoma with secondary effusion localization (29, 30). Given its propensity to involve body cavities such as the pleural space or peritoneum, PEL is also referred to as a body cavity lymphoma.

Epidemiology and clinical features

PEL accounts for 0.5% of all lymphoma cases and 1–8% of HIV-associated NHL cases. It has rarely been described in patients with immunodeficiency secondary to organ transplantation or in patients older than 80 years (30).

Symptoms reflect the extent and distribution of disease, and fever, fatigue and dyspnea are often present (31). Most cases (85%) present with pleural effusion and ascites are present in approximately half (50%) (32). Hepatomegaly and splenomegaly are present in two-thirds of cases (30). Kaposi's sarcoma with cutaneous or mucosal localization is present in many (25–100%), and concomitant multicentric Castleman's disease may be present in 9–50% (32). Peripheral lymphadenopathy is rare.

Anemia, thrombocytopenia, and hypoalbuminemia with elevated LDH are common.

Radiology

Imaging reveals pleural effusion, and close evaluation of the CT chest reveals pleural effusion without pulmonary lesions or a detectable mass. Pleural thickening may be present.

Pathology

Pleural fluid is exudative and often bloody (1). Cytologic examination of pleural fluid is diagnostic. The malignant cells range from large immunoblastic or plasmablastic cells to those with more anaplastic characteristics (1). The immunophenotype often reflects that of a mature B cell shifting toward terminal plasma cell differentiation (Figure 20.4). The presence of HHV-8 in the nuclei of the malignant cell is a key diagnostic criterion for PEL (30). In 70% of cases, coinfection with EBV is present, but staining for latent membrane protein is negative (1).

Prognosis and treatment

Median overall survival after diagnosis without treatment is 2–3 months (33). While there may be response to chemotherapy, remissions are often short-lived, and median survival is often extended by only an average of 6 months. Median survival in HIV-related PEL is 6.2 months with a 39% 1-year survival rate (32). Prognostic factors associated with impaired clinical outcomes in HIV-related PEL include poor performance status and absence of antiretroviral therapy before diagnosis (32).

Given the rareness of the disease, there are very few retrospective studies and no prospective trials, hence treatment data is limited. Treatment includes antiretroviral therapy, cytotoxic chemotherapy, radiation therapy, antiviral therapy, and combination of these modalities. Optimized antiretroviral therapy alone can have antitumoral activity and may lead to remission (34).

Post-transplantation lymphoproliferative disorders

Post-transplant lymphoproliferative disorders (PTLD) are one of the most serious complications in those undergoing transplantation (solid organ or allogeneic hematopoietic stem cell transplantation [HSCT]). These may be either lymphoid and/or plasmacytic proliferations that are a sequela of immunosuppression. EBV infection is thought to play a central role in the pathogenesis in many of those affected. The majority of lymphoma in transplant recipients is NHL, and extranodal involvement is more common when compared to the general population (35).

Epidemiology and clinical features

PTLD constitutes 10% of all malignancies in the solid organ transplant population whereas it accounts for very few secondary cancers following HSCT (36). Incidence of PTLD varies among transplant centers likely based on different patient populations, allograft types, and immunosuppressive regimens. In a case series from Europe and the United States, approximately 85% of PTLD was found to be of B-cell origin and >80% was associated with EBV infection (36). Risk factors include degree of immunosuppression, EBV serologic status of the recipient, time post-transplant, recipient age, and ethnicity (37, 38). PTLD may occur at any time after transplantation, but the majority (80%) of these cases occur in the first year following transplant (36, 39).

The clinical presentation of PTLD can be variable and depends on the area of involvement. Nonspecific respiratory symptoms include cough, shortness of breath or chest pain, along with more systemic symptoms such as fever, weight loss, and fatigue.

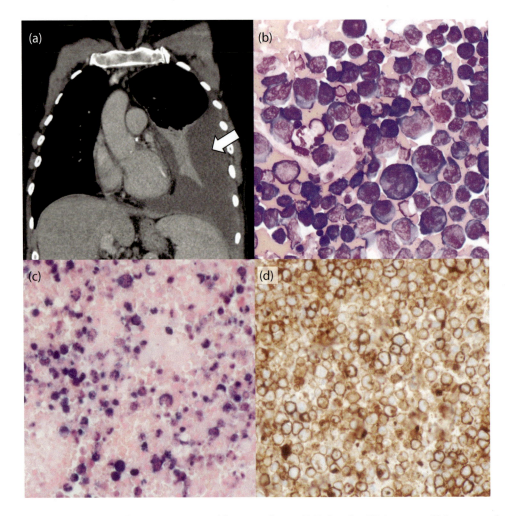

FIGURE 20.4 Primary effusion lymphoma. A 63-year-old man with HIV/AIDS and a CD4 count of 24 presented with chest tightness and shortness of breath of 3 months duration. (a): A CT scan showed large left pleural effusion, with no pulmonary nodules or mediastinal adenopathy. (b): An ultrasound-guided thoracentesis was performed, with cytology showing large blast-like atypical lymphoid cells consistent with primary effusion lymphoma (original magnification of 50×). (c): Lymphoid cells showing diffuse positivity for EBV (original magnification of 40×) using Epstein–Barr virus-encoded RNA in situ hybridization stain (EBER-ISH). (d): Lymphoid cells stain positive for activated B-cell marker –CD30, another common feature in primary effusion lymphoma (original magnification of 40×). (Pathology images courtesy of Xiaohong I. Wang, MD, University of Texas Health–McGovern Medical School, Houston.)

Nodal involvement can present with symptoms arising from compression of various organs, so respiratory symptoms due to underlying pleural effusion or lung collapse may arise. Laboratory findings may include anemia, thrombocytopenia, leukopenia, elevated serum lactate dehydrogenase, hypercalcemia, hyperuricemia, and monoclonal protein in serum or urine. Increasing EBV viral loads might provide an indirect clue for the development of PTLD. Many centers have also incorporated EBV monitoring into their routine evaluation of patients at high risk for PTLD, but the significance of various EBV tests and importance in different transplant populations need further study (40).

Radiology
Imaging is usually the first step in diagnostic workup. Presentation on chest radiograph may include a solitary mass, multiple non-cavitating nodules, and hilar adenopathy (41). Pulmonary nodules are usually multiple and well defined. Other findings include pleural-based masses, consolidation, or hilar/mediastinal lymphadenopathy. PET-CT scan has very good sensitivity and specificity for PTLD.

Pathology
The diagnosis of PTLD is based on the histological examination of tumor tissue via surgical excision or core needle biopsy. If feasible, the former is often preferred to ensure that enough tissue is available for full histopathological evaluation. Differentiating atypical infection, rejection, or a reactive process from PTLD is important. The pathological diagnosis is centered around the WHO classification, which includes four major categories of PTLD: early lesions, polymorphic PTLD, monomorphic PTLD, and classical Hodgkin lymphoma type PTLD (36). Immunophenotyping, detection of EBV-encoded RNA in situ hybridization and molecular genetic studies of antigen receptor genes for clonality are used for classification and vary among the four types. In practice, differentiating between the various types may not always be possible so these also likely represent a pathological spectrum.

Prognosis and treatment
Overall survival rates range from 25 to 35% and prognosis can vary by clonality and extent of disease. Prognosis for PTLD is considerably worse than that for NHL in non-immunocompromised

patients. Outcomes for polymorphic disease are better when compared to monomorphic disease, from which T-cell lymphomas (diagnosed based on predominant cell type within monomorphic disease) have an extremely poor prognosis (42).

Treatment decisions are made based on histological subtype, grade, stage, and site of the tumor as well as assessment of the patient's clinical status including organ dysfunction and performance status. Eradication of the PTLD and preservation of graft function are the main goals of therapy. Treatment includes reduction or discontinuation of immunosuppressive therapy, which may result in regression or complete resolution (43). Additional therapies include immunotherapy with the CD20 monoclonal antibody rituximab, chemotherapy, radiation therapy, or a combination of these.

Conclusion

Although primary pulmonary lymphoproliferative disorders are a rare group of disease, pulmonologists should be aware of these entities. Delays in diagnosis or unnecessary additional testing frequently occur when these disorders are not included in the differential. Advances in modalities to obtain tissue, such as navigational or robotic bronchoscopy, and techniques to analyze specimens with both immunohistochemistry and molecular testing, may facilitate diagnosis, but certain pathologies may require larger samples with surgical intervention. The differentiation of these processes from benign, reactive, inflammatory, or other cancer pathologies is crucial, for it will impact both prognosis and treatment. Referral to and consultation with specialized centers may be prudent until more evidence of these disorders is available.

References

1. Borie R, Wislez M, Antoine M, Cadranel J. Lymphoproliferative disorders of the lung. Respiration. 2017; 94: 157–75.
2. Pina-Oviedo S, Weissferdt A, Kalhor N, Moran CA. Primary pulmonary lymphomas. Adv Anat Pathol. 2015;22:355–75.
3. Isaacson P, Wright DH. Extranodal malignant lymphoma arising from mucosa-associated lymphoid tissue. Cancer. 1984; 53:2515–24.
4. Khalil MO, Morton LM, Devesa SS, Check DP, Curtis RE, Weisenburger DD, Dores GM. Incidence of marginal zone lymphoma in the United States, 2001-2009 with a focus on primary anatomic site. Br J Haematol. 2014;165:67–77.
5. Suarez F, Lortholary O, Hermine O, Lecuit M. Infection-associated lymphomas derived from marginal zone B cells: A model of antigen-driven lymphoproliferation. Blood. 2006;107:3034–44.
6. Tang VK, Vijhani P, Cherian SV, Ambelil M, Estrada YMRM. Primary pulmonary lymphoproliferative neoplasms. Lung India. 2018;35:220–30.
7. Kurtin PJ, Myers JL, Adlakha H, Strickler JG, Lohse C, Pankratz VS, Inwards DJ. Pathologic and clinical features of primary pulmonary extranodal marginal zone B-cell lymphoma of MALT type. Am J Surg Pathol. 2001;25:997–1008.
8. Satani T, Yokose T, Kaburagi T, Asato Y, Itabashi M, Amemiya R. Amyloid deposition in primary pulmonary marginal zone B-cell lymphoma of mucosa-associated lymphoid tissue. Pathol Int. 2007;57:746–50.
9. Bae YA, Lee KS, Han J, Ko YH, Kim BT, Chung MJ, Kim TS. Marginal zone B-cell lymphoma of bronchus-associated lymphoid tissue: Imaging findings in 21 patients. Chest. 2008;133:433–40.
10. Bashoura L, Eapen GA, Faiz SA. Pulmonary manifestations of lymphoma and leukemia. Clin Chest Med. 2017;38:187–200.
11. Yoon RG, Kim MY, Song JW, Chae EJ, Choi CM, Jang S. Primary endobronchial marginal zone B-cell lymphoma of bronchus-associated lymphoid tissue: CT findings in 7 patients. Korean J Radiol. 2013;14:366–74.
12. Wei Z, Li J, Cheng Z, Yuan L, Liu P. A single center experience: Rituximab plus cladribine is an effective and safe first-line therapy for unresectable bronchial-associated lymphoid tissue lymphoma. J Thorac Dis. 2017;9:1081–92.
13. Bi L, Li J, Dan W, Lu Z. Pulmonary MALT lymphoma: A case report and review of the literature. Exp Ther Med. 2015;9:147–50.
14. Borie R, Wislez M, Thabut G, Antoine M, Rabbat A, Couderc LJ, Monnet I, Nunes H, Blanc FX, Mal H, Bergeron A, Dusser D, Israel-Biet D, Crestani B, Cadranel J. Clinical characteristics and prognostic factors of pulmonary MALT lymphoma. Eur Respir J. 2009;34:1408–16.
15. Hare SS, Souza CA, Bain G, Seely JM, Frcpc, Gomes MM, Quigley M. The radiological spectrum of pulmonary lymphoproliferative disease. Br J Radiol. 2012;85:848–64.
16. Remstein ED, Kurtin PJ, Einerson RR, Paternoster SF, Dewald GW. Primary pulmonary MALT lymphomas show frequent and heterogeneous cytogenetic abnormalities, including aneuploidy and translocations involving API2 and MALT1 and IGH and MALT1. Leukemia. 2004;18:156–60.
17. Santopietro M, Kovalchuk S, Battistini R, Puccini B, Annibali O, Romano I, Zoli V, Avvisati G, Bosi A, Rigacci L. Treatment and prognosis of primary pulmonary lymphoma: A long-term follow-up study. Eur J Haematol. 2021;106:49–57.
18. Cadranel J, Wislez M, Antoine M. Primary pulmonary lymphoma. Eur Respir J. 2002;20:750–62.
19. Neri N, Jesus Nambo M, Aviles A. Diffuse large B-cell lymphoma primary of lung. Hematology. 2011;16:110–12.
20. Liebow AA, Carrington CR, Friedman PJ. Lymphomatoid granulomatosis. Hum Pathol. 1972;3:457–558.
21. Lee JS, Tuder R, Lynch DA. Lymphomatoid granulomatosis: Radiologic features and pathologic correlations. AJR Am J Roentgenol. 2000;175:1335–9.
22. Beaty MW, Toro J, Sorbara L, Stern JB, Pittaluga S, Raffeld M, Wilson WH, Jaffe ES. Cutaneous lymphomatoid granulomatosis: Correlation of clinical and biologic features. Am J Surg Pathol. 2001;25:1111–20.
23. Gupta S, Gupta OP. Lymphomatoid granulomatosis of the oropharynx. Ear Nose Throat J. 1980;59:152–4.
24. Hicken P, Dobie JC, Frew E. The radiology of lymphomatoid granulomatosis in the lung. Clin Radiol. 1979;30:661–4.
25. Melani C, Jaffe ES, Wilson WH. Pathobiology and treatment of lymphomatoid granulomatosis, a rare EBV-driven disorder. Blood. 2020;135:1344–52.
26. Katzenstein AL, Carrington CB, Liebow AA. Lymphomatoid granulomatosis: A clinicopathologic study of 152 cases. Cancer. 1979; 43:360–73.
27. Katzenstein AL, Doxtader E, Narendra S. Lymphomatoid granulomatosis: Insights gained over 4 decades. Am J Surg Pathol. 2010;34:e35–48.
28. Roschewski M, Wilson WH. Lymphomatoid granulomatosis. Cancer J. 2012;18:469–74.
29. Cesarman E, Chang Y, Moore PS, Said JW, Knowles DM. Kaposi's sarcoma-associated herpesvirus-like DNA sequences in AIDS-related body-cavity-based lymphomas. N Engl J Med. 1995; 332:1186–91.
30. Borie R, Cadranel J, Guihot A, Marcelin AG, Galicier L, Couderc LJ. Pulmonary manifestations of human herpesvirus-8 during HIV infection. Eur Respir J. 2013;42:1105–18.
31. Boulanger E, Agbalika F, Maarek O, Daniel MT, Grollet L, Molina JM, Sigaux F, Oksenhendler E. A clinical, molecular and cytogenetic study of 12 cases of human herpesvirus 8 associated primary effusion lymphoma in HIV-infected patients. Hematol J. 2001;2:172–9.
32. Boulanger E, Gerard L, Gabarre J, Molina JM, Rapp C, Abino JF, Cadranel J, Chevret S, Oksenhendler E. Prognostic factors and outcome of human herpesvirus 8-associated primary effusion lymphoma in patients with AIDS. J Clin Oncol. 2005; 23:4372–80.
33. Komanduri KV, Luce JA, McGrath MS, Herndier BG, Ng VL. The natural history and molecular heterogeneity of HIV-associated primary malignant lymphomatous effusions. J Acquir Immune Defic Syndr Hum Retrovirol. 1996;13:215–26.

34. Oksenhendler E, Clauvel JP, Jouveshomme S, Davi F, Mansour G. Complete remission of a primary effusion lymphoma with antiretroviral therapy. Am J Hematol. 1998;57:266.
35. Penn I. Cancers complicating organ transplantation. N Engl J Med. 1990;323:1767–9.
36. Parker A, Bowles K, Bradley JA, Emery V, Featherstone C, Gupte G, Marcus R, Parameshwar J, Ramsay A, Newstead C, Haemato-oncology Task Force of the British Committee for Standards in H, British Transplantation S. Diagnosis of post-transplant lymphoproliferative disorder in solid organ transplant recipients–BCSH and BTS Guidelines. Br J Haematol. 2010;149:675–92.
37. Smith JM, Rudser K, Gillen D, Kestenbaum B, Seliger S, Weiss N, McDonald RA, Davis CL, Stehmen-Breen C. Risk of lymphoma after renal transplantation varies with time: An analysis of the United States Renal Data System. Transplantation. 2006;81:175–80.
38. Caillard S, Lelong C, Pessione F, Moulin B, French PWG. Post-transplant lymphoproliferative disorders occurring after renal transplantation in adults: Report of 230 cases from the French registry. Am J Transplant. 2006;6:2735–42.
39. Opelz G, Henderson R. Incidence of non-Hodgkin lymphoma in kidney and heart transplant recipients. Lancet. 1993;342:1514–16.
40. Tsai DE, Douglas L, Andreadis C, Vogl DT, Arnoldi S, Kotloff R, Svoboda J, Bloom RD, Olthoff KM, Brozena SC, Schuster SJ, Stadtmauer EA, Robertson ES, Wasik MA, Ahya VN. EBV PCR in the diagnosis and monitoring of posttransplant lymphoproliferative disorder: Results of a two-arm prospective trial. Am J Transplant. 2008;8:1016–24.
41. Thompson GP, Utz JP, Rosenow EC, Myers JL, Swensen SJ. Pulmonary lymphoproliferative disorders. Mayo Clin Proc. 1993;68:804–17.
42. Savage P, Waxman J. Post-transplantation lymphoproliferative disease. QJM. 1997;90:497–503.
43. Starzl TE, Nalesnik MA, Porter KA, Ho M, Iwatsuki S, Griffith BP, Rosenthal JT, Hakala TR, Shaw BW, Jr., Hardesty RL, et al. Reversibility of lymphomas and lymphoproliferative lesions developing under cyclosporin-steroid therapy. Lancet. 1984;1:583–7.

21

DIFFUSE IDIOPATHIC PULMONARY NEUROENDOCRINE CELL HYPERPLASIA

Amitha M. Avasarala, Sameer K. Avasarala, Sanjay Mukhopadhyay, Subha Ghosh, and Atul C. Mehta

Contents

Introduction 153
Epidemiology 153
Pathology and etiopathogenesis...154
Clinical features..155
Laboratory investigations...155
Imaging...155
Pulmonary function testing 156
Bronchoscopy 156
Differential diagnosis...157
Treatment 157
Conclusion..157
References...158

Abbreviations

DIPNECH	diffuse idiopathic pulmonary neuroendocrine cell hyperplasia
PNEC	pulmonary neuroendocrine cells
NEB	neuroendocrine body
WHO	World Health Organization
NORD	National Organization for Rare Disorders
CT	computed tomography
CGRP	calcitonin gene-related peptide
GRP	gastrin-releasing peptide
SYP	synaptophysin
MEN 1	multiple endocrine neoplasia

KEY POINTS

- Diffuse idiopathic pulmonary neuroendocrine cell hyperplasia (DIPNECH) is a rare lung disorder characterized by diffuse proliferation of pulmonary neuroendocrine cells that often affects middle-aged to elderly women.
- DIPNECH may be a pre-neoplastic condition with potential for development of carcinoid tumors in some of the affected patients.
- Computed tomography imaging findings may include multiple nodules, atelectasis, bronchiectasis, bronchial wall thickening, and mosaic attenuation.
- Histologically, DIPNECH presents as a generalized proliferation of neuroendocrine cells, tiny nodular aggregates, or linear proliferation of neuroendocrine cells.

Introduction

Pulmonary neuroendocrine cells (PNECs) are specialized epithelial cells that produce a wide variety of neuropeptides, amines, and neurotransmitters. They arise from bronchial mucosal Kulchitsky cells (1). Clusters of PNECs are called neuroendocrine bodies (NEB) and are usually located in airway branch points in normal lungs (2). Diffuse idiopathic pulmonary neuroendocrine cell hyperplasia (DIPNECH) is defined by the World Health Organization (WHO) as "generalized proliferation of pulmonary neuroendocrine cells that may be confined to the mucosa of airways (with or without luminal protrusion), may invade locally to form tumorlets, or may develop into carcinoid tumors" (3). In 1992, Aguayo et al. published the first case series of six patients with DIPNECH, who presented with symptoms of cough and dyspnea on exertion, none of whom had a history of cigarette smoking or concomitant lung disease (4). The last three decades have witnessed a rising recognition of this disease in part due to more liberal utilization of advanced chest imaging. Attempts are being made to better understand its pathophysiology and its association with more familiar illnesses of neuroendocrine cell origin. DIPNECH lies within the spectrum of pulmonary neuroendocrine proliferations and is considered by the WHO to represent a precursor ("preinvasive lesion") to carcinoid tumors in the lungs (5).

Epidemiology

DIPNECH has thus far only been reported in case reports and small case series. It has been recognized by the National Organization for Rare Disorders (NORD) as a rare disease. To date, only several hundred cases of DIPNECH have been reported. Most patients are diagnosed in the fifth or sixth decade of life. Approximately 90% of patients are women, usually middle-aged to elderly, and most are nonsmokers. Smoking is not reported as a risk factor (6–8). Due to its benign clinical course, delays in diagnosis ranging from months to years are relatively common. With increasing awareness of this disease and more widespread use of cross-sectional imaging modalities of the chest, an increase in its incidence is expected.

Pathology and etiopathogenesis

Pulmonary neuroendocrine cells have multiple functions including airway oxygen sensing, pulmonary blood flow regulation, and bronchial tone control (9, 10). These cells are round to oval or spindle-shaped and contain eosinophilic cytoplasm with round to oval nuclei that have a granular, "salt-and-pepper" chromatin pattern (11). Neuroendocrine bodies contain various amines and peptides, including serotonin (5-HT), calcitonin gene-related peptide (CGRP), calcitonin, substance P, somatostatin, chromogranin A, gastrin-releasing peptide (GRP), and synaptophysin (SYP) (Figure 21.1). Various physiological stimuli, such as hypoxia, lead to the release of these contents. These peptides stimulate fibroblast proliferation, bronchoconstriction, and chemotaxis of airway cells, which may lead to small airway fibrosis (12). One of the factors that complicates this diagnosis is that PNEC hyperplasia occurs as a secondary phenomenon in many other lung diseases, including emphysema, chronic bronchitis, interstitial pneumonitis, eosinophilic granuloma, and pulmonary neoplasms with neuroendocrine features (small cell lung carcinoma) (13). It has long been recognized that airway inflammation can lead to secondary neuroendocrine hyperplasia and the formation of incidental carcinoid tumorlets (Figure 21.2).

Three patterns of PNEC proliferation have been reported that occur in different clinical settings:

1. Reactive PNEC, which is usually a secondary response to chronic hypoxia in the setting of pulmonary pathologies such as emphysema and airway inflammation.
2. PNEC proliferation occurring in the background lung of carcinoid tumors, also known as carcinoid tumorlets.
3. DIPNECH, a generalized PNEC proliferation of the peripheral (small) airways.

Histopathologic confirmation forms the cornerstone of the diagnosis of DIPNECH. Surgical lung biopsy is the usual diagnostic modality and considered the gold standard. It offers the ability to demonstrate key histopathological findings and confirm the diffuse nature of the disease (14).

Although it is universally accepted that the pathologic hallmark of DIPNECH is a proliferation of neuroendocrine cells in small airways, the pathologic diagnosis of DIPNECH is plagued by several problems. The easiest part of the diagnosis is the demonstration of the neuroendocrine nature of the cells, which can be done by the traditional neuroendocrine markers synaptophysin, chromogranin, or CD56 or the novel nuclear neuroendocrine marker INSM1 (15, 16). The first problem is showing evidence of "diffuse" disease because there is no well-defined cut-off that marks the boundary between incidental disease and DIPNECH. In prototypical cases, there are numerous foci of neuroendocrine cell proliferation within bronchioles in the surgical biopsy, testifying to the diffuse nature of the process.

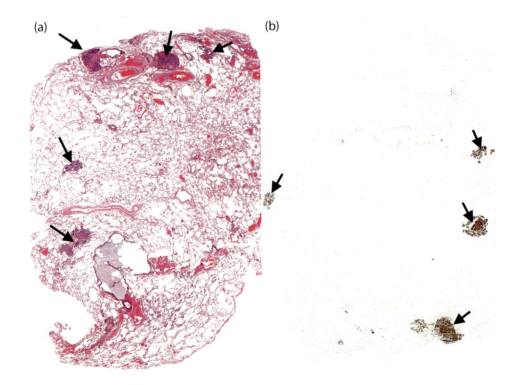

FIGURE 21.1 Pathology of DIPNECH. Low magnification photomicrographs from a surgical lung specimen to show diffuse nature of process. (a): Arrows indicate foci of neuroendocrine cell hyperplasia. Hematoxylin-eosin, 0.4×. (b): In this photomicrograph, the slide is stained with the neuroendocrine marker chromogranin, which confirms the neuroendocrine nature of these cells (chromogranin, 0.4×).

Diffuse Idiopathic Pulmonary Neuroendocrine Cell Hyperplasia

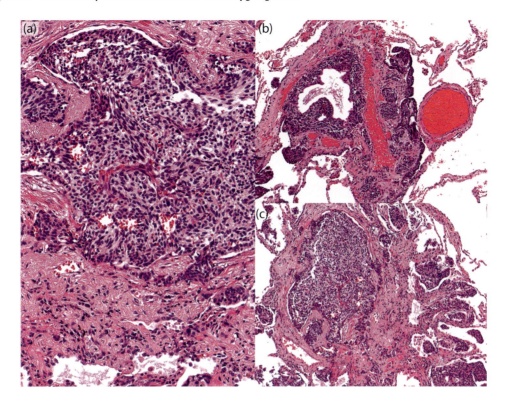

FIGURE 21.2 Pathologic features of DIPNECH at higher magnification. (a): Proliferation of cytologically bland neuroendocrine cells. These cells are morphologically identical to carcinoid tumor, but the lesions are much smaller (hematoxylin-eosin, 20×). (b): Neuroendocrine cells are present within ("undermining") bronchiolar mucosa without forming nodular growths. Some would regard this growth pattern as being typical of true neuroendocrine cell hyperplasia (hematoxylin-eosin, 10×). (c). Neuroendocrine cells are forming a nodule. Many experts refer to such nodules as carcinoid tumorlets. They are commonly found in the background lung of resected carcinoid tumors (hematoxylin-eosin, 10×).

Secondly, it is a challenge to prove the process is idiopathic. Incidental foci of neuroendocrine cell hyperplasia are common in inflamed and fibrotic lungs. This reactive process possesses a challenge in labeling neuroendocrine cell hyperplasia as secondary, or truly idiopathic. Generally, the less the background lung pathology and the more diffuse the neuroendocrine proliferation, the clearer the support for an idiopathic process.

The third challenge is the distinction between DIPNECH and carcinoid tumorlets. The WHO manual suggests that neuroendocrine cells that "invade locally" by "crossing the basement membrane" are tumorlets and defines these in a way that seems to indicate that they should be considered part of the spectrum of DIPNECH (3). However, this view is not universally accepted by experts in pulmonary pathology. Some experts use the term "carcinoid tumorlets" for the multiple tiny neuroendocrine nodules that commonly occur in the background lung of asymptomatic patients with carcinoid tumor, reserving the term DIPNECH only for patients with evidence of airflow obstruction (17). Others have proposed alternative criteria (18).

Clinical features

There appear to be two distinctive groups of patients with DIPNECH, asymptomatic and symptomatic. Asymptomatic patients are usually identified through surgical referral for resection of an incidental pulmonary nodule or nodules of unclear etiology. Symptomatic patients typically present with nonspecific symptoms such as a chronic nonproductive cough, wheezing, and dyspnea. Progression of the clinical course in symptomatic patients is characterized by the development of carcinoid tumors or progressive airflow obstruction. These patients are frequently misdiagnosed as having asthma or chronic bronchitis and remain asymptomatic for many years (19, 20). An initial clinical diagnosis of asthma was noted in 41% of patients in a 32-patient case series (6).

Laboratory investigations

The diagnosis of DIPNECH is challenging as there are no diagnostic blood or serologic investigations to confirm or deny the diagnosis of DIPNECH. The literature suggests expressions of certain neuroendocrine markers (chromogranin A, CD56, synaptophysin, and CD10), markers of proliferation and death (retinoblastoma), and predictive markers (mTIRp, P70S6K, and SSTR2) that suggest the presence of DIPNECH (21). Studies investigating the differential expression of key antigens involved in controlling cell kinetics suggest a distinction between the "reactive" process of PNEC proliferation that occurs as part of the normal response to pulmonary injury compared to those seen in DIPNECH (8, 22). DIPNECH may also be found in patients with coexisting multi-organ endocrinopathies, including those with multiple endocrine neoplasia (MEN1) syndrome and acromegaly (20, 23).

Imaging

In general, chest imaging in patients with DIPNECH typically demonstrate multiple pulmonary nodules, which are best appreciated on high-resolution computed tomography. In a case series of

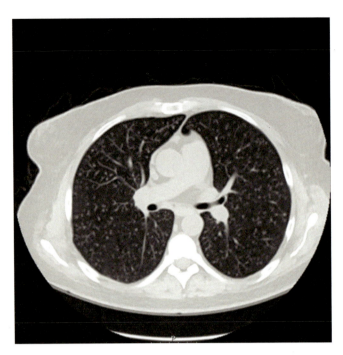

FIGURE 21.3 A contrasted computed chest CT scan of a patient with histopathological confirmation of DIPNECH. The axial image is most significant with diffuse pulmonary micronodules. Although this finding is not specific for DIPNECH, it is one of the common radiographic patterns than can be seen.

11 patients, pulmonary nodules were present in all, and multiple nodules (≥5) were present in 7/11 patients (65%) (Figure 21.3) (24). Computed tomography (CT) findings typically include those of airway-related diseases such as multiple nodules, atelectasis, bronchiectasis, bronchial wall thickening, and mosaic attenuation. A case series of 32 patients with DIPNECH suggests that the diagnosis is not easily made by radiologists: The differential was only mentioned by the interpreting radiologist in 31% of cases. Eighty-five percent of the patients with repeat imaging in a 3-year interval showed an increase in the size of the largest nodule (6). Mosaic attenuation occurs due to vasoconstriction in the lung areas with small airway obstructions. Expiratory CT scans can be used to confirm air trapping, a radiological clue to constrictive bronchiolitis, in patients with mosaic attenuations. Coronal minimum intensity projection image better depicts mosaic attenuation, and maximum intensity projection reformation is useful for detecting nodules (25, 26). Multiple nodules may also indicate metastatic pulmonary disease, especially in those with prior history of malignancy (27). Although none of these radiographic findings are pathognomonic, the association of multiple, small nodules with concomitant CT features of constrictive bronchiolitis can support the diagnosis of DIPNECH.

Pulmonary function testing

Due to progressive airway narrowing secondary to mechanical obstruction, an obstructive pattern of pulmonary function tests (PFTs) is the most prominent finding in patients. Lung function tests may also indicate a mixed obstructive/restrictive or reveal normal patterns in a number of patients (21, 22). Not all cases of DIPNECH that are pathologically encountered are associated with clinical evidence of airflow obstruction in airways. Reduction in the diffusing capacity for carbon monoxide has also been reported (28).

Bronchoscopy

Bronchoscopy is primarily used as a diagnostic tool to help rule out differential diagnoses in patients suspected to have DIPNECH. This is in stark contrast to other pulmonary neuroendocrine neoplasms in which bronchoscopy has been proven to be useful for both diagnosis and treatment (29). A variety of methods can be used to debulk tumors that cause central airway obstruction (30). Endobronchial samples can be obtained and linear endobronchial ultrasound can helpful in providing staging information (31).

In certain situations, samples obtained from bronchoscopy can provide diagnostic information for patients being evaluated for DIPNECH. Limitations in size of the sample acquired combined with the heterogenous involvement of the parenchyma and airways can lead to a sizeable false negative rate with bronchoscopy sampling. It is for these reasons that surgical lung biopsy is heavily relied upon to acquire diagnostic tissue samples in patients suspected to have DIPNECH (8).

A histological finding of DIPNECH is the identification of tumorlets of irregular neuroendocrine cells that infiltrate into the basement membrane of bronchioles (32). Although endobronchial carcinoid shows clear evidence of disease on white light bronchoscopy, the airway examination of a patient with DIPNECH will likely be normal. Bronchoalveolar lavage does not provide specific information but can be useful to rule out other differential diagnoses. The diagnosis is unlikely to be made on tissue samples acquired from traditional transbronchial biopsies, although some case reports exist highlight success in diagnosis with transbronchial biopsies. In some instances, presumptive diagnoses of DIPNECH can be made on the findings from a transbronchial biopsy — identifying a (portion) small airway with neuroendocrine proliferation compatible with DIPNECH. Advanced imaging and guidance mechanisms have allowed for more precise sampling of the lung parenchyma, small nodules that represent DIPNECH can be targeted (Figure 21.4).

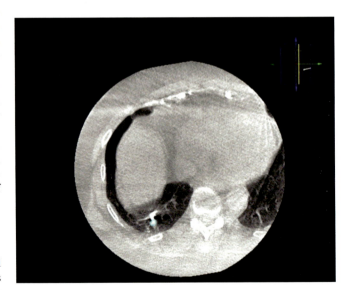

FIGURE 21.4 A small (<10 mm) right lower lobe peripheral nodule was successfully sampled using electromagnetic navigational technology with cone-beam CT guidance. Histopathological analysis of transbronchial biopsies obtained from this procedure showed findings consistent with DIPNECH.

Diffuse Idiopathic Pulmonary Neuroendocrine Cell Hyperplasia

Much like the diagnostic process of interstitial lung diseases, these histopathological findings must be in line with compatible clinical, functional, and radiological findings (33, 34). There have been case reports describing the use of transbronchial cryobiopsy as a successful sampling modality (35, 36).

Differential diagnosis

When present, symptoms are nonspecific. The differential diagnoses are vast and primarily include any etiology for constrictive bronchiolitis (Table 21.1). These range from connective tissue disorders, toxic fume/mineral dust exposure, drug reactions, or diseases such as ulcerative colitis. Clinically, DIPNECH is an asthma mimic considering the protracted course and symptomatic resemblance. Delay in diagnosis is common and can range from less than 1 month to more than 20 years, with an average delay of around 1 year as reported in one case series (6).

Treatment

Unfortunately, data on long-term treatment options and prognosis in patients with DIPNECH are limited. No consensus guidelines exist. Management strategies heavily depend on inferences drawn from case reports and case series.

Treatment methods range from a conservative "wait and watch" approach to major surgical interventions. A variety of pharmacotherapeutics that have been used in other disease states have been assessed as treatment strategies in patients with DIPNECH. Unsuccessful attempts at the use of cytotoxic agents in two patients with DIPNECH, one of whom ultimately died of progressive respiratory failure while receiving treatment with fluorouracil, were reported in the initial description of DIPNECH (4). Neuroendocrine cells produce bombesin-like peptide that are bronchoconstrictors, leading to the use of steroids for anti-inflammatory effect (33). Azithromycin is used for its similar anti-inflammatory effect. Myint et al., reported the effective management of DIPNECH with m-TOR inhibitors such as sirolimus or rapamycin (37). Somatostatin is a direct inhibitor the cell cycle and exerts antitumor activity. One study of 42 patients treated with somatostatin analogs reported improvement of symptoms in more than half of the patients and an improvement in PFTs in most patients. Imaging however revealed no change in size or number of nodules with the use of somatostatin analogs (38). Per one case report, double lung transplantation led to stable conditions in both patients (39).

Conclusion

DIPNECH is rare and an often under-recognized disease characterized by small airway obstruction. Presentation and clinical course vary greatly between patients. There are no pathognomonic laboratory or imaging findings that clinch the diagnosis. The diagnosis hinges on key histopathological findings, which are subject to intricacies of interpretation.

Although rare, it is suspected that rates of DIPNECH diagnosis will increase due to the more widespread use of CT. However, there remain significant voids in our understanding of this illness's etiopathogenesis and clinical course, leading to an absence of consistently effective and established management strategies. Further clinical trials and a database to systematically investigate the nuances that surround the disease are needed.

TABLE 21.1: Characteristics of Pulmonary Neuroendocrine Disorders

	DIPNECH	Carcinoid Tumors	Large Cell Neuroendocrine Carcinoma	Small Cell Neuroendocrine Carcinoma
Definition and Pathologic Features	Widespread neuroendocrine cell hyperplasia in mucosa of peripheral airways.	Well-differentiated neoplasms with neuroendocrine histologic features, >5mm in size, with <2 mitoses per 2 mm^2, and no necrosis. Atypical carcinoids have 2–10 mitoses per 2 mm^2 or punctate necrosis.	High-grade non-small cell lung carcinoma with neuroendocrine histologic features, staining for at least one neuroendocrine marker, and >10 mitoses per 2 mm^2.	High-grade neuroendocrine carcinoma, with scant cytoplasm and absence of prominent nucleoli.
Risk Factors	Seen in older females (50–70), Predominantly nonsmokers.	Wide age range, 4–95 years old. Affects Caucasians primarily. No known association with cigarette smoking.	Predominantly seen in men with an average age of 65 years. Associated with heavy smoking history.	Seen usually in older men (60–70 years). Almost exclusively in smokers.
Clinical Features	Nonproductive cough, less commonly hemoptysis, dyspnea, and chest pain.	Recurrent infections, cough, hemoptysis, wheezing, rarely paraneoplastic syndromes, and carcinoid syndrome.	Chest pain, hemoptysis, and cough, less likely dyspnea, weight loss and fever.	Cough, hemoptysis, chest pain, dyspnea, fatigue, weight loss, and anorexia. Symptoms along with paraneoplastic syndromes.
Imaging Findings	CT findings of multifocal pulmonary micronodules with features of constrictive bronchiolitis, bronchiectasis, and bronchial wall thickening.	Chest radiographs may show a centrally located, well defined solitary nodule or mass. CT findings with soft tissue nodule, bronchiectasis, mucoid impaction, atelectasis, and air trapping. Bronchus sign (bronchus leading directly to tumor) may also be seen. Metastases to liver, bone, and adrenals.	Large peripheral pulmonary mass, commonly associated with necrosis, lymphadenopathy, and metastases.	Large central or mediastinal mass with mediastinal and hilar lymphadenopathy, bronchial encasement, obstruction or compression, post obstructive pneumonia, atelectasis, and pleural nodules. May exhibit bronchus cut-off sign. Metastases to liver, adrenals, and bones.

(Continued)

TABLE 21.1: Characteristics of Pulmonary Neuroendocrine Disorders (*Continued*)

	DIPNECH	Carcinoid Tumors	Large Cell Neuroendocrine Carcinoma	Small Cell Neuroendocrine Carcinoma
Diagnosis	Based on imaging findings, along with clinical features. Open lung or thoracoscopic biopsy is the gold standard.	Biopsy via bronchoscopy, image-guided percutaneous needle biopsy, or thoracotomy.	Biopsy or preferably excision.	Biopsy via image-guided bronchoscopy and surgical biopsy. Biopsy of suspected metastasis can expedite diagnosis.
Treatment	No known curative therapy. Inhaled and systemic corticosteroids, somatostatin analogs, and surgical procedures.	Surgical resection with mediastinal lymph node resection is curative in most patients with low-stage disease. Role and efficacy of adjuvant chemotherapy is unclear. Immunotherapy, chemotherapy, or radiolabeled agents may be used for unresectable and metastatic tumors.	No well-defined efficacious treatments. Some patients respond to cisplatin-based chemotherapy; efficacy of radiation is unknown.	Systemic chemotherapy, with etoposide, increasingly with immunotherapy. Prophylactic cranial irradiation.
Prognosis	Good, 83% of patients alive at 5 years.	Typical carcinoids: 5-year survival rate 87–100%. Atypical carcinoids: 44–88%.	Poor, 5-year survival rate 15–57%.	Poor, 5-year survival rate 5% for patients with extensive local or metastatic disease.

References

1. Dincer HE, Podgaetz E, Andrade RS. Pulmonary neuroendocrine tumors: Part I. Spectrum and characteristics of tumors. J Bronchology Interv Pulmonol. 2015 Jul;22(3):267–73.
2. Garg A, Sui P, Verheyden JM, Young LR, Sun X. Consider the Lung as a Sensory Organ: A Tip from Pulmonary Neuroendocrine Cells. In: Current Topics in Developmental Biology [Internet]. Academic Press Inc.; 2019 [cited 2021 Apr 29]. p. 67–89. Available from: https://pubmed.ncbi.nlm.nih.gov/30797518/
3. Travis WD, Brambilla E, Burke AP, Marx A, Nicholson AG. Introduction to the 2015 World Health Organization classification of tumors of the lung, pleura, thymus, and heart. J Thorac Oncol. 2015;10:1240–2.
4. Aguayo SM, Miller YE, Waldron JAJ, Bogin RM, Sunday ME, Staton GWJ, et al. Brief report: Idiopathic diffuse hyperplasia of pulmonary neuroendocrine cells and airways disease. N Engl J Med. 1992 Oct;327(18):1285–8.
5. Flint K, Ye C, Henry TL. Diffuse idiopathic pulmonary neuroendocrine cell hyperplasia (DIPNECH) with liver metastases. BMJ Case Rep. 2019 Jun;12(6).
6. Little BP, Junn JC, Zheng KS, Sanchez FW, Henry TS, Veeraraghavan S, et al. Diffuse idiopathic pulmonary neuroendocrine cell hyperplasia: Imaging and clinical features of a frequently delayed diagnosis. AJR Am J Roentgenol. 2020 Dec;215(6):1312–20.
7. Benson REC, Rosado-de-Christenson ML, Martínez-Jiménez S, Kunin JR, Pettavel PP. Spectrum of pulmonary neuroendocrine proliferations and neoplasms. Radiogr a Rev Publ Radiol Soc North Am Inc. 2013 Oct;33(6):1631–49.
8. Wirtschafter E, Walts AE, Liu ST, Marchevsky AM. Diffuse idiopathic pulmonary neuroendocrine cell hyperplasia of the lung (DIPNECH): Current Best evidence. Lung. 2015 Oct;193(5):659–67.
9. Linnoila RI. Functional facets of the pulmonary neuroendocrine system. Lab Invest. 2006 May;86(5):425–44.
10. Song H, Yao E, Lin C, Gacayan R, Chen M-H, Chuang P-T. Functional characterization of pulmonary neuroendocrine cells in lung development, injury, and tumorigenesis. Proc Natl Acad Sci U S A. 2012 Oct;109(43):17531–6.
11. Tazelaar H. Pathology of Lung Malignancies. UptoDate. 2020;
12. Degan S, Lopez GY, Kevill K, Sunday ME. Gastrin-releasing peptide, immune responses, and lung disease. Ann N Y Acad Sci. 2008 Nov;1144:136–47.
13. Domnik NJ, Cutz E. Pulmonary neuroepithelial bodies as airway sensors: Putative role in the generation of dyspnea. Curr Opin Pharmacol. 2011 Jun;11(3):211–7.
14. Miller RR, Müller NL. Neuroendocrine cell hyperplasia and obliterative bronchiolitis in patients with peripheral carcinoid tumors. Am J Surg Pathol. 1995 Jun;19(6):653–8.
15. Dermawan JK, Mukhopadhyay S. Insulinoma-associated protein 1 (INSM1) differentiates carcinoid tumourlets of the lung from pulmonary meningothelial-like nodules. Histopathology. 2018;72:1067–9.
16. Mukhopadhyay S, Dermawan JK, Lanigan CP, Farver CF. Insulinoma-associated protein 1 (INSM1) is a sensitive And highly specific marker of neuroendocrine differentiation in primary lung neoplasms: An immunohistochemical study of 345 cases, including 292 whole-tissue sections. Mod Pathol an Off J United States Can Acad Pathol Inc. 2019 Jan;32(1):100–9.
17. Aubry M-C, Thomas CFJ, Jett JR, Swensen SJ, Myers JL. Significance of multiple carcinoid tumors and tumorlets in surgical lung specimens: Analysis of 28 patients. Chest. 2007 Jun;131(6):1635–43.
18. Marchevsky AM, Walts AE. Diffuse idiopathic pulmonary neuroendocrine cell hyperplasia (DIPNECH). Semin Diagn Pathol. 2015 Nov;32(6):438–44.
19. Ryu JH, Azadeh N, Samhouri B, Yi E. Recent advances in the understanding of bronchiolitis in adults. F1000Research. 2020;9.
20. Davies SJ, Gosney JR, Hansell DM, Wells AU, du Bois RM, Burke MM, et al. Diffuse idiopathic pulmonary neuroendocrine cell hyperplasia: An under-recognised spectrum of disease. Thorax. 2007 Mar;62(3):248–52.
21. Mengoli MC, Rossi G, Cavazza A, Franco R, Marino FZ, Migaldi M, et al. Diffuse idiopathic pulmonary neuroendocrine cell hyperplasia (DIPNECH) syndrome and carcinoid tumors With/Without NECH: A clinicopathologic, radiologic, and immunomolecular comparison study. Am J Surg Pathol. 2018 May;42(5):646–55.
22. Trisolini R, Valentini I, Tinelli C, Ferrari M, Guiducci GM, Parri SNF, et al. DIPNECH: Association between histopathology and clinical presentation. Lung. 2016 Apr;194(2):243–7.
23. Fessler MB, Cool CD, Miller YE, Schwarz MI, Brown KK. Idiopathic diffuse hyperplasia of pulmonary neuroendocrine cells in a patient with acromegaly. Respirology. 2004 Jun;9(2):274–7.
24. Foran PJ, Hayes SA, Blair DJ, Zakowski MF, Ginsberg MS. Imaging appearances of diffuse idiopathic pulmonary neuroendocrine cell hyperplasia. Clin Imaging. 2015;39(2):243–6.
25. Chassagnon G, Favelle O, Marchand-Adam S, De Muret A, Revel MP. DIPNECH: When to suggest this diagnosis on CT. Clin Radiol. 2015 Mar;70(3):317–25.
26. Lee JS, Brown KK, Cool C, Lynch DA. Diffuse pulmonary neuroendocrine cell hyperplasia: Radiologic and clinical features. J Comput Assist Tomogr. 2002;26(2):180–4.

27. Fabbri N, Rocca T, Navarra G, Adani GL, Rinaldi R, Carcoforo P. "Carcinoid tumorlets". Case report and review of the literature. Ann Ital Chir. 1998;69(4):509–11.
28. Samhouri BF, Azadeh N, Halfdanarson TR, Yi ES, Ryu JH. Constrictive bronchiolitis in diffuse idiopathic pulmonary neuroendocrine cell hyperplasia. ERJ Open Res. 2020 Oct;6(4).
29. Gao Y, Moua T, Midthun DE, Mullon JJ, Decker PA, Ryu JH. Diagnostic yield and bleeding complications associated with bronchoscopic biopsy of endobronchial carcinoid tumors. J Bronchology Interv Pulmonol. 2020 Jul;27(3):184–9.
30. Reuling EMBP, Dickhoff C, Plaisier PW, Coupé VMH, Mazairac AHA, Lely RJ, et al. Endobronchial treatment for bronchial carcinoid: Patient selection and predictors of outcome. Respiration. 2018;95(4):220–7.
31. Vial MR, Nasim F, La Garza H De, Ost DE, Casal RF, Eapen GA, et al. Endobronchial ultrasound- guided transbronchial needle aspiration for mediastinal lymph node staging in patients with typical pulmonary carcinoids. Lung Cancer. 2020 Sep;147:198–203.
32. Rossi G, Cavazza A, Spagnolo P, Sverzellati N, Longo L, Jukna A, et al. Diffuse idiopathic pulmonary neuroendocrine cell hyperplasia syndrome. Eur Respir J. 2016 Jun;47(6):1829–41.
33. Nassar AA, Jaroszewski DE, Helmers RA, Colby T V, Patel BM, Mookadam F. Diffuse idiopathic pulmonary neuroendocrine cell hyperplasia: A systematic overview. Am J Respir Crit Care Med. 2011 Jul;184(1):8–16.
34. Richeldi L, Launders N, Martinez F, Walsh SLF, Myers J, Wang B, et al. The characterisation of interstitial lung disease multidisciplinary team meetings: A global study. ERJ Open Res. 2019 Apr;5(2).
35. Sauer R, Griff S, Blau A, Franke A, Mairinger T, Grah C. Diffuse idiopathic pulmonary neuroendocrine cell hyperplasia diagnosed by transbronchial lung cryobiopsy: A case report. J Med Case Rep. 2017 Apr;11(1):95.
36. Patel R, Collazo-Gonzalez C, Andrews A, Johnson J, Rumbak M, Smith M. Diffuse idiopathic pulmonary neuroendocrine cell hyperplasia diagnosed by tranbronchoscopic cryoprobe biopsy technique. Respirology Case Reports. 2017;5(6):e0275.
37. Myint ZW, McCormick J, Chauhan A, Behrens E, Anthony LB. Management of diffuse idiopathic pulmonary neuroendocrine cell hyperplasia: Review and a single center experience. Lung. 2018 Oct;196(5):577–81.
38. Al-Toubah T, Strosberg J, Halfdanarson TR, Oleinikov K, Gross DJ, Haider M, et al. Somatostatin analogs improve respiratory symptoms in patients with diffuse idiopathic pulmonary neuroendocrine cell hyperplasia. Chest. 2020 Jul;158(1):401–5.
39. Zhou H, Ge Y, Janssen B, Peterson A, Takei H, Haque A, et al. Double lung transplantation for diffuse idiopathic pulmonary neuroendocrine cell hyperplasia. J Bronchology Interv Pulmonol. 2014 Oct;21(4):342–5.

22

PULMONARY AMYLOIDOSIS

Parijat Sen and Said Chaaban

Contents

Introduction 160
Nodular pulmonary amyloidosis 160
Tracheobronchial amyloidosis 163
Conclusion 166
Acknowledgments 166
References 166

KEY POINTS

- Pulmonary amyloidosis presents in one of five forms: Diffuse alveolar-septal, nodular, tracheobronchial, mediastinal nodal, and pleural.
- Most of the time, it is associated with systemic amyloidosis and treatment is geared toward systemic therapies of such.
- Local treatments can be bronchoscopic (excision, ablation, balloon dilation, stent placement) or radiation (external beam).

Introduction

The term amyloid, which means "starch-like" or "cellulose-like" was first coined in 1853 by Rudolf Virchow. Amyloids are the result of the abnormal folding of autologous proteins. The most commonly involved fibril proteins are immunoglobin light chains (AL), serum amyloid (AA), and transthyretin (ATTR) (1–3). Consequently, amyloidosis refers to the deposition of these insoluble products in the extracellular matrix, which leads to organ dysfunction. The clinical presentation of patients with amyloidosis differs depending on the involved organ and the deposition pattern. The World Health Organization has classified amyloidosis into subtypes (Table 22.1) based on the variable protein constituents (3).

Types of pulmonary amyloidosis

Amyloidosis of the pulmonary system can present either as an isolated form or as part of systemic disease (1). The isolated disease is very rare (4). The factors that may lead to deposition in the lungs are not clear. Pulmonary amyloidosis is usually recognized post-mortem, on autopsy, and rarely diagnosed clinically (5–7). Novel techniques such as positron emission tomography using radiolabeled fluorine-18 may help in the recognition of pulmonary involvement ante-mortem in individual cases (5, 8).

Lung involvement in amyloidosis has been described in five different forms: Diffuse- alveolar septal amyloidosis, nodular pulmonary amyloidosis, tracheobronchial amyloidosis, mediastinal lymph node amyloidosis, and pleural amyloidosis (1, 3).

Diffuse alveolar-septal amyloidosis

Diffuse alveolar-septal amyloidosis, also known as diffuse parenchymal amyloidosis, occurs as a result of the deposition of amyloid proteins in the alveolar septa and vessel walls. As mentioned previously, it more commonly presents as part of a systemic disease such as systemic AL amyloidosis and, to a lesser extent, systemic AA, systemic ATTR wild type, and systemic hereditary ATTR; however, isolated cases of diffuse alveolar septal amyloidosis have been reported (6, 9).

Lung involvement could range from 30–90% (5, 10). A nationwide survey of 741 patients in Japan with systemic AL amyloidosis, showed that only 1.6% (12 patients) were diagnosed with lung biopsy (1) (Figures 22.1–22.3).

On high-resolution computed tomography of the chest, reticular opacities with interlobular septal thickening are usually present. While micro-nodules are common findings, ground-glass opacities, traction bronchiectasis, and honeycombing are far less common. Bullae and cysts have been described, especially if associated with Sjögren's syndrome (6, 11–13). Concomitant mediastinal lymphadenopathy is also a common feature and it is present in 50% of the cases. Thus, although the concomitant presence of adenopathy, micro-nodules (<1.5 cm), interlobular septal thickening, and reticular opacities should raise the suspicion for the diagnosis, these findings are not pathognomonic (6, 14) and the differential diagnosis includes multiple other etiologies such as metastasis, hypersensitivity pneumonitis, coal workers pneumoconiosis, and miliary tuberculosis. This dictates a difficulty in reaching a diagnosis solely based on imaging.

As for the clinical manifestations, patients are usually symptomatic from other organ involvement rather than from lung involvement (15). However, if lung is the predominantly involved organ, then patients with diffuse parenchymal amyloidosis have a severe presentation with progressive dyspnea that is not attributed to cardiac cause (6, 11).

Nodular pulmonary amyloidosis

Nodular pulmonary amyloidosis (NPA) is a form of localized amyloidosis where one or multiple nodular deposits of amyloid are found in the lungs. These typically consist of AL or mixed light and heavy chain (AL/AH) deposits. Occasionally, NPA may be secondary to localized AA, ATTR or Aβ2M/AL. Rarely, it may be a manifestation of systemic AL disease. The mean age of the patients is 67 years, and the male:female ratio is 3:2 (9).

Localized AL amyloid differs from its systemic counterpart by the morphological appearance of the amyloid, and the presence of clonal plasma cells and giant cells. In localized amyloidosis

Pulmonary Amyloidosis

TABLE 22.1: Major Subtypes of Systemic Amyloidosis and Their Features

Type	Systemic AL Amyloidosis (Primary Amyloidosis)	Systemic AA Amyloidosis (Secondary Amyloidosis)	Systemic Wild-Type ATTR Amyloidosis (Senile Systemic Amyloidosis)	Systemic Hereditary ATTR Amyloidosis
Prevalence	60%	10%	8%	10% (1)
Acquired/Hereditary (2)	Acquired	Acquired	Acquired	Hereditary
Underlying disorder (2, 55)	Monoclonal plasma cell proliferative disorder	Secondary to chronic inflammation conditions	Wild-type transthyretin (9)	Mutations in the transthyretin gene
Pathophysiology (2)	Monoclonal immunoglobulin light chain	Tissue deposition of serum amyloid A	Deposition of unmutated transthyretin in tissues (myocardium)	Abnormal TTR
Symptoms	Nonspecific symptoms: Fatigue and weight loss	Depending on organ involved	Heart failure Arrythmia	Heart failure Arrythmia
Organ involved	Organs involved: Nephrotic syndromes, restrictive cardiomyopathy, peripheral neuropathy, hepatomegaly	Affects a variety of organs	Heart Renal (rare involvement)	Heart Renal (rare involvement)
Treatment	Chemotherapy followed by autologous stem cell transplant	Treat underlying disease	Heart failure (9) Chemotherapy or autologous stem cell transplant is contraindicated	Liver transplant (9) Chemotherapy or autologous stem cell transplant is contraindicated
Treatment target (2)	Difference between involved and uninvolved light chain <40 mg/dL	Serum Amyloid A <4 mg/L	Optimum heart failure control	Optimum heart failure, autonomic neuropathy, and peripheral neuropathy control

kappa light chains are more frequent than the lambda form, in contrast to the systemic form, where lambda chains constitute the overwhelming majority of case (16). This has led many to believe that the pathogenesis of localized AL amyloidosis may differ from that of the systemic type. Light chains that compose amyloid deposits in localized NPA are the same as those expressed by the lymphoma cells. In the past, NPA and primary pulmonary lymphoma with amyloid production were thought to be fundamentally different processes, but now many believe that most cases of NPA are the result of an underlying lymphoproliferative disorder of the MALT lymphoma type (17–19). Such lymphomas are typically indolent and mildly symptomatic, making them hard to diagnose but sensitive methods may reveal a clonal B-cell population in most cases (18–20). The finding of monotypic lymphoid cells on immunohistochemical analysis confirms the diagnosis of lymphoma.

NPA may be asymptomatic particularly if there are few nodules. In other instances, obstructive and/or restrictive pulmonary manifestations such as dry cough, shortness of breath, hemoptysis, and weight loss may be present (21, 22). However, most often the diagnosis is incidentally found on radiology or post-mortem. NPA may be associated with Sjögren's syndrome, hematologic malignancies, plasma cell dyscrasias and, thus, manifest symptoms typical of these diseases (23).

The most common computed tomography (CT) scan findings are nodules and/or cysts. The cysts seen may have variable wall

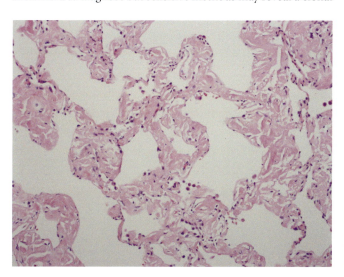

FIGURE 22.1 Hematoxylin and eosin stain of diffuse alveolar septal amyloidosis (10×).

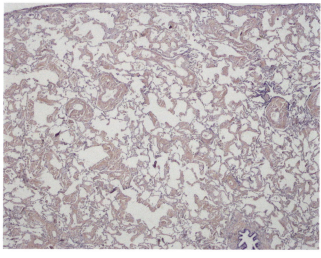

FIGURE 22.2 Diffuse alveolar septal amyloidosis under Congo red stain.

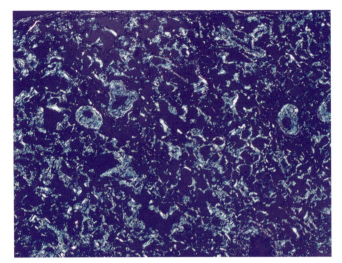

FIGURE 22.3 Diffuse alveolar septal amyloidosis with Congo red stain under polarized light showing apple green birefringence.

thickness, are predominately found in the lower lobes, and are more frequently seen with Sjögren's syndrome. These features make the cysts in NPA easily distinguishable from emphysema (21). Over time, the cysts may increase in size. As for the nodules, approximately half of them calcify but rarely do they cavitate (24) (Figures 22.4 and 22.5).

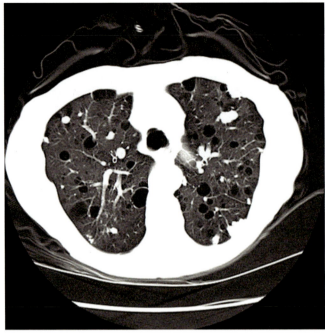

FIGURE 22.4 CT scan showing multiple pulmonary nodules and lung cysts in a patient with Sjögren's syndrome who had nodular pulmonary amyloidosis. (Image reprinted with permission from Reference [56].)

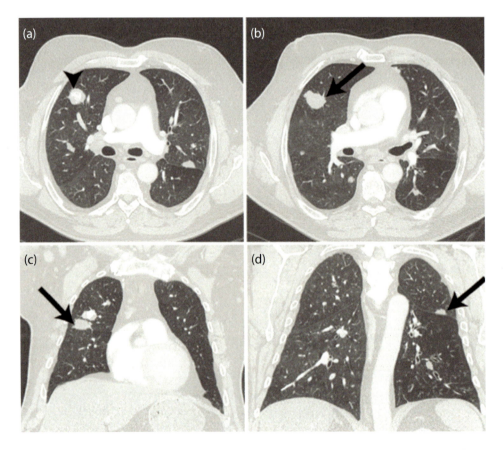

FIGURE 22.5 High-resolution chest computed tomography scans in the axial (a and b) and coronal (c and d) views of a patient with nodular pulmonary amyloidosis. (Image reprinted with permission from Reference [57].)

Pulmonary Amyloidosis

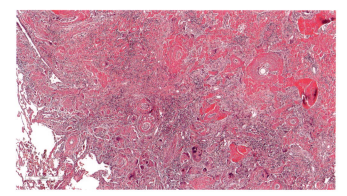

FIGURE 22.6 Nodular amyloidosis. Note nodular mass of amorphous eosinophilic material in lung parenchyma. Multinucleated giant cells are often prominent, as in this case, and can be mistaken for a granuloma (hematoxylin-eosin, 200×).

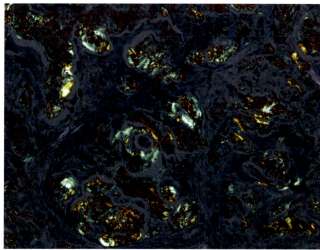

FIGURE 22.8 Appearance of nodular amyloid on Congo red stain when viewed under polarized light. Note apple-green birefringence (Congo red stain, 400×).

On gross pathology, there is typically one nodule but, rarely, additional nodules can be present. These nodules vary in size from 0.4 to 5 cm in their greatest dimension (15). Also, they are well circumscribed and are composed of homogeneous, densely eosinophilic material. Small aggregates of lymphocytes and plasma cells are usually found within or adjacent to the nodules. Foreign body giant cells, calcifications, and bony or cartilaginous areas may also be seen (9). If amyloid is suspected, Congo red staining must be done. Amyloid tissue stains with it and under polarized microscopy demonstrate the typical apple green birefringence (Figures 22.6–22.8).

Further studies include amyloid subtyping in an attempt to diagnose any underlying localized lymphoproliferative disorder. Amyloid subtyping usually reveals monoclonal immunoglobulin (Ig) light chains. In rare cases of nodular pulmonary amyloidosis, serum amyloid A or transthyretin may also be detected. Immunohistochemistry can help identify the clonality of the lympho-plasmacytic components.

One of the differentials for NPA is pulmonary hyalinizing granuloma, which often presents as an incidental solitary nodule or as multiple nodules on chest imaging studies. Histologically, it differs from NPA in its appearance; while amyloid is homogeneous in appearance, pulmonary hyalinizing granuloma is composed of thick collagen bundles arranged in lamellae (25, 26). More importantly, Congo red staining is negative in the latter. Another differential of NPA is light chain deposition disease of lung, which presents with bilateral cystic lung disease and manifests with progressively worsening symptoms often necessitating lung transplant (27). Also, the light chain fragments (typically lambda) in this disease are granular in nature and do not form the beta-pleated sheets seen in amyloid. Besides, they do not stain with Congo red stain or show birefringence.

Treatment of NPA depends on the extent of disease, its progression, and its association with other systemic conditions. Asymptomatic patients may be continued to be followed with PFTs and imaging. In case of obstructive symptoms, isolated localized NPA may need surgical resection (laser excision) (28, 29). In the presence of systemic disease, particularly systemic AL amyloidosis or progression of symptoms, systemic chemotherapy may be considered. A combination regimen of cyclophosphamide, bortezomib, and dexamethasone (CyBorD) has shown promise in stabilization of symptoms (30, 31).

Tracheobronchial amyloidosis

Tracheobronchial amyloidosis (TBA) is one of the rarer forms of pulmonary amyloidosis. Less than 150 cases of tracheobronchial amyloidosis have been described in literature. Boston University, in a 15-year experience, reported only 10 patients with this form of pulmonary amyloidosis (32). The age at presentation is usually between the fifth and sixth decade of life, though often the diagnosis is only established years after the onset of symptoms.

Unlike, nodular, and diffuse alveolar septal amyloidosis, TBA is mostly localized to the airways and is not associated with systemic amyloidosis (6, 33). Though rare, cases in association with systemic AL, AA disease, and multiple myeloma (MM) have been described, and the development of TBA is attributed to the deposition of monoclonal Ig light chains produced locally by small number of lymphoplasma cells (34). However, it's hard to establish given that the number of these cells are very low.

The most common symptom of TBA is cough, particularly when there is laryngeal involvement. Other symptoms include dyspnea (specifically with stenosis), hoarseness of voice,

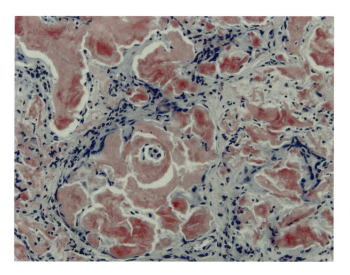

FIGURE 22.7 Appearance of nodular amyloid on Congo red stain. Note salmon pink color (Congo red stain, 400C×).

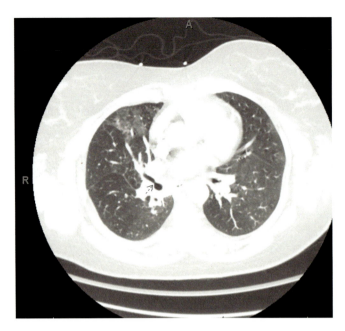

FIGURE 22.9 CT chest showing endobronchial lesion of tracheobronchial amyloidosis.

hemoptysis, and recurrent post-obstructive pneumonias (9, 15). The pulmonary function test is often normal in case of distal airway involvement. In case of more proximal airway involvement, there may be a decrease in flows, which along with wheezing may lead to it being misdiagnosed as asthma (9, 32). Attention should be paid to flow volume loops for evidence of fixed obstruction, particularly in tracheal stenosis from amyloid. CT scans may show thickening of tracheobronchial wall (Figure 22.9) with or without calcification (32, 35). A distinguishing feature from tracheobronchopathia osteochondroplastica (TPO) that also demonstrates airway calcification is that TPO typically spares the posterior wall as opposed to amyloidosis (9, 35).

On bronchoscopy, the commonest finding is thickening and/or irregularity of the bronchial mucosa as a result of submucosal deposits (9). Other findings may include multifocal irregular grayish white plaques or even raised mass-like lesions of amyloid material (Figure 22.10), which can be confused with malignancy (6, 36). Biopsy for histopathologic diagnosis remains the mainstay of diagnosis, but one must be careful about bleeding as these lesions are friable in nature. Histopathology typically reveals submucosal deposits of amorphous, eosinophilic material (Figure 22.11) surrounding submucosal glands and occasionally shows cartilage plates and small vessels as well (9, 15, 34). The material stains with Congo red under polarized microscopy shows apple green birefringence (15, 34). Immunofluorescence typically shows lambda light chains as AL is the most common type of amyloidosis in these cases.

The management of TBA depends on the constellation of symptoms and disease complications. Obstructive symptoms such as dyspnea, atelectasis, and pneumonia secondary to major airway involvement/stenosis often require local therapies. Endoscopic interventions such as mechanical debridement, laser ablation, balloon dilatation, and stent placements are required in case of a focal involvement of a major airway. However, the problem of these endoscopic managements is the high risk of recurrence and thus the need for frequent repetitive procedures (32, 37, 38). Another therapeutic option is external beam radiation where CT simulation is used to plan the radiation field followed by a targeted radiation aimed at suppressing the locally responsible clonal B cells within the tissue (38, 39). This method has been reported to be successful in terms of reduction in lesion size but that is associated with airway edema (32, 40). Complications of using external beam radiation include local effects of radiation such as radiation pneumonitis, cutaneous manifestations, as well as a minor risk of secondary cancer (41).

Systemic chemotherapy and steroids have been studied in refractory TBA and in TBA associated with systemic AL amyloidosis with only modest benefits seen at best (32, 42). Rituximab, a monoclonal anti-CD20 molecule, has been also studied, but the results were not encouraging. One needs to demonstrate local B-cell clonal proliferation before considering Rituximab therapy and even then, other considerations remain such as: Stage of differentiation for B cells, as amyloidosis often involves plasma cells which do not express CD-20, as well as efficacy of intravenous

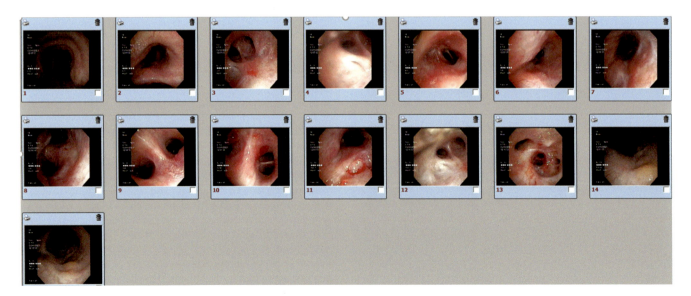

FIGURE 22.10 Bronchoscopic images showing nodular lesions of tracheobronchial amyloidosis. Notice the presence of lesions in the posterior wall, which helps distinguish it from tracheobronchopathia osteochondroplastica.

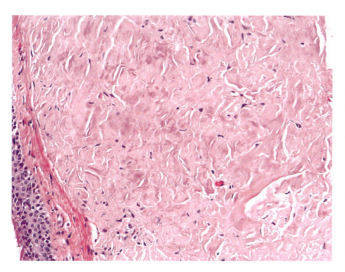

FIGURE 22.11 Tracheobronchial amyloidosis. Note the mass of amorphous eosinophilic material in tracheal mucosa (hematoxylin-eosin, 200×).

Rituximab penetrating the amyloid deposits. Other potential therapies holding promise such as intravenous antibodies directed against serum amyloid P component to eliminate tissue amyloid deposits still need clinical trials (43).

Pleural effusions in amyloidosis

Pleural effusions have been described in up to 30% of patients with systemic amyloidosis (44, 45). The pleural effusions in amyloidosis are usually a consequence of heart failure and, thus, are transudative in nature (46). Other less common causes of pleural effusions in amyloidosis include nephrotic syndrome, liver failure, and direct deposition into the pleura (44). Involvement of the pleura happens as a result of the direct infiltration of the parietal pleural and is usually part of AL (45, 46). The amyloid deposits lead to the disruption of the parietal pleura, which subsequently leads to fluid accumulation in the pleural space (46). Consequently, a unilateral exudative pleural effusion with lymphocytic predominance is evident (Figure 22.12). In rare instances, chylous effusions may develop when there is lymphatic infiltration (46–48). This entity is usually missed or misdiagnosed due to the lack of specificity of the clinical and radiological findings. (49)

Diagnosis is usually established via biopsy obtained either by thoracoscopy or by open-lung biopsy (44). On thoracoscopy, note is made of hyperemia of the pleural surface and inflammation with nodular lesions or brown lesions of the parietal pleura (49). Special stains such as crystal violet or Congo red applied to the tissue is needed for definitive diagnosis (44). Apple green birefringence appearance under polarized light seen with Congo red stain is the gold standard for diagnosis (49).

Initial management would include large volume thoracentesis with attempts for diuresis. This could be challenging as patients may suffer from autonomic neuropathy, decreased cardiac output, and kidney involvement. When thoracentesis becomes needed on a weekly basis, alternative approaches such as pleurodesis, chest tube thoracostomy, video assisted thoracoscopy with talc insufflation, or tunneled pleural catheter insertion can be entertained (46).

Mediastinal amyloidosis

Mediastinal and hilar lymphadenopathy are most commonly seen in systemic AL amyloidosis, but rarely seen in localized disease (12, 13, 50). Lymph node involvement can be localized to one station or spread over multiple stations. The localized amyloidoma may happen in any of the compartments of the mediastinum (13). Amyloidomas are well-circumscribed amorphous eosinophilic amyloid proteins, surrounded by an inflammatory cell infiltrate that is made up of plasma cells and lymphocytes, which often leads to a granulomatous reaction (8).

Mediastinal and hilar adenopathy can be present as a solitary finding or as association with parenchymal disease as seen in 50% of the cases (12). Presentation is mainly asymptomatic, however symptoms may arise depending on the anatomical location of the lesion. On imaging, variable forms of calcification are recognized and those include punctate, diffuse, or eggshell (13, 51). Biopsy of the lymph nodes may be diagnostic and the biopsy could be done either via mediastinoscopy or endobronchial ultrasound-guided transbronchial fine needle aspiration (51). The yield of the latter is unknown as the data is limited.

Pulmonary hypertension related to amyloidosis

Amyloid commonly deposits in the pulmonary vessels, but rarely gives rise to pulmonary hypertension (PH). If present, PH usually belongs to group 2, which is secondary to restrictive cardiomyopathy, or group 3, which is secondary to underlying diffuse lung disease, and rarely to group 1, which is secondary to pulmonary arterial hypertension. The latter happens only if the amyloid was deposited in the media layer of pulmonary vessels. PH may also occur in systemic AL amyloidosis but rarely in in AA amyloidosis. Infrequently, this deposition in blood vessel may manifest as bronchial bleeding secondary to arterial dissection, pulmonary hematomas, or arteriovenous fistulas (9, 52, 53).

Pulmonary function testing is notable for restriction with reduced diffusing capacity. Hypoxia is present on exertion and is recorded on a multi-oximetry evaluation of a 6-minute walk testing (9).

While lung involvement is recognized in 50–92% of the patients with systemic amyloidosis post mortem, bronchoscopic transbronchial biopsy can be done to help in diagnosis antemortem in selective cases. Caution is advised when attempting transbronchial biopsy, as patients with AL amyloidosis are at a higher bleeding risk that may predispose to a significant pulmonary hemorrhage (1, 8, 54).

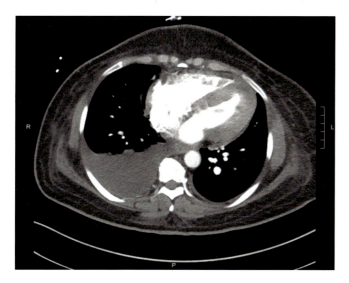

FIGURE 22.12 Moderate right-sided pleural effusion in a patient with AL amyloidosis-associated nephrotic syndrome.

On autopsy, the lungs are rubbery with a sponge-like appearance. It usually involves all lobes and in some cases, the visceral pleura can be involved as well.

Management is to target and treat the underlying disease. In AL amyloidosis, treatment aims at reducing the concentration of free light chains. This is not only associated with an improved organ function but also with prolonged survival (1). Chemotherapeutic regimens used are extrapolated from regimens initially developed for MM. It should be noted that patients with AL amyloidosis are at a higher risk of death after treatment as compared to MM patients. Close monitoring is essential and the frequent evaluation of effectiveness of the chemotherapeutic regimens is important (3).

Autologous stem cell transplant could be considered essentially only in patients with a diffusion capacity >50% (9). The impact of this treatment on pulmonary involvement has not been reported. Lung transplantation could be considered in cases where there is an isolated involvement of the lung.

Conclusion

Pulmonary amyloidosis is a rare entity that often presents as sequelae of multi-organ involvement in systemic amyloidosis. There are some forms of pulmonary amyloidosis that may be isolated and localized, mostly associated with local B-cell proliferations and Ig production. Pulmonary amyloidosis may mimic multiple conditions, particularly interstitial lung diseases and malignancy, and diagnosis is confirmed by histopathology, particularly with specific stains like Congo red. Management often revolves around management of underlying systemic diseases. In some conditions, they can be locally managed through bronchoscopic procedures or radiation.

Acknowledgments

- Dr. Sanjay Mukopadhyay, MD, Director, Pulmonary Pathology, Cleveland Clinic, Cleveland, OH
- Dr. Abdul Kareem Uduman, MD, Faculty, Division of Pulmonary and Critical Care Medicine, Henry Ford Hospital, Detroit, MI
- Dr. Suha Jabak, MD, Fellow, American University of Beirut, Beirut, Lebanon
- Dr. Atreyee Basu, MD, Fellow, Cardio-Thoracic Pathology, Department of Pathology, NYU Langone Health, NY

References

1. Yamada, M., et al., Amyloidosis of the respiratory system: 16 patients with amyloidosis initially diagnosed ante mortem by pulmonologists. ERJ Open Research, 2020. **6**(3).
2. Wechalekar, A.D., J.D. Gillmore, and P.N. Hawkins, Systemic amyloidosis. The Lancet, 2016. **387**(10038): p. 2641–2654.
3. de Almeida, R.R., et al., Respiratory tract amyloidosis. state-of-the-art review with a focus on pulmonary involvement. Lung, 2015. **193**(6): p. 875–883.
4. Chu, H., et al., Clinical characteristics of amyloidosis with isolated respiratory system involvement: A review of 13 cases. Ann Thorac Med, 2012. **7**(4): p. 243.
5. Ussavarungsi, K., et al., Clinical relevance of pulmonary amyloidosis: An Analysis of 76 autopsy-derived cases. Eur Respir J, 2017. **49**(2).
6. Utz, J.P., S.J. Swensen, and M.A. Gertz, Pulmonary amyloidosis. The Mayo clinic experience from 1980 to 1993. Ann Intern Med, 1996. **124**(4): p. 407–413.
7. Kim, C.H., et al., Pulmonary diffuse alveolar septal amyloidosis: Diagnosed by transbronchial lung biopsy. Korean J Intern Med, 1990. **5**(1): p. 63.
8. Narechania, S., et al., A 70-year-old man with large cervical and mediastinal lymphadenopathies. Chest, 2015. **148**(1): p. e8–e13.
9. Milani, P., et al., The lung in amyloidosis. Eur Respir Rev, 2017. **26**(145).
10. Smith, R.R., et al., Type and distribution of pulmonary parenchymal and vascular amyloid: Correlation with cardiac amyloidosis. Am J Med, 1979. **66**(1): p. 96–104.
11. Pickford, H., S. Swensen, and J. Utz, Thoracic cross-sectional imaging of amyloidosis. Am J Roentgenol, 1997. **168**(2): p. 351–355.
12. Aylwin, A.C., P. Gishen, and S.J. Copley, Imaging appearance of thoracic amyloidosis. J Thorac Imaging, 2005. **20**(1): p. 41–46.
13. Czeyda-Pommersheim, F., et al., Amyloidosis: Modern cross-sectional imaging. Radiographics, 2015. **35**(5): p. 1381–1392.
14. Jeong, Y.J., et al., Amyloidosis and lymphoproliferative disease in Sjögren syndrome: Thin-section computed tomography findings and histopathologic comparisons. J Comput Assist Tomogr, 2004. **28**(6): p. 776–781.
15. Khoor, A. and T.V. Colby, Amyloidosis of the lung. Arch Pathol Lab Med, 2017. **141**(2): p. 247–254.
16. Westermark, P., Localized AL amyloidosis: A suicidal neoplasm? Upsala J Med Sci, 2012. **117**(2): p. 244–250.
17. Dacic, S., T.V. Colby, and S.A. Yousem, Nodular amyloidoma and primary pulmonary lymphoma with amyloid production: A differential diagnostic problem. Modern Pathol, 2000. **13**(9): p. 934–940.
18. Grogg, K.L., et al., Nodular pulmonary amyloidosis is characterized by localized immunoglobulin deposition and is frequently associated with an indolent B-cell lymphoproliferative disorder. Am J Surg Pathol, 2013. **37**(3): p. 406–412.
19. Lim, J., et al., Pulmonary marginal zone lymphoma of MALT type as a cause of localised pulmonary amyloidosis. J Clin Pathol, 2001. **54**(8): p. 642–646.
20. Miyamoto, T., et al., Monoclonality of infiltrating plasma cells in primary pulmonary nodular amyloidosis: Detection with polymerase chain reaction. J Clin Pathol, 1999. **52**(6): p. 464–467.
21. Zamora, A.C., et al., Amyloid-associated cystic lung disease. Chest, 2016. **149**(5): p. 1223–1233.
22. Core, J.M., et al., Nodular pulmonary amyloidosis: A complex disease with malignancy association. Case Reports, 2017. p. bcr-2017-220428.
23. Gómez Correa, G.A., et al., Nodular pulmonary amyloidosis: A manifestation of Sjögren's syndrome. Case Reports in Pulmonology, 2018.
24. Lachmann, H. and P. Hawkins, Amyloidosis and the lung. Chron Respir Dis, 2006. **3**(4): p. 203–214.
25. Engleman, P., et al., Pulmonary hyalinizing granuloma. Am Rev Respir Dis, 1977. **115**(6): p. 997–1008.
26. Yousem, S.A. and L. Hochholzer, Pulmonary hyalinizing granuloma. Am J Clin Pathology, 1987. **87**(1): p. 1–6.
27. Colombat, M., et al., Pulmonary cystic disorder related to light chain deposition disease. Am J Respir Crit Care Med, 2006. **173**(7): p. 777–780.
28. Fujiwara, S., et al., A case of isolated nodular pulmonary amyloidosis. Kyobu Geka. Japanese Journal of Thoracic Surgery, 1986. **39**(12): p. 986–989.
29. Nugent, A., et al., Pulmonary amyloidosis: Treatment with laser therapy and systemic steroids. Respir Med, 1996. **90**(7): p. 433–435.
30. Mahmood, S., et al., Update on treatment of light chain amyloidosis. Haematologica, 2014. **99**(2): p. 209.
31. Palladini, G., et al., A European collaborative study of cyclophosphamide, bortezomib, and dexamethasone in upfront treatment of systemic AL amyloidosis. Blood, J Am Soc Hematol, 2015. **126**(5): p. 612–615.
32. O'Regan, A., et al., Tracheobronchial amyloidosis. The Boston University experience from 1984 to 1999. Medicine, 2000. **79**(2): p. 69–79.
33. Da Costa, P. and B. Corrin, Amyloidosis localized to the lower respiratory tract: Probable immunoamyloid nature of the tracheobronchial and nodular pulmonary forms. Histopathology, 1985. **9**(7): p. 703–710.

34. Borie, R., et al., Tracheobronchial amyloidosis: Evidence for local B-cell clonal expansion. Eur Respir J, 2012. **39**(4): p. 1042–1045.
35. Crestani, B., et al., Tracheobronchial amyloidosis with hilar lymphadenopathy associated with a serum monoclonal immunoglobulin. Eur Respir J, 1993. **6**(10): p. 1569–1571.
36. Prince, J.S., et al., Nonneoplastic lesions of the tracheobronchial wall: Radiologic findings with bronchoscopic correlation. Radiographics, 2002. **22**(suppl_1): p. S215–S230.
37. Hui, A., et al., Amyloidosis presenting in the lower respiratory tract. Clinicopathologic, radiologic, immunohistochemical, and histochemical studies on 48 cases. Arch Pathol Lab Med, 1986. **110**(3): p. 212–218.
38. Capizzi, S.A., E. Betancourt, and U.B. Prakash. Tracheobronchial Amyloidosis. in Mayo Clinic Proceedings. 2000. Elsevier.
39. Monroe, A.T., et al., Tracheobronchial amyloidosis: A case report of successful treatment with external beam radiation therapy. Chest, 2004. **125**(2): p. 784–789.
40. Shinoi, K., Y. Shiraishi, and J.I. Yahata, Amyloid tumor of the trachea and lung, resembling bronchial asthma: Case report. Dis Chest, 1962. **42**(4): p. 442–445.
41. Ng, A.K., et al., Second malignancy after Hodgkin disease treated with radiation therapy with or without chemotherapy: Long-term risks and risk factors. Blood, J Am Soc Hematol, 2002. **100**(6): p. 1989–1996.
42. Jaccard, A., et al., High-dose melphalan versus melphalan plus dexamethasone for AL amyloidosis. New Engl J Med, 2007. **357**(11): p. 1083–1093.
43. Bodin, K., et al., Antibodies to human serum amyloid p component eliminate visceral amyloid deposits. Nature, 2010. **468**(7320): p. 93–97.
44. Kavuru, M.S., et al., Amyloidosis and pleural disease. Chest, 1990. **98**(1): p. 20–23.
45. Berk, J.L., et al., Persistent pleural effusions in primary systemic amyloidosis: Etiology and prognosis. Chest, 2003. **124**(3): p. 969–977.
46. Berk, J.L., Pleural effusions in systemic amyloidosis. Current Opinion in Pulmonary Medicine, 2005. **11**(4): p. 324–328.
47. Maskell, N. and R. Butland, BTS guidelines for the investigation of a unilateral pleural effusion in adults. Thorax, 2003. **58**(Suppl 2): p. ii8.
48. Scala, R., et al., Amyloidosis involving the respiratory system: 5-year's experience of a multi-disciplinary group's activity. Annals of Thoracic Medicine, 2015. **10**(3): p. 212.
49. Dai, Y., et al., Pleural amyloidosis with recurrent pleural effusion and pulmonary embolism: A case report. Medicine, 2019. **98**(3).
50. Plöckinger, B., M. Müller, and F. Eckersberger, Isolated amyloidosis of hilar lymph nodes. Langenbecks Archiv fur Chirurgie, 1993. **378**(3): p. 167–170.
51. Ordemann, J., et al., Isolated amyloid tumor in the mediastinum: Report of a case. Surgery Today, 2003. **33**(3): p. 202–204.
52. Eder, L., et al., Pulmonary hypertension and amyloidosis—an uncommon association: A case report and review of the literature. J Gen Intern Med, 2007. **22**(3): p. 416–419.
53. Cirulis, M.M., et al., Pulmonary arterial hypertension in primary amyloidosis. Pulmonary Circulation, 2016. **6**(2): p. 244–248.
54. Govender, P., et al., Transbronchial biopsies safely diagnose amyloid lung disease. Amyloid, 2017. **24**(1): p. 37–41.
55. Sipe, J.D., et al., Amyloid fibril proteins and amyloidosis: Chemical identification and clinical classification International Society of Amyloidosis 2016 nomenclature guidelines. Amyloid, 2016. **23**(4): p. 209–213.
56. Sen P, Chang B. Medical image of the week: Pulmonary amyloidosis in primary Sjögren's syndrome. Southwest J Pulm Crit Care. 2018;**16**(6):336–7.
57. Al-Umairi RS, Al-Lawati F, Al-Busaidi FM. Nodular pulmonary amyloidosis mimicking metastatic pulmonary nodules: A case report and review of the literature. Sultan Qaboos Univ Med J. 2018 Aug;**18**(3):e393–e396.

23

PRIMARY TRACHEAL TUMORS

Moiz Salahuddin and Carlos A. Jimenez

Contents

Introduction...168
Tracheal anatomy and embryology...168
Clinical presentation...169
Diagnostic studies...169
Management and treatment...170
Survival and follow-up..170
Types of tracheal tumors..170
Conclusion...176
References...176

KEY POINTS

- Primary tracheal tumors arise from the wall of the trachea and are commonly malignant tumors.
- Primary tracheal tumors are extremely rare, with an incidence of 2.6 per 1 million cases, and account for 0.2% of malignant tumors of the respiratory tract.
- The most common malignant tracheal tumor is squamous cell carcinoma, followed by adenoid cystic carcinoma.
- Commonly reported benign tracheal tumors are squamous papilloma and nerve sheath tumors.
- Surgical resection for local disease is the best option for cure. If it is unresectable, then radiation and/or therapeutic bronchoscopy can be considered.
- Patients with malignant tracheal tumors have an overall 5-year survival rate of 52%.

Introduction

Primary tracheal tumors include benign and malignant conditions originating from the wall of the trachea. These tumors are rare and have an approximate annual incidence of 1 in 10,000–1 million people (1, 2). The largest population-based study on tracheal tumors was the Surveillance, Epidemiology, and End Results (SEER) study, which found an incidence of 2.6 per 1 million cases (3). Tracheal tumors account for 0.2% of malignant tumors of the respiratory tract and 0.01% of all malignant tumors (4). Due to the low incidence of primary tracheal tumors, data are sparse and are mainly from case reports or retrospective reviews collected over many decades.

Any pathology involving the tracheal structures or causing their extrinsic compression (i.e., from surrounding mediastinal structures) can disturb tracheal function and lead to symptoms. For example, systemic diseases such as relapsing polychondritis, polyangiitis with granulomatosis, or sarcoidosis can affect the trachea. Some diseases are limited to the trachea (e.g., tracheal stenosis, tracheal webs, and tracheal tumors). Tumors affecting the trachea mostly originate in surrounding structures, such as the lung, thyroid, esophagus, and larynx, and extend directly into the trachea (5). Tracheal tumors can also occur due to metastatic spread from melanoma or any solid organ malignancy; spread from breast, colon, and renal tumors is the most frequent.

In this chapter, we will discuss primary tracheal tumors that originate from the tracheal wall. We will also discuss tracheal anatomy and delve into the clinical presentation, evaluation, management, and prognosis of tracheal tumors. Finally, we will address some of the more common primary tracheal tumors.

Tracheal anatomy and embryology

The trachea is a cylindrical tube through which air enters the bronchi and, ultimately, the alveoli. Its cervical portion extends from the larynx caudally at the level of C6 and runs anteriorly ending at the level of the sternal notch. Distal to the sternal notch, the thoracic portion of the trachea moves posteriorly and ends in the main carina (6). The main carina is where the trachea divides into the left and right main stem bronchi at the level of the fourth thoracic vertebra, posterior to the sternal angle and the division of the main pulmonary artery trunk (7). The average tracheal diameter is 23 mm in men and 20 mm in women (8). The trachea contains about 18–22 cartilages along its length. The average length of the trachea is 10–12 cm (8). The tracheal wall is approximately 3 mm thick; therefore, if any area looks larger than that on computed tomography (CT) imaging, one should be concerned about tracheal pathology (6, 8). The posterior wall of the trachea is in contact with the anterior wall of the esophagus. The trachea and main carina have sensitive receptors that trigger coughing to protect the airway in case of aspiration.

The tracheal wall consists of four histological layers: The mucosa, the submucosa, the musculo-cartilaginous layer, and the adventitia (8). The mucosa is lined by pseudostratified ciliary columnar epithelial cells, the primary function of which is the clearance of secretions. The submucosa consists of connective tissue with goblet cells, brush cells, and neuroendocrine cells (7).

The anterior and lateral aspects of the trachea have C-shaped cartilaginous rings that prevent the trachea's collapse and a posterior membranous wall that moves and narrows its lumen to facilitate the movement of secretions outwards during coughing (6, 8). The trachea has stem cells that regenerate the epithelium. Recently, a multipotent stem cell that can differentiate into secretory cells and ciliated epithelial cells was described. These cells can survive a severe ischemic injury, and the study of their characteristics and function may provide unique insights into tracheal pathology (7).

The arteries that nourish the trachea enter the tracheal wall laterally at different segments. The cervical trachea is supplied by branches of the inferior thyroid artery, a branch of the thyrocervical trunk (6, 8, 9). The thoracic trachea's blood supply comes from the bronchial arteries that are usually branches of the aorta (6, 8). The lymphatic drainage flows to the pretracheal or paratracheal lymph nodes. The trachea receives innervation from the pulmonary plexus. The recurrent laryngeal nerve travels on the left lateral aspect of the cervical trachea, and its impingement can lead to left vocal cord paralysis (6, 9).

At the fourth week of gestation, an outgrowth of the foregut endoderm leads to a respiratory diverticulum. The interaction between the respiratory diverticulum and the surrounding mesoderm, which is driven by multiple signaling pathways, leads to the differentiation of the trachea and the formation of the right and left lung buds. The tracheal epithelium and glands are derived from the endoderm of the foregut, and the tracheal smooth muscle, connective tissue, and cartilage are derived from visceral mesoderm. As the respiratory diverticulum grows, mesodermal folds — called the tracheoesophageal ridges — form and separate the trachea from the esophagus. By the 10th week of gestation, the tracheal endoderm proliferates and then recanalizes the lumen (7). The etiology and rarity of primary tracheal tumors compared with primary lung tumors cannot be explained embryologically, as the lungs are derived from the trachea.

Clinical presentation

Primary tracheal tumors can present with symptoms such as cough, hemoptysis, wheezing, or dyspnea on exertion. The severity of the symptoms depends on the degree of involvement of the tracheal lumen. Often, tracheal tumors are detected incidentally in patients undergoing chest imaging for unrelated reasons. The diagnosis is often delayed as patients may be asymptomatic early in the course of the disease. Alternatively, patients may have symptoms that are insidious in onset at which time more common causes of chronic cough or shortness of breath are often pursued, resulting in delayed diagnosis. The average time from symptom onset to the diagnosis of a primary tracheal tumor is approximately 12 months, but some studies report delays of up to 20 months (10, 11). Patients are more often diagnosed between the fourth and sixth decades of life, and men are more commonly affected than women (2).

Malignant tumors tend to grow more quickly than benign tumors, leading to quicker symptom progression. Malignant tumors are also more likely to present with hemoptysis, whereas benign tumors are more likely to present with cough and dyspnea (12). Cough is a common initial symptom, especially in those with larger tumors. Tracheal tumors should be in the differential diagnoses of patients with chronic cough who do not improve with empirical treatment of upper airway cough syndrome, gastroesophageal reflux disease, chronic obstructive pulmonary disease, or asthma (13).

Any mucosal breakdown in the tracheobronchial tree can lead to hemoptysis, and a tracheal tumor with mucosal invasion can also cause the condition. Hemoptysis due to tracheal tumors is generally low in volume and contains fresh blood that usually is not mixed with sputum. Large tracheal tumors can cause obstruction of the tracheal lumen. When an obstruction exceeds 50% of the tracheal diameter at any point along its length, air flow limitation and related symptoms, including dyspnea on exertion, orthopnea, wheezing, and stridor, may occur. The degree of symptoms is usually inversely proportional to the residual tracheal lumen diameter. Stridor at rest is usually observed when the tracheal lumen is <5 mm in diameter. Other less common symptoms that may be present are hoarseness, dysphagia, sore throat, wheezing, and weight loss (11, 13). Tumors may be located in either the cervical or the thoracic portion of the trachea, but they occur more frequently in the cervical portion (11).

Diagnostic studies

Tracheal tumors may be detected incidentally on a chest CT scan or during bronchoscopy. When a patient presents with persistent symptoms of shortness of breath, chronic cough, hemoptysis, or stridor and no other clear etiology is found, the presence of a tracheal tumor should be considered. A chest radiograph may be the first diagnostic image available. It is abnormal for approximately 50% of tracheal tumors, but small tracheal lesions may be undetected (13). An irregular tracheal lumen will be seen if the tracheal lesion is larger than 1 cm. A CT scan of the chest should be obtained if any abnormality is observed in the trachea on a chest radiograph or if the chest radiograph is normal but there is a high suspicion of a tracheal lesion. A CT scan of the chest would show a tracheal mass or an irregular thickening in the tracheal mucosa. The differential diagnosis for tracheal abnormalities seen on CT scans includes tracheal tumors, mucoid impactions, blood clots, metastatic disease, granulation tissue, and tracheal webs.

All patients with a suspected tracheal lesion on a CT scan of the chest should undergo bronchoscopy. Malignant tumors may erode the tracheal mucosa; however, the appearance of a tracheal mass on bronchoscopy would not help differentiate between a malignant or benign condition. Therefore, these lesions should be biopsied to obtain a pathological diagnosis. Tracheal tumors that are not highly vascularized and are not significantly obstructing the tracheal lumen can be biopsied using flexible bronchoscopy. However, rigid bronchoscopy is the preferred approach when these lesions cause significant tracheal obstruction or appear to be highly vascularized. During bronchoscopy, the tracheal length affected by the tumor should be measured as the affected length is one of the factors that could determine if surgical resection is feasible.

Although video laryngoscopy can be effectively used to assess cervical tracheal tumors, it may miss up to 75% of tracheal tumors (13). Thus, to make a definitive diagnosis, bronchoscopy should be performed. Preoperative positron emission tomography (PET) scans may help assess the extent of disease, regional and distant metastatic lesions, and resection feasibility. PET uptake is typically high in squamous cell carcinoma (SCC) and variable in adenoid cystic carcinoma (ACC) and mucoepidermoid carcinoma (14).

Pulmonary function tests may show changes suggestive of central airway obstruction, including fixed airway obstruction and variable intra- or extrathoracic obstruction patterns, on the flow volume loops. These findings cannot be used to make any specific diagnosis, but patients should be further evaluated to explain the cause of the abnormality. In patients with diagnosed tracheal tumors, pulmonary function tests may help assess the degree of respiratory limitation due to the tracheal obstruction and monitor the response to treatment.

Management and treatment

There is no TNM (tumor, nodes, metastases) staging system for primary tracheal tumors. A few studies have attempted to develop one; however, due to the low prevalence of these tumors, TNM proposals are difficult to develop and validate (15, 16). There is no evidence to support invasive mediastinal staging with endobronchial ultrasound or mediastinoscopy, although this strategy could be considered an important tool for the evaluation of patients who are not ideal candidates for surgical resection. A PET scan should be performed to identify local and regional spread.

The primary treatment for tracheal tumors consists of surgery and/or radiation therapy. Patients who undergo surgery for primary tracheal tumors have better outcomes than those who receive radiation therapy alone (3). For primary malignant tracheal tumors, complete surgical resection should be considered when possible. The maximum resectable length is 4–5 cm of the trachea or eight tracheal rings, which allows an end-to-end anastomosis with acceptable tension (9). Decisions on resectability are based on imaging studies and the expertise of the surgical team. Approximately 50–70% of patients have resectable disease at diagnosis. For patients with malignant tumors, systematic lymph node dissection is avoided to preserve the tracheal blood supply. The resection is judged to be complete when airway margins are disease-free (17). The operative mortality rate is approximately 7% but may have declined to 3% in recent years (3, 10, 17).

Radiation therapy with curative intent is the treatment alternative if the patient is not a candidate for surgical resection due to the patient's extent of disease or inability to tolerate the surgical procedure. It was recently shown that the median overall survival was 48 months for patients with malignant tracheal tumors treated with primary radiation therapy compared with 180 months for patients whose tumors were surgically resected. However, the patients who underwent primary radiation therapy were more likely than those who underwent surgery to have comorbidities and a worse performance status to begin with (4). Adjuvant radiation therapy should be considered when surgical resection margins have malignant involvement. In patients who do not undergo resection, radiation therapy is associated with improved survival in those with regional disease and squamous cell histology (11, 17, 18).

Patients who are not candidates for surgical resection could be evaluated for therapeutic bronchoscopy. The objective of the therapeutic bronchoscopy is to palliate symptoms; it is rarely curative. Rigid bronchoscopy is the optimal approach when a bronchoscopic intervention for a tracheal tumor is planned. Various methods such as electrocautery snare, cryotherapy, micro-debridement, argon plasma coagulation, and coring the tumor with the rigid bronchoscope itself can be used for endoscopic resection. However, because most tracheal tumors have extraluminal components that cannot be resected endoscopically, these methods of resection may not provide definitive therapy for tumor control. In such cases, adjuvant radiotherapy could be added. Due to substantial tracheal obstruction in some cases, tracheal stenting with silicone or metallic stents may be necessary to improve dyspnea.

All benign tracheal tumors should be considered for surgical resection. These benign tumors are unlikely to recur and usually do not need adjuvant therapies. Patients with these tumors can be monitored for recurrence with surveillance CT or bronchoscopy. If patients are not good candidates for surgery, then endoscopic resection using rigid bronchoscopy can be considered as an alternative.

Survival and follow-up

Patients with malignant tracheal tumors have an overall 5-year survival rate of 52% and an overall 10-year survival rate of 29% (3, 19). Patients with localized disease have better outcomes than those with regional or distant disease. Other factors associated with poor prognosis include older age, SCC, and presence of regional or distant metastatic disease. Factors associated with good prognosis include ACC or sarcoma and tumors where surgical resection has negative margins (2, 3). Overall survival has improved over the last four decades, likely due to early detection, improvements in CT imaging and bronchoscopy, and improved surgery and radiation techniques for patients with advanced disease (3, 17). However, it must be kept in mind that, due to the rarity of these diseases, survival outcomes presented in the literature are derived from small cohorts and therefore may not be generalizable to all patients.

Patients undergoing surgical resection should be monitored periodically to identify disease recurrence. For slow-growing tumors, long periods of surveillance are suggested. The authors recommend a CT scan of the chest once a year for the first 3 years, followed by once every 2 years up to 10 years following surgical resection. If there is any abnormality found on CT imaging, a bronchoscopic exam is warranted to evaluate the findings. PET scans may not help detect early or slow-growing tumors; therefore, we do not recommend PET scanning for surveillance imaging. If patients have symptoms suggestive of recurrence, such as dyspnea, wheezing, coughing, or hemoptysis, then they should have a CT scan of the chest and a bronchoscopy.

Types of tracheal tumors

Most primary tracheal tumors (55–90%) are malignant. Approximately 50–70% of primary tracheal tumors are SCC (2, 3). ACC is the second-most-common tracheal tumor (approximately 10–15% of cases) (2, 3). However, there may be variations based on demographics and population, as a study in China showed that ACC was the most common primary tracheal tumor (50.7%), followed by SCC (30.4%) (11). Aside from SCC and ACC, the other types of malignant primary tracheal tumors are mucoepidermoid carcinomas, sarcomas, carcinoid tumors, and lymphomas (12, 20). Table 23.1 lists the different types of tracheal tumors. Figures 23.1–23.3 show the radiologic and bronchoscopic appearances of some rare tracheal tumors.

Malignant tumors
Squamous cell carcinoma
SCC is the most common type of primary tracheal tumor. Histologically, SCCs of the trachea appear similar to those of the lung or larynx, but they occur much less frequently. They are usually not related to human papillomavirus (HPV) infection, which causes benign squamous papillomas and only rarely leads to malignant transformation and SCC. Histologically, these tumors are characterized by squamous differentiation with or without keratinization (19, 20).

Primary Tracheal Tumors

TABLE 23.1: Types of Tracheal Tumors

Common Malignant Tumors
Squamous cell carcinomas
Adenoid cystic carcinomas

Rare Malignant Tumors
Mucoepidermoid carcinomas
Adenocarcinomas
Sarcomas
Carcinoid tumors
Lymphomas
Chondrosarcomas
Small cell carcinomas
Melanomas

Common Benign Tumors
Tracheobronchopathia osteochondroplastica lesions
Squamous papillomas
Schwannomas/paragangliomas
Glomus tumors

Rare Benign Tumors
Hamartomas
Chondromas
Hemangiomas
Pleomorphic adenomas
Myxomas
Fibrous histiocytomas
Granular cell tumors
Leiomyomas

SCC of the trachea is more commonly seen in men than in women (4:1 ratio), smokers, and patients above the age of 60 (4, 13). Prior radiotherapy to the chest and neck may also be a predisposing factor (13). SCC usually grows as a polypoid and ulcerative mass that projects into the lumen of the trachea. It is commonly seen in the thoracic and distal third of the trachea (13, 20) and can appear multifocal in a small number of patients.

Surgery for curative or limited resection is an option for approximately 40% of patients. About 25% receive adjuvant chemoradiation therapy and 15% receive radiation therapy alone. The 5-year overall survival is 25%, but patients with metastatic disease have a 5-year survival rate of only 4%. Patients of older age and with poor performance status may have the worst outcomes (21).

Adenoid cystic carcinoma

ACCs are well-differentiated, malignant tumors that arise from the glandular epithelial cells of the trachea. Histologically, they appear as epithelial and myoepithelial cells in variable morphologic configurations, including tubular, cribriform, and solid patterns (19). They are not linked to cigarette smoking and there are no clear risk factors associated with them.

The average age at diagnosis is 48 years. Cough and dyspnea are the most common symptoms (10, 13). ACCs are slightly more common in women than men (1.2:1 ratio) (13). The tumors present as a polypoidal lesions in the trachea and often spread submucosally with extensions along vascular and neural structures leading to locally advanced disease (11). Approximately two-thirds of patients with ACC present with locally advanced disease (22).

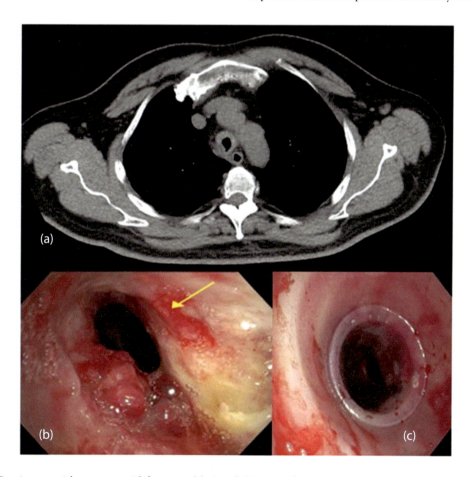

FIGURE 23.1 Carcinoma with sarcomatoid features. (a): Axial CT scan showing circumferential wall thickening and 50% narrowing of the tracheal lumen. (b): Bronchoscopic view of the distal tracheal tumor causing narrowing of the lumen. (c): Silicone stent placement to improve tracheal tumor obstruction. The carina is seen distally.

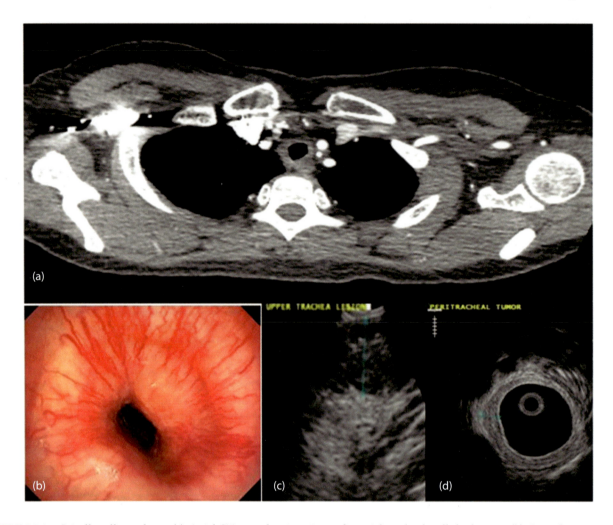

FIGURE 23.2 Spindle cell neoplasm. (a): Axial CT scan showing circumferential tracheal wall thickening. (b): Bronchoscopic view of the mid-tracheal narrowing. Mucosal neovascularization is seen. (c): Convex probe endobronchial ultrasound view of the lesion showing the depth of its invasion into the tracheal wall. (d): Radial probe endobronchial ultrasound view of the lesion showing the depth of its invasion into the tracheal wall.

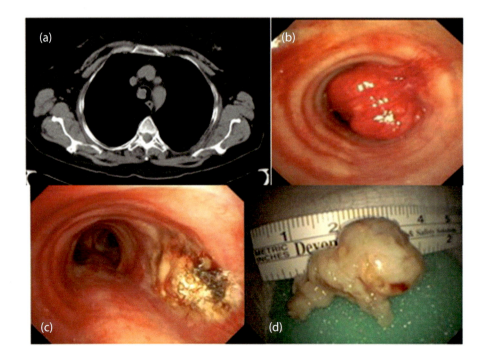

FIGURE 23.3 Tracheal adenocarcinoma. (a): Axial CT scan shows a large polypoid mass obstructing 80% of the mid-tracheal lumen. (b): Bronchoscopic view of the tracheal tumor showing a highly vascularized polypoid mass with a stalk. (c): Bronchoscopic endoluminal resection of the tumor and subsequent treatment with argon plasma coagulation. The trachea is fully patent and the main carina is visible distally. (d): Tumor size and appearance after endoluminal resection.

Primary Tracheal Tumors

Surgical resection is recommended if technically feasible and is associated with better survival outcomes — a 5-year survival of 86.4% and 10-year survival of 55.6% — than those seen in patients who do not undergo surgical resection (10). Complete surgical resection is not always achievable, and up to 60% of cases have positive resection margins (10). Therefore, adjuvant radiotherapy is commonly offered to these patients. In one study, the 10-year overall survival in selected patients who underwent radiotherapy alone was 83% (22). Patients with ACC have better survival than patients with other malignant primary tracheal tumors (4, 13). Figures 23.4 and 23.5 show the radiologic and bronchoscopic appearances of ACC.

Mucoepidermoid carcinomas

Tracheal mucoepidermoid carcinomas are pathologically similar to salivary gland mucoepidermoid tumors. They arise from the bronchial glands in the central airways and are more common in the bronchi than in the trachea. The fusion protein MECT1-MAML2 leads to dysregulation of the cell cycle and subsequent tumorigenesis in salivary and bronchopulmonary mucoepidermoid carcinomas (23). There are no known risk factors for development of these tumors, and there is no sex predilection.

Mucoepidermoid carcinomas are usually pedunculated lesions with well-circumscribed margins. Based on their mitotic activity and nuclear pleomorphism, they are divided into low- and high-grade types. Low-grade tumors are localized without regional spread whereas high-grade tumors frequently have regional and distant spread (24). In most cases, low-grade tumors can be resected with clear margins, and patients with these tumors have an excellent prognosis. High-grade tumors are aggressive and are usually nonresectable, and affected patients have poor survival rates (23). Factors such as younger age at diagnosis, low-grade

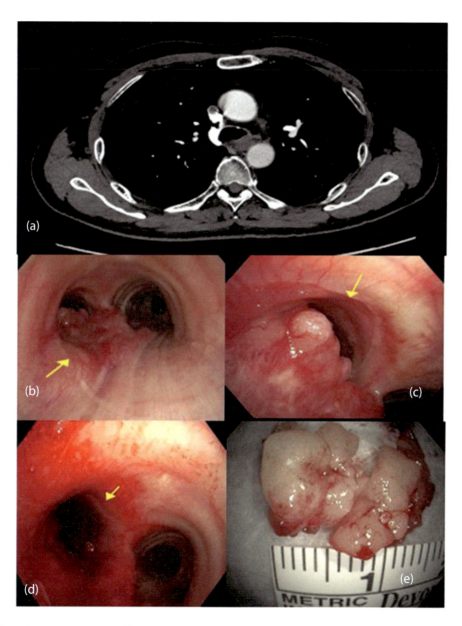

FIGURE 23.4 Adenoid cystic carcinoma. (a): Axial CT scan showing a posterolateral, distal tracheal mass. (b): Bronchoscopic view of an exophytic mass occupying the distal trachea and extending to the carina and left main stem bronchus. (c): Close-up bronchoscopic view of the mass extending into the left main stem bronchus. (d): Bronchoscopic view after endobronchial tumor resection. (e): Tumor size and appearance after endobronchial resection.

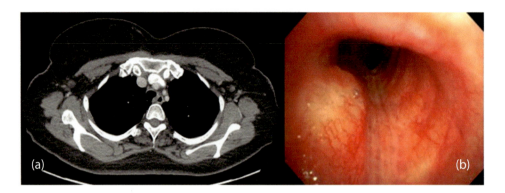

FIGURE 23.5 Adenoid cystic carcinoma. (a): Axial CT scan shows a partially obstructed lesion in the left posterolateral wall of the mid-trachea. (b): Bronchoscopic view of the lesion in the mid-trachea. The mucosa is relatively intact with the lesion appearing mostly submucosal.

tumor histology, no lymph node involvement, and the ability to achieve complete surgical resection are independent favorable prognostic factors.

Benign tumors
Squamous papillomas
Squamous papillomas occur in the trachea and are caused by HPV infections. Persistent infections of the respiratory mucosal epithelium caused by low-risk HPV strains 6 or 11 lead to metaplasia and benign growths (25). Often, there are multiple lesions located in different sites of the tracheobronchial tree. There is a risk of malignant transformation in 3–7% of cases. The risk for malignant transformation is higher in patients infected with HPV strains 16 or 18; therefore, virus typing should be done to determine the prognosis and appropriate frequency of follow-up. Tracheal papillomas appear as multiple exophytic growths that are located in different sites of the tracheobronchial tree, and these lesions can obstruct the tracheal lumen (20).

HPV lesions are highly infectious and thus can recur after treatment. Because of the high risk of recurrence, and because these lesions are mainly benign, local treatment with bronchoscopy is the preferred treatment. Patients sometimes need multiple endoscopic treatments because of recurrent disease (26). These lesions may need to be biopsied again to exclude malignant transformation when there is a substantial change in size. Forceps biopsies may not be large enough and do not include the basement membrane, making it hard to differentiate between in situ and invasive SCC (27). Tracheal papillomatosis also affects the lung parenchyma in 1% of cases, causing lung parenchyma necrosis, cavitation, or consolidation. Figure 23.6 shows the radiological and bronchoscopic appearance of recurrent tracheal papillomatosis.

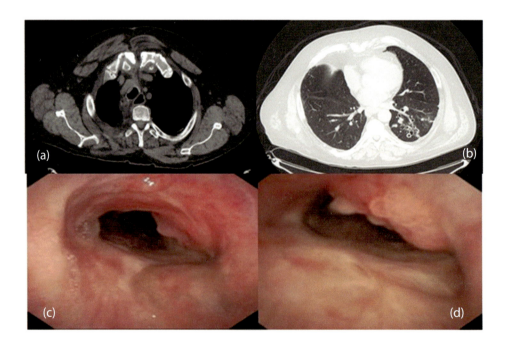

FIGURE 23.6 Squamous papillomas. (a): Axial CT scan showing an anterolateral lesion in the mid-trachea. (b): Axial CT scan showing left lower-lobe cystic lesions with infiltrates related to papillomatosis. (c) and (d): Bronchoscopic view of an anterior mid-tracheal lesion.

Primary Tracheal Tumors

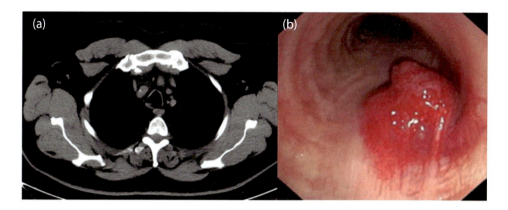

FIGURE 23.7 Glomus tumor. (a): Axial CT scan showing a polypoid lesion in the posterolateral wall of the mid-trachea. (b): Bronchoscopic view of a well-defined mid-tracheal mass.

Glomus tumors

Glomus tumors arise from the glomus bodies, which are specialized smooth muscle cells around arteriovenous anastomoses. They can occur in any part of the body but rarely occur in the trachea. These tumors are very rare; only a few case reports describe this entity. Glomus tumors arise more commonly from the posterior wall of the lower two-thirds of the trachea. They are mostly benign but can have malignant transformation (28). Once resected, the chance of recurrence is very low (29, 30). Figure 23.7 shows the radiologic and bronchoscopic appearance of a glomus tumor.

Schwannomas and paragangliomas

These are benign tumors that grow from the peripheral nerve sheath. They are usually isolated, well-encapsulated tumors and may appear highly vascularized. Schwannomas are rarely associated with von Recklinghausen disease. Based on limited data, these may have a female preponderance (31, 32). They are more commonly located in the distal trachea (31, 32). Surgical resection should be offered as recurrence is very rare. With bronchoscopic endoluminal resection, nearly 25% of patients may have recurrence (32).

Tracheobronchopathia osteochondroplastica

Tracheobronchopathia osteochondroplastica (TPO) lesions are benign nodules that appear on the anterior cartilaginous rings of the trachea. They are usually found in patients older than 50 years of age (33). TPO lesions are among the most common tracheal lesions a pulmonologist may come across. The incidence in reported to be around 0.1%. Usually, these lesions are seen on CT scans of the chest or bronchoscopy as small, submucosal nodules or irregularities in the anterior tracheal wall with normal mucosal coverings (34). Figure 23.8 shows a typical finding of small TPO lesions. Their appearance on bronchoscopy is classic, and biopsy or pathological confirmation is usually unnecessary. These lesions can be difficult to biopsy as they are hard and made of cartilage or bone (33).

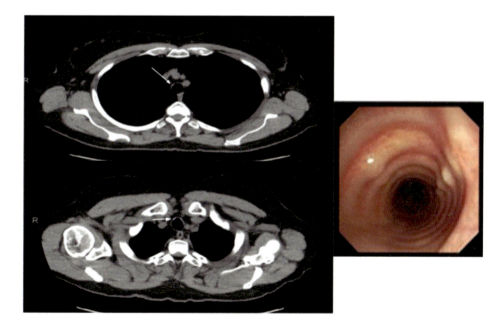

FIGURE 23.8 Tracheobronchopathia osteochondroplastica lesions. (a): Axial CT showing an irregularity on the right-anterior tracheal wall. (b): Axial CT showing a separate small nodule in the right-anterior tracheal wall. (c): Bronchoscopic view of the classic appearance of tracheobronchopathia osteochondroplastica lesions.

TPO lesions are usually an incidental finding and seldom cause symptoms. Very rarely, affected patients have cough, wheezing, or hemoptysis (33, 35). TPO lesions usually do not grow or else grow extremely slowly, and therefore interventions and follow-up are not needed (36). In a minority of patients, TPO lesions may grow and obstruct the tracheal lumen; in such cases, therapeutic bronchoscopic interventions are required to improve tracheal patency (35).

Conclusion

Primary tracheal tumors are rare. Patients are minimally symptomatic early in the course of the disease and usually develop symptoms because of obstruction of the tracheal lumen. Symptoms and findings on diagnostic imaging and bronchoscopy are not specific, and only pathological examination can establish a correct diagnosis. Localized malignant tumors should be considered for surgical resection. Benign tumors rarely recur after surgical resection, but malignant tumors may recur and have local or distant spread. Benign tumors have a good prognosis. Malignant tumors with clean surgical margins have a favorable outcome, whereas unresectable or incompletely resected tumors have worse outcomes; affected patients usually require adjuvant radiation therapy to improve survival

References

1. Ellman P, Whittaker H. Primary carcinoma of the trachea. Thorax. 1947;2 (3):153–62.
2. Honings J, van Dijck JA, Verhagen AF, van der Heijden HF, Marres HA. Incidence and treatment of tracheal cancer: A nationwide study in the Netherlands. Ann Surg Oncol. 2007;14 (2):968–76.
3. Urdaneta AI, Yu JB, Wilson LD. Population based cancer registry analysis of primary tracheal carcinoma. Am J Clin Oncol. 2011;34 (1):32–7.
4. Mallick S, Benson R, Giridhar P, Rajan Singh A, Rath GK. Demography, patterns of care and survival outcomes in patients with malignant tumors of trachea: A systematic review and individual patient data analysis of 733 patients. Lung Cancer. 2019;132:87–93.
5. Madariaga MLL, Gaissert HA. Overview of malignant tracheal tumors. Ann Cardiothorac Surg. 2018;7 (2):244–54.
6. Furlow PW, Mathisen DJ. Surgical anatomy of the trachea. Ann Cardiothorac Surg. 2018;7 (2):255–60.
7. Brand-Saberi BEM, Schafer T. Trachea: Anatomy and physiology. Thorac Surg Clin. 2014;24 (1):1–5.
8. Minnich DJ, Mathisen DJ. Anatomy of the trachea, carina, and bronchi. Thorac Surg Clin. 2007;17 (4):571–85.
9. Mehran RJ. Fundamental and practical aspects of airway anatomy: From glottis to segmental bronchus. Thorac Surg Clin. 2018;28 (2):117–25.
10. Ran J, Qu G, Chen X, Zhao D. Clinical features, treatment and outcomes in patients with tracheal adenoid cystic carcinoma: A systematic literature review. Radiat Oncol. 2021;16 (1):38.
11. Zhengjaiang L, Pingzhang T, Dechao Z, Reddy-Kolanu G, Ilankovan V. Primary tracheal tumours: 21 years of experience at Peking Union Medical College, Beijing, China. J Laryngol Otol. 2008;122 (11):1235–40.
12. Gaissert HA, Grillo HC, Shadmehr MB, Wright CD, Gokhale M, Wain JC, et al. Uncommon primary tracheal tumors. Ann Thorac Surg. 2006;82 (1):268–72; discussion 72-3.
13. Webb BD, Walsh GL, Roberts DB, Sturgis EM. Primary tracheal malignant neoplasms: The University of Texas MD Anderson Cancer Center experience. J Am Coll Surg. 2006;202 (2):237–46.
14. Jindal T, Kumar A, Kumar R, Dutta R, Meena M. Role of positron emission tomography-computed tomography in bronchial mucoepidermoid carcinomas: A case series and review of the literature. J Med Case Rep. 2010;4:277.
15. Bhattacharyya N. Contemporary staging and prognosis for primary tracheal malignancies: A population-based analysis. Otolaryngol Head Neck Surg. 2004;131 (5):639–42.
16. Macchiarini P. Primary tracheal tumours. Lancet Oncol. 2006;7 (1):83–91.
17. Gaissert HA, Grillo HC, Shadmehr MB, Wright CD, Gokhale M, Wain JC, et al. Long-term survival after resection of primary adenoid cystic and squamous cell carcinoma of the trachea and carina. Ann Thorac Surg. 2004;78 (6):1889–96; discussion 96-7.
18. Xie L, Fan M, Sheets NC, Chen RC, Jiang GL, Marks LB. The use of radiation therapy appears to improve outcome in patients with malignant primary tracheal tumors: A SEER-based analysis. Int J Radiat Oncol Biol Phys. 2012;84 (2):464–70.
19. Junker K. Pathology of tracheal tumors. Thorac Surg Clin. 2014;24 (1):7–11.
20. Moores D, Mane P. Pathology of primary tracheobronchial malignancies other than adenoid cystic carcinomas. Thorac Surg Clin. 2018;28 (2):149–54.
21. Hararah MK, Stokes WA, Oweida A, Patil T, Amini A, Goddard J, et al. Epidemiology and treatment trends for primary tracheal squamous cell carcinoma. Laryngoscope. 2020;130 (2):405–12.
22. Hogerle BA, Lasitschka F, Muley T, Bougatf N, Herfarth K, Adeberg S, et al. Primary adenoid cystic carcinoma of the trachea: Clinical outcome of 38 patients after interdisciplinary treatment in a single institution. Radiat Oncol. 2019;14 (1):117.
23. Salem A, Bell D, Sepesi B, Papadimitrakopoulou V, El-Naggar A, Moran CA, et al. Clinicopathologic and genetic features of primary bronchopulmonary mucoepidermoid carcinoma: The MD Anderson Cancer Center experience and comprehensive review of the literature. Virchows Arch. 2017;470 (6):619–26.
24. Abu Saleh WK, Aljabbari O, Ramchandani M. Mucoepidermoid carcinoma of the tracheobronchial tree. Methodist Debakey Cardiovasc J. 2015;11 (3):192–4.
25. Popper HH, Wirnsberger G, Juttner-Smolle FM, Pongratz MG, Sommersgutter M. The predictive value of human papilloma virus (HPV) typing in the prognosis of bronchial squamous cell papillomas. Histopathology. 1992;21 (4):323–30.
26. Ogata-Suetsugu S, Izumi M, Takayama K, Nakashima T, Inoue H, Nakanishi Y. A case of multiple squamous cell papillomas of the trachea. Ann Thorac Cardiovasc Surg. 2011;17 (2):212–4.
27. Glispie DM, Sweis AM, Sims HS. Laryngology clinic: Solitary tracheal papilloma. Ear Nose Throat J. 2020;99 (3):194–5.
28. Braham E, Zairi S, Mlika M, Ayadi-Kaddour A, Ismail O, El Mezni F. Malignant glomus tumor of trachea: A case report with literature review. Asian Cardiovasc Thorac Ann. 2016;24 (1):104–6.
29. Gowan RT, Shamji FM, Perkins DG, Maziak DE. Glomus tumor of the trachea. Ann Thorac Surg. 2001;72 (2):598–600.
30. Sakr L, Palaniappan R, Payan MJ, Doddoli C, Dutau H. Tracheal glomus tumor: A multidisciplinary approach to management. Respir Care. 2011;56 (3):342–6.
31. Ge X, Han F, Guan W, Sun J, Guo X. Optimal treatment for primary benign intratracheal schwannoma: A case report and review of the literature. Oncol Lett. 2015;10 (4):2273–6.
32. Hamouri S, Novotny NM. Primary tracheal schwannoma a review of a rare entity: Current understanding of management and followup. J Cardiothorac Surg. 2017;12 (1):105.
33. Abu-Hijleh M, Lee D, Braman SS. Tracheobronchopathia osteochondroplastica: A rare large airway disorder. Lung. 2008;186 (6):353–9.
34. Jabbardarjani HR, Radpey B, Kharabian S, Masjedi MR. Tracheobronchopathia osteochondroplastica: Presentation of ten cases and review of the literature. Lung. 2008;186 (5):293–7.
35. Cho HK, Jeong BH, Kim H. Clinical course of tracheobronchopathia osteochondroplastica. J Thorac Dis. 2020;12 (10):5571–9.
36. Leske V, Lazor R, Coetmeur D, Crestani B, Chatte G, Cordier JF, et al. Tracheobronchopathia osteochondroplastica: A study of 41 patients. Medicine (Baltimore). 2001;80 (6):378–90.

PART G
Rare Pleural Disorders

24

UNUSUAL CAUSES OF PLEURAL EFFUSION

Niranjan Setty, Nai-Chien Huan, and Rajesh Thomas

Contents

Introduction	177
Pleural effusion of extra-vascular origin	177
Eosinophilic pleural effusions	185
Pleural effusions secondary to atypical infections	185
Pleural effusions related to connective tissue diseases and vasculitis	185
Pleural effusion related to the endocrine and reproductive systems	185
Unusual miscellaneous causes	188
Acknowledgment	189
References	189

KEY POINTS

- Congestive heart failure, parapneumonic effusion, malignant pleural effusion and pulmonary embolism are the most common causes of pleural effusions.
- Uncommon causes collectively form a significant minority of all pleural effusions.
- Diagnosing an unusual cause of a pleural effusion requires a high index of clinical suspicion.
- An early correct diagnosis is important as disease-specific management is usually required for treatment.

Introduction

There are more than 60 known causes of pleural effusion. Congestive heart failure (CHF), parapneumonic effusion, malignant effusion and pulmonary embolism are the commonest aetiologies (1–3). Pleural effusions of unusual causes collectively form a large minority, and they often require disease-specific management. However, not all 'unusual' pleural effusions are, depending on region, endemicity and disease setting, truly rare. In this chapter, we will provide an overview of the pathogenesis, clinical presentation, pleural fluid characteristics, image findings and management of pleural effusions of unusual causes. The unusual pleural effusions described in this chapter have been grouped broadly based on their etiology and pathogenetic mechanisms.

Pleural effusion of extra-vascular origin

Pleural effusions, both exudates and transudates, can arise from extra-vascular origins (PEEVO). The pathogenetic mechanisms of pleural fluid formation in these conditions is different to 'usual' pleural effusions that develop secondary to hydrostatic and oncotic pressure imbalance, inflammation, infection or abnormalities in lymphatic drainage pathways.

Exudative PEEVO

Chylothorax and pseudochylothorax are uncommon exudative PEEVOs. Both conditions are typically characterized by accumulation of white, opaque pleural fluid — chyle and pseudochyle, respectively — but they have different aetiologies and pathophysiological mechanisms (4).

Chylothorax
Cause and pathogenesis

Accumulation of chyle in the pleural space usually occurs because of disruption and damage to the transporting thoracic duct or draining lymphatics (4, 5). Conditions that cause chylothorax are summarised in Table 24.1 (6–16). Traumatic injury or tear of the thoracic duct, either iatrogenic or non-iatrogenic (Figure 24.1), is the commonest cause. Other pathogenetic mechanisms include thoracic duct obstruction, weakening of thoracic duct wall, anatomic anomalies of the duct and lymphatic system, excessive lymph production and defects in chyle transportation systems (4). Malignancy, of both lymphoproliferative and non-lymphoproliferative types, is the most common non-traumatic cause for a chylothorax (17).

Clinical presentation

The clinical features of a chylothorax depend on its underlying cause and rate of chyle accumulation in the pleural cavity. Traumatic chylothorax post-trauma or -surgery can develop rapidly within a few days causing acute-onset shortness of breath. Depending on the site of thoracic duct leakage, chylothorax may be right-sided (in 50% of cases), left-sided (33%) or bilateral (17%) (18, 19). The thoracic duct crosses anatomically from the right to the left side at the level of the fifth thoracic vertebra as it ascends the thorax; as a result, a chylothorax is usually left-sided when thoracic duct damage occurs above the level of fifth thoracic vertebra and right-sided when the duct is damaged below this level (18, 19). With non-traumatic chylothorax, patients typically present with a more gradual onset of fatigue, weight loss, malnutrition and breathlessness. Patients with chylothorax are also at a risk of developing opportunistic infections due to malnourishment and loss of immunoglobulins (20).

Pleural fluid characteristics

Chylothorax should be suspected in any patient with pleural fluid that appears milky or turbid. However, the milky appearance of

DOI: 10.1201/9781003089384-24

TABLE 24.1: Causes of Chylothorax

Non-Traumatic	Traumatic
Malignancy	***Iatrogenic***
Lymphoma	Thoracic surgery, e.g., lung resection, esophagectomy and mediastinal mass resection.
Leukaemia	
Other malignancies, e.g., lung cancer, sarcoma, and mediastinal tumors	Heart surgery
	Head and neck surgery
	Heart and/or lung transplantation
	Pacemaker insertion
	Central line insertion
	Embolization of pulmonary arteriovenous malformation
Infection (rare, and mainly in endemic regions)	***Non-iatrogenic***
Tuberculosis	Penetrating injuries to neck, chest and/or abdomen
Filariasis	Road traffic accidents
Histoplasmosis	Gunshot wounds
Paragonimiasis	Childbirth
	Repeated trauma from heavy exercise
Other unusual causes	
Sarcoidosis	
Systemic lupus erythematosus	
Lymphangioleiomyomatosis	
Intestinal lymphangiectasia	
Amyloidosis	
Protein-losing enteropathy	
Hepatic cirrhosis	
Tuberous sclerosis	
Castleman disease	
Superior vena cava obstruction	
Thoracic radiation	
Turner syndrome	
Noonan syndrome	
Idiopathic	

Sources: From (6–16).

pleural fluid may be seen only in half of the patients with chylothorax (Figure 24.2). A high index of suspicion for chylothorax is necessary in bloody or serosanguinous effusions of unclear etiology, particularly in patients who had undergone recent chest, neck or abdominal surgery prior to presentation (21). Ingestion of a high-fat meal may help to increase the milky appearance of the chylous fluid (21).

Pleural fluid analysis for cholesterol and triglyceride levels and for the presence of chylomicrons can easily confirm chylous effusion (Table 24.2) (4). A pleural fluid triglyceride level >110 mg/dL is highly suggestive of chylous effusion; triglyceride level <50 mg/dL is supportive evidence for an alternative non-chylous etiology for the effusion (4, 22, 23). The presence of chylomicrons by lipid electrophoresis analysis is diagnostic of chylous effusion when the triglyceride level is 50–110 mg/dL and in other indeterminate cases (22). Pleural fluid cholesterol level (>200 mg/dL) is useful to evaluate for pseudochylothorax that, with its milky-appearing pleural fluid, can mimic chylothorax (4, 22, 23).

Evaluation

Following a diagnosis of chylothorax, further imaging is useful to determine its underlying cause and to identify the site of chyle leakage and thoracic duct damage. Computed tomography (CT) scan of the thorax, abdomen and pelvis can identify mediastinal tumors and lymphadenopathy secondary to lymphoproliferative disease and metastatic malignancy; benign lymphadenopathy, e.g., tuberculosis; goitre and expansile neck lesions; thoracic duct anomalies; cystic lung diseases, e.g., lymphangioleiomyomatosis; and misplaced central vascular lines and pacemaker wires (4). Lymphangiography, lymphoscintigraphy and magnetic resonance lymphangiography may be useful to identify thoracic duct tear (24–29) and to assess anatomical anomalies seen in lymphangiectasia, lymphangiomatosis, and rare lymphatic conduction disorders; it is also useful when planning surgical interventions to correct lymphatic leakage and when chylothorax recurs after thoracic duct ligation (27–29).

Management

Management measures are aimed at correcting the primary cause and in large or refractory effusions, fluid control interventions to provide dyspnoea relief and minimise nutritional loss (Table 24.3) (4, 30–35). Surgical or radiological interventions may be necessary when, despite conservative and dietary measures, large volume chyle drainage (>1.5 L/day) persists for >2 weeks. Surgical ligation of the thoracic duct just above the right hemi-diaphragm is successful in >90% of patients (33, 34). In patients who are unfit

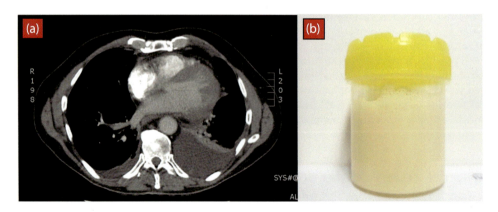

FIGURE 24.1 Spontaneous, idiopathic, bilateral chylothoraces caused by intense long-distance running. (a): CT scan (axial view) of thorax demonstrating bilateral pleural effusions, larger on the left side, in a patient who presented with chest pain and breathlessness a day after completing intense long-distance running. (b): Diagnostic thoracentesis revealed pleural fluid with typical milky appearance of chylothorax with biochemistry confirming elevated triglycerides and presence of chylomicrons. Extensive evaluation did not reveal a malignancy or another cause for the chylothorax. The chylothorax resolved with low fat dietary modification and conservative measures.

Unusual Causes of Pleural Effusion

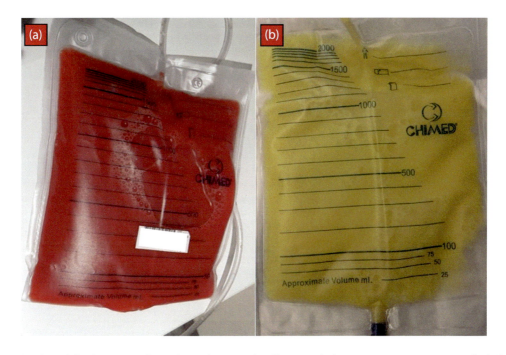

FIGURE 24.2 The pleural fluid may not always have the typical milky or turbid appearance in a patient with chylothorax. A high index of suspicion is needed in non-milky effusions of unclear etiology in patients with a recent history of chest, neck, or abdominal surgery. Ingestion of a high-fat meal may help to increase the milky appearance of the chylous fluid. (a): Pleural fluid with haemorrhagic appearance in a patient with chylothorax secondary to Kaposi sarcoma and mediastinal disease. (b): Pleural fluid with opaque, deep yellow appearance in a patient with chylothorax caused by lymphoma.

TABLE 24.2: Pleural Fluid Biochemistry in Chylothorax and Pseudochylothorax

	Triglyceride	Cholesterol	Chylomicrons	Cholesterol Crystals
Chylothorax	>110 mg/dL (1.24 mmol/L)	<200 mg/dL (<5.18 mmol/L)	Present	Absent
Pseudochylothorax	<50 mg/dL (<0.56 mmol/L)	>200 mg/dL (>5.18 mmol/L)	Absent	Present

Source: From (4).

for surgery, pleuro-peritoneal shunt and radiologically guided thoracic duct occlusion using gel foams and coils are useful measures (35).

Pseudochylothorax

Pseudochylothorax, also known as cholesterol effusion, cholesterol pleurisy and chyliform effusion, develops in the setting of a chronic effusion encased by inflamed, fibrotic and thickened pleural peel (4).

Cause and pathogenesis

The exact incidence of pseudochylothorax is unclear (36, 37). It is most commonly seen with chronic tuberculous and rheumatoid pleural effusions; several rare causes are also described (Table 24.4) (4, 38–43). The cholesterol crystals, characteristic of pseudochylothorax, are thought to be released into the pleural space following lysis of erythrocytes and neutrophils in a chronic, entrapped effusion (4, 44).

TABLE 24.3: Management of Chylothorax

1. **Treatment of primary disease**
2. **Conservative measures to reduce chyle formation**
   - Dietary modification using low-fat diet
   - Total parenteral nutrition
3. **Local control of chylous pleural effusion**
   - Repeat thoracentesis
   - Intercostal tube drainage and chemical pleurodesis
   - Indwelling pleural catheter in intractable cases
   - Pleuroperitoneal pump
4. **Interventions to correct chyle leak**
   - Surgical ligation of thoracic duct
   - Intrapleural fibrin glue
   - Image-guided thoracic duct occlusion using gel foam and coil

Sources: From (4, 30–35).

TABLE 24.4: Causes of Pseudochylothorax

Common causes
- Chronic tuberculous pleural effusion
- Chronic rheumatoid pleural effusion

Rare causes
- Paragonimiasis
- Echinococcosis
- Syphilis
- Lung cancer
- Hodgkin disease
- Iatrogenic
- Liver cirrhosis
- Heart and renal failure

Sources: From (4, 38–43).

Clinical presentation and evaluation

Patients with a pseudochylothorax, even with a large effusion, may have only minimal symptoms (4). Chest radiography and CT scan will reveal a thickened pleura surrounding a unilateral pleural effusion that is often longstanding (Figure 24.3) (4). CT imaging may also identify the underlying cause of the pseudochylothorax, e.g., lung nodules and interstitial abnormalities typical of rheumatoid arthritis and rheumatoid effusion (Figure 24.4) or lung infiltrates and mediastinal adenopathy in tuberculosis (4). Bedside thoracic ultrasound may reveal cholesterol crystals, characterized by increased echogenic densities within a hypo-echoic, exudative-appearing pleural fluid.

Pleural fluid characteristics

The fluid in pseudochylothorax typically has a high cholesterol level (>200 mg/dL), low triglycerides (<50 mg/dL) and no chylomicrons, thus distinguishing it from chylothorax (4). Microscopic analysis of the pleural fluid demonstrates characteristic rhomboid-shaped cholesterol crystals (Figure 24.4) (4, 44).

Management

In endemic settings, the pleural fluid should be tested after diagnostic thoracentesis for tuberculosis and paragonimiasis (45). Therapeutic thoracentesis is needed only in symptomatic patients; many patients remain asymptomatic even in the presence of a large effusion (4). Thoracentesis can be technically difficult in these patients due to the hardened, and often, heavily calcified pleural peel; it should be performed cautiously due to the high risk of causing negative pressure pulmonary oedema in the entrapped lung (4).

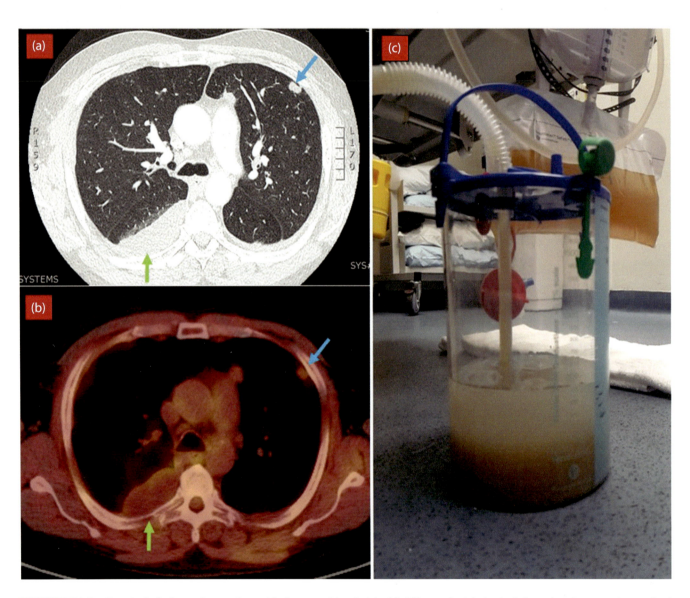

FIGURE 24.3 Pseudochylothorax in a patient with rheumatoid arthritis. (a): CT scan (axial view) of chest showing a moderate sized right-sided pleural effusion (green arrow) with pleural thickening and a rheumatoid lung nodule (blue arrow). (b): ^{18}FDG-PET scan (fused image, axial view) chest showing only low-avidity of the pleura (green arrow) and lung nodule (blue arrow). (c): Pleural fluid drainage revealed fluid with a milky appearance, suggestive of chyle; however, biochemistry showing low triglycerides, high cholesterol and absent chylomicrons was consistent with pseudo-chyle. Cytology evaluation of fluid demonstrated cholesterol crystals to confirm pseudochylothorax.

Unusual Causes of Pleural Effusion

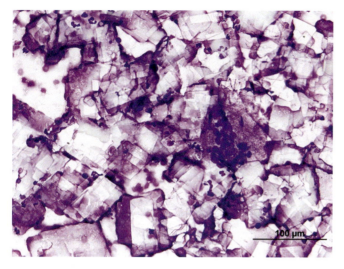

FIGURE 24.4 Cholesterol crystals pleural fluid in rheumatoid effusion demonstrating a multinucleate giant cell and numerous cholesterol crystals (Diff-Quick original magnification 40×). (Image courtesy of Dr. Amber Louw, Department Of Anatomical Pathology, PathWest Laboratory Medicine, QEII Medical Centre, Perth, Australia.)

Pleural effusion secondary to esophageal and gastric perforation
Cause and pathogenesis

Pleural effusion following perforation of the upper gastrointestinal tract may be secondary to (i) traumatic causes, e.g., penetrating injury and ingestion of corrosive acid; (ii) iatrogenic causes, e.g., post-endoscopic dilatation and other interventions; and (iii) spontaneous causes, e.g., excessive vomiting (Boerhaave syndrome) (Figure 24.5) and esophageal and gastric cancers (46, 47). The pleural effusion can be directly caused by esophageal and gastric contents through a direct communication when there is a concomitant tear in the mediastinal pleura, or can be formed indirectly due to irritation, inflammation or infection of the adjacent pleural membrane.

Clinical presentation and evaluation

Patients commonly present with features of pleural infection. In many cases, a clinical history pointing toward a gastro-esophageal origin is absent and a high index of suspicion is needed in severely ill patients with an undiagnosed pleural effusion (46). The effusion is more commonly left-sided from distal esophageal rupture but may be seen on the right side with upper and mid-esophageal tears (48). Features of pneumo-mediastinum, mediastinitis, esophageal-pleural fistula and gas in the pleural space, when present on CT scan of the chest, should raise suspicion for gastro-esophageal rupture (Figure 24.6a–b). CT scan with oral contrast swallow and endoscopy are useful to identify the site and size of the fistula and plan further management (Figure 24.6c).

Pleural fluid characteristics

Urgent diagnostic thoracentesis is necessary to confirm the gastro-esophageal origin of the effusion and to guide management. The pleural fluid macroscopical appearance may be sero-sanguineous or purulent and may even contain food material. Fluid analysis typically reveals an exudate with high lactate dehydrogenase (LDH) (>1,000 IU/L), amylase (pleural fluid-serum amylase ratio of >15) and lipase levels (48, 49). Biochemical testing for amylase sub-type can differentiate esophageal (associated with salivary amylase) from pancreatic amylase-rich effusions (see Pancreatopleural Fistula and Pancreatic Pseudocyst). Presence of food material macro- or microscopically, when present, is diagnostic (50).

Management

Gastro-esophageal perforation is a life-threatening condition (mortality of up to 40%) (51, 52). Urgent assessment by a gastroenterologist and surgeon is critical. Endoscopic localization of the perforation site followed by repair of the tear are necessary, however, many patients are unsuitable for aggressive interventions due to advanced age, frailty, malignancy and co-morbidities. Management directed at the pleural effusion itself is like that for a pleural infection and involves therapeutic fluid drainage and appropriate broad-spectrum antibiotics. Intra-pleural fibrinolytic therapy may be considered for complex, multi-loculated effusions in suitable cases after careful risk assessment for bleeding in the setting of esophageal perforation.

Bilothorax

Bilothorax, also known as thoracobilia, cholethorax, thoracobiliary fistula and pleurobilia, is characterized by accumulation of bile in the pleural space (53). The term 'bilothorax' was first described in a person who developed a traumatic bilo-pleural fistula causing bile accumulation in the pleural cavity (54). Approximately 60 cases of bilothorax are reported in THE literature.

Cause and pathogenesis

Conditions that could cause bilothorax include diaphragmatic and pleural trauma; subphrenic and hepatic infection, collection or abscess; biliary obstruction; and iatrogenic complications of percutaneous trans-hepatic biliary drainage (55–59). Bile is thought to enter the pleural cavity either indirectly via a lymphatic route through pleuro-peritoneal lymphatic connections or directly across diaphragmatic defect(s) and communications.

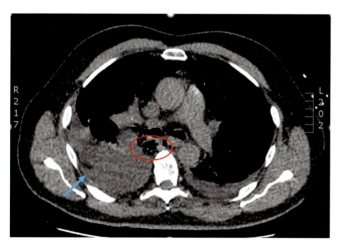

FIGURE 24.5 Boerhaave syndrome causing spontaneous esophageal tear and right-sided pleural effusion. CT scan (axial view) of thorax showing right pleural effusion (blue arrow) and extraluminal tracking of air (circled area) from esophagus to the pleura following barogenic esophageal tear.

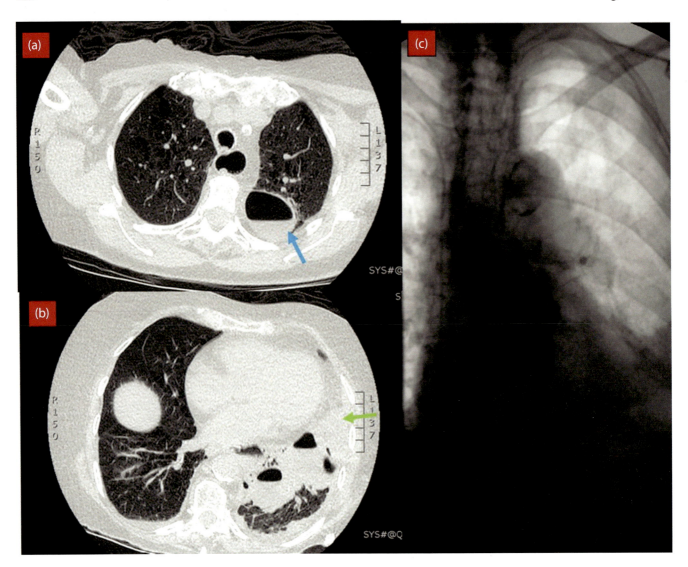

FIGURE 24.6 (a and b): CT scan of chest (axial views) demonstrating gas filled, multi-loculated left-sided fluid collections extending into the oblique fissure (blue arrow) and basal pleural cavity (green arrow) in a patient with Boerhaave syndrome and esophageal rupture. (c): CT scan with contrast swallow shows extravasation of contrast at the left margin of mid-esophagus into the left pleural space.

Clinical presentation and evaluation

Patients usually present acutely with features of a large pleural effusion. A recent history of upper gastrointestinal and biliary surgery or presence of underlying biliary and hepatic risk factors should raise a high index of suspicion. However, bilothorax is a rare condition and usually, it is suspected only following thoracentesis of bile-coloured pleural fluid. Standard CT scan, ultrasound and ERCP are useful to identify hepatobiliary injury and the communication between the biliary tree and pleural cavity.

Pleural fluid characteristics

A raised pleural fluid bilirubin level and a pleural fluid-serum bilirubin ratio >1 are diagnostic of bilothorax (60).

Management

Patients with bilothorax are at a high risk of developing empyema (61). Prompt diagnosis, therapeutic fluid drainage and early broad-spectrum antibiotics, in addition to definitive management of primary abdominal disease, are critical management measures needed to improve outcomes.

Pancreatico-pleural fistula and pancreatic pseudocyst

Cause and pathogenesis

Both acute and chronic pancreatitis may be complicated by a pleural effusion. Pleural effusion in pancreatic diseases can develop due to reactive pleural fluid formation secondary to inflammation and irritation of pleura adjacent to the inflamed pancreas; following development of pancreatico-pleural fistula; and by rupture of pancreatic pseudocyst into the pleural cavity (62).

Clinical presentation and evaluation

In the acute setting, the clinical findings of pancreatitis often predominate and mimics pleural infection/sepsis with high inflammatory markers on serology. Pancreatic pleural effusion must

Unusual Causes of Pleural Effusion

always be considered in high-risk patients, particularly in those with acute pancreatitis or a history of alcohol-related and other causes of chronic pancreatitis. CT scan, ERCP (63) and magnetic resonance cholangio-pancreatography (MRCP) (64, 65) are useful to diagnose and manage pancreatitis and pseudocysts and additionally, can demonstrate any communication between the pancreas and pleural cavity (62, 66).

Pleural fluid characteristics
Ultrasound evaluation usually demonstrates hypoechoic fluid with exudative appearance, and in many cases, features of a complex effusion with septations and multi-loculations. Pleural fluid LDH is raised on biochemical assessment. High pleural fluid amylase (usually >100,000 IU/L) and lipase levels are diagnostic of pancreatic pleural effusion (62, 66).

Management
Depending on its severity and extent, management is aimed primarily at medical, endoscopic and surgical repair of pancreatitis and the pancreatic fistula. Exocrine suppression with somatostatin analogues, e.g., octreotide (67) combined with ERCP stenting of the pancreatic duct fistula may be successful in >80% of cases (68). Surgery is needed in those who fail initial conservative and endoscopic interventions. Therapeutic pleural drainage for local fluid control is performed in large, symptomatic and/or complex effusions.

Transudative PEEVO
Hepatic hydrothorax (HH) and continuous ambulatory peritoneal dialysis (CAPD)-related pleural effusions are relatively more common transudative PEEVOs; urinothorax, glycinothorax and effusions secondary to duro-pleural fistula and CVC placement are rare causes. Like most other transudative effusions, management is aimed at definitive treatment of the underlying primary etiology.

Hepatic hydrothorax
Pathogenesis and clinical presentation
The classic presentation of HH is that of a new onset transudative pleural effusion, that is usually right-sided, in a patient with pre-existing liver disease and portal hypertension (69, 70). The effusion is formed of ascitic fluid that has moved via diaphragmatic pores into the pleural space; in some cases, significant ascites may not be easily noticeable when a large amount of ascitic fluid has escaped into the pleural cavity (Figure 24.7).

Management
Management of refractory HH is difficult and complicated. Curing the underlying chronic liver disease and portal hypertension is usually not possible. Standard medical treatment with salt and fluid restriction and diuretic therapy may not be successful in up to 26% of cases (69). In HH that is refractory to medical treatment, interventional procedures have variable success and

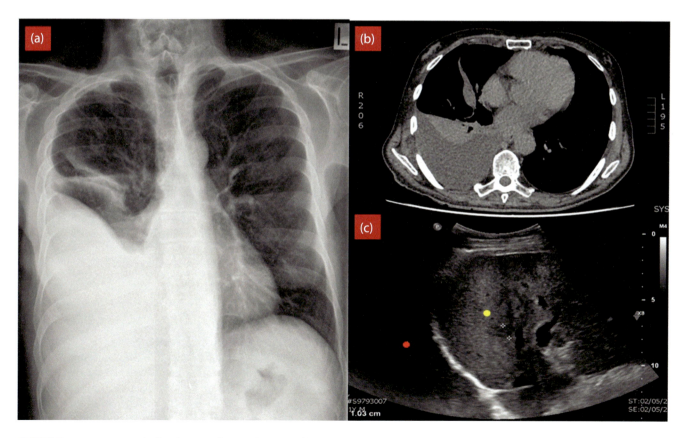

FIGURE 24.7 Hepatic hydrothorax. Chest radiograph (a) and CT (axial view) of chest (b) showing a large right-sided pleural effusion in a patient with chronic liver cirrhosis secondary to hepatitis C and alcohol abuse. (c): Ultrasound of liver shows coarse liver architecture of cirrhosis (yellow dot) and an anechoic transudate-like right pleural effusion (red dot) above the liver and diaphragm. There was minimal fluid below the diaphragm as most of the ascitic fluid had escaped into the pleural cavity.

include (i) repeated needle thoracentesis; (ii) intercostal tube drainage with chemical pleurodesis; (iii) trans-jugular intra-hepatic porto-systemic shunt (response rate of up to 74%); and (iv) video-assisted thoracoscopic surgery (VATS) to repair diaphragmatic defects followed by talc insufflation for pleurodesis. Post-operative continuous positive airway pressure (CPAP) and therapeutic ascitic drainage to decompress the abdomen may improve pleural apposition and pleurodesis success (69, 71–74). Interventions for HH are complicated due to the higher bleeding and infection risks in liver disease; it is particularly important to minimise pleural interventions to reduce risk of pleural infection in those patients likely to undergo liver transplantation.

Continuous ambulatory peritoneal dialysis-related pleural effusion

Pathogenesis and clinical presentation

Continuous ambulatory peritoneal dialysis (CAPD)-related pleural effusion, usually right-sided, is seen in 2% of all patients undergoing CAPD (75) and should be suspected in any patient undergoing CAPD who presents with a pleural effusion (75, 76). It is often associated with reduced dialysis adequacy and ultrafiltration rate. Patients may be asymptomatic in 25% of cases (75–77). The main pathogenetic mechanism for development of pleural effusion is by migration of dialysate fluid across the diaphragm via congenital and acquired diaphragmatic defects (78); this may be exacerbated by impaired lymphatic drainage or when the pleuro-peritoneal pressure gradient is increased by the volume of dialysate fluid in the abdomen (75).

Pleural fluid characteristics

The pleural fluid is transudative with an increased glucose level (pleural fluid-serum glucose ratio of >1) (75–77). Differential diagnoses for a transudative effusion in this setting include congestive cardiac failure, pulmonary embolism and fluid overload commonly seen in end-stage renal disease; however, it is distinguishable from CAPD-related pleural effusion because the pleural fluid glucose is usually not increased in the former cases.

Management

Temporary cessation of CAPD and conversion to haemodialysis is successful in half of the cases (75, 77). In patients in whom CAPD cannot be stopped, local interventions for effusion control include chest tube drainage and bedside chemical pleurodesis or VATS to repair the diaphragmatic defects and talc pleurodesis. Post-surgery, >80% of cases may successfully return to long-term CAPD (79, 80).

Urinothorax and glycinothorax

Pathogenesis and clinical presentation

Urinothorax refers to the presence of urine in the pleural space (81–83) and can develop following obstructive uropathy, urethral stricture or fibrosis, and compression by bladder, urethral or renal tumors (81, 82).

Glycinothorax develops when bladder irrigation fluid that is rich in glycine accumulates in the pleural cavity. It is usually associated with rupture of the urinary bladder wall during urethral surgery or bladder irrigation followed by migration of the irrigation fluid into the pleural space via diaphragmatic pores and lymphatic connections (84).

Pleural fluid characteristics

The pleural fluid is transudative in urinothorax (81, 82) and glycinothorax (84). A pleural fluid-serum creatinine ratio >1 is suggestive of urinothorax (82); a pleural fluid-serum glycine ratio of >300 is diagnostic of glycinothorax (84).

Management

Urgent correction of the underlying urological cause is necessary in urinothorax and glycinothorax. Bladder irrigation is also ceased immediately in case of glycinothorax (84).

Central Venous catheter-related pleural effusion

Pathogenesis

Central venous catheter (CVC)-related pleural effusions can develop following (i) mal-placement of CVC, e.g., after inadvertent puncture of the pleural membrane during CVC insertion and (ii) migration, e.g., following erosion of the venous catheter tip into the pleural space secondary to infection or inflammation (85, 86). The true incidence of mal-placed and migrated CVC is unknown. Catheter migration and mal-placement are more likely to occur with the left internal jugular and subclavian veins than on the right side due to the anatomically horizontal course of the left brachiocephalic vein (87, 88).

Pleural fluid characteristics

The pleural fluid will reflect the composition of fluid infused via the CVC, e.g., milky appearance with TPN and transudative fluid with saline infusion.

Clinical presentation and management

Extra-vascular migration of CVC into the pleural space is difficult to diagnose clinically or by chest radiography (89); CT scan is usually required to demonstrate the abnormal position of the CVC tip. Prompt removal of the CVC is necessary; cardiothoracic and vascular surgeons may also need to be involved.

Duro-pleural fistula-related pleural effusion

Pathogenesis

An abnormal or iatrogenic communication between the pleural and dural spaces results in leakage of cerebrospinal fluid (CSF) into the pleural cavity and effusion formation. A duro-pleural fistula (DPF) can occur secondary to (i) blunt trauma to the vertebrae and spinal cord; (ii) space-occupying lesions of the spinal cord; (iii) complications following surgical interventions such as laminectomy and trans-thoracic discectomy; and (iv) iatrogenic causes, e.g., mal-positioned or mal-functioning ventriculo-peritoneal shunt and therapeutic ventriculo-pleural shunt for hydrocephalus management (Figure 24.8) (90–94).

Pleural fluid characteristics

The pleural fluid is transudative and pauci-cellular. A high pleural fluid beta-2 transferrin level is strongly suggestive of dural origin (95–97).

Clinical presentation and management

A diagnosis of DPF requires a high index of suspicion. Patients with DPF have neurological symptoms such as headache, nausea and vomiting, in addition to breathlessness caused by the effusion. When suspected, radionuclide diethylenetriamine penta-acetate myelography may demonstrate the fistulous communication between dural and pleural spaces. Conservative management with close monitoring is usually preferred and spontaneous resolution is seen in many cases (92); neurosurgical intervention may be necessary in refractory cases. Correction or removal of ventriculo-peritoneal and ventriculo-pleural shunts may be needed in iatrogenic cases with refractory symptomatic effusion.

Unusual Causes of Pleural Effusion

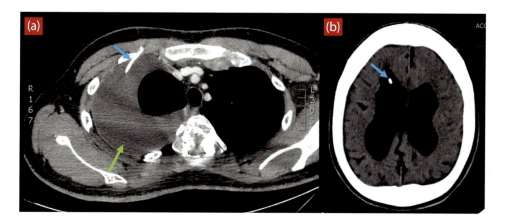

FIGURE 24.8 Duro-pleural fistula (DPF)-related pleural effusion in a patient with spina bifida and hydrocephalus presenting with progressive breathlessness. He had previously undergone bladder entero-cystoplasty surgery for neurogenic bladder. This was complicated by post-operative abdominal infection that necessitated conversion of a long-standing ventriculo-peritoneal shunt to a ventriculo-pleural shunt leading to cerebrospinal fluid accumulation in the pleural space and a DPF-related pleural effusion. No pleural intervention was performed as to avoid risk of pleural and meningeal infection. (a): CT scan (axial view) of chest showing right-sided pleural effusion (green arrow) and the ventriculo-pleural shunt catheter in the pleural space (blue arrow). (b): CT scan (axial view) of head showing hydrocephalus and tip of the ventriculo-pleural shunt in the right cerebral ventricle.

Eosinophilic pleural effusions

Pleural fluid eosinophils >10% of the fluid cell count is characteristic of an eosinophilic pleural effusion (97, 98). The eosinophils are recruited into the pleural space from bone marrow and peripheral blood with recruitment mediated by interleukin (IL)-3, IL-5 and granulocyte-monocyte cell-stimulating factor (GM-CSF) (98). Blood and air in the pleural space are the most common causes of pleural eosinophilia; less common causes are drug-related, asbestos exposure, atypical infections, pleural malignancy and pulmonary embolism (99).

Drug-related eosinophilic pleural effusions

Many drugs, particularly anti-epileptic and anti-psychotic drugs, are reported to cause eosinophilic pleural effusions (100–102). There may be a long latency after initial drug administration before effusion develops. Patients present with nonspecific symptoms such as breathlessness, cough, chest pain and fever. Cessation of the suspected drug is followed by gradual resolution of the effusion (Figure 24.9) and symptoms (103). Glucocorticoids may be useful in refractory cases (104–106).

Other unusual causes of eosinophilic pleural effusions

Eosinophilic pleural effusions may complicate eosinophilic pulmonary diseases, e.g., acute eosinophilic pneumonia and eosinophilic granulomatosis with polyangiitis (EGPA) (107).

No underlying cause is found in up to 35% of patients with eosinophilic effusions; drugs, unknown asbestos exposure and occult infection are thought to be responsible for many of the idiopathic cases (97, 99, 101, 108).

Pleural effusions secondary to atypical infections

Pleural infections caused by atypical organisms are unusual other than in endemic area. Causative organisms include: (i) bacteria, e.g., *Mycobacteria*; (ii) fungi, e.g., *Aspergillus* (109, 110), *Blastomyces* (111, 112), *Cryptococcus* (113, 114), *Coccidioides* (115, 116) and *Histoplasma* (117–119); (iii) parasites, e.g., *Entamoeba* (120, 121), *Echinococcus* (122, 123) and *Paragonimus* (124–126); and (iv) other atypical organisms, e.g., *Actinomyces* (127–129) and *Nocardia* (130–133). Principles of management are like that for common bacterial pleural infections and include early diagnosis, appropriate anti-microbial therapy and pleural drainage.

Pleural effusions related to connective tissue diseases and vasculitis

Many patients with a connective tissue disease (CTD) develop pleural effusions. The effusion may be either directly related to the CTD or a complication to CTD management such as drug reaction or pleural infection secondary to immune suppression. Pleural effusion caused directly by the CTD itself is uncommon and is typically seen with rheumatoid arthritis (causing pseudochylothorax and rheumatoid empyema) (134–136), systemic lupus erythematosus (fibrinous pleuritis) (137–139), Sjögren syndrome (140, 141) and systemic sclerosis (causing lymphocytic effusions and chylothorax) (142), EGPA (eosinophilic effusion) (143–145), and familial Mediterranean fever (causing acute pleuro-pericarditis) (145). Management is directed at the primary disease and may involve more aggressive immunosuppressive therapy; pleural drainage and pleurodesis is of benefit in recurrent or symptomatic effusions despite optimal immunosuppressive therapy.

Pleural effusion related to the endocrine and reproductive systems

Patients with endocrine, e.g., hypothyroidism, and reproductive system disorders rarely develop pleural effusions associated with their primary disease (146, 147). Patients with Meigs syndrome present with a triad of pleural effusion, ascites and benign ovarian tumor (Figure 24.10). Pleural effusion typically resolves after resection of the tumor. Ovarian hyperstimulation syndrome is an unusual iatrogenic complication associated with ovarian hyperstimulation for assisted reproduction (Figure 24.11) (Table 24.5) (148–152).

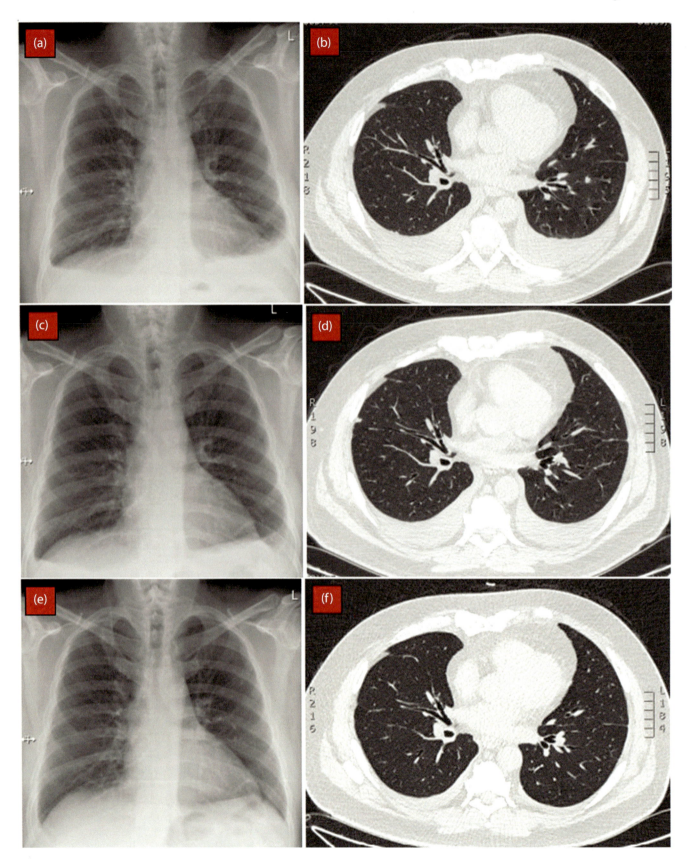

FIGURE 24.9 Dasatinib-related pleural effusion. (a and b): Chest radiograph (a) and CT (axial view) of chest (b) demonstrating new-onset, bilateral, moderate-sized pleural effusions in a patient undergoing treatment with dasatinib for chronic myeloid leukaemia. Pleural fluid analysis showed a lymphocyte-predominant exudate. Extensive evaluation did not reveal another cause for the effusion and a diagnosis of dasatinib-related pleural effusion was made by exclusion. (c–f): Dasatinib was replaced by imatinib for the management of CLL. Serial imaging shows the spontaneous improvement in pleural effusion at 2 months (c and d) and 3 months (e and f) after cessation of dasatinib.

Unusual Causes of Pleural Effusion

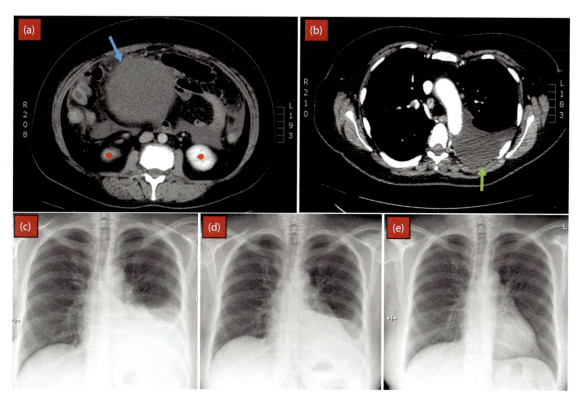

FIGURE 24.10 A case of Meigs syndrome. (a and b): CT scan (axial views) of lower abdomen (a) and chest (b) showing a large mass (blue arrow; red dots identify the lower pole of both kidneys) arising from the pelvis and a left-sided moderate-sized pleural effusion (green arrow) in a patient with Meigs syndrome. (c–e): Serial chest radiographs showing improvement and resolution of the effusion following surgical resection of the ovarian fibroma.

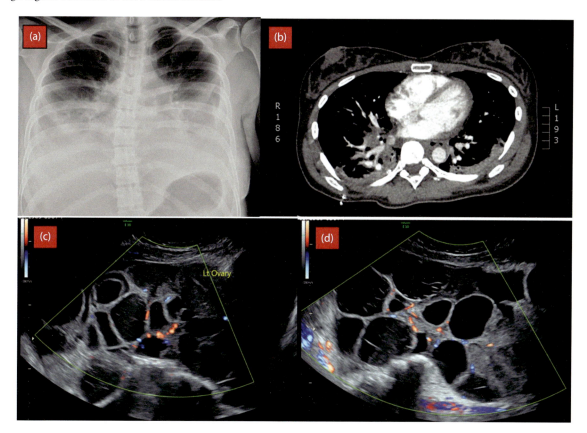

FIGURE 24.11 Ovarian hyperstimulation syndrome. (a and b): Chest radiograph and CT scan of chest demonstrating bilateral pleural effusions in a young woman presenting with acute respiratory distress after undergoing ovarian stimulation for assisted reproduction. (c and d): Ultrasound of pelvis showed the right and left ovaries (c and d, respectively) were massively enlarged with multiple haemorrhagic follicles.

TABLE 24.5: Pleural Effusion Related to Endocrine and Reproductive System

	Pathogenesis	Clinical Features	Management
Ovarian Hyperstimulation Syndrome (OHSS) A serious complication of controlled ovarian hyperstimulation for assisted reproduction. *Features* Enlarged ovaries, ascites, pleural effusion, hypovolemia, haemoconcentration and oliguria. *Risk factors* Previous episode of OHSS, polycystic ovary syndrome and high serum estradiol level. *Predictors of OHSS* Number of collected oocytes, number of transferred embryos and peak serum oestradiol level.	HCG-driven surge in luteinization and ovarian production of vascular endothelial growth factor (VEGF) and cytokines, e.g., IL-8 and IL-6. • Causes angiogenesis, proliferation and capillary leak. • Leading to vascular leak into third space.	Depends on severity and acuity of onset. Usual symptoms are nausea, vomiting, abdominal distension and breathlessness. Rarely, severe end-organ dysfunction can occur with organ-specific symptoms/signs.	*Diagnosis and treatment* • Ultrasound of pelvis, abdomen and thorax to confirm diagnosis and guide management. • Diagnostic thoracentesis and paracentesis. • Therapeutic thoracentesis and paracentesis when symptomatic from effusion and ascites, respectively. *Supportive measures* • Maintain hydration and electrolyte balance • Thrombo-prophylaxis *Prevention* • Personalized ovary stimulation dosing, treatment of polycystic ovary disease and close monitoring of oestradiol level.
Hypothyroidism Pleural effusion is a rare complication. May also be associated with ascites and pericardial effusion.	Develops due to increased capillary permeability mediated by vascular endothelial growth factor.	Symptoms may be those related to hypothyroidism and/or secondary to the pleural effusion, ascites, and pericardial effusion.	*Diagnosis and treatment* • X-ray and CT imaging of thorax. • Blood thyroid profile. • Diagnostic thoracentesis: Fluid may be either a transudate or exudate. • Diagnosis of exclusion • Therapeutic thoracentesis if symptomatic due to effusion. • Thyroxine replacement is the definitive treatment.

Sources: From (146–152).

Unusual miscellaneous causes

Yellow nail syndrome
Pathogenesis
Yellow nail syndrome (YNS) is a rare condition characterized by the triad of lymphoedema, yellow nails without cuticle and lung disease, including pleural effusion, bronchiectasis and recurrent pulmonary infections (153). Functional and anatomical abnormalities of the lymphatic system are thought to cause YNS (154–156). It may be familial in a small number of cases (157), and is also associated with malignancy, immunodeficiency disorders, CTDs, endocrine diseases and drugs (153).

Pleural fluid characteristics
Pleural effusion develops in 36–50% of patients with YNS (158) with a characteristic lymphocytic-predominant exudate; in two-thirds of cases, the effusion is bilateral (153).

Management
There is no definitive treatment for YNS. Symptomatic pleural effusions require therapeutic pleural drainage and pleurodesis (153).

Immunoglobulin G4 disease-related pleural effusion
Pathogenesis and clinical presentation
Immunoglobulin G4 (IgG4)-related disease is a systemic, fibro-inflammatory disorder that can involve the pancreas (159), salivary glands (160), skin, biliary tree, blood vessels, lymph nodes, meninges, kidneys, pericardium and, rarely, the lungs and pleura (161). It is characterized pathologically by tissue infiltration by IgG4-positive plasma cells, obliterative phlebitis and storiform fibrosis (Figure 24.12) (162). IgG4-related pleural effusion (161) can occur in isolation or with thoracic and extra-thoracic manifestations (163, 164). Other pleural manifestations of IgG4 disease include pleural mass, pleuritis and pleural fibrosis.

Pleural fluid characteristics
The pleural fluid is a lymphocyte-predominant exudate with increased number of plasma cells; pleural biopsy also shows infiltration by IgG4-positive plasma cells (Figure 24.12) (161). Pleural fluid adenosine deaminase (ADA) level is often raised (>40 U/mL) in patients with IgG4-related pleural effusion (165, 166). Serum IgG4 levels are also usually, but not always, elevated (163, 164).

Management
Patients with isolated IgG4-related pleural effusion and an indolent course can be monitored closely (161). Patients with recurrent symptomatic effusion and those with extra-pleural involvement of vital organs, e.g., pericarditis, aortitis and interstitial nephritis, require early initiation of immunosuppressive therapy to prevent end-organ damage (167). Glucocorticoids effectively reduce the size of IgG4-related pleural effusion and improve respiratory symptoms and rituximab and steroid-sparing immunosuppressive agents may be effective in refractory cases not responding to steroid therapy and in recurrent disease (168, 169).

Unusual Causes of Pleural Effusion

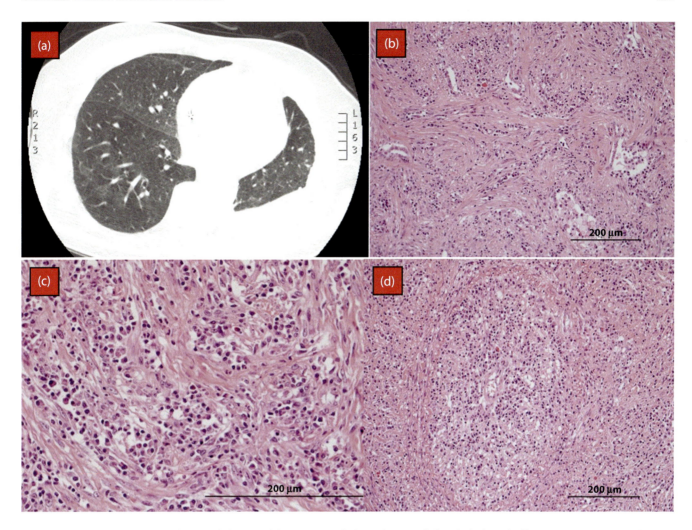

FIGURE 24.12 IgG4-related pleural disease. (a): CT scan of chest showing left-sided pleural effusion in a patient with IgG4 disease. (b–d): Microscopy of pleural biopsy showing classical features of IgG4 disease including storiform fibrosis, lymphoplasmacytic infiltrate and obliterative fibrosis. (b): Storiform pattern of fibrosis (hematoxylin and eosin stain [H&E], original magnification 20×). (c): Numerous plasma cells and lymphocytes scattered between collagen fibers (H&E, original magnification 40×). (d): Obliteration of the lumen of vessels by fibro-collagen infiltrated by plasma cells (H&E, original magnification 20×). (Images courtesy of Dr Amber Louw, Department of Anatomical Pathology, PathWest Laboratory Medicine, QEII Medical Centre, Perth, Australia.)

Acknowledgment

RT has received career research fellowship funding from National Health & Medical Research Council (NH & MRC) and Cancer Council Western Australia.

References

1. Sassoon CSH. Textbook of Pleural Diseases (Light RW, Lee YCG, editors). Respiratory Care. 2004:1257–70.
2. Feller-Kopman D, Light R. Pleural disease. N Engl J Med. 2018;378 (8):740–51.
3. Walker S, Maskell N. Identification and management of pleural effusions of multiple aetiologies. Curr Opin Pulm Med. 2017;23 (4):339–45.
4. Hillerdal G. Chylothorax and pseudochylothorax. Eur Respir J. 1997;10 (5):1157–62.
5. Macfarlane JR, Holman CW. Chylothorax. Am Rev Respir Dis. 1972;105 (2):287–91.
6. Ferguson MK, Little AG, Skinner DB. Current concepts in the management of postoperative chylothorax. Ann Thorac Surg. 1985;40 (6):542–5.
7. Terzi A, Furlan G, Magnanelli G, Terrini A, Ivic N. Chylothorax after pleuro-pulmonary surgery: A rare but unavoidable complication. Thorac Cardiovasc Surg. 1994;42 (2):81–4.
8. Bacon BT, Mashas W. Chylothorax caused by blunt trauma: Case review and management proposal. Trauma Case Rep. 2020;28:100308.
9. Miao L, Zhang Y, Hu H, Ma L, Shun Y, Xiang J, et al. Incidence and management of chylothorax after esophagectomy. Thorac Cancer. 2015;6 (3):354–8.
10. Bryant AS, Minnich DJ, Wei B, Cerfolio RJ. The incidence and management of postoperative chylothorax after pulmonary resection and thoracic mediastinal lymph node dissection. Ann Thorac Surg. 2014;98 (1):232–5; discussion 5–7.
11. Ziedalski TM, Raffin TA, Sze DY, Mitchell JD, Robbins RC, Theodore J, et al. Chylothorax after heart/lung transplantation. J Heart Lung Transplant. 2004;23 (5):627–31.

12. Wemyss-Holden SA, Launois B, Maddern GJ. Management of thoracic duct injuries after oesophagectomy. Br J Surg. 2001;88 (11):1442–8.
13. Cho HJ, Kim DK, Lee GD, Sim HJ, Choi SH, Kim HR, et al. Chylothorax complicating pulmonary resection for lung cancer: Effective management and pleurodesis. Ann Thorac Surg. 2014;97 (2):408–13.
14. Liu CY, Hsu PK, Huang CS, Sun YH, Wu YC, Hsu WH. Chylothorax complicating video-assisted thoracoscopic surgery for non-small cell lung cancer. World J Surg. 2014;38 (11):2875–81.
15. Weening AA, Schurink B, Ruurda JP, van Hillegersberg R, Bleys R, Kruyt MC. Chyluria and chylothorax after posterior selective fusion for adolescent idiopathic scoliosis. Eur Spine J. 2018;27 (9):2088–92.
16. Thomas R, Christopher DJ, Roy A, Rose A, Chandy ST, Cherian RA, et al. Chylothorax following innominate vein thrombosis: A rare complication of transvenous pacemaker implantation. Respiration. 2005;72 (5):546–8.
17. Valentine VG, Raffin TA. The management of chylothorax. Chest. 1992;102 (2):586–91.
18. Restoy E, Cueto FB, Arenas EE, Duch AA. Spontaneous bilateral chylothorax: Uniform features of a rare condition. Eur Respir J. 1988;1:872–3.
19. Flaherty S, Ellison R, Grishkin B. Bilateral chylothorax Following thymectomy: resolution Following unilateral drainage. Military Medicine. 1994;159 9:627–8.
20. Nair SK, Petko M, Hayward MP. Aetiology and management of chylothorax in adults. Eur J Cardio-Thorac Surg: Official Journal of the European Association for Cardio-Thoracic Surgery. 2007;32 2:362–9.
21. Maldonado F, Hawkins FJ, Daniels CE, Doerr CH, Decker PA, Ryu JH. Pleural fluid characteristics of chylothorax. Mayo Clin Proc. 2009;84 (2):129–33.
22. Staats BA, Ellefson RD, Budahn LL, Dines DE, Prakash UB, Offord K. The lipoprotein profile of chylous and nonchylous pleural effusions. Mayo Clin Proc. 1980;55 (11):700–4.
23. Mine S, Udagawa H, Kinoshita Y, Makuuchi R. Post-esophagectomy chylous leakage from a duplicated left-sided thoracic duct ligated successfully with left-sided video-assisted thoracoscopic surgery. Interact Cardiovasc Thorac Surg. 2008;7 (6):1186–8.
24. Alejandre-Lafont E, Krompiec C, Rau WS, Krombach GA. Effectiveness of therapeutic lymphography on lymphatic leakage. Acta Radiol. 2011;52 (3):305–11.
25. Plotnik AN, Foley PT, Koukounaras J, Lyon SM. How i do it: Lymphangiography. J Med Imaging Radiat Oncol. 2010;54 (1):43–6.
26. Kos S, Haueisen H, Lachmund U, Roeren T. Lymphangiography: Forgotten tool or rising star in the diagnosis and therapy of postoperative lymphatic vessel leakage. Cardiovasc Intervent Radiol. 2007;30 (5):968–73.
27. Matsumoto T, Yamagami T, Kato T, Hirota T, Yoshimatsu R, Masunami T, et al. The effectiveness of lymphangiography as a treatment method for various chyle leakages. Br J Radiol. 2009;82 (976):286–90.
28. Momose M, Kawakami S, Koizumi T, Yoshida K, Kanda S, Kondo R, et al. Lymphoscintigraphy using technetium-99m HSA-DTPA with SPECT/CT in chylothorax after childbirth. Radiat Med. 2008;26 (8):508–11.
29. Yu DX, Ma XX, Wang Q, Zhang Y, Li CF. Morphological changes of the thoracic duct and accessory lymphatic channels in patients with chylothorax: Detection with unenhanced magnetic resonance imaging. Eur Radiol. 2013;23 (3):702–11.
30. Akaogi E, Mitsui K, Sohara Y, Endo S, Ishikawa S, Hori M. Treatment of postoperative chylothorax with intrapleural fibrin glue. Ann Thorac Surg. 1989;48 (1):116–8.
31. DePew ZS, Iqbal S, Mullon JJ, Nichols FC, Maldonado F. The role for tunneled indwelling pleural catheters in patients with persistent benign chylothorax. Am J Med Sci. 2013;346 (5):349–52.
32. Oishi H, Hoshikawa Y, Sado T, Watanabe T, Sakurada A, Kondo T, et al. A case of successful therapy by intrapleural injection of fibrin glue for chylothorax after lung transplantation for lymphangioleiomyomatosis. Ann Thorac Cardiovasc Surg. 2017;23 (1):40–4.
33. Zoetmulder F, Rutgers E, Baas P. Thoracoscopic ligation of a thoracic duct leakage. Chest. 1994;106 (4):1233–4.
34. Kent RB, 3rd, Pinson TW. Thoracoscopic ligation of the thoracic duct. Surg Endosc. 1993;7 (1):52–3.
35. Murphy MC, Newman BM, Rodgers BM. Pleuroperitoneal shunts in the management of persistent chylothorax. Ann Thorac Surg. 1989;48 (2):195–200.
36. Lama A, Ferreiro L, Toubes ME, Golpe A, Gude F, Alvarez-Dobano JM, et al. Characteristics of patients with pseudochylothorax—a systematic review. J Thorac Dis. 2016;8 (8):2093–101.
37. Garcia-Zamalloa A. Pseudochylothorax, an unknown disease. Chest. 2010;137 (4):1004–5; author reply 5.
38. Thewjitcharoen Y, Poopitaya S. Paragonimiasis presenting with unilateral pseudochylothorax: Case report and literature review. Scand J Infect Dis. 2006;38 (5):386–8.
39. Ryu JH, Tomassetti S, Maldonado F. Update on uncommon pleural effusions. Respirology. 2011;16 (2):238–43.
40. Streit A, Guerrera F, Kouki M, Siat J, Lyberis P, Filosso PL, et al. Pseudochylothorax: An unusual mode of revelation of pleural metastasis from solid tumor. Tumori. 2018;104 (6):NP46–NP9.
41. Amini S, Kahramfar Z, Rahimi B. A case of extrapulmonary intrathoracic hydatidosis with pseudochylothorax. Clin Case Rep. 2018;6 (8):1507–9.
42. Hibino M, Hikino K, Oe M, Kondo T. Cholesterol crystals in pleural effusion. Intern Med. 2013;52 (23):2685.
43. Zhou Q, Fan J, Peng H, Chen P. [Secondary infection of traumatic pulmonary cyst misdiagnosed as cholesterol encapsulated pleural effusion: A rare case and review of literature]. Zhong Nan Da Xue Xue Bao Yi Xue Ban. 2017;42 (5):591–5.
44. Hamm H, Pfalzer B, Fabel H. Lipoprotein analysis in a chyliform pleural effusion: Implications for pathogenesis and diagnosis. Respiration. 1991;58 (5–6):294–300.
45. Debieuvre D, Gury JP, Ory JP, Jobard JM. [Association of pseudochylothorax and pleural tuberculosis. Apropos of a case]. Rev Pneumol Clin. 1994;50 (4):175–7.
46. Light RW. Exudative pleural effusions secondary to gastrointestinal diseases. Clin Chest Med. 1985;6 (1):103–11.
47. Nguyen Ho L, Tran Van N, Le TV. Boerhaave's syndrome - tension hydropneumothorax and rapidly developing hydropneumothorax: Two radiographic clues in one case. Respirol Case Rep. 2016;4 (4):e00160.
48. Sahn SA. Pleural effusions of extravascular origin. Clin Chest Med. 2006;27 (2):285–308.
49. Good JT, Jr., Antony VB, Reller LB, Maulitz RM, Sahn SA. The pathogenesis of the low pleural fluid pH in esophageal rupture. Am Rev Respir Dis. 1983;127 (6):702–4.
50. Drury M, Anderson W, Heffner JE. Diagnostic value of pleural fluid cytology in occult Boerhaave's syndrome. Chest. 1992;102 (3):976–8.
51. Nirula R. Esophageal perforation. Surg Clin North Am. 2014;94 (1):35–41.
52. Puerta Vicente A, Priego Jiménez P, Cornejo López M, García-Moreno Nisa F, Rodríguez Velasco G, Galindo Álvarez J, et al. Management of esophageal perforation: 28-year experience in a major referral center. Am Surg. 2018;84 (5):684–9.
53. Amir-Jahed AK, Sadrieh M, Farpour A, Azar H, Namdaran F. Thoracobilia: A surgical complication of hepatic echinococcosis and amebiasis. Ann Thorac Surg. 1972;14 (2):198–205.
54. Williams SW, Majewski PL, Norris JE, Cole BC, Doohen DJ. Biliary decompression in the treatment of bilothorax. Am J Surg. 1971;122 (6):829–31.
55. Jenkinson MR, Campbell W, Taylor MA. Bilothorax as a rare sign of intra-abdominal bile leak in a patient without peritonitis. Ann R Coll Surg Engl. 2013;95 (7):118–9.
56. Basu S, Bhadani S, Shukla VK. A dangerous pleural effusion. Ann R Coll Surg Engl. 2010;92 (5):W53–4.
57. Sano A, Yotsumoto T. Bilothorax as a complication of percutaneous transhepatic biliary drainage. Asian Cardiovasc Thorac Ann. 2016;24 (1):101–3.
58. Dahiya D, Kaman L, Behera A. Biliopleural fistula following gun shot injury in right axilla. BMJ Case Reports. 2015;2015.

59. Frampton AE, Williams A, Wilkerson PM, Paterson IM. Thoracobilia: A rare complication of gallstone disease. Annals of the Royal College of Surgeons of England. 2010;92 5:W1–3.
60. Saraya T, Light RW, Sakuma S, Nakamoto Y, Wada S, Ishida M, et al. A new diagnostic approach for bilious pleural effusion. Respir Investig. 2016;54 (5):364–8.
61. Oparah SS, Mandal AK. Traumatic thoracobiliary (pleurobiliary and bronchobiliary) fistulas: Clinical and review study. J Trauma. 1978;18 (7):539–44.
62. Ali T, Srinivasan N, Le V, Chimpiri AR, Tierney WM. Pancreaticopleural fistula. Pancreas. 2009;38 (1):e26–31.
63. Safadi BY, Marks JM. Pancreatic-pleural fistula: The role of ERCP in diagnosis and treatment. Gastrointest Endosc. 2000;51 (2):213–5.
64. Materne R, Vranckx P, Pauls C, Coche E, Deprez PH, Van beers BE. Pancreaticopleural fistula: Diagnosis with magnetic resonance pancreatography. Chest. 2000;117 3:912–4.
65. Vyas S, Gogoi D, Sinha SK, Singh P, Yadav TD, Khandelwal N. Pancreaticopleural fistula: An unusual complication of pancreatitis diagnosed with magnetic resonance cholangiopancreatography. JOP. 2009;10 (6):671–3.
66. Machado NO. Pancreaticopleural fistula: Revisited. Diagn Ther Endosc. 2012;2012:815476.
67. Gans SL, van Westreenen HL, Kiewiet JJ, Rauws EA, Gouma DJ, Boermeester MA. Systematic review and meta-analysis of somatostatin analogues for the treatment of pancreatic fistula. Br J Surg. 2012;99 (6):754–60.
68. Alexakis N, Sutton R, Neoptolemos JP. Surgical treatment of pancreatic fistula. Dig Surg. 2004;21 (4):262–74.
69. Singh A, Bajwa A, Shujaat A. Evidence-based review of the management of hepatic hydrothorax. Respiration. 2013;86 (2):155–73.
70. Huang PM, Chang YL, Yang CY, Lee YC. The morphology of diaphragmatic defects in hepatic hydrothorax: Thoracoscopic finding. J Thorac Cardiovasc Surg. 2005;130 (1):141–5.
71. Jung Y. Surgical treatment of hepatic hydrothorax: A "Four-step approach". Ann Thorac Surg. 2016;101 (3):1195–7.
72. Cerfolio RJ, Bryant AS. Efficacy of video-assisted thoracoscopic surgery with talc pleurodesis for porous diaphragm syndrome in patients with refractory hepatic hydrothorax. Ann Thorac Surg. 2006;82 (2):457–9.
73. Mouroux J, Perrin C, Venissac N, Blaive B, Richelme H. Management of pleural effusion of cirrhotic origin. Chest. 1996;109 (4):1093–6.
74. Takahashi K, Chin K, Sumi K, Nakamura T, Matsumoto H, Niimi A, et al. Resistant hepatic hydrothorax: A successful case with treatment by nCPAP. Respir Med. 2005;99 (3):262–4.
75. Szeto CC, Chow KM. Pathogenesis and management of hydrothorax complicating peritoneal dialysis. Curr Opin Pulm Med. 2004;10 (4):315–9.
76. Lew SQ. Hydrothorax: Pleural effusion associated with peritoneal dialysis. Perit Dial Int. 2010;30 (1):13–8.
77. Bae EH, Kim CS, Choi JS, Kim SW. Pleural effusion in a peritoneal dialysis patient. Chonnam Med J. 2011;47 (1):43–4.
78. Tsunezuka Y, Hatakeyama S, Iwase T, Watanabe G. Video-assisted thoracoscopic treatment for pleuroperitoneal communication in peritoneal dialysis. Eur J Cardiothorac Surg. 2001;20 (1):205–7.
79. Mak SK, Nyunt K, Wong PN, Lo KY, Tong GM, Tai YP, et al. Long-term follow-up of thoracoscopic pleurodesis for hydrothorax complicating peritoneal dialysis. Ann Thorac Surg. 2002;74 (1):218–21.
80. Tang S, Chui WH, Tang AW, Li FK, Chau WS, Ho YW, et al. Video-assisted thoracoscopic talc pleurodesis is effective for maintenance of peritoneal dialysis in acute hydrothorax complicating peritoneal dialysis. Nephrol Dial Transplant. 2003;18 (4):804–8.
81. Austin A, Jogani SN, Brasher PB, Argula RG, Huggins JT, Chopra A. The urinothorax: A comprehensive review with case series. Am J Med Sci. 2017;354 (1):44–53.
82. Toubes ME, Lama A, Ferreiro L, Golpe A, Alvarez-Dobano JM, Gonzalez-Barcala FJ, et al. Urinothorax: A systematic review. J Thorac Dis. 2017;9 (5):1209–18.
83. Barker L. Glycinothorax revisited. Anaesthesia. 2000;55 (7):706–7.
84. Pittman JA, Dirnhuber M. Glycinothorax: A new complication of transurethral surgery. Anaesthesia. 2000;55 (2):155–7.
85. Bach A. Complications of central venous catheterization. Chest. 1993;104 (2):654–5.
86. Lang-Jensen T, Nielsen R, Sorensen MB, Jacobsen E. Primary and secondary displacement of central venous catheters. Acta Anaesthesiol Scand. 1980;24 (3):216–8.
87. Paw HG. Bilateral pleural effusions: Unexpected complication after left internal jugular venous catheterization for total parenteral nutrition. Br J Anaesth. 2002;89 (4):647–50.
88. Thomas CJ, Butler CS. Delayed pneumothorax and hydrothorax with central venous catheter migration. Anaesthesia. 1999;54 (10):987–90.
89. Duntley P, Siever J, Korwes ML, Harpel K, Heffner JE. Vascular erosion by central venous catheters. Clinical features and outcome. Chest. 1992;101 (6):1633–8.
90. Lloyd C, Sahn SA. Subarachnoid pleural fistula due to penetrating trauma: Case report and review of the literature. Chest. 2002;122 (6):2252–6.
91. Saini P, Callejas L, Gudi M, Grosu HB. Recurrent pleural effusion due to duropleural fistula. J Bronchology Interv Pulmonol. 2014;21 (3):265–6.
92. Sarwal V, Suri RK, Sharma OP, Baruah A, Singhi P, Gill S, et al. Traumatic subarachnoid-pleural fistula. Ann Thorac Surg. 1996;62 (6):1622–6.
93. Jahn K, Winkler K, Tiling R, Brandt T. Intracranial hypotension syndrome due to duropleural fistula after thoracic diskectomy. J Neurol. 2001;248 (12):1101–3.
94. Maskin LP, Raimondi A, Hlavnicka A, Diaz MF, Roura N, Wainsztein N. Duropleural fistula revealed by neurological manifestations: An unusual cause of pleural effusion. Anaesth Intensive Care. 2010;38 (1):201–3.
95. Huggins JT, Sahn SA. Duro-pleural fistula diagnosed by beta2-transferrin. Respiration. 2003;70 (4):423–5.
96. Maeda D, Kosuda S, Kusano S, Fujikawa Y. Pleural cerebrospinal fluid input and output kinetics dynamically demonstrated by in-111 DTPA myelography in a patient with pleural cerebrospinal fluid fistulae. Clin Nucl Med. 2004;29 (12):836–7.
97. Kalomenidis I, Light RW. Eosinophilic pleural effusions. Curr Opin Pulm Med. 2003;9 (4):254–60.
98. Martinez-Garcia MA, Cases-Viedma E, Cordero-Rodriguez PJ, Hidalgo-Ramirez M, Perpina-Tordera M, Sanchis-Moret F, et al. Diagnostic utility of eosinophils in the pleural fluid. Eur Respir J. 2000;15 (1):166–9.
99. Oba Y, Abu-Salah T. The prevalence and diagnostic significance of eosinophilic pleural effusions: A meta-analysis and systematic review. Respiration. 2012;83 (3):198–208.
100. Krenke R, Light RW. Drug-induced eosinophilic pleural effusion. Eur Respir Rev. 2011;20 (122):300–1.
101. Krenke R, Nasilowski J, Korczynski P, Gorska K, Przybylowski T, Chazan R, et al. Incidence and aetiology of eosinophilic pleural effusion. Eur Respir J. 2009;34 (5):1111–7.
102. Alagha K, Tummino C, Sofalvi T, Chanez P. Iatrogenic eosinophilic pleural effusion. Eur Respir Rev. 2011;20 (120):118–20.
103. Huggins JT, Sahn SA. Drug-induced pleural disease. Clin Chest Med. 2004;25 (1):141–53.
104. Felz MW, Haviland-Foley DJ. Eosinophilic pleural effusion due to dantrolene: resolution With steroid therapy. South Med J. 2001;94 (5):502–4.
105. Strong DH, Westcott JY, Biller JA, Morrison JL, Effros RM, Maloney JP. Eosinophilic "empyema" associated with crack cocaine use. Thorax. 2003;58 (9):823–4.
106. Sen N, Ermis H, Karatasli M, Habesoglu MA, Eyuboglu FO. Propylthiouracil-associated eosinophilic pleural effusion: A case report. Respiration. 2007;74 (6):703–5.
107. Boyer D, Vargas SO, Slattery D, Rivera-Sanchez YM, Colin AA. Churg-strauss syndrome in children: A clinical and pathologic review. Pediatrics. 2006;118 (3):e914–20.
108. Kalomenidis I, Light RW. Pathogenesis of the eosinophilic pleural effusions. Curr Opin Pulm Med. 2004;10 (4):289–93.
109. Hillerdal G. Pulmonary aspergillus infection invading the pleura. Thorax. 1981;36 (10):745–51.

110. Wex P, Utta E, Drozdz W. Surgical treatment of pulmonary and pleuro-pulmonary aspergillus disease. Thorac Cardiovasc Surg. 1993;41 (1):64–70.
111. Failla PJ, Cerise FP, Karam GH, Summer WR. Blastomycosis: Pulmonary and pleural manifestations. South Med J. 1995;88 (4):405–10.
112. Nelson O, Light RW. Granulomatous pleuritis secondary to blastomycosis. Chest. 1977;71 (3):433–4.
113. Chechani V, Kamholz SL. Pulmonary manifestations of disseminated cryptococcosis in patients with AIDS. Chest. 1990;98 (5):1060–6.
114. Young EJ, Hirsh DD, Fainstein V, Williams TW. Pleural effusions due to cryptococcus neoformans: A review of the literature and report of two cases with cryptococcal antigen determinations. Am Rev Respir Dis. 1980;121 (4):743–7.
115. Drutz DJ. Urban coccidioidomycosis And histoplasmosis: Sacramento And Indianapolis. N Engl J Med. 1979;301 (7):381–2.
116. Lonky SA, Catanzaro A, Moser KM, Einstein H. Acute coccidioidal pleural effusion. Am Rev Respir Dis. 1976;114 (4):681–8.
117. Goodwin RA, Jr., Des prez RM. State of the art: Histoplasmosis. Am Rev Respir Dis. 1978;117 (5):929–56.
118. Brewer PL, Himmelwright JP. Pleural effusion due to infection with histoplasma capsulatum. Chest. 1970;58 (1):76–9.
119. Schub HM, Spivey CG, Jr., Baird GD. Pleural involvement in histoplasmosis. Am Rev Respir Dis. 1966;94 (2):225–32.
120. Lyche KD, Jensen WA. Pleuropulmonary amebiasis. Semin Respir Infect. 1997;12 (2):106–12.
121. Cameron EW. The treatment of pleuropulmonary amebiasis with metronidazole. Chest. 1978;73 (5):647–50.
122. Rakower J, Milwidsky H. Hydatid pleural disease. Am Rev Respir Dis. 1964;90:623–31.
123. Jacobson ES. A case of secondary echinococcosis diagnosed by cytologic examination of pleural fluid and needle biopsy of pleura. Acta Cytol. 1973;17 (1):76–9.
124. Yokogawa M, Kojima S, Araki K, Tomioka H, Yoshida S. Immunoglobulin e: Raised levels in sera and pleural exudates of patients with paragonimiasis. Am J Trop Med Hyg. 1976;25 (4):581–6.
125. Minh VD, Engle P, Greenwood JR, Prendergast TJ, Salness K, St Clair R. Pleural paragonimiasis in a southeast Asia refugee. Am Rev Respir Dis. 1981;124 (2):186–8.
126. Oh IJ, Kim YI, Chi SY, Ban HJ, Kwon YS, Kim KS, et al. Can pleuropulmonary paragonimiasis be cured by only the 1st set of chemotherapy? Treatment outcome and clinical features of recently developed pleuropulmonary paragonimiasis. Intern Med. 2011;50 (13):1365–70.
127. Brown JR. Human actinomycosis. A study of 181 subjects. Hum Pathol. 1973;4 (3):319–30.
128. Karetzky MS, Garvey JW. Empyema due to actinomyces naeslundi. Chest. 1974;65 (2):229–30.
129. Varkey B, Landis FB, Tang TT, Rose HD. Thoracic actinomycosis. Dissemination to skin, subcutaneous tissue, and muscle. Arch Intern Med. 1974;134 (4):689–93.
130. Uttamchandani RB, Daikos GL, Reyes RR, Fischl MA, Dickinson GM, Yamaguchi E, et al. Nocardiosis in 30 patients with advanced human immunodeficiency virus infection: Clinical features and outcome. Clin Infect Dis. 1994;18 (3):348–53.
131. Wilson JW. Nocardiosis: Updates and clinical overview. Mayo Clin Proc. 2012;87 (4):403–7.
132. Kramer MR, Uttamchandani RB. The radiographic appearance of pulmonary nocardiosis associated with AIDS. Chest. 1990;98 (2):382–5.
133. Agterof MJ, van der Bruggen T, Tersmette M, ter Borg EJ, van den Bosch JM, Biesma DH. Nocardiosis: A case series and A mini review of clinical and microbiological features. Neth J Med. 2007;65 (6):199–202.
134. Basoglu A, Celik B, Yetim TD. Massive spontaneous hemopneumothorax complicating rheumatoid lung disease. Ann Thorac Surg. 2007;83 (4):1521–3.
135. Walker WC, Wright V. Rheumatoid pleuritis. Ann Rheum Dis. 1967;26 (6):467–74.
136. Balbir-Gurman A, Yigla M, Nahir AM, Braun-Moscovici Y. Rheumatoid pleural effusion. Semin Arthritis Rheum. 2006;35 (6):368–78.
137. Purnell DC, Baggenstoss AH, Olsen AM. Pulmonary lesions in disseminated lupus erythematosus. Ann Intern Med. 1955;42 (3):619–28.
138. Turner-Stokes L, Turner-Warwick M. Intrathoracic manifestations of SLE. Clin Rheum Dis. 1982;8 (1):229–42.
139. Sharma S, Smith R, Al-Hameed F. Fibrothorax and severe lung restriction secondary to lupus pleuritis and its successful treatment by pleurectomy. Can Respir J. 2002;9 (5):335–7.
140. Teshigawara K, Kakizaki S, Horiya M, Kikuchi Y, Hashida T, Tomizawa Y, et al. Primary Sjögren's syndrome complicated by bilateral pleural effusion. Respirology. 2008;13 (1):155–8.
141. Alvarez-Sala R, Sanchez-Toril F, Garcia-Martinez J, Zaera A, Masa JF. Primary sjögren syndrome and pleural effusion. Chest. 1989;96 (6):1440–1.
142. Thompson AE, Pope JE. A study of the frequency of pericardial and pleural effusions in scleroderma. Br J Rheumatol. 1998;37 (12):1320–3.
143. Lanham JG, Elkon KB, Pusey CD, Hughes GR. Systemic vasculitis with asthma and eosinophilia: A clinical approach to the churg-strauss syndrome. Medicine (Baltimore). 1984;63 (2): 65–81.
144. Erzurum SC, Underwood GA, Hamilos DL, Waldron JA. Pleural effusion in churg-strauss syndrome. Chest. 1989;95 (6):1357–9.
145. Sohar E, Gafni J, Pras M, Heller H. Familial mediterranean fever. A survey of 470 cases and review of the literature. Am J Med. 1967;43 (2):227–53.
146. Hsu CY, Gong ST. Myxedematous pleural effusion. Chest. 1992;101 (1):291–2.
147. Gottehrer A, Roa J, Stanford GG, Chernow B, Sahn SA. Hypothyroidism and pleural effusions. Chest. 1990;98 (5):1130–2.
148. Polishuk WZ, Schenker JG. Ovarian overstimulation syndrome. Fertil Steril. 1969;20 (3):443–50.
149. Loret de Mola JR. Pathophysiology of unilateral pleural effusions in the ovarian hyperstimulation syndrome. Hum Reprod. 1999;14 (1):272–3.
150. Rizk B, Aboulghar M, Smitz J, Ron-El R. The role of vascular endothelial growth factor and interleukins in the pathogenesis of severe ovarian hyperstimulation syndrome. Hum Reprod Update. 1997;3 (3):255–66.
151. Tummon I, Gavrilova-Jordan L, Allemand MC, Session D. Polycystic ovaries and ovarian hyperstimulation syndrome: A systematic review*. Acta Obstet Gynecol Scand. 2005;84 (7): 611–6.
152. Asch RH, Li HP, Balmaceda JP, Weckstein LN, Stone SC. Severe ovarian hyperstimulation syndrome in assisted reproductive technology: Definition of high risk groups. Hum Reprod. 1991;6 (10):1395–9.
153. Valdes L, Huggins JT, Gude F, Ferreiro L, Alvarez-Dobano JM, Golpe A, et al. Characteristics of patients with yellow nail syndrome and pleural effusion. Respirology. 2014;19 (7):985–92.
154. Bull RH, Fenton DA, Mortimer PS. Lymphatic function in the yellow nail syndrome. Br J Dermatol. 1996;134 (2):307–12.
155. Solal-Celigny P, Cormier Y, Fournier M. The yellow nail syndrome. Light and electron microscopic aspects of the pleura. Arch Pathol Lab Med. 1983;107 (4):183–5.
156. D'Alessandro A, Muzi G, Monaco A, Filiberto S, Barboni A, Abbritti G. Yellow nail syndrome: Does protein leakage play a role? Eur Respir J. 2001;17 (1):149–52.
157. Hoque SR, Mansour S, Mortimer PS. Yellow nail syndrome: Not a genetic disorder? Eleven new cases and a review of the literature. Br J Dermatol. 2007;156 (6):1230–4.
158. Maldonado F, Ryu JH. Yellow nail syndrome. Curr Opin Pulm Med. 2009;15 (4):371–5.
159. Hamano H, Kawa S, Horiuchi A, Unno H, Furuya N, Akamatsu T, et al. High serum IgG4 concentrations in patients with sclerosing pancreatitis. N Engl J Med. 2001;344 (10):732–8.
160. Yamamoto M, Ohara M, Suzuki C, Naishiro Y, Yamamoto H, Takahashi H, et al. Elevated IgG4 concentrations in serum of

160. patients with Mikulicz's disease. Scand J Rheumatol. 2004;33 (6):432–3.
161. Murata Y, Aoe K, Mimura Y. Pleural effusion related to IgG4. Curr Opin Pulm Med. 2019;25 (4):384–90.
162. Deshpande V, Zen Y, Chan JK, Yi EE, Sato Y, Yoshino T, et al. Consensus statement on the pathology of IgG4-related disease. Mod Pathol. 2012;25 (9):1181–92.
163. Stone JH, Zen Y, Deshpande V. IgG4-related disease. N Engl J Med. 2012;366 (6):539–51.
164. Kamisawa T, Zen Y, Pillai S, Stone JH. IgG4-related disease. Lancet. 2015;385 (9976):1460–71.
165. Matsui S, Hebisawa A, Sakai F, Yamamoto H, Terasaki Y, Kurihara Y, et al. Immunoglobulin G4-related lung disease: Clinicoradiological and pathological features. Respirology. 2013;18 (3):480–7.
166. Nagayasu A, Kubo S, Nakano K, Nakayamada S, Iwata S, Miyagawa I, et al. IgG4-related pleuritis with elevated adenosine deaminase in pleural effusion. Intern Med. 2018;57 (15):2251–7.
167. Khosroshahi A, Wallace ZS, Crowe JL, Akamizu T, Azumi A, Carruthers MN, et al. International consensus guidance statement on the management and treatment of IgG4-related disease. Arthritis Rheumatol. 2015;67 (7):1688–99.
168. Carruthers MN, Topazian MD, Khosroshahi A, Witzig TE, Wallace ZS, Hart PA, et al. Rituximab for IgG4-related disease: A prospective, open-label trial. Ann Rheum Dis. 2015;74 (6):1171–7.
169. Ebbo M, Grados A, Samson M, Groh M, Loundou A, Rigolet A, et al. Long-term efficacy and safety of rituximab in IgG4-related disease: Data from a French nationwide study of thirty-three patients. PLoS One. 2017;12 (9):e0183844.

25

THORACIC ENDOMETRIOSIS

Ravi Kanth Velagapudi and John P. Egan

Contents

Introduction 194
Pathophysiology 194
Clinical presentation 194
Diagnosis of thoracic endometriosis 195
Management of thoracic endometriosis 197
Conclusion 197
Acknowledgment 197
References 197

KEY POINTS

- Thoracic endometriosis can present with varying clinical manifestations like hemoptysis, pneumothorax, and chest pain.
- Procedures like VATS (video-assisted thoracoscopy) and medical thoracoscopy can serve as both diagnostic and therapeutic.
- Pharmacologic agents to reduce endogenous estrogen production can be used alone or in conjunction with a surgical approach to treat thoracic endometriosis.

Introduction

Endometriosis is defined as the presence of endometrial-like tissue (stroma and glands) outside of the uterine cavity (1, 2). The presence of endometrial tissue in the thoracic cavity is called thoracic endometriosis (TE). It is estimated that 10% of women of reproductive age have endometriosis (1). The thoracic cavity is the most common location for extra abdominopelvic endometriosis (3).

Catamenial pneumothorax (CP) is the most common manifestation of TE and accounts for up to one-third of spontaneous pneumothorax occurring in women of reproductive age (4). Other less common manifestations include hemoptysis, hemothorax, catamenial chest pain, and lung nodules.

Pathophysiology

Several hypotheses have been proposed for TE. One of the earliest and well-accepted theories is retrograde menstruation, which is defined as spillage of viable endometrial tissue from the uterus into pelvic cavity (2). Lymphovascular spread and transdiaphragmatic spread through congenital or acquired diaphragmatic defects are some of the other hypothesized mechanisms by which endometrial tissue could spread to thoracic cavity (5, 6). Anatomical asymmetry in the abdominopelvic cavity and the existence of peritoneal currents are thought to be the reason for the predominant right-sided involvement of thoracic endometriosis (2, 7). Another proposed theory is microembolization after trauma or uterine procedures (8, 9).

Implanted endometrium may or may not undergo cyclic hormonal changes as does normal endometrial tissue (5). However, as learned from *in vitro* studies, certain growth factors like epidermal growth factor, insulin-like growth factor, and macrophage-derived growth factor may play a role in the proliferation of ectopic endometrial tissue, in addition to estrogen (1, 5). Therefore, the ectopic endometrial lesions in the presence of a complex hormonal and proinflammatory environment tend to continue proliferation and angiogenesis (1).

Clinical presentation

The clinical manifestations of TE encompass a wide spectrum of disease and patients can present with more than one clinical entity. An increasing amount of literature demonstrates nonpneumothorax related manifestations of thoracic endometriosis (Table 25.1). Manifestations of TE may or may not be catamenial. The term catamenial refers to a clinical manifestation occurring around the time of menses, typically 24 hours before and 72 hours after the onset of menses (10).

Pneumothorax

Pneumothorax is the most common clinical manifestation of TE accounting for 70% of cases (11). CP is defined as pneumothorax occurring between 1 day prior to the onset of menses and up to 3 days after the onset (4). Less commonly, it can occur in intermenstrual period as well (8). Roussett-Jablosnki et al. studied pneumothorax and its temporal relationship with the menstrual cycle and described four different categories (Table 25.2) (8).

Symptoms of patients presenting with spontaneous pneumothorax include cough, chest pain, and shortness of breath. Joseph et al. reported that 97.5% of CP cases occur on the right side (9). Up-to one in every four women with CP can have a history of recurrent thoracic or scapular pain during their menstrual periods and about half of the patients reported a history of having an obstetric or gynecologic procedure (8). History of obstetric or gynecologic procedures could add weight to the theory of microembolization leading to vascular spread of endometriosis (8). Though CP is associated with pelvic endometriosis, it is not associated with infertility (12).

Thoracic Endometriosis

TABLE 25.1: Clinical Manifestations of Thoracic Endometriosis

Clinical Manifestation	Percentage of Cases Contributing to Overall TE Cases
Pneumothorax	72%
Hemoptysis	14%
Hemothorax/Hemorrhagic pleural effusion	12%
Lung nodules/mass	2%
Catamenial chest pain	N/A
Hydropneumothorax	N/A
Diaphragmatic hernia	N/A
Pneumopericardium (42)	N/A

Note: Incidences of some of the common clinical manifestations are reported in this table. Incidences of other rare clinical manifestations of TE are not available (N/A) (13).

Catamenial hemothorax/hemorrhagic pleural effusion

Though a rare cause of pleural effusion, catamenial hemothorax composes up to 15% of all thoracic endometriosis syndromes (9). Like CP, catamenial hemothorax also predominantly involves the right hemithorax in up to 70% of cases, with 20% occurring bilaterally (13). Pleural fluid analysis itself was not sufficient for establishing the diagnosis of TE in patients presenting with hemothorax or hemorrhagic effusion (14). Recurrence rates are lower in catamenial hemothorax compared to CP (15).

For recurrent hemothorax or pleural effusion related to TE, VATS guided wedge resection, pleurectomy, and chemical pleurodesis were reported in the literature (14, 16). Another less invasive approach that can be considered is medical thoracoscopy (MT) followed by diagnostic biopsies and indwelling pleural catheter placement or chemical pleurodesis.

Catamenial hemoptysis

Catamenial hemoptysis is described as hemoptysis occurring during the menses resulting from the presence of endobronchial or parenchymal endometrial tissue (17). Catamenial hemoptysis was noted to occur in relatively younger patients compared to the other clinical manifestations of TE (17). Kim C-J et al. reported that 84% of the patients with catamenial hemoptysis underwent a gynecologic procedure prior to onset of symptoms. Imaging showed ground-glass opacities predominantly in the lower lobes, further confirming the theory of microembolization of endometrial tissue (17).

TABLE 25.2: Categories of Spontaneous Pneumothorax in Women of Reproductive Age

1.	Catamenial and TE-related pneumothorax	Pneumothorax occurring in temporal relation with menses and with evidence of TE
2.	Catamenial but non-TE-related pneumothorax	Pneumothorax occurring in temporal relation with menses but without evidence of TE
3.	Noncatamenial but TE-related pneumothorax	No temporal relation of pneumothorax with menses but with evidence of TE
4.	Idiopathic pneumothorax	Predominant group, with neither temporal relation with menses nor evidence of TE

Diaphragmatic rupture

Diaphragmatic rupture can be primarily due to diaphragmatic lesions in TE or secondarily as a consequence of diaphragmatic repair for TE (10). Around two-thirds of reproductive-age women presenting with diaphragmatic rupture were found to have endometriosis during VATS (10). Occurrence of diaphragmatic rupture more than 6 months after undergoing VATS for CP could be attributed to TE rather than a complication of surgery (18).

Lung nodules

Lung nodules are not a common presentation of TE (13). They can be present asymptomatically or identified in patients with catamenial hemoptysis (13, 17). Lung nodules on a chest computed tomography (CT) scan can change in size and appearance depending on the temporal relation with the menstrual cycle (19).

Diagnosis of thoracic endometriosis

High clinical suspicion and isolation of endometrial tissue plays a key role in the diagnosis of TE. The choice of clinical modality for diagnosis predominantly depends on the patient's clinical presentation.

Radiologic studies

Radiologic studies help determine the next step in many cases. While chest x-ray can easily detect pneumothorax and hemothorax, chest CT can be helpful in further characterizing the parenchymal lesions and presence of diaphragmatic implants that appear as hypo-attenuating areas (20). Posterosuperior diaphragm is the most common location for the diaphragmatic implants because endometrial cells travel through the paracolic gutter and implant on the right hemi-diaphragm (20). In contrast, the presence of phrenocolic and falciform ligaments prevent the endometrial cells from coming into contact with the left hemi-diaphragm (21). Parenchymal endometriosis can present as single or multiple lung nodules that vary in size and characteristics in temporal relation with the menstrual cycle (19, 20). Formation of thin-walled cavities and bullae have also been described in literature (20).

Chest magnetic resonance imaging (MRI) maybe a useful imaging modality particularly in individuals with isolated catamenial chest pain who are being considered for VATS. When performed during menses, MRI of chest can help in identifying diaphragmatic and pleural implants when CT chest had been nondiagnostic (22, 23).

Laboratory testing

There is no specific laboratory test to diagnose TE. Significantly higher levels of cancer antigen (CA) 125 were found in females with TE compared to those who are disease free (24). Also, measurement of CA-125 levels can predict recurrence with high specificity and poor sensitivity (24). A high level of CA-125 in a woman presenting with spontaneous pneumothorax could raise the suspicion of TE in the right clinical context (24).

Video-assisted thoracoscopic surgery

Video-assisted thoracoscopic surgery (VATS) can serve as both a diagnostic and therapeutic procedure. Various findings during VATS have been described in the literature including diaphragmatic defects, diaphragmatic implants, visceral and parietal pleural implants, parenchymal implants, blebs, and bullae (13). Although roughly half of the patients with CP who underwent

VATS were found to have diaphragmatic defects, no statistical association was found between the presence of diaphragmatic defect and development of CP (13). It was also noted that the odds ratio of having a hemothorax is five times higher in patients who were found to have visceral and parietal pleural implants during VATS (13). In one case series, roughly half of the patients with CP were found to have TE (25). The presence of the endometrial implants predominantly in posterosuperior diaphragm might limit the ability to visualize some TE lesions during VATS (3, 20).

Medical thoracoscopy

Utility of MT for TE is not well described in literature, it can be performed as a less invasive alternative for VATS (26). MT is currently undergoing a resurgence as the field of interventional pulmonology continues to grow. The reasons for this include the procedures safety profile, accuracy in diagnosing malignant pleural effusions, and cost effectiveness (27, 28). It also allows for excellent visualization of the pleural cavity with either a rigid or semi-rigid video telescope (Figure 25.1).

Following are the utilities of medical thoracoscopy in thoracic endometriosis:

1. Tissue acquisition for diagnosis (Figure 25.2).
2. Inspection of the pleural and diaphragmatic surfaces to determine if the lung is entrapped (Figure 25.3).
3. Pleural adhesions (Figure 25.4) can be removed using biopsy forceps resulting in a partial decortication.
4. A definitive procedure for recurring pleural effusion to achieve pleurodesis is either through talc instillation or placement of a tunneled pleural catheter (TPC).

While MT with placement of a TPC in conjunct with hormonal therapy may result in a good outcome (26), the gold standard for diagnosis and management of TE remains VATS. However, further studies on the utility of MT in the diagnosis and management of TE are probably warranted.

Bronchoscopy

Role of bronchoscopy in TE is limited and specific. In a case of catamenial hemoptysis, bronchoscopy with airway examination can help identify the anatomical region that is bleeding, which

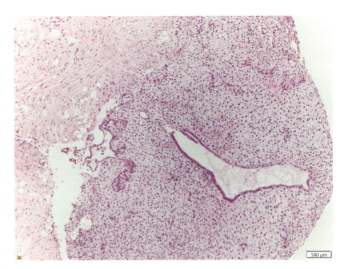

FIGURE 25.2 Hematoxylin and eosin (H&E)-stained section of a pleural biopsy with a focus of endometrial-type glands and stroma, diagnostic of endometriosis.

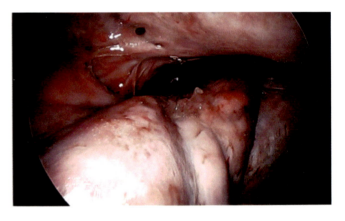

FIGURE 25.3 Inspection of visceral and parietal pleura during medical thoracoscopy showing trapped lung following partial decortication.

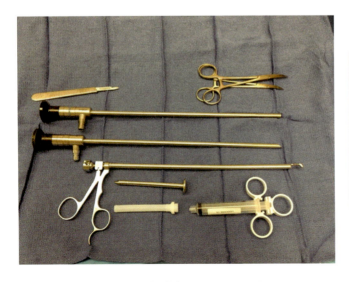

FIGURE 25.1 Rigid medical thoracoscopy equipment.

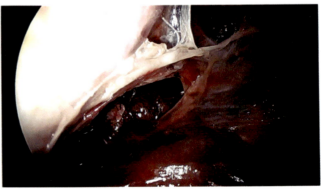

FIGURE 25.4 Pleural adhesions noted during medical thoracoscopy that were removed, resulting in a partial decortication.

can be followed by VATS wedge resection or endobronchial laser ablation (29–31). Performing bronchoscopy during menses increases the likelihood of successfully identifying endobronchial endometrial tissue (32).

Histopathologic and immunohistochemical analysis
The tissue samples can be obtained by various methods as mentioned above, which includes VATS, endobronchial biopsies with bronchoscopy, and pleural biopsies obtained by MT. Classic histopathologic features including the presence of endometrial glands, stroma, and hemosiderin laden macrophages are not always present in TE, making the diagnosis challenging (33). Absence of these histopathologic findings does not rule out TE (34). An immunohistochemical analysis positive for estrogen and progestin receptors is not always suggestive of TE as almost 60% of men with spontaneous pneumothorax were also found to be estrogen- and progestin-receptor positive on resected VATS specimens (33). However, positive estrogen and progestin receptor in an aggregated pattern along with positive CD-10 could aid in diagnosis of TE and indicate a high risk of recurrence (33).

Management of thoracic endometriosis

Medical management
Anti-gonadotropic agents work by decreasing endogenous estrogen production, therefore promoting atrophy of endometrial tissue (35, 36). Hormonal therapy alone is associated with higher recurrence after discontinuation, therefore anti-gonadotropin agents are frequently prescribed both pre- and postoperatively (36). The recommended duration for an antigonadotropin agent is at least 6–12 months with a multidisciplinary approach and timely reassessments (4). Some of the antigonadotrophic agents include cyclic or continuous oral contraceptives, dienogest, danazol, cyproterone acetate, and gonadotropin releasing hormone (GnRH) agonist like leuprolide (15, 37). While there are no head-to-head comparison studies, one study showed that cyclic oral contraceptives had higher recurrence rates compared with continuous oral contraceptives and GnRH agonists (15). Compared to surgical pleurodesis, hormonal treatment has a higher recurrence (9).

Surgical management
VATS remains the first line of diagnostic and therapeutic procedure for TE, especially in CP. VATS allows the surgeon to inspect and identify blebs or bullae, air leaks, signs of TE on visceral and parietal pleura, and defects in the diaphragm. Therefore, it helps in performing resection of blebs or bullae, pulmonary wedge resection, pleurectomy for lesions on parietal pleura, and diaphragmatic resection (38). Depending on the size and location of the endometrial infiltrates, a wedge resection, segmental versus subsegmental resection, or a lobectomy can be performed (39, 40). High rates of recurrence (32–55%) were reported in patients with CP related to TE despite undergoing surgery followed by hormonal therapy (15, 35). VATS performed in women with catamenial chest pain refractory to conservative management showed symptomatic improvement (10). Pleurodesis can also be achieved by chemical pleurodesis, pleural abrasion, or parietal pleurectomy. However, patients who underwent talc pleurodesis had lower rates of recurrence compared to pleural abrasion (35).

Patients with pelvic pain, chest/shoulder pain, CP, catamenial hemothorax, and history of endometriosis in varying combinations, can undergo a combination of laparoscopy for treatment of abdominopelvic endometriosis and thoracoscopy for treatment of TE (41). This approach could potentially reduce the number of times a patient needs to undergo a procedure and provide diagnostic and therapeutic value to both abdominopelvic and thoracic endometriosis at once.

Conclusion
The clinical presentation of TE is broad, and diagnosis can be challenging. High clinical suspicion and thorough gynecological history is paramount to establishing a diagnosis. VATS remains the gold standard for diagnosis and treatment. Hormonal treatment can be used as an adjuvant to surgical treatment. However, treating solely with anti-gonadotropic agents has a higher likelihood of recurrence. Though not well described in literature, MT could be helpful in diagnosis and management of TE-related hemothorax. A multidisciplinary approach involving a gynecologist, thoracic surgeon, radiologist, pulmonologist, and interventional pulmonologist is crucial to properly navigating workup and management of this complex disease process.

Acknowledgment
John Egan reports personal fees from Auris Health, outside the submitted work.

References
1. Zondervan KT, Becker CM, Missmer SA (2020) Endometriosis. N Engl J Med 382:1244–1256
2. Chapron C, Marcellin L, Borghese B, Santulli P (2019) Rethinking mechanisms, diagnosis and management of endometriosis. Nat Rev Endocrinol 15:666–682
3. Nezhat C, Lindheim SR, Backhus L, et al (2019) Thoracic endometriosis syndrome: A review of diagnosis and management. JSLS J Soc Laparoendosc Surg 23:e2019.00029
4. Fournel L, Bobbio A, Robin E, Canny-Hamelin E, Alifano M, Regnard J-F (2018) Clinical presentation and treatment of catameinal pneumothorax and endometriosis-related pneumothorax. Expert Rev Respir Med 12:1031–1036
5. Olive DL, Schwartz LB (1993) Endometriosis. N Engl J Med 328:1759–1769
6. Alifano M, Trisolini R, Cancellieri A, Regnard JF (2006) Thoracic endometriosis: Current knowledge. Ann Thorac Surg 81:761–769
7. Bricou A, Batt RE, Chapron C (2008) Peritoneal fluid flow influences anatomical distribution of endometriotic lesions: Why sampson seems to be right. Eur J Obstet Gynecol Reprod Biol 138:127–134
8. Rousset-Jablonski C, Alifano M, Plu-Bureau G, et al (2011) Catamenial pneumothorax and endometriosis-related pneumothorax: Clinical features and risk factors. Hum Reprod 26:2322–2329
9. Joseph J, Sahn SA (1996) Thoracic endometriosis syndrome: New observations from an analysis of 110 cases. Am J Med 100:164–170
10. Bobbio A, Canny E, Mansuet Lupo A, et al (2017) Thoracic endometriosis syndrome other than pneumothorax: Clinical and pathological findings. Ann Thorac Surg 104:1865–1871
11. Andres MP, Arcoverde FVL, Souza CCC, Fernandes LFC, Abrão MS, Kho RM (2020) Extrapelvic endometriosis: A systematic review. J Minim Invasive Gynecol 27:373–389
12. Ottolina J, De Stefano F, Viganò P, Ciriaco P, Zannini P, Candiani M (2017) Thoracic endometriosis syndrome: Association with pelvic endometriosis and fertility status. J Minim Invasive Gynecol 24:461–465
13. Channabasavaiah AD, Joseph JV (2010) Thoracic endometriosis. Medicine (Baltimore) 89:183–188

14. Nair SS (2016) Thoracic endometriosis syndrome: A veritable Pandora's box. J Clin DIAGNOSTIC Res. https://doi.org/10.7860/JCDR/2016/17668.7700
15. Fukuda S, Hirata T, Neriishi K, et al (2018) Thoracic endometriosis syndrome: Comparison between catamenial pneumothorax or endometriosis-related pneumothorax and catamenial hemoptysis. Eur J Obstet Gynecol Reprod Biol 225:118–123
16. Sharma N, Todhe P, Ochieng P, Ramakrishna S (2020) Refractory thoracic endometriosis. BMJ Case Rep 13:e235965
17. Kim C-J, Nam H-S, Lee C-Y, et al (2010) Catamenial hemoptysis: A nationwide analysis in korea. Respiration 79:296–301
18. Larraín D, Suárez F, Braun H, Chapochnick J, Diaz L, Rojas I (2018) Thoracic and diaphragmatic endometriosis: Single-institution experience using novel, broadened diagnostic criteria. J Turkish-German Gynecol Assoc 19:116–121
19. Chung SY, Kim SJ, Kim TH, et al (2005) Computed tomography findings of pathologically confirmed pulmonary parenchymal endometriosis. J Comput Assist Tomogr 29:815–818
20. Rousset P, Rousset-Jablonski C, Alifano M, Mansuet-Lupo A, Buy J-N, Revel M-P (2014) Thoracic endometriosis syndrome: CT and MRI features. Clin Radiol 69:323–330
21. Gui B, Valentini AL, Ninivaggi V, et al (2017) Shining light in a dark landscape: MRI evaluation of unusual localization of endometriosis. Diagnostic Interv Radiol 23:272–281
22. Marchiori E, Hochhegger B, Zanetti G (2015) Thoracic endometriosis: The role of imaging. Arch Bronconeumol (English Ed) 51:202
23. Marchiori E, Zanetti G, Rafful PP, Hochhegger B (2012) Pleural endometriosis and recurrent pneumothorax: The role of magnetic resonance imaging. Ann Thorac Surg 93:696–697
24. Bagan P, Berna P, Assouad J, Hupertan V, Le Pimpec Barthes F, Riquet M (2008) Value of cancer antigen 125 for diagnosis of pleural endometriosis in females with recurrent pneumothorax. Eur Respir J 31:140–142
25. Korom S, Canyurt H, Missbach A, et al (2004) Catamenial pneumothorax revisited: Clinical approach and systematic review of the literature. J Thorac Cardiovasc Surg 128:502–508
26. Velagapudi RK, Egan JP (2021) Thoracic endometriosis: A clinical review and update of current and evolving diagnostic and therapeutic techniques. Curr Pulmonol Reports 10:22–29
27. Wan Y-Y, Zhai C-C, Lin X-S, et al (2019) Safety and complications of medical thoracoscopy in the management of pleural diseases. BMC Pulm Med 19:125
28. McDonald CM, Pierre C, de Perrot M, et al (2018) Efficacy and cost of awake thoracoscopy and video-assisted thoracoscopic surgery in the undiagnosed pleural effusion. Ann Thorac Surg 106:361–367
29. Marques VD, de Mattos LA, Pimenta AM, et al (2020) Resection of pulmonary endometriosis by VATS using bronchoscopy as a preoperative strategy. Ann Thorac Surg. https://doi.org/10.1016/j.athoracsur.2020.03.074
30. Huang H, Li C, Zarogoulidis P, et al (2013) Endometriosis of the lung: Report of a case and literature review. Eur J Med Res 18:13
31. Gates J, Sharma A, Kumar A (2018) Rare case of thoracic endometriosis presenting with lung nodules and pneumothorax. BMJ Case Rep Bcr-2018-224181
32. Wang H-C, Kuo P-H, Kuo S-H, Luh K-T (2000) Catamenial hemoptysis from tracheobronchial endometriosis. Chest 118:1205–1208
33. Kawaguchi Y, Hanaoka J, Ohshio Y, et al (2018) Diagnosis of thoracic endometriosis with immunohistochemistry. J Thorac Dis 10:3468–3472
34. Scarnecchia E, Inzirillo F, Declich P, Della Pona C (2019) Thoracic endometriosis-related non-catamenial pneumothorax with peculiar histological findings. Gen Thorac Cardiovasc Surg 1:3
35. Alifano M, Jablonski C, Kadiri H, et al (2007) Catamenial and non-catamenial, endometriosis-related or nonendometriosis-related pneumothorax referred for surgery. Am J Respir Crit Care Med 176:1048–1053
36. (2014) Thoracic endometriosis syndrome: Case report and review of the literature. Perm J 61–65
37. Vercellini P, De Giorgi O, Mosconi P, Stellato G, Vicentini S, Crosignani PG (2002) Cyproterone acetate versus a continuous monophasic oral contraceptive in the treatment of recurrent pelvic pain after conservative surgery for symptomatic endometriosis. Fertil Steril 77:52–61
38. Alifano M, Roth T, Broët SC, Schussler O, Magdeleinat P, Regnard J-F (2003) Catamenial pneumothorax. Chest 124:1004–1008
39. Terada Y, Chen F, Shoji T, Itoh H, Wada H, Hitomi S (1999) A case of endobronchial endometriosis treated by subsegmentectomy. Chest 115:1475–1478
40. Kristiansen K, Fjeld NB (1993) Pulmonary endometriosis causing haemoptysis: Report of a case treated with lobectomy. Scand J Thorac Cardiovasc Surg 27:113–115
41. Nezhat C, Nicoll LM, Bhagan L, et al (2009) Endometriosis of the diaphragm: Four cases treated with a combination of laparoscopy and thoracoscopy. J Minim Invasive Gynecol 16:573–580
42. Kienlen A, Fernandez C, Henni-Laleg Z, Andre M, Gazaille V, Coolen-Allou N (2018) Endométriose thoracique compliquée de pneumopéricarde et pneumothorax itératifs sur dystrophie bulleuse. Rev Pneumol Clin 74:104–108

26

TUMORS OF THE PLEURA

Nai-Chien Huan and Rajesh Thomas

Contents

Introduction 199
Classification of pleural tumors 199
Conclusion 208
Acknowledgments 209
References 209

KEY POINTS

- Metastatic pleural disease is more frequently seen than primary pleural tumors and typically presents as a malignant pleural effusion.
- Malignant pleural mesothelioma is the most common primary pleural tumor.
- Benign pleural tumors and non-neoplastic conditions (termed tumor-like) can mimic pleural malignancy.
- Malignant pleural mesothelioma remains an incurable disease although advancements in immunotherapy are subjects of ongoing trials.
- The management of malignant pleural effusions has improved significantly in the past decade with evidence-based use of indwelling pleural catheters (IPC) and combined approaches with IPC and talc pleurodesis.

Introduction

Pleural malignancies can be broadly classified into primary pleural tumors and secondary pleural metastases. Malignant pleural mesothelioma (MPM) is the most common primary pleural tumor; other primary pleural tumors are rare. Metastatic pleural disease is more frequently seen than primary pleural tumors. It complicates most thoracic and extra-thoracic cancers, and typically presents as a malignant pleural effusion (MPE) (1). Benign pleural tumors and non-neoplastic conditions of the pleura (termed tumor-like) can mimic pleural malignancy and pose diagnostic challenges (2). In this chapter, we provide an overview of the classification, epidemiology, pathogeneses, clinical presentations and management of pleural tumors, in particular MPM. We will provide expert commentary and evidence-based recommendations, and highlight important knowledge gaps and future directions in the assessment and management of pleural tumors.

Classification of pleural tumors

Primary malignant pleural tumors

Primary malignant pleural tumors can be classified, based on their morphology, histology and cell origin, into a) mesothelial malignancy, e.g., MPM; b) mesenchymal tumors; and c) tumors related to lymphoproliferative disorders (3). MPM is the classic, albeit rare, form of primary pleural cancer; other primary pleural malignancies are extremely rare.

Pleural mesothelial tumors

Malignant mesothelioma develops in the pleura in >90% of cases; peritoneal and pericardial involvement by mesothelioma at onset is less common. MPM is a heterogeneous disease with predominant histological subtypes of epithelioid (60–70%), sarcomatoid/desmoplastic (10%) and biphasic/mixed (20%) mesothelioma (4).

Epidemiology and pathogenesis

Exposure to asbestos, particularly blue asbestos (crocidolite), is the commonest and most important risk factor for MPM. It is associated with long latency periods of up to 30–40 years following initial exposure (5). The incidence of mesothelioma varies by regions, depending on the pattern and extent of local asbestos extraction and usage (5). Asbestos use was banned in many Western countries in the 1980s and 1990s (6, 7); as a result, mesothelioma rates declined in the United States between 1973 and 2002 (8). Its incidence in England peaked in 2015 (9), and in Western Europe, it is expected to peak by 2021 (6). However, asbestos is still widely used in less-developed countries and it is predicted that the incidence of mesothelioma in developing countries will continue to rise in the coming decades (7).

Once inhaled, asbestos fibers are resistant to degradation and are thought to reach the pleura via the pulmonary lymphatics; here, the fibers cause local inflammatory reactions, leading to hyaline fibrosis along the pleural surface (10). Only a small proportion of people exposed to asbestos develop malignant mesothelioma. Genetic associations, e.g., BRCA-associated protein 1 (BAP-1) (11), and mutations to DNA repair genes, e.g., cyclin dependent kinase inhibitors 2A (CDKN2A) (12), PABL (13) and FANCI (14), may have important roles in predisposing individuals who were exposed to asbestos to a higher risk of developing mesothelioma. Most cases of epithelioid MPM and biphasic MPM are associated with loss of BAP-1, which is less common in the sarcomatoid and desmoplastic variants of mesothelioma (11, 14–16).

Clinical presentation

The clinical manifestations of MPM are often insidious (5). In the early stages, patients may be asymptomatic or have nonspecific symptoms. More than 90% of patients present with a pleural effusion and breathlessness. Breathlessness can be disabling in

DOI: 10.1201/9781003089384-26

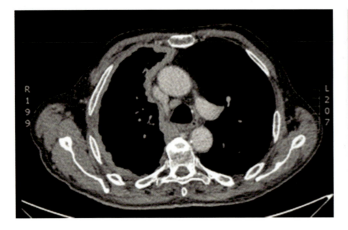

FIGURE 26.1 Circumferential, nodular pleural thickening. CT scan of chest (axial view) showing right-sided, circumferential, nodular pleural thickening causing contraction of hemi-thorax in a patient with mesothelioma.

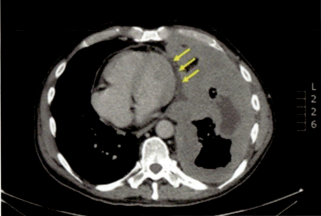

FIGURE 26.3 Pericardial tumor infiltration and effusion. CT of chest (axial view) showing a circumferential pleural tumor in a patient with mesothelioma presenting with atrial flutter and pericardial tamponade. The CT performed (after drainage of the pericardial effusion) shows tumor infiltration of the pericardium (yellow arrow) and a small residual pericardial effusion.

advanced disease, even in the absence of effusion, due to severe restrictive disease caused by the circumferential mesothelioma rind (Figure 26.1) (5, 6). Dysphagia from esophageal compression by tumor is very distressing and significantly affects a patients' quality of life (QoL) (17, 18). Lethargy, anorexia and weight loss develop as the cancer progresses but are under-reported. Severe chest pain can develop due to local invasion of the chest wall, bone and nerves. Lymphangitis (Figure 26.2), pericardial effusion (Figure 26.3) and ascites are late manifestations following lymphatic, pericardial and trans-diaphragmatic spread, respectively. Distant metastases are common but are usually asymptomatic and only detected on post-mortem examination (19).

A previous history of asbestos exposure or pleural plaques on imaging (Figure 26.4) should raise suspicion for mesothelioma in a patient presenting with a pleural effusion; however, in many instances, patients may not be able to specify an instance of asbestos exposure.

Imaging

Imaging is very useful in patients with suspected MPM to determine disease extent and staging, to guide pleural biopsy, and to assess response to treatment (5). Chest radiography is usually the initial imaging performed and typically demonstrates unilateral pleural thickening, irregularity or effusion (1, 20). A contrast CT scan of the thorax (with pleural phase enhancement protocol) is highly informative in the evaluation of suspected MPM (21). It is particularly useful to demonstrate early pleural abnormalities due to mesothelioma. Characteristic CT findings, in addition to the effusion, are diffuse, nodular or circumferential pleural thickening (Figure 26.1). Involvement of the mediastinal pleura is an early and specific sign in this setting (Figure 26.5). Presence of air in the pleural cavity (pleural-air contrast) may enhance detection of subtle pleural abnormalities (22).

Rib crowding, unilateral volume loss of the hemithorax (Figures 26.1 and 26.2), pleural mass (Figure 26.6d), pericardial effusion, contralateral pleural effusion, pulmonary metastatic nodules (Figure 26.2), lymphangitis, rib and chest wall erosion (Figure 26.6b and d), mediastinal adenopathy, esophageal

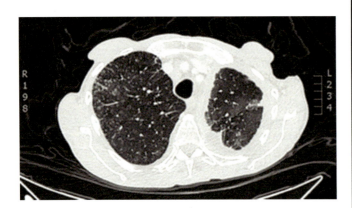

FIGURE 26.2 Lymphangitis. CT scan of chest (axial view) showing bilateral nodular and linear infiltrates secondary to lymphangitis in a patient with advanced mesothelioma. Note the circumferential nodular pleural thickening on the left side, causing a contracted hemithorax.

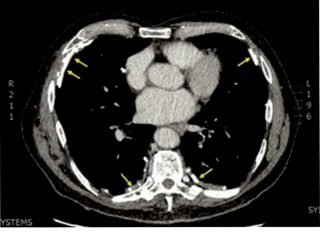

FIGURE 26.4 Pleural plaques. CT chest (axial view) showing multiple, bilateral calcified pleural plaques (yellow arrows) in a patient with previous asbestos exposure.

Tumors of the Pleura

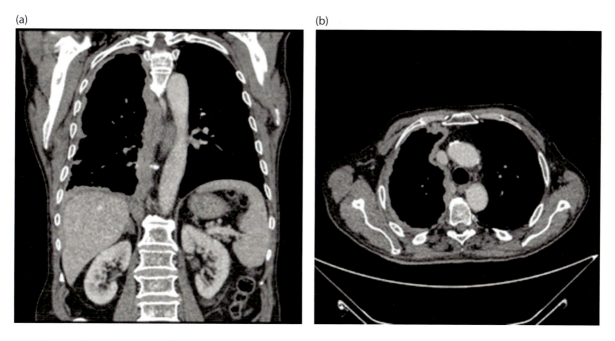

FIGURE 26.5 Mediastinal pleural thickening. Coronal (a) and axial (b) CT images showing severe mediastinal pleural thickening in an 81-year-old patient with biopsy-proven malignant pleural mesothelioma.

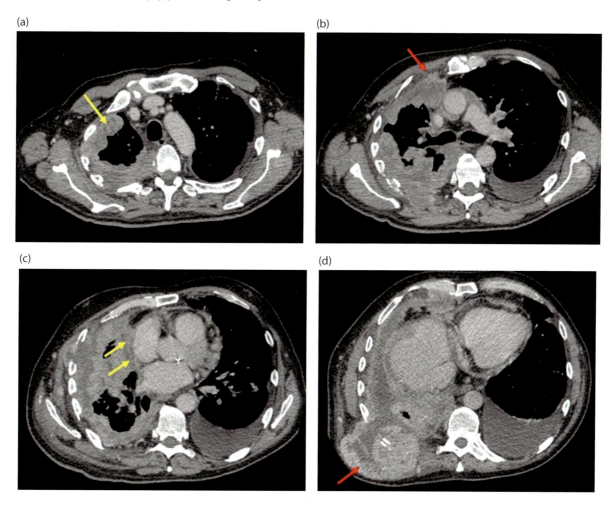

FIGURE 26.6 Advanced malignant pleural mesothelioma. (a): CT scan of thorax (axial views) in a patient with severe breathlessness and chest pain due to malignant pleural mesothelioma showing severe contraction of right hemithorax due to thick nodular visceral and parietal pleural thickening (yellow arrow). (b and d): Infiltration of chest wall (red arrows). (c): Infiltration of intercostal spaces and pericardium (yellow arrows).

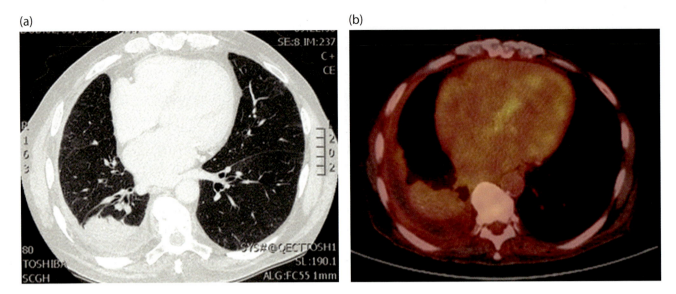

FIGURE 26.7 Round atelectasis. CT chest (a) showing a right sub-pleural mass-like lesion due to round atelectasis in a patient with previous asbestos exposure. Linear bands seen radiating from the superior aspect of the mass into adjacent lung tissue resemble the feet of a crow, aptly termed the 'crow feet' sign. There is adjacent right-sided pleural effusion. Both the lesion and pleural effusion are not avid on PET scan (b), consistent with a benign pathology.

compression and mediastinal invasion also become apparent on CT as the disease progresses (20). CT imaging is also useful to identify benign asbestos-related abnormalities, e.g., pleural plaques (Figures 26.4 and 26.8), round atelectasis (Figures 26.7 and 26.8) and asbestosis.

Thoracic ultrasound is very useful to assess pleural effusions, to demonstrate pleural thickening, irregularity and nodularity, and to help safely perform pleural biopsy and effusion drainage (Figure 26.9b and c). ^{18}Flouro-deoxy glucose positron emission tomography (^{18}FDG-PET) is not specific enough to diagnose mesothelioma but can be useful to guide pleural biopsies when the initial pleural fluid cytology is not diagnostic (Figure 26.9a) (5). ^{18}FDG-PET in patients who have undergone talc pleurodesis may mimic malignancy by demonstrating hypermetabolic pleural uptake that is indistinguishable from that from malignancy (5). Magnetic resonance imaging (MRI) with gadolinium contrast enhancement is not widely used or well-validated but can help to assess tumor extension into the chest wall and diaphragm in selected cases (5). The role of MRI in assessing treatment response and monitoring disease progress is an area of active research.

Diagnosis

Pleural fluid cytology Pleural fluid cytology following thoracentesis of a pleural effusion is usually the first diagnostic procedure when MPM is suspected (2, 5). Differentiating malignant mesothelial cells from benign or reactive mesothelial cells, based

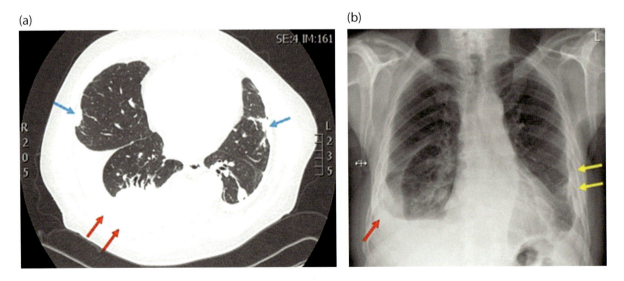

FIGURE 26.8 Benign asbestos-related lung disease. Pleural effusion (red arrows on images a and b), calcified pleural plaques (blue arrows on image a), right-sided round atelectasis, and left-sided pleural thickening (yellow arrows on image b) in a patient with prior asbestos exposure. Pleural fluid and biopsy were negative for malignancy.

Tumors of the Pleura

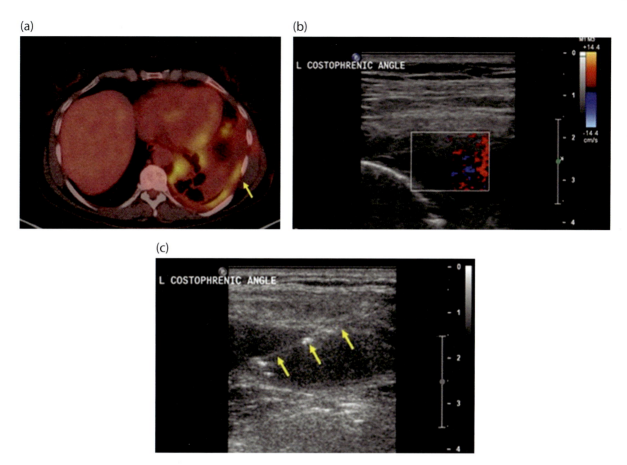

FIGURE 26.9 Ultrasound-guided pleural biopsy. The FDG-avid area on PET scan (yellow arrow on image a) of left pleural thickening in the left costophrenic recess was identified using ultrasound (b) for ultrasound-guided needle biopsy (yellow arrows) in a patient with mesothelioma (c).

on fluid cytology and immunohistochemistry alone is challenging. Nevertheless, pleural fluid cytology for diagnosis of mesothelioma is accepted by international guidelines and expert centres report a diagnostic sensitivity of up to 70% (23–25). Cytology is more reliable and allows use of ancillary tests such as immunohistochemistry (IHC) and genetic and molecular studies if the pleural fluid cellular material is concentrated in cyto-blocks.

IHC testing with mesothelial markers, e.g., calretinin and cytokeratin, is useful to establish the mesothelial lineage of abnormal pleural cells. Additional carcinoma markers, e.g., TTF-1 and CEA, if negative, help to rule out epithelial malignancies such as carcinoma. Newer, advanced techniques that detect molecular and genetic abnormalities associated with mesothelioma can enhance diagnostic certainty. Loss of BAP-1 gene, homozygous deletion of chromosome 9p21 (which encodes for CDKN2A and can be detected using fluorescence in situ hybridization [FISH] [26]) and methylthioadenosine phosphorylase ([MTAP] detected by IHC assessment and used as a surrogate marker for CDKN2A) in abnormal pleural mesothelial cells are highly predictive of mesothelioma (27, 28). Its absence, however, does not rule out a diagnosis of mesothelioma. Excellent reviews of IHC evaluation and application of molecular markers are available in the literature (28).

Pleural biopsy In a significant number of cases, even after expert cytology evaluation, tissue biopsy may be necessary to confirm the diagnosis of mesothelioma; this is more so in the setting of sarcomatoid mesothelioma wherein the pleural fluid is often paucicellular (5). Pleural biopsy can reveal invasion of subpleural fat and muscle tissue, the hallmark feature to distinguish malignant from benign pleural disease. Pleural tissue can be obtained by minimally invasive techniques such as percutaneous closed pleural biopsy ('blind' biopsy with Abrams needle or guided by ultrasound/CT imaging) and by more invasive medical thoracoscopy or video-assisted thoracoscopy surgery (VATS) for biopsy under direct vision.

'Blind' biopsy using an Abrams needle has a low sensitivity (27–60%) for pleural malignancy because tumor involvement of the pleura is patchy; it may be more useful in the presence of diffuse pleural thickening (29–32). Ultrasound or CT-guided closed pleural biopsy is reliable in the presence of nodular pleural thickening (87% diagnostic yield) and requires fewer needle passes. This is important in mesothelioma because of the high risk of tumor seeding (needle tract metastasis [NTM]) along the needle tract.

Medical thoracoscopy (or pleuroscopy) and VATS are more invasive but provide larger pleural tissue from multiple sites with diagnostic yields of 92% and >95%, respectively (33). It also simultaneously allows complete drainage of effusion (33–36) and pleurodesis in the same setting (37). Medical thoracoscopy can be performed under intravenous sedation but when the pleura is highly thickened, as seen with sarcomatoid mesothelioma or benign asbestos-related pleural effusion, rigid forceps or cryobiopsy may be needed to provide adequate diagnostic tissue.

VATS is more advantageous when the pleural space is complex and highly septated by adhesions and/or when additional biopsy from the lung and mediastinum is required. Moreover, both procedures allow careful and thorough assessment of pleural cavity for staging purposes. Direct visual examination for invasion of diaphragm and visceral pleura provides important prognostic data for patients with MPM (38). However, surgical approaches do have a higher risk of tract metastasis in mesothelioma (39).

Mesothelin Soluble mesothelin is a glycoprotein biomarker that is useful when diagnostic uncertainty of mesothelioma persists (40). A raised pleural fluid and/or serum mesothelin level is indicative of mesothelioma (and rarely, another malignancy) even if initial biopsy is negative for malignancy. A normal mesothelin level, however, does not definitively exclude mesothelioma.

Management
Management of mesothelioma
MPM is an incurable disease. The reported median survival varies between 3–12 months (1, 5, 41) depending on key factors such as cell type (better with epithelioid subtype), performance status (PS) (better when PS <1) (5) and weight loss (a strong predictor of poor survival) (42). There are no curative treatment options which, at best, only prolong survival by a few months.

Radical surgery does not improve survival or QoL and is not recommended. Extra-pleural pneumonectomy and pleurectomy/decortication were shown to have higher mortality and morbidity in the mesothelioma and radical surgery (MARS) (43) and Meso-VATS trials, respectively (44, 45), compared to standard pleurodesis treatment (46, 47).

The main role of radiotherapy in mesothelioma is palliative; it is useful to control pain caused by focal chest-wall involvement and reduce esophageal obstruction and dysphagia due to mediastinal extension of tumor. Multiple RCTs have shown little benefit with prophylactic radiotherapy to prevent NTM (48–50), however, palliative dose radiotherapy can achieve good pain control in the 10% of patients with mesothelioma who develop tract metastasis following pleural interventions (51). Higher 'curative' dose radiotherapy is difficult to provide safely due to the large pleural surface area involved (41). High dose radiotherapy has been used for adjuvant and neo-adjuvant treatment as part of multimodal therapy but hasn't been shown in randomized studies to improve survival.

Systemic therapy for mesothelioma provides modest survival benefits. Chemotherapy with cisplatin-pemetrexed (or cisplatin-raltitrexed) combination, compared to cisplatin alone, improves overall median survival by 2.8 months, however, only ~25% of patients respond to therapy (52, 53). The combination bevacizumab-pemetrexed-cisplatin treatment improves survival further compared to pemetrexed-cisplatin alone (19 months vs. 16 months) (54). Most recently, dual immunotherapy (ipilimumab + nivolumab) has been shown to improve survival, particularly in sarcomatoid mesothelioma, compared to standard pemetrexed-cisplatin chemotherapy (18 months vs. 14 months) (55). Combination immunotherapy-chemotherapy as a first-line systemic mesothelioma treatment followed by second-line immunotherapy are subjects of ongoing clinical studies (56).

Management of malignant pleural effusion
Recurrent MPE is a typical feature of MPM (and metastatic pleural disease). Fluid drainage is usually performed for palliation of symptoms, particularly breathlessness and chest pain, and to improve QoL (20). Recent advances have led to a more evidence-based and patient-focused approach to management of MPEs (57–59). It is now recognized that pleural drainage improves breathlessness in three out of four, but not all, patients (60). A patient with severe breathlessness at baseline and an abnormal shaped or paralysed diaphragm is more likely to benefit from pleural drainage than a less symptomatic patient with a normal diaphragm (60).

Pleural interventions should be tailored according to a) patient factors, e.g., symptoms, prognosis, performance status and wishes of the patient; and b) effusion factors, e.g., size, loculation and rate of re-accumulation of effusion, and degree of lung entrapment. The LENT score (pleural fluid lactate dehydrogenase, Eastern Cooperative Oncology Group performance score, serum neutrophil/lymphocyte ratio, tumor subtype) is a validated tool to predict survival in a patient with MPE and may be useful in guiding pleural interventions based on patients' expected survival (61).

Repeated therapeutic thoracentesis, using either needle or small-bore intercostal catheter, is reserved mainly for frail patients with a very short life expectancy and for patients with only slow recurrence of effusion (20, 41). Pleurodesis to prevent recurrence of effusion after drainage can be successfully achieved in ~70% of patients using talc poudrage during video-assisted thoracoscopic surgery (VATS) or thoracoscopy and by bedside instillation through an intercoastal catheter of talc or another sclerosant (20, 62). However, pleurodesis fails in ~50% by 6 months. It is also contraindicated when the underlying lung is entrapped. Indwelling pleural catheter is another first-line intervention recommended by guidelines for MPE management (63). The major advantages of IPC over standard pleurodesis include (i) ambulatory management of MPE; (ii) effective control of effusion (and improvement of symptoms and QoL) in patients with entrapped lung; (iii) shorter hospitalization for IPC insertion and during the remaining life span of the cancer patient (shorter by 3.6 days); and (iv) reduced number of repeat pleural interventions (4% vs. 22% with talc pleurodesis) (57, 64).

Talc instillation via IPC combines the advantages of IPC and standard pleurodesis and allows the IPC to be removed earlier whilst improving symptoms and QoL (58).

Pleural mesenchymal tumors
Primary pleural mesenchymal tumors are rare; they are classified based on their cell of origin into (a) fibroblastic tumors, e.g., malignant solitary fibrous tumor (MSFT), desmoid-type fibromatosis (DTF), and calcifying fibrous tumor (CFT) (3, 65); (b) vascular tumors, e.g., primary pleural angiosarcoma (PPA) and primary pleural epithelioid hemangio-endothelioma (EHE); and (c) tumors of uncertain differentiation (65).

Fibroblastic tumors
Malignant solitary fibrous tumor MSFT comprise only 5–10% of all solitary fibrous tumors (see below) (66). Patients may be asymptomatic (when the tumor is detected incidentally on imaging) or may exhibit symptoms, e.g., chest pain and shortness of breath, due to local compressive effect. Approximately 10% of patients may present with paraneoplastic syndromes such as hypertrophic pulmonary osteoarthropathy (HPOA) (67) or uniquely, with recurrent hypoglycaemia due to tumoral production of insulin-like growth factor (65, 67).

Large tumor size (>10 cm) and sarcomatous or de-differentiated histology are poor prognostic markers (66, 68–71). Surgical resection is recommended in localized MSFT; systemic treatment with chemotherapy and anti-angiogenic agents such as pazopanib and sunitinib may have a role in advanced or recurrent disease (67).

Desmoid-type fibromatosis DTF is a very rare form of a locally aggressive tumor with limited metastatic tendency (65). Active surveillance by MRI is recommended as initial management and surgery is reserved for progressive disease (72).

Calcifying fibrous tumor Calcifying fibrous tumors (CFT) typically affect middle-aged females (73) and present as well-defined, calcified lesions that are localized to the visceral pleura without invading the adjacent lung parenchyma (74). Surgical excision is recommended if the tumor causes symptoms. Local recurrence can occur in 15% of cases, but there is little risk of metastasis (65, 75).

Vascular tumors

Primary pleural angiosarcoma and primary pleural epithelioid hemangio-endothelioma Primary pleural angiosarcoma (PPA) and primary pleural EHE are aggressive diseases but, with <60 cases combined reported in the literature, are exceedingly rare (76, 77). The patient may present with chest pain, dyspnoea, haemoptysis, cough and weight loss (76). There is no known association with asbestos exposure although it mimics mesothelioma with common findings of a bloody pleural effusion and diffuse pleural thickening (78, 79).

Histopathological findings on pleural biopsy in PPA are of large, anaplastic, epithelioid malignant cells with abundant eosinophilic cytoplasm and vaso-formation (65). EHE is characterized histologically by a distinct angiocentric growth of epithelioid endothelial cells (77). Surgery and combination treatments with chemo- and radio-therapy have been tried; however, these are rapidly progressive and fatal diseases with a median survival of <12 months (76, 77, 80).

Mesenchymal tumors of uncertain differentiation

Mesenchymal tumors of uncertain differentiation include pleural synovial sarcoma and desmoplastic small round cell tumor of the pleura (3, 65). Primary pleural sarcoma is very rare; the more common sarcoma involvement of the pleura involves local spread from chest wall sarcoma, usually chondro-sarcoma that represents 4–10% of all cases of sarcomas (5, 65). Other causes of chest wall sarcoma include Ewing's sarcoma, primitive neuroectodermal tumor, malignant fibrous histiocytoma and fibrosarcoma. Surgery with adjuvant radiotherapy in some cases is the mainstay of treatment for localized pleural sarcoma (81); surgery may involve extensive resection and chest wall reconstruction (65, 81).

Primary pleural tumors related to lymphoproliferative disorders

Pleural disease due to lymphoproliferative disorders commonly occurs secondary to nodal, extra-nodal and bone marrow involvement by diffuse large B-cell lymphoma (DLBCL), chronic lymphocytic leukaemia (CLL) and follicular lymphoma (Figure 26.10) (82, 83). Primary pleural lymphoma is a rare disease and is of two types: Primary effusion lymphoma (PEL) and diffuse large B-cell lymphoma associated with chronic inflammation (DLBCL-CI) (65).

Pathogenesis

The pathogenesis of primary pleural lymphoma is not fully understood but likely involves a complex interplay between host immune factors and viral infections leading to malignant transformation. PEL and DLBCL-CI are associated with human herpes virus-8 (HHV-8) and Epstein–Barr virus (EBV) infections, respectively (83).

Primary effusion lymphoma

PEL is associated with severe immunosuppression, particularly human immune-deficiency virus (HIV). Approximately 4% of all HIV-related non-Hodgkin lymphoma (84) are due to PEL. Typical patient groups affected by PEL are young adult males (6:1 male predominance) (85) affected by HIV and with a CD4 cell count of <200/microliter (70–80% of all PELs), elderly immunosuppressed patients and immunosuppressed solid organ transplant recipients (65, 86, 87). The pleura is affected in >75% of cases; in remaining cases, the pericardium, peritoneum and multi-system cavities are involved (65). The typical presentation is that of an immune-compromised or HIV-positive patient presenting with breathlessness and a pleural effusion (88); B-symptoms of fever, night sweats and weight loss may also be present (88).

Pleural fluid and biopsy demonstrate a variable morphology on cyto-pathology and is characterized by large immunoblastic, plasmablastic or anaplastic large cell lymphoma and Reed-Sternberg cells (88). Confirmation by polymerase chain reaction testing of HHV-8 infection in the nuclei of malignant cells is diagnostic (88, 89). Chemotherapy with CHOP (cyclophosphamide, doxorubicin, vincristine and prednisone) and EPOCH (etoposide, prednisolone, vincristine, cyclophosphamide and doxorubicin) regimes, stem cell transplant, radiation therapy and targeted therapy with bortezomib are all treatments available (88, 90). Unfortunately, relapse is common, and prognosis is poor. The overall survival is 18 months in patients with single-cavity disease and 4 months in to those with multi-cavity disease (88).

Diffuse large B-cell lymphoma associated with chronic inflammation

DLBCL-CI is an EBV-related malignancy that arises most commonly in the pleura and is characterized by chronic inflammation and limited vascularization (91). There may be >10 years of latency between the onset of inflammation and development of lymphoma (65). It affects older people (median age of 65 years) and males (10:1 male predominance) (65, 92, 93). The classic presentation is that of pleural lymphoma developing in a patient with a remote history of pyothorax complicating old chronic tuberculous pleuritis (91, 92). Presenting symptoms include chest-wall pain, fever and other B symptoms. Serosal thickening, necrosis and local invasion into surrounding structures (lungs, pericardium, liver, mediastinum) are typical findings; distant metastasis is rare (65). The histological features are similar to other types of DLBCL. Chemotherapy is possible, however, prognosis is poor and the median survival is <1 year (65).

Secondary pleural metastasis

Metastatic pleural disease leading to MPE is more frequent than primary pleural tumors. Secondary pleural cancers usually spread from the lung, mediastinum or extra-thoracic malignancy (Figure 26.11). Pleural involvement may occur secondary to a) direct local pleural invasion (from adjacent structures such as chest wall, mediastinum and lung); b) lymphatic spread; c) hematogenous dissemination; and d) tumor emboli with pleural seeding (commonly seen with lung cancers) (5). Most cases present with an MPE formed due to imbalance between formation and absorption of malignant pleural fluid. Excessive pleural fluid formation in metastatic pleural disease is mediated by secretion of cytokines by tumor cells, e.g., vascular endothelial growth factor (VEGF), that causes angiogenesis, increased vascular permeability and leakage (5, 94). Obstruction of pleural lymphatic channels by tumor cells leads to reduced absorption of pleural fluid (5, 94).

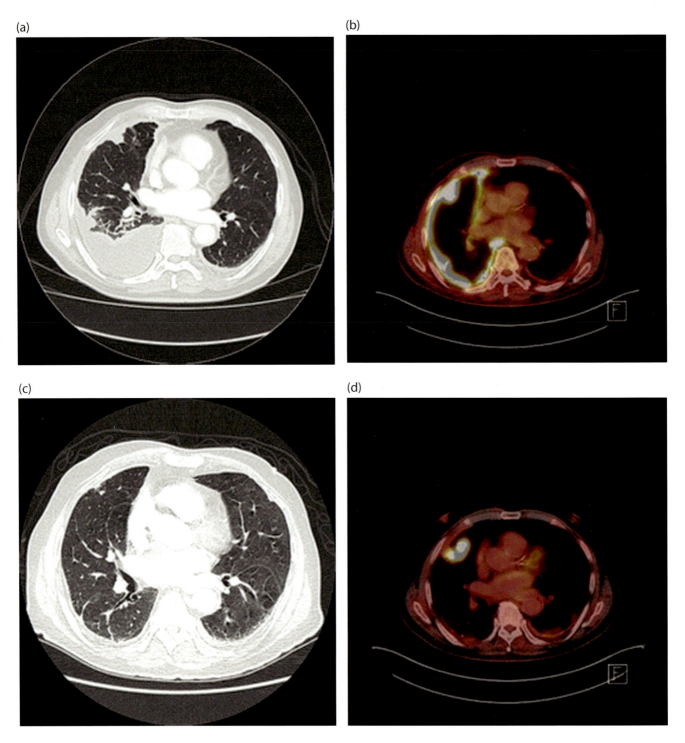

FIGURE 26.10 Pleural lymphoma. (a): CT scan of the thorax showing a right-sided pleural effusion in a patient who initially presented with breathlessness. (b): ^{18}FDG-PET shows intense uptake throughout the right pleural cavity. (c): Pleural biopsy confirmed non-Hodgkin lymphoma of the pleura. Imaging performed 2 months post-treatment with R-cHOP (cyclophosphamide, doxorubicin, vincristine, and prednisone) regime demonstrates complete resolution of the pleural effusion and significant reduction in PET-avid tumor burden (d).

Patients with secondary pleural metastases classically demonstrate a unilateral, moderate-large pleural effusion associated with irregular, pleural nodular changes and/or pleural thickening on CT or thoracic ultrasonography (TUS) (2). The presence of a moderate/massive unilateral pleural effusion without contralateral mediastinal shift on chest radiograph should raise suspicion of a) a presence of concurrent lung collapse secondary to endobronchial tumor; b) a fixed mediastinum due to extensive tumoral infiltration of mediastinal structures; and c) extensive tumoral infiltration of the ipsilateral lung that may mimic MPM on chest radiograph (5). Treatment is aimed at the underlying primary tumor and effusion management for symptom control.

Tumors of the Pleura

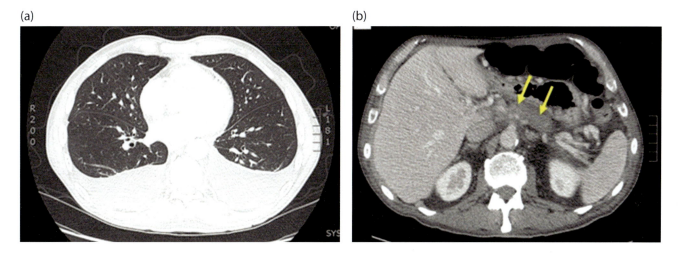

FIGURE 26.11 Metastatic pancreatic cancer with bilateral pleural metastases. CT of the abdomen showing bilateral, large pleural effusions (a) secondary to metastases from pancreatic carcinoma, seen as a low-attenuation density within the pancreatic body (yellow arrows, image b).

Benign pleural tumors
Solitary fibrous tumor (SFT)

Solitary fibrous tumors (SFTs) are the most common benign neoplasm of the pleura and account for 5% of all pleural tumors (66, 95). It is a slow-growing tumor of fibroblastic origin that is usually detected incidentally as an asymptomatic mass on imaging (Figure 26.12). SFTs occasionally grow to a large size to cause compressive symptoms. Unusual paraneoplastic presentations, e.g., HPOA and hypoglycaemia related to secretion of insulin-like growth factor by the tumor cells, may be seen rarely. SFT classically appears as a well-circumscribed pleural mass and may demonstrate additional findings of central necrosis, bleeding and calcification (96). Microscopy showing elongated and spindle shaped cells that are erratically separated by collagen bands (described as a 'patternless pattern') is a characteristic feature (97). A three-tier Demicco risk stratification model (based on age, tumor size, and mitotic figures per 10 high-power fields) is used to classify SFT into low-, moderate- and high-risk sub-groups (98). Most SFTs are low-risk and benign, but they can grow locally to a large size necessitating surgical removal (98).

Pleural lipoma

Pleural lipoma is a benign pleural tumor arising from pleural adipocytes. It has a homogenous, low-density appearance and does not demonstrate contrast enhancement on computed tomography (CT) scan. Rarely, it can undergo malignant transformation into liposarcoma; on CT scan, this has a characteristic heterogenous appearance with enhancing septa within the lipoma (96). A small, asymptomatic lipoma does not need to be removed and can be monitored with serial imaging; surgical excision is recommended for large lipomas and for lipomas causing compressive symptoms.

Tumor-like lesions of the pleura

Tumor-like lesions of the pleura are non-neoplastic lesions that mimic a malignancy on imaging (2) and cause diagnostic

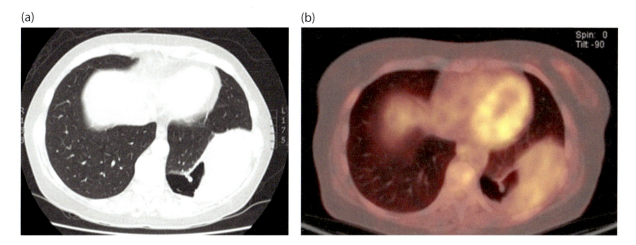

FIGURE 26.12 Solitary fibrous tumor. (a): CT scan of chest showing a 12 cm large left-sided pleural mass in a 48-year-old woman presenting with chest pain. (b): The mass shows uniform, mildly increased FDG activity on ^{18}FDG-PET. Ultrasound-guided core biopsy of the mass revealed features of solitary fibrous tumor, classified as intermediate risk based on the Demicco risk stratification model. She subsequently underwent curative left lower lobectomy.

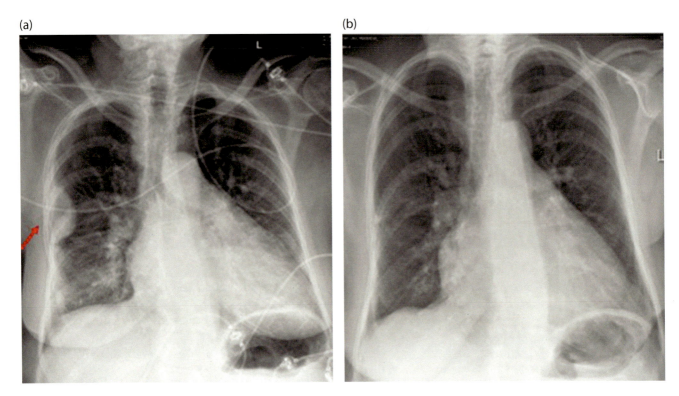

FIGURE 26.13 Tumor-like lesion of the pleura. (a): Chest radiograph showing a loculated right pleural effusion resembling a pleural based mass (red arrow) in a patient with congestive cardiac failure. (b): Repeat chest radiograph 2 months after treatment of heart failure shows complete resolution of right pleural lesion.

challenges (2). Tumor-like lesions of the pleura may be either focal or diffuse and include pleural plaques, diffuse pleural thickening, pleural splenosis and other focal tumor-like lesions of the pleura.

Pleural plaque

Pleural plaque is a common manifestation of asbestos inhalation and a useful marker of previous asbestos exposure (5, 99). It is seen in 3–14% of dockyard workers and 58% of insulation workers. The plaque does not cause any symptoms even when it presents as a focal tumor-like lesion (99, 100). There is no risk of malignant transformation (2), however, it is now recognized that patients with pleural plaques have an increased risk of developing malignant mesothelioma and bronchogenic carcinoma compared to people without pleural plaques (101, 102).

Diffuse pleural thickening

Diffuse pleural thickening can also mimic pleural malignancy and develop secondary to pleural infections such as bacterial empyema and tuberculous effusion, asbestos exposure, connective tissue disease and post-haemothorax (2, 103). Diffuse pleural thickening can be easily differentiated from more focal pleural plaques by features such as blunting of costophrenic angle (not seen with isolated pleural plaques); greater extent of pleural involvement; and fading margins (discrete margins present with plaques) (2, 101). Differentiating it from pleural malignancy, particularly in the absence of a history of pleural infection and haemothorax or in the presence of a history of asbestos exposure, usually requires pleural biopsy.

Pleural splenosis

Pleural splenosis refers to auto-transplantation of splenic tissue to the pleural cavity, usually following splenic and diaphragmatic penetrating injury. It can manifest as focal tumor-like pleural lesions (104, 105) and should be suspected in the setting of solitary or multiple pulmonary nodules and a history of splenic trauma. Scintigraphy with ^{99m}Tc heat-damaged tagged erythrocytes confirms the diagnosis (105, 106).

Other focal tumor-like lesions of the pleura

Other conditions that can present as a focal tumor-like pleural lesion are pleural pseudo-tumors and extra-pleural hematomas. Pleural pseudo-tumor refers to a loculated pleural fluid collection within the lung fissure with the appearance of a lenticular or biconvex opacity on chest radiographs (Figure 26.13) (2, 107). A CT scan can differentiate it from a tumor by identifying the fluid density and fissural position of the opacity. Extra-pleural hematoma commonly develops acutely or sub-acutely following blunt chest-wall trauma, penetrating or iatrogenic chest wall injury, and aortic rupture (107, 108). Early recognition is vital as expansion of the hematoma can lead to circulatory and airway compromise.

Conclusion

A variety of primary and secondary tumors can affect the pleura. Benign conditions can mimic pleural malignancy and causes diagnostic dilemma. A thorough history, physical examination and imaging are crucial and cytological/histopathological assessment of pleural fluid and pleural biopsy is needed in most cases to guide proper management.

Acknowledgments

RT has received career research fellowship funding from National Health & Medical Research Council (NH & MRC) and Cancer Council Western Australia.

References

1. Koegelenberg CFN, Shaw JA, Irusen EM, Lee YCG. Contemporary best practice in the management of malignant pleural effusion. Ther Adv Respir Dis. 2018;12:1753466618785098.
2. Walker CM, Takasugi JE, Chung JH, Reddy GP, Done SL, Pipavath SN, et al. Tumorlike conditions of the pleura. Radiographics. 2012;32 (4):971–85.
3. Galateau-Salle F, Churg A, Roggli V, Travis WD, World Health Organization Committee for Tumors of the p. The 2015 World Health Organization classification of tumors of the pleura: Advances since the 2004 classification. J Thorac Oncol. 2016;11 (2):142–54.
4. Zhang YZ, Brambilla C, Molyneaux PL, Rice A, Robertus JL, Jordan S, et al. Presence of pleomorphic features but not growth patterns improves prognostic stratification of epithelioid malignant pleural mesothelioma by 2-tier nuclear grade. Histopathology. 2020;77 (3):423–36.
5. Scherpereel A, Opitz I, Berghmans T, Psallidas I, Glatzer M, Rigau D, et al. ERS/ESTS/EACTS/ESTRO guidelines for the management of malignant pleural mesothelioma. Eur Respir J. 2020;55 (6).
6. Antman KH. Natural history and epidemiology of malignant mesothelioma. Chest. 1993;103 (4 Suppl):373S–6S.
7. Le GV, Takahashi K, Park EK, Delgermaa V, Oak C, Qureshi AM, et al. Asbestos use and asbestos-related diseases in Asia: Past, present and future. Respirology (Carlton, Vic). 2011;16 (5):767–75.
8. Teta MJ, Mink PJ, Lau E, Sceurman BK, Foster ED. US mesothelioma patterns 1973-2002: Indicators of change and insights into background rates. Eur J Cancer Prev. 2008;17 (6):525–34.
9. Hodgson JT, McElvenny DM, Darnton AJ, Price MJ, Peto J. The expected burden of mesothelioma mortality in Great Britain from 2002 to 2050. Br J Cancer. 2005;92 (3):587–93.
10. Hillerdal G. The pathogenesis of pleural plaques and pulmonary asbestosis: Possibilities and impossibilities. Eur J Respir Dis. 1980;61 (3):129–38.
11. Panou V, Gadiraju M, Wolin A, Weipert CM, Skarda E, Husain AN, et al. Frequency of germline mutations in cancer susceptibility genes in malignant mesothelioma. J Clin Oncol. 2018;36 (28):2863–71.
12. Kettunen E, Savukoski S, Salmenkivi K, Bohling T, Vanhala E, Kuosma E, et al. CDKN2A copy number and p16 expression in malignant pleural mesothelioma in relation to asbestos exposure. BMC Cancer. 2019;19 (1):507.
13. Yang YW, Marrufo A, Chase J, Woodard GA, Jablons DM, Lemjabbar-Alaoui H. Ponatinib is a potential therapeutic approach for malignant pleural mesothelioma. Exp Lung Res. 2021;47 (1):9–25.
14. Betti M, Aspesi A, Sculco M, Matullo G, Magnani C, Dianzani I. Genetic predisposition for malignant mesothelioma: A concise review. Mutat Res Rev Mutat Res. 2019;781:1–10.
15. Carbone M, Ferris LK, Baumann F, Napolitano A, Lum CA, Flores EG, et al. BAP1 cancer syndrome: Malignant mesothelioma, uveal and cutaneous melanoma, and MBAITs. J Transl Med. 2012;10:179.
16. Carbone M, Yang H, Pass HI, Krausz T, Testa JR, Gaudino G. BAP1 and cancer. Nat Rev Cancer. 2013;13 (3):153–9.
17. Santos Seoane SM, Yano Escudero R, Arenas Garcia V. An unexpected cause of dysphagia: Pleural mesothelioma. Rev Esp Enferm Dig. 2019;111 (6):494–5.
18. Hayama M, Maeda H. A rare cause of dysphagia: Malignant pleural mesothelioma in the posterior mediastinum. Ann Thorac Surg. 2010;90 (4):1358–61.
19. Finn RS, Brims FJH, Gandhi A, Olsen N, Musk AW, Maskell NA, et al. Postmortem findings of malignant pleural mesothelioma: A two-center study of 318 patients. Chest. 2012;142 (5):1267–73.
20. Bibby AC, Dorn P, Psallidas I, Porcel JM, Janssen J, Froudarakis M, et al. ERS/EACTS statement on the management of malignant pleural effusions. European Respiratory Journal. 2018;52 (1).
21. Patel AM, Berger I, Wileyto EP, Khalid U, Torigian DA, Nachiappan AC, et al. The value of delayed phase enhanced imaging in malignant pleural mesothelioma. J Thorac Dis. 2017;9 (8):2344–9.
22. Fysh ETH, Thomas R, Tobin C, Kuok YJ, Lee YCG. Air in the pleural cavity enhances detection of pleural abnormalities by CT scan. Chest. 2018;153 (6):e123–e8.
23. Mott FE. Mesothelioma: A review. Ochsner J. 2012;12 (1):70–9.
24. Heffner JE, Klein JS. Recent advances in the diagnosis and management of malignant pleural effusions. Mayo Clin Proc. 2008;83 (2):235–50.
25. Paintal A, Raparia K, Zakowski MF, Nayar R. The diagnosis of malignant mesothelioma in effusion cytology: A reappraisal and results of A multi-institution survey. Cancer Cytopathol. 2013;121 (12):703–7.
26. Steven A, Fisher SA, Robinson BW. Immunotherapy for lung cancer. Respirology (Carlton, Vic). 2016;21 (5):821–33.
27. Hasteh F, Lin GY, Weidner N, Michael CW. The use of immunohistochemistry to distinguish reactive mesothelial cells from malignant mesothelioma in cytologic effusions. Cancer Cytopathol. 2010;118 (2):90–6.
28. Hwang HC, Sheffield BS, Rodriguez S, Thompson K, Tse CH, Gown AM, et al. Utility of BAP1 immunohistochemistry and p16 (CDKN2A) FISH in the diagnosis of malignant mesothelioma in effusion cytology specimens. Am J Surg Pathol. 2016;40 (1):120–6.
29. Mestitz P, Purves MJ, Pollard AC. Pleural biopsy in the diagnosis of pleural effusion; A report of 200 cases. Lancet. 1958;2 (7061):1349–53.
30. Von Hoff DD, LiVolsi V. Diagnostic reliability of needle biopsy of the parietal pleura. A review of 272 biopsies. Am J Clin Pathol. 1975;64 (2):200–3.
31. Poe RH, Israel RH, Utell MJ, Hall WJ, Greenblatt DW, Kallay MC. Sensitivity, specificity, and predictive values of closed pleural biopsy. Arch Intern Med. 1984;144 (2):325–8.
32. Escudero Bueno C, Garcia Clemente M, Cuesta Castro B, Molinos Martin L, Rodriguez Ramos S, Gonzalez Panizo A, et al. Cytologic and bacteriologic analysis of fluid and pleural biopsy specimens with Cope's needle. Study of 414 patients. Arch Intern Med. 1990;150 (6):1190–4.
33. Rahman NM, Ali NJ, Brown G, Chapman SJ, Davies RJ, Downer NJ, et al. Local anaesthetic thoracoscopy: British Thoracic Society pleural disease guideline 2010. Thorax. 2010;65 Suppl 2:ii54–60.
34. Son HS, Lee SH, Darlong LM, Jung JS, Sun K, Kim KT, et al. Is there a role for a needle thoracoscopic pleural biopsy under local anesthesia for pleural effusions? Korean J Thorac Cardiovasc Surg. 2014;47 (2):124–8.
35. Haridas N, K PS, T PR, P TJ, Chetambath R. Medical thoracoscopy vs closed pleural biopsy in pleural effusions: A randomized controlled study. J Clin Diagn Res. 2014;8 (5):MC01–4.
36. Zahid I, Sharif S, Routledge T, Scarci M. What is the best way to diagnose and stage malignant pleural mesothelioma? Interact Cardiovasc Thorac Surg. 2011;12 (2):254–9.
37. Greillier L, Cavailles A, Fraticelli A, Scherpereel A, Barlesi F, Tassi G, et al. Accuracy of pleural biopsy using thoracoscopy for the diagnosis of histologic subtype in patients with malignant pleural mesothelioma. Cancer. 2007;110 (10):2248–52.
38. Pinelli V, Laroumagne S, Sakr L, Marchetti GP, Tassi GF, Astoul P. Pleural fluid cytological yield and visceral pleural invasion in patients with epithelioid malignant pleural mesothelioma. J Thorac Oncol. 2012;7 (3):595–8.
39. Bolukbas S, Eberlein M, Kudelin N, Demes M, Stallmann S, Fisseler-Eckhoff A, et al. Factors predicting poor survival after lung-sparing radical pleurectomy of IMIG stage III malignant pleural mesothelioma. Eur J Cardiothorac Surg. 2013;44 (1):119–23.
40. Hollevoet K, Reitsma JB, Creaney J, Grigoriu BD, Robinson BW, Scherpereel A, et al. Serum mesothelin for diagnosing malignant pleural mesothelioma: An individual patient data meta-Analysis. J Clin Oncol: Offic J Am Soc Clin Oncol. 2012;30 (13):1541–9.

41. Thomas R, Rahman NM, Maskell NA, Lee YCG. Pleural effusions and pneumothorax: Beyond simple plumbing: Expert opinions on knowledge gaps and essential next steps. Respirology. 2020;25 (9):963–71.
42. Brims FJ, Meniawy TM, Duffus I, de Fonseka D, Segal A, Creaney J, et al. A novel clinical prediction model for prognosis in malignant pleural mesothelioma using decision tree analysis. J Thorac Oncol. 2016;11 (4):573–82.
43. Treasure T, Tan C, Lang-Lazdunski L, Waller D. The MARS trial: Mesothelioma and radical surgery. Interact Cardiovasc Thorac Surg. 2006;5 (1):58–9.
44. Rintoul RC, Ritchie AJ, Edwards JG, Waller DA, Coonar AS, Bennett M, et al. Efficacy And cost of video-assisted thoracoscopic partial pleurectomy versus talc pleurodesis in patients with malignant pleural mesothelioma (MesoVATS): An open-label, randomised, controlled trial. Lancet. 2014;384 (9948):1118–27.
45. Rintoul RC. The MesoVATS trial: Is there a future for video-assisted thoracoscopic surgery partial pleurectomy? Future Oncol. 2015;11 (24 Suppl):15–7.
46. Rena O, Casadio C. Extrapleural pneumonectomy for early stage malignant pleural mesothelioma: A harmful procedure. Lung Cancer. 2012;77 (1):151–5.
47. Burt BM, Cameron RB, Mollberg NM, Kosinski AS, Schipper PH, Shrager JB, et al. Malignant pleural mesothelioma and the Society of Thoracic Surgeons database: An Analysis of surgical morbidity and mortality. J Thorac Cardiovasc Surg. 2014;148 (1):30–5.
48. Clive AO, Taylor H, Dobson L, Wilson P, de Winton E, Panakis N, et al. Prophylactic radiotherapy for the prevention of procedure-tract metastases after surgical and large-bore pleural procedures in malignant pleural mesothelioma (SMART): A multicentre, open-label, phase 3, randomised controlled trial. Lancet Oncol. 2016;17 (8):1094–104.
49. Arnold DT, Clive AO. Prophylactic radiotherapy for procedure tract metastases in mesothelioma: A review. Curr Opin Pulm Med. 2017;23 (4):357–64.
50. O'Rourke N, Garcia JC, Paul J, Lawless C, McMenemin R, Hill J. A randomised controlled trial of intervention site radiotherapy in malignant pleural mesothelioma. Radiother Oncol. 2007;84 (1):18–22.
51. Thomas R, Budgeon CA, Kuok YJ, Read C, Fysh ETH, Bydder S, et al. Catheter tract metastasis associated with indwelling pleural catheters. Chest. 2014;146 (3):557–62.
52. Woods B, Paracha N, Scott DA, Thatcher N. Raltitrexed plus cisplatin is cost-effective compared with pemetrexed plus cisplatin in patients with malignant pleural mesothelioma. Lung Cancer. 2012;75 (2):261–7.
53. Goudar RK. Review of pemetrexed in combination with cisplatin for the treatment of malignant pleural mesothelioma. Ther Clin Risk Manag. 2008;4 (1):205–11.
54. Zalcman G, Mazieres J, Margery J, Greillier L, Audigier-Valette C, Moro-Sibilot D, et al. Bevacizumab for newly diagnosed pleural mesothelioma in the mesothelioma avastin cisplatin pemetrexed study (MAPS): A randomised, controlled, open-label, phase 3 trial. Lancet. 2016;387 (10026):1405–14.
55. Baas P, Scherpereel A, Nowak AK, Fujimoto N, Peters S, Tsao AS, et al. First-line nivolumab plus ipilimumab in unresectable malignant pleural mesothelioma (CheckMate 743): A multicentre, randomised, open-label, phase 3 trial. Lancet. 2021;397 (10272):375–86.
56. Forde PM, Anagnostou V, Sun Z, Dahlberg SE, Kindler HL, Niknafs N, et al. Durvalumab with platinum-pemetrexed for unresectable pleural mesothelioma: Survival, genomic and immunologic analyses from the phase 2 PrE0505 trial. Nat Med. 2021;27 (11):1910–20.
57. Davies HE, Mishra EK, Kahan BC, Wrightson JM, Stanton AE, Guhan A, et al. Effect of an indwelling pleural catheter vs chest tube and talc pleurodesis for relieving dyspnea in patients with malignant pleural effusion: The TIME2 randomized controlled trial. Jama. 2012;307 (22):2383–9.
58. Bhatnagar R, Keenan EK, Morley AJ, Kahan BC, Stanton AE, Haris M, et al. Outpatient talc administration by indwelling pleural catheter for malignant effusion. The New England Journal of Medicine. 2018;378 (14):1313–22.
59. Rahman NM, Pepperell J, Rehal S, Saba T, Tang A, Ali N, et al. Effect of opioids vs NSAIDs and larger vs smaller chest tube size on pain control and pleurodesis efficacy among patients with malignant pleural effusion: The TIME1 randomized clinical trial. Jama. 2015;314 (24):2641–53.
60. Muruganandan S, Azzopardi M, Thomas R, Fitzgerald DB, Kuok YJ, Cheah HM, et al. The pleural effusion and symptom evaluation (PLEASE) study of breathlessness in patients with a symptomatic pleural effusion. Eur Respir J. 2020;55 (5).
61. Clive AO, Kahan BC, Hooper CE, Bhatnagar R, Morley AJ, Zahan-Evans N, et al. Predicting survival in malignant pleural effusion: Development and validation of the LENT prognostic score. Thorax. 2014;69 (12):1098–104.
62. Bhatnagar R, Luengo-Fernandez R, Kahan BC, Rahman NM, Miller RF, Maskell NA. Thoracoscopy and talc poudrage compared with intercostal drainage and talc slurry infusion to manage malignant pleural effusion: The TAPPS RCT. Health Technol Assess. 2020;24 (26):1–90.
63. Feller-Kopman DJ, Reddy CB, DeCamp MM, Diekemper RL, Gould MK, Henry T, et al. Management of malignant pleural effusions. An official ATS/STS/STR clinical practice guideline. Am J Respir Crit Care Med. 2018;198 (7):839–49.
64. Fysh ET, Thomas R, Read CA, Kwan BC, Yap E, Horwood FC, et al. Protocol of the Australasian malignant pleural effusion (AMPLE) trial: A multicentre randomised study comparing indwelling pleural catheter versus talc pleurodesis. BMJ Open. 2014;4 (11):e006757.
65. Attanoos RL, Pugh MR. The diagnosis of pleural tumors other than mesothelioma. Arch Pathol Lab Med. 2018;142 (8):902–13.
66. England DM, Hochholzer L, McCarthy MJ. Localized benign and malignant fibrous tumors of the pleura. A clinicopathologic review of 223 cases. Am J Surg Pathol. 1989;13 (8):640–58.
67. Martin-Broto J, Mondaza-Hernandez JL, Moura DS, Hindi N. A comprehensive review on solitary fibrous tumor: new insights for new horizons. Cancers (Basel). 2021;13 (12).
68. Chamberlain MH, Taggart DP. Solitary fibrous tumor associated with hypoglycemia: An example of the Doege-Potter syndrome. J Thorac Cardiovasc Surg. 2000;119 (1):185–7.
69. Balduyck B, Lauwers P, Govaert K, Hendriks J, De Maeseneer M, Van Schil P. Solitary fibrous tumor of the pleura with associated hypoglycemia: Doege-Potter syndrome: A case report. J Thorac Oncol. 2006;1 (6):588–90.
70. Liu B, Liu L, Li Y. Giant solitary fibrous tumor of the pleura: A case report. Thorac Cancer. 2015;6 (3):368–71.
71. Ricciuti B, Metro G, Leonardi GC, Sordo RD, Colella R, Puma F, et al. Malignant giant solitary fibrous tumor of the pleura metastatic to the thyroid gland. Tumori. 2016;102 (Suppl. 2).
72. Penel N, Kasper B, van Der Graaf WTA. Desmoid-type fibromatosis: Toward a holistic management. Curr Opin Oncol. 2021;33 (4):309–14.
73. Suh JH, Shin OR, Kim YH. Multiple calcifying fibrous pseudotumor of the pleura. J Thorac Oncol. 2008;3 (11):1356–8.
74. Lee SC, Tzao C, Ou SM, Hsu HH, Yu CP, Cheng YL. Solitary fibrous tumors of the pleura: Clinical, radiological, surgical and pathological evaluation. Eur J Surg Oncol. 2005;31 (1):84–7.
75. Chorti A, Papavramidis TS, Michalopoulos A. Calcifying fibrous tumor: Review of 157 patients reported in international literature. Medicine (Baltimore). 2016;95 (20):e3690.
76. Kao YC, Chow JM, Wang KM, Fang CL, Chu JS, Chen CL. Primary pleural angiosarcoma as A mimicker of mesothelioma: A case report **VS**. Diagn Pathol. 2011;6:130.
77. Wethasinghe J, Sood J, Walmsley R, Milne D, Jafer A, Gordon-Glassford N. Primary pleural epithelioid hemangioendothelioma mimicking as a posterior mediastinal tumor. Respirol Case Rep. 2015;3 (2):75–7.
78. Anderson T, Zhang L, Hameed M, Rusch V, Travis WD, Antonescu CR. Thoracic epithelioid malignant vascular tumors: A clinicopathologic study of 52 cases with emphasis on pathologic grading and molecular studies of WWTR1-CAMTA1 fusions. Am J Surg Pathol. 2015;39 (1):132–9.
79. Zhang PJ, Livolsi VA, Brooks JJ. Malignant epithelioid vascular tumors of the pleura: Report of a series and literature review. Hum Pathol. 2000;31 (1):29–34.

80. Ha SY, Choi IH, Han J, Choi YL, Cho JH, Lee KJ, et al. Pleural epithelioid hemangioendothelioma harboring CAMTA1 rearrangement. Lung Cancer. 2014;83 (3):411–5.
81. Guinee DG, Allen TC. Primary pleural neoplasia: Entities other than diffuse malignant mesothelioma. Arch Pathol Lab Med. 2008;132 (7):1149–70.
82. Das DK, Gupta SK, Ayyagari S, Bambery PK, Datta BN, Datta U. Pleural effusions in non-Hodgkin's lymphoma. A cytomorphologic, cytochemical and immunologic study. Acta Cytol. 1987;31 (2):119–24.
83. Swerdlow SH, Campo E, Pileri SA, Harris NL, Stein H, Siebert R, et al. The 2016 revision of the World Health Organization classification of lymphoid neoplasms. Blood. 2016;127 (20):2375–90.
84. Kaplan LD. Human herpesvirus-8: Kaposi sarcoma, multicentric Castleman disease, and primary effusion lymphoma. Hematology Am Soc Hematol Educ Program. 2013;2013:103–8.
85. Castillo JJ, Shum H, Lahijani M, Winer ES, Butera JN. Prognosis in primary effusion lymphoma is associated with the number of body cavities involved. Leuk Lymphoma. 2012;53 (12):2378–82.
86. Luppi M, Barozzi P, Santagostino G, Trovato R, Schulz TF, Marasca R, et al. Molecular evidence of organ-related transmission of Kaposi sarcoma-associated herpesvirus or human herpesvirus-8 in transplant patients. Blood. 2000;96 (9):3279–81.
87. Dotti G, Fiocchi R, Motta T, Facchinetti B, Chiodini B, Borleri GM, et al. Primary effusion lymphoma after heart transplantation: A new entity associated with human herpesvirus-8. Leukemia. 1999;13 (5):664–70.
88. Narkhede M, Arora S, Ujjani C. Primary effusion lymphoma: Current perspectives. Onco Targets Ther. 2018;11:3747–54.
89. Brimo F, Michel RP, Khetani K, Auger M. Primary effusion lymphoma: A series of 4 cases and review of the literature with emphasis on cytomorphologic and immunocytochemical differential diagnosis. Cancer. 2007;111 (4):224–33.
90. Dunleavy K, Wilson WH. How i treat HIV-associated lymphoma. Blood. 2012;119 (14):3245–55.
91. Kanno H, Naka N, Yasunaga Y, Iuchi K, Yamauchi S, Hashimoto M, et al. Production of the immunosuppressive cytokine interleukin-10 by Epstein–Barr-virus-expressing pyothorax-associated lymphoma: Possible role in the development of overt lymphoma in immunocompetent hosts. Am J Pathol. 1997;150 (1):349–57.
92. Loong F, Chan AC, Ho BC, Chau YP, Lee HY, Cheuk W, et al. Diffuse large B-cell lymphoma associated with chronic inflammation as an incidental finding and new clinical scenarios. Mod Pathol. 2010;23 (4):493–501.
93. Keung YK, Cobos E, Morgan D, McConnell TS. Non-pyothorax-associated primary pleural lymphoma with complex karyotypic abnormalities. Leuk Lymphoma. 1996;23 (5–6):621–4.
94. Feller-Kopman D, Light R. Pleural disease. N Engl J Med. 2018;378 (8):740–51.
95. Cardillo G, Lococo F, Carleo F, Martelli M. Solitary fibrous tumors of the pleura. Curr Opin Pulm Med. 2012;18 (4):339–46.
96. Sureka B, Thukral BB, Mittal MK, Mittal A, Sinha M. Radiological review of pleural tumors. Indian J Radiol Imaging. 2013;23 (4):313–20.
97. Chang YL, Lee YC, Wu CT. Thoracic solitary fibrous tumor: Clinical and pathological diversity. Lung Cancer. 1999;23 (1):53–60.
98. Demicco EG, Park MS, Araujo DM, Fox PS, Bassett RL, Pollock RE, et al. Solitary fibrous tumor: A clinicopathological study of 110 cases and proposed risk assessment model. Mod Pathol. 2012;25 (9):1298–306.
99. Nishimura SL, Broaddus VC. Asbestos-induced pleural disease. Clin Chest Med. 1998;19 (2):311–29.
100. Peacock C, Copley SJ, Hansell DM. Asbestos-related benign pleural disease. Clin Radiol. 2000;55 (6):422–32.
101. Lynch DA, Gamsu G, Aberle DR. Conventional and high resolution computed tomography in the diagnosis of asbestos-related diseases. Radiographics. 1989;9 (3):523–51.
102. Fletcher DE. A mortality study of shipyard workers with pleural plaques. Br J Ind Med. 1972;29 (2):142–5.
103. Copley SJ, Wells AU, Rubens MB, Chabat F, Sheehan RE, Musk AW, et al. Functional consequences of pleural disease evaluated with chest radiography and CT. Radiology. 2001;220 (1):237–43.
104. Normand JP, Rioux M, Dumont M, Bouchard G, Letourneau L. Thoracic splenosis after blunt trauma: Frequency and imaging findings. Am J Roentgenol. 1993;161 (4):739–41.
105. Yammine JN, Yatim A, Barbari A. Radionuclide imaging in thoracic splenosis and a review of the literature. Clin Nucl Med. 2003;28 (2):121–3.
106. Armas RR. Clinical studies with spleen-specific radiolabeled agents. Semin Nucl Med. 1985;15 (3):260–75.
107. Chung JH, Carr RB, Stern EJ. Extrapleural hematomas: Imaging appearance, classification, and clinical significance. J Thorac Imaging. 2011;26 (3):218–23.
108. Rashid MA, Wikstrom T, Ortenwall P. Nomenclature, classification, and signficance of traumatic extrapleural hematoma. J Trauma. 2000;49 (2):286–90.

INDEX

Note: Locators in *italics* represent figures and **bold** indicate tables in the text.

A

AAT, *see* Alpha-1 antitrypsin
AATD, *see* Alpha-1 antitrypsin deficiency
ABPA, *see* Allergic bronchopulmonary aspergillosis
ABPM, *see* Allergic bronchopulmonary mycosis
Abrams needle, 203
ACB, *see* Accessory cardiac bronchus
ACC, *see* Adenoid cystic carcinoma
Accessory cardiac bronchus (ACB), 9
Acromegaly, 155
Activin-receptor like kinase 1 gene (ACVRL1), 57
ACT trial, *see* Alpha Coded Testing trial
Acute bronchiolitis, 45
Acute eosinophilic pneumonia (AEP), 91
    clinical features, 92, **92**
    diagnosis, 93
    histopathology, 93
    imaging, 93
    treatment and prognosis, 93
ACVRL1, *see* Activin-receptor like kinase 1 gene
Adenoid cystic carcinoma (ACC), 169, 171–173, *173*, *174*
Adult pulmonary alveolar proteinosis, *see* Pulmonary alveolar proteinosis
AEP, *see* Acute eosinophilic pneumonia
Airway disease, 88
    ABPA in patients with, 51
        asthma, 51
        cystic fibrosis, 52
Airway obstruction, 6
Allergic bronchopulmonary aspergillosis (ABPA), 51
    with central bronchiectasis (ABPA-CB), 52
    without central bronchiectasis (ABPA-S), 52
    clinical features of, 52
    diagnosis of, 52
        bronchoscopy, 53
        imaging, 53–54
        laboratory findings, 53
        peripheral eosinophilia, 53
        serum IgE, 53
        skin testing, 53
    diagnostic criteria, **53**
    management of, 54
        antifungal therapies, 54
        inhaled corticosteroids, 54
        systemic corticosteroids, 54
        systemic steroids versus antifungals, 54
        targeted biologics, 54–55
    in patients with airway diseases, 51
        asthma, 51
        cystic fibrosis, 52
Allergic bronchopulmonary mycosis (ABPM), 51
Allergic sensitization (AS), 51
Alpha-1 antitrypsin (AAT), 20
Alpha-1 antitrypsin deficiency (AATD)
    augmentation therapy, 27
    clinical features of, 24–27
        liver disease, 25
        lung disease, 25
        panniculitis, 25, *26*
        vasculitis, 25
    diagnosis, 26–27
    diagnostic delay interval for, **22**
    emerging therapies for, 28, **28**
    epidemiology of, 21
    genetics and pathogenesis of, 21–24
    history of, 20–21
    lung transplantation, 27–28
    lung volume reduction in, 28
    natural history of, 25
    phenotypes, **22**
    treatment, 27
Alpha-1 antitrypsin glycoprotein, *23*
Alpha Coded Testing (ACT) trial, 27
Alveolar macrophages, 110
Amitani disease, 77
AMLs, *see* Angiomyolipomas
Amyloid, 160
Amyloidomas, 165
Amyloidosis, 160
ANCA, *see* Antineutrophil cytoplasm antibody
Ancylostoma, 96
Angiomyolipomas (AMLs), 116, 118
Anomalous pulmonary venous drainage, 9–10
Antifungal therapies, 54
Anti-GBM disease, 68
Anti-inflammatory agents, 104
Antineutrophil cytoplasm antibody (ANCA), 35
    -associated vasculitis (AAV), 35, 64, 67–68
Apical caps and PPFE, **81**
Aplasia, 4
Arteriovenous malformation (AVM), 10, *11*
AS, *see* Allergic sensitization
Asbestos fibers, 199
Ascaris, 96
Ascaris lumbricoides, 96
Aspergillus fumigatus, 51, 53
Asthma, 51
Asthma Control Test scores, 54
Augmentation therapy, 27
Autoimmune PAP, 112
AVM, *see* Arteriovenous malformation
Azathioprine, 68, 89, 105, 129
Azithromycin, 157

B

BADE, *see* Bronchiolitis, alveolar ductitis, and centrilobular emphysema
BAL, *see* Bronchoalveolar lavage
BALT, *see* Bronchus-associated lymphoid tissue
BCs, *see* Bronchogenic cysts
Benign asbestos-related lung disease, *202*
Benign central airway disorders
    central airway obstruction, miscellaneous causes of, 38–39
    granulomatosis with polyangiitis (GPA), 35
        clinical presentation, 35
        diagnosis, 35–36
        pathology, 36–37
        risk factors, 35
        treatment, 37
    idiopathic subglottic stenosis, 33
        clinical features, 33–34
        diagnosis, 34
        etiology, 33
        pathophysiology and risk factors, 33
        treatment, 34–35
    relapsing polychondritis (RP), 37
        clinical presentation, 38
        management, 38
    tracheobronchomalacia (TBM), 37
        clinical features, 37
        diagnosis, 37
        etiology, 37
        management, 37
Benign pleural tumors
    pleural lipoma, 207
    solitary fibrous tumor (SFT), 207, *207*
Benign tumors
    glomus tumors, 175, *175*
    paragangliomas, 175
    schwannomas, 175
    squamous papillomas, 174, *174*
    tracheobronchopathia osteochondroplastica (TPO), 175–176, *175*
Benralizumab, 55
Bertill-Laurell, Carl, 20
Berylliosis, 106, *108*
BHD, *see* Birt–Hogg–Dubé syndrome
Bilothorax, 181
    cause and pathogenesis, 181
    clinical presentation and evaluation, 182
    management, 182
    pleural fluid characteristics, 182
Biogenesis of lysosome-related organelles complexes (BLOCs), 18
Biomarkers, 81
Biopsy, 7
Birbeck granules, 138
Birt–Hogg–Dubé syndrome (BHD), 132
    clinical findings, **135**
    clinical presentation, 133–134
    diagnostic evaluation, 134–135
    epidemiology and genetics, 132–133
    monitoring and management, 135
    pathology, 133
Black pleural sign, 15
Bland alveolar hemorrhage, 64
BLOCs, *see* Biogenesis of lysosome-related organelles complexes
B lymphocyte, 95
Boerhaave syndrome, 181, *181*
BOOP, *see* Bronchiolitis obliterans organizing pneumonia

Index

BOS, *see* Bronchiolitis obliterans syndrome
Boston criteria, 88, **89**
BPS, *see* Bronchopulmonary sequestration
BRAF, *see* Braf proto-oncogene
Braf proto-oncogene (BRAF), 138
BRAFV600E gene mutation, 138, 140, 141
Bronchiectasis
    cystic, *54*
    differential diagnosis of, **52**
Bronchiolitis, 42
    background, definition, and classification, 42–43
    chest CT findings in, *44*
    chest imaging, 43, *44*
    clinical presentation, 43
    diagnosis, 43–44
    histopathologic features of, *45*
    management, 44
    specific forms of, 44
        acute bronchiolitis, 45
        bronchiolitis, alveolar ductitis, and centrilobular emphysema (BADE), 47
        constrictive bronchiolitis, 45–46
        diffuse aspiration bronchiolitis (DAB), 47
        diffuse panbronchiolitis (DPB), 47
        follicular bronchiolitis, 46–47
        mineral dust airway disease (MDAD), 47
        respiratory bronchiolitis (RB), 44–45, *45*
    suspicion of, 47
Bronchiolitis, alveolar ductitis, and centrilobular emphysema (BADE), 47
Bronchiolitis obliterans organizing pneumonia (BOOP), 45
Bronchiolitis obliterans syndrome (BOS), 45
Bronchoalveolar lavage (BAL), 16, 65, 66, 89, 92, 98, 102, 104, 106, 110, 111, 127, 138, 141, 142
Bronchodilators, 123
Bronchogenic cysts (BCs), 6
Bronchoprovocation, 103
Bronchopulmonary anomalies, 3, 4–9
    accessory cardiac bronchus (ACB), 9
    bronchogenic cysts (BCs), 6
    combined pulmonary parenchymal-vascular anomalies, 11
        bronchopulmonary sequestration (BPS), 12–13, *12*
        hypogenetic lung syndrome (HLS), 11–12, *11*
    congenital bronchial atresia (CBA), 4–6, *5*
    congenital lobar overinflation (CLO), 6–7, *7*
    congenital pulmonary airway malformation (CPAM), 7, *8*
    pulmonary agenesis (PA), aplasia, and hypoplasia, 4
    tracheal bronchus (TB), 8
    tracheal diverticulum (TD), 8–9
Bronchopulmonary sequestration (BPS), 12–13, *12*
Bronchoscopy, 34, 36, 53, 92, 127, 156–157, 196–197
    demonstrating lobar and segmental stenosis, *38*

demonstrating mucosal involvement, *38*
showing simple web-like stenosis., *34*
showing ulceration and airway pseudotumors, *36*
Bronchus-associated lymphoid tissue (BALT), 128, 145
Brugia malayi, 96

C

CA-125, *see* Cancer antigen 125
Calcifying fibrous tumor (CFT), 205
Cancer antigen 125 (CA-125), 121, 195
Cannibalistic, 104
CAPD-related pleural effusion, *see* Continuous ambulatory peritoneal dialysis-related pleural effusion
Carcinoid tumorlets, 155
Carcinoma
    adenoid cystic carcinoma (ACC), 171–173
    mucoepidermoid carcinomas, 173–174
    with sarcomatoid features, *171*
    squamous cell carcinoma (SCC), 170–171
Cardiopulmonary exercise testing (CPET), 74
Catamenial hemoptysis, 195
Catamenial hemothorax, 195
Catamenial pneumothorax (CP), 194
CBA, *see* Congenital bronchial atresia
CD1a-, 140, 141
CD4+ T cells, 106
CD4, 85
CD20, 113, 148, 164
CD34+, 91
CD68+, 140, 141
CD68, 141
CD79a, 148
Central nervous system (CNS), 141
Central venous catheter (CVC)-related pleural effusions
    clinical presentation and management, 184
    pathogenesis, 184
    pleural fluid characteristics, 184
CEP, *see* Chronic eosinophilic pneumonia
Cerebrospinal fluid (CSF), 184
CFT, *see* Calcifying fibrous tumor
CH, *see* Cystic hygroma
Charcot-Leyden crystals, 91
Chest CT, 4, 5, 6
Chest radiography, 10, 11, 59, 79
Cholesterol effusion, *see* Pseudochylothorax
Cholesterol pleurisy, *see* Pseudochylothorax
Cholethorax, *see* Bilothorax
CHOP therapy, *see* Cyclophosphamide, doxorubicin, vincristine, and prednisone therapy
Chronic beryllium disease, *see* Berylliosis
Chronic eosinophilic pneumonia (CEP), 93
    clinical features, **92**, 93–94
    diagnosis, 94
    histopathology, 94
    imaging, 94
    steroid-sparing therapy, 95
    treatment and prognosis, 94–95
Chronic lymphocytic leukaemia (CLL), 205
Chronic obstructive pulmonary disease (COPD), 20
Chronic pulmonary aspergillosis (CPA), 51

Chronic thromboembolic pulmonary hypertension (CTEPH), 73
Chyliform effusion, *see* Pseudochylothorax
Chyloptysis, 118
Chylothorax, 116, 177
    cause, 177, **178**
    clinical presentation, 177
    evaluation, 178
    management, 178–179, **179**
    pathogenesis, 177
    pleural fluid characteristics, 177–178
Cladribine, 138
CLL, *see* Chronic lymphocytic leukaemia
CLO, *see* Congenital lobar overinflation
Club cells, 43
CNS, *see* Central nervous system
Coagulopathy, transfusion and correction of, 66
Cobalt, 102
Common variable immunodeficiency (CVID), 46
Congenital bronchial atresia (CBA), 4–6, *5*
Congenital cystic adenomatoid malformation, *see* Congenital pulmonary airway malformation
Congenital lobar emphysema, *see* Congenital lobar overinflation
Congenital lobar overinflation (CLO), 6–7, *7*
Congenital pulmonary airway malformation (CPAM), 7, *8*
Congenital tracheal diverticulum, 8
Congo red stain, *129*, 130, *161*, *162*, *163*
Connective tissue diseases (CTDs), 45, 64
    pleural effusions related to, 185
Constrictive bronchiolitis, 45–46, 107
Continuous ambulatory peritoneal dialysis (CAPD)-related pleural effusion, 183
    management, 184
    pathogenesis and clinical presentation, 184
    pleural fluid characteristics, 184
Continuous positive airway pressure (CPAP), 184
COPD, *see* Chronic obstructive pulmonary disease
Corticosteroids, 66, 68, 105, 142
COVID-19 pneumonia, 111
CP, *see* Catamenial pneumothorax
CPA, *see* Chronic pulmonary aspergillosis
CPAM, *see* Congenital pulmonary airway malformation
CPAP, *see* Continuous positive airway pressure
CPET, *see* Cardiopulmonary exercise testing
Crazy paving pattern, 111, *111*
C-reactive protein (CRP), 92, 140
CRP, *see* C-reactive protein
Cryobiopsy, 104
Cryptogenic constrictive bronchiolitis, 46
CSF, *see* Cerebrospinal fluid
C-shaped cartilaginous rings, 168
CTDs, *see* Connective tissue diseases
CTEPH, *see* Chronic thromboembolic pulmonary hypertension
Curacao criteria, **58**
Cutis laxa, **18**
CVC-related pleural effusions, *see* Central venous catheter-related pleural effusions

CVID, *see* Common variable
 immunodeficiency
CyBorD, *see* Cyclophosphamide, bortezomib,
 and dexamethasone
Cyclophosphamide, 66, 68, 95, 129
Cyclophosphamide, bortezomib, and
 dexamethasone (CyBorD), 163
Cyclophosphamide, doxorubicin, vincristine,
 and prednisone (CHOP)
 therapy, 148
Cyclosporine, 105
Cystic bronchiectasis, *54*
Cystic fibrosis, 52
Cystic hygroma (CH), 10–11
Cystic lung diseases, 132
 differential diagnosis of, **122**

D

DAB, *see* Diffuse aspiration bronchiolitis
DAH, *see* Diffuse alveolar hemorrhage
Dasatinib-related pleural effusion, *186*
DC, *see* Dyskeratosis congenita
Deployed military personnel, lung disease in, 107
Desmoid-type fibromatosis, 205
Developmental lung anomalies (DLAs), 3
 bronchopulmonary anomalies, 4–9
  accessory cardiac bronchus (ACB), 9
  bronchogenic cysts (BCs), 6
  congenital bronchial atresia (CBA), 4–6, *5*
  congenital lobar overinflation (CLO), 6–7, *7*
  congenital pulmonary airway
   malformation (CPAM), 7, *8*
  pulmonary agenesis (PA), aplasia, and
   hypoplasia, 4
  tracheal bronchus (TB), *8*
  tracheal diverticulum (TD), 8–9
 combined pulmonary parenchymal-
  vascular anomalies
  bronchopulmonary sequestration
   (BPS), 12–13, *12*
  hypogenetic lung syndrome (HLS), 11–12, *11*
 embryology of lungs, 3–4
 vascular anomalies, 9
  central pulmonary artery, proximal
   interruption of, 9
  cystic hygroma (CH), 10–11
  left pulmonary artery (LPA), anomalous
   origination of, 9
  partial anomalous pulmonary venous
   return (PAPVR), 9–10, *10*
  pulmonary arteriovenous malformation
   (AVM), 10, *11*
  pulmonary vein varix, 10
Diaphragmatic rupture, 195
Diethylcarbamazine, 96
Difficult-to-control asthma, 51
Diffuse alveolar damage, 64
Diffuse alveolar hemorrhage (DAH)
 ANCA-associated vasculitis, 67–68
 anti-GBM disease, 68
 classification, 64
 clinical features, 64–65
 diagnostic approach and management of, 67

diagnostic workup, 65
 bronchoscopy, 66–67
 imaging, 66
 laboratory testing, 65–66
 lung biopsy, 67
idiopathic pulmonary hemosiderosis
 (IPH), 68
immune-mediated and non-immune-
 mediated causes of, **65**
isolated pauci-immune pulmonary
 capillaritis, 68
management, 66
 coagulopathy, transfusion and
  correction of, 66
 hemostatic agents, specific, 66
 oxygenation, maintaining, 66
pathophysiology, 64
systemic lupus erythematosus, 68
treating the underlying condition leading
 to, 66
Diffuse alveolar-septal amyloidosis, 160
Diffuse aspiration bronchiolitis (DAB), 43, 47
Diffuse idiopathic pulmonary neuroendocrine
 cell hyperplasia (DIPNECH), 46, 153
 bronchoscopy, 156–157
 clinical features, 155
 differential diagnosis, 157
 epidemiology, 153–154
 etiopathogenesis, 154–155
 histopathological confirmation, *156*
 imaging, 155–156
 laboratory investigations, 155
 pathology, 154–155, *154*, *155*
 pulmonary function tests (PFTs), 156
 treatment, 157
Diffuse large B-cell lymphoma (DLBCL), 205
Diffuse large B-cell lymphoma associated
 with chronic inflammation
 (DLBCL-CI), 205
Diffuse panbronchiolitis (DPB), 43, 47
Diffuse pleural thickening, 208
Diffusion capacity of carbon monoxide
 (DLCO), 36, 43, 92
DIPNECH, *see* Diffuse idiopathic pulmonary
 neuroendocrine cell hyperplasia
DLAs, *see* Developmental lung anomalies
DLBCL, *see* Diffuse large B-cell lymphoma
DLBCL-CI, *see* Diffuse large B-cell
 lymphoma associated with chronic
 inflammation
DLCO, *see* Diffusion capacity of carbon
 monoxide
DPB, *see* Diffuse panbronchiolitis
DPF, *see* Duro-pleural fistula
Drug-induced eosinophilic lung disease, 96, **97**
 imaging, 98
 treatment, 98
Drug-related eosinophilic pleural
 effusions, 185
Duro-pleural fistula (DPF), 184
Duro-pleural fistula-related pleural
 effusion, *185*
 clinical presentation and management, 184
 pathogenesis, 184
 pleural fluid characteristics, 184
Dyskeratosis congenita (DC), 16–18, *17*
Dyspnea, 58, 118

E

EACA, *see* Epsilon aminocaproic acid
EBTB, *see* Endobronchial tuberculosis
EBUS, *see* Endobronchial ultrasound
EBV, *see* Epstein–Barr virus
ECD, *see* Erdheim–Chester disease
ECMO, *see* Extracorporeal membranous
 oxygenation
ECP, *see* Extracorporeal photopheresis
EGPA, *see* Eosinophilic granulomatosis with
 polyangiitis
Elastosis, 78
Electron probe micro-analyzer (EPMA), 102, 104
ELS, *see* Extralobar sequestration
Embryology of lungs, 3–4
Endobronchial tuberculosis (EBTB), 38
Endobronchial ultrasound (EBUS), 6
Endocrine and reproductive systems
 pleural effusions related to, 185
Endoscopy, 34
Eosinophilic granulomatosis with polyangiitis
 (EGPA), 67, 95, 96
 clinical features, **92**, 95
 diagnosis, 95
 Five Factor Score in, **96**
 histopathology, 95
 imaging, 95
 treatment and prognosis, 95–96
Eosinophilic lung diseases, 91, **92**
 acute eosinophilic pneumonia (AEP), 91
  clinical features, 92, **92**
  diagnosis, 93
  histopathology, 93
  imaging, 93
  treatment and prognosis, 93
 chronic eosinophilic pneumonia
  (CEP), 93
  clinical features, **92**, 93–94
  diagnosis, 94
  histopathology, 94
  imaging, 94
  steroid-sparing therapy, 95
  treatment and prognosis, 94–95
 drug-induced, 96, **97**
  imaging, 98
  treatment, 98
 eosinophilic granulomatosis with
  polyangiitis (EGPA), 95, 96
  clinical features, **92**, 95
  diagnosis, 95
  Five Factor Score in, **96**
  histopathology, 95
  imaging, 95
  treatment and prognosis, 95–96
 parasitic infection causing eosinophilic
  pneumonia, 96
 tropical pulmonary eosinophilia, 96
Eosinophilic pleural effusions, 185
 drug-related eosinophilic pleural
  effusions, 185
 unusual causes of, 185
Eosinophils, 95
EPMA, *see* Electron probe micro-analyzer
Epsilon aminocaproic acid (EACA), 66
Epstein–Barr virus (EBV), 147, 205
Erdheim–Chester disease (ECD), 138

Index

diagnosis and clinical manifestations, 140–141
incidence and risk factors, 138–140
management, 141
pathogenesis, 140
pulmonary disease, 141
Eriksson, Sten, 20
Erythrocyte sedimentation rates (ESR), 92
ESR, see Erythrocyte sedimentation rates
Exposure, removal of, 104
Extracorporeal membranous oxygenation (ECMO), 66, 93
Extracorporeal photopheresis (ECP), 46
Extralobar sequestration (ELS), 12
Exudative PEEVO, 177
    bilothorax, 181
        cause and pathogenesis, 181
        clinical presentation and evaluation, 182
        management, 182
        pleural fluid characteristics, 182
    chylothorax
        cause and pathogenesis, 177
        clinical presentation, 177
        evaluation, 178
        management, 178–179
        pleural fluid characteristics, 177–178
    pancreatico-pleural fistula and pancreatic pseudocyst
        cause and pathogenesis, 182
        clinical presentation and evaluation, 182–183
        management, 183
        pleural fluid characteristics, 183
    pleural effusion secondary to esophageal and gastric perforation
        cause and pathogenesis, 181
        clinical presentation and evaluation, 181
        management, 181
        pleural fluid characteristics, 181
    pseudochylothorax, 179
        cause and pathogenesis, 179
        clinical presentation and evaluation, 180
        management, 180
        pleural fluid characteristics, 180

F

F allele, 26
Familial pulmonary alveolar proteinosis, **18**
FB, see Follicular bronchiolitis
FDA, see Food and Drug Administration
FDG, see Fluorodeoxyglucose
18FDG-PET, see 18Flouro-deoxy glucose positron emission tomography
Fetal lung, development of, 3–4
Fibroblastic tumors
    calcifying fibrous tumor (CFT), 205
    desmoid-type fibromatosis, 205
    malignant solitary fibrous tumor, 204–205
Fibrofolliculomas, 133, *134*
Fibrotic scarring stenosis, 37
"Finger-in-glove" appearance, 5
"Finger-in-glove" sign, 54
FISH, see Fluorescence in situ hybridization
Flavor-worker's lung, 107

FLCN, see Folliculin gene
Flock-worker's lung, 106–107
Fluorescence in situ hybridization (FISH), 203
Fluorodeoxyglucose (FDG), 130, 146
18Flouro-deoxy glucose positron emission tomography (18FDG-PET), 202
FNIP1, see Folliculin-interacting protein 1
FNIP2, see Folliculin-interacting protein 2
Focal tumor-like lesions of the pleura, 208
Follicular bronchiolitis (FB), 43, 46–47, 129
Follicular lymphoma, 205
Folliculin disease, 132
Folliculin gene (FLCN), 132, *133*
Folliculin-interacting protein 1 (FNIP1), 132
Folliculin-interacting protein 2 (FNIP2), 132
Food and Drug Administration (FDA), 20
Forced vital capacity (FVC), 81, 112
FVC, see Forced vital capacity

G

Galactin-10, 91
GAP score, see Gender-age-physiology score
Gastroesophageal reflux disorder (GERD), 33
Gaucher disease, **18**
Gender-age-physiology (GAP) score, 81
Gene therapy, 114
Genetic infiltrative lung diseases, 15
    dyskeratosis congenita (DC), 16–18, *17*
    genetic infiltrative disorders of lung, 15
    Hermansky–Pudlak syndrome (HPS), 18, *18*
    neurofibromatosis (NF), 16, *17*
    pulmonary alveolar microlithiasis (PAM), 15–16, *16*
GERD, see Gastroesophageal reflux disorder
GGO, see Ground-glass opacities
Giant cell interstitial pneumonitis (GIP), 102, 104, *104*, 106
GIP, see Giant cell interstitial pneumonitis
Global Obstructive Lung Disease (GOLD), 26
Glomus tumors, 175, *175*
Glucocorticoid pulse therapy, 95
Glucocorticoids, 89, 114
Glucocorticoid therapy, 94
Glycinothorax
    management, 184
    pathogenesis and clinical presentation, 184
    pleural fluid characteristics, 184
GM-CSF, see Granulocyte-macrophage colony-stimulating factor
GOLD, see Global Obstructive Lung Disease
GPA, see Granulomatosis with polyangiitis
Graft-versus-host disease (GVHD), 45
Granulocyte-macrophage colony-stimulating factor (GM-CSF), 110, 112–113
Granulomatosis with polyangiitis (GPA), 35, 67
    clinical presentation, 35
    diagnosis, 35–36
    pathology, 36–37
    risk factors, 35
    treatment, 37
Ground-glass opacities (GGO), 68

H

Haemophilus influenzae, 45
HAM, see High attenuation mucus

Hard metal lung disease (HMLD), 101
    characteristics, **102**
    clinical features, 103
    establishing diagnosis, 103
    exposure associated with, 102–103, **103**
    pathogenesis, 102
    pathophysiology and risk factors, 102
    reactive airway disease, 103
    treatment, 103
Helicobacter pylori, 145
Hematopoietic stem cell transplant (HSCT), 45, 68, 72
Hematoxylin, *161*
Hematoxylin and eosin (H&E)-stained section of pleural biopsy, *196*
Hemoptysis, 169
Hemorrhagic pleural effusion, 195
Hemostatic agents, specific, 66
Hepatic hydrothorax (HH), 183, *183*
    management, 183–184
    pathogenesis and clinical presentation, 183
Hepatic veno-occlusive disease (HVOD), 74
Hereditary hemorrhagic telangiectasia (HHT), 57
    clinical features of, **58**
    clinical presentation, 58–59
    diagnostic evaluation, 59–60
    hereditary hemorrhagic telangiectasia, 57–58
    management of complications of, **61**
    monitoring and management, 60–61
    prevalence and risk factors, 57
    pulmonary arteriovenous malformation in, *59*
    skin telangiectasias in patient with, *60*
Hereditary PAP, 112
Hermansky–Pudlak syndrome (HPS), 18, *18*
HH, see Hepatic hydrothorax
HHT, see Hereditary hemorrhagic telangiectasia
HHV-8, see Human herpes virus-8
High attenuation mucus (HAM), 54
High-resolution computed tomography (HRCT), 53, 79, 104, 111, 119, 126, 127, 132
HIV, see Human immune-deficiency virus
HLA haplotypes, see Human leukocyte antigen haplotypes
HLS, see Hypogenetic lung syndrome
HMLD, see Hard metal lung disease
HP, see Hypersensitivity pneumonitis
HPOA, see Hypertrophic pulmonary osteoarthropathy
HPS, see Hermansky–Pudlak syndrome
HPV infection, see Human papillomavirus infection
HRCT, see High-resolution computed tomography
HSCT, see Hematopoietic stem cell transplant
Human herpes virus-8 (HHV-8), 205
Human immune-deficiency virus (HIV), 205
Human leukocyte antigen (HLA) haplotypes, 86
Human papillomavirus (HPV) infection, 170
HVOD, see Hepatic veno-occlusive disease
Hydroxychloroquine, 129
Hyperlucent lung syndrome, see Swyer–James–MacLeod syndrome

Index

Hypersensitivity pneumonitis (HP), 101, *105*
Hypertrophic pulmonary osteoarthropathy (HPOA), 204
Hypogammaglobulinemia, 125, 129
Hypogenetic lung syndrome (HLS), 11–12, *11*
Hypoplasia, 4
Hypoxemia, 112

I

IAFE, *see* Intra-alveolar fibrosis and elastosis
IBD, *see* Inflammatory bowel disease
ICS, *see* Inhaled corticosteroids
Idiopathic interstitial pneumonia (IIP), 79, 125
Idiopathic pulmonary hemosiderosis (IPH), 64, 68
Idiopathic pulmonary upper-lobe fibrosis (idiopathic PULF), 77
Idiopathic subglottic stenosis, 33
    clinical features, 33–34
    diagnosis, 34
    etiology, 33
    pathophysiology and risk factors, 33
    treatment, 34–35
IgG4 isotype, 85
IgG4-RD, *see* Immunoglobulin G4-related disease
IIP, *see* Idiopathic interstitial pneumonia
ILD, *see* Interstitial lung disease
ILS, *see* Intralobar sequestration
Immunoglobulin G4-related disease (IgG4-RD), 85, 188, *189*
    clinical presentation, 86
    CT imaging, 86, *87*
    diagnosis, 88–89
    imaging patterns of pulmonary involvement in, **86**
    incidence, 85
    intrathoracic involvement, imaging patterns of, 86
        airway disease, 88
        mediastinal disease, 88
        parenchymal disease, 86–88
        pleural disease, 88
    management, 188
    pathogenesis and clinical presentation, 188
    pathogenesis and risk factors, 85–86
    pleural fluid characteristics, 188
    treatment, 89
        immunosuppressant therapy, 89–90
        relapse and prognosis, 90
Immunosuppressant therapy, 89–90
Indium tin oxide lung disease, 107
Inflammatory bowel disease (IBD), 33, 38
Influenza virus, 45
Inhaled corticosteroids (ICS), 54, 95
Interferon-alpha (IFN-α), 141
Interferon-gamma (IFN-γ), 85
Interleukin-10, 85
Interleukin-6, 140
Interlobular septum, *71*
International Society for Human and Animal Mycology (ISHAM), 53
Interstitial lung disease (ILD), 77, 101, 106
Interstitial pulmonary fibrosis (IPF), 78
Intra-alveolar fibrosis and elastosis (IAFE), 77
Intra-alveolar haemorrhage, *64*
Intralesional injection, of steroids, 35
Intralobar sequestration (ILS), 12
Intrapulmonary bronchogenic cyst, 6
Intrathoracic involvement, imaging patterns of, 86
    airway disease, 88
    mediastinal disease, 88
    parenchymal disease, 86–88
    pleural disease, 88
Invasive pulmonary aspergillosis (IPA), 51
IPA, *see* Invasive pulmonary aspergillosis
IPF, *see* Interstitial pulmonary fibrosis
IPH, *see* Idiopathic pulmonary hemosiderosis
ISHAM, *see* International Society for Human and Animal Mycology
Isolated pauci-immune pulmonary capillaritis, 68
Itraconazole, 54

K

Kaposi's sarcoma, 149
KL-6, 81

L

LAM, *see* Lymphangioleiomyomatosis
Langerhans cells, 137, 138
Large airway involvement, 36
Latent transforming growth factor beta binding protein 4 (LTBP-4), 81
LCDD, *see* Light chain deposition disease
Left pulmonary artery (LPA), 9
LENT score, 204
Light chain deposition disease (LCDD), 130
LIP, *see* Lymphocytic interstitial pneumonia
Lipoid granulomatose, 138
Liver disease, 25
Loeffler's syndrome, 96
Loop-sheet polymerization, 23
LPA, *see* Left pulmonary artery
LTBP-4, *see* Latent transforming growth factor beta binding protein 4
Lung auscultation, 43
Lung biopsy, 66
Lung bud, 3
Lung disease, 25
Lung nodules, 195
Lung transplantation, 16, 104, 114
Lung volume reduction surgery (LVRS), 27, 28
LVRS, *see* Lung volume reduction surgery
Lymphangiography, 178
Lymphangioleiomyomatosis (LAM), 116, 123
    clinical manifestations, 118
    diagnosis, 118, *120*
        differential diagnosis, 122
        prognosis, 122
        treatment, 122–123
    pathogenesis, 116–117
    pathology, 117–118
Lymphangiomas, 118
Lymphangitis, 200, *200*
Lymphocytic interstitial pneumonia (LIP), 125
    clinical conditions associated with, **126**
    epidemiology and clinical features of, 125
    follicular bronchiolitis (FB), 129
    histopathological features of, 127
    management of, 128
    pulmonary amyloidosis and light chain deposition disease, 129
    radiological features of, 126
Lymphoid hyperplasia, 106
Lymphomatoid granulomatosis, *148*
Lymphoproliferative disorders, 126
    in immunocompromised patient, 149
    post-transplantation lymphoproliferative disorders (PTLD), 149–151
        primary effusion lymphoma (PEL), 149, *150*
    primary pleural tumors related to, 205
        diffuse large B-cell lymphoma associated with chronic inflammation (DLBCL-CI), 205
        pathogenesis, 205
        primary effusion lymphoma (PEL), 205
Lymphoscintigraphy, 178

M

Macrolides, 44
Magnetic resonance angiography (MRA), 60
Magnetic resonance lymphangiography, 178
Malignant pleural effusion (MPE), 199, 204
    management of, 204
Malignant pleural mesothelioma (MPM), 199, *201*
Malignant solitary fibrous tumor, 204–205
Malignant tumors, 169
    adenoid cystic carcinoma (ACC), 171–173, *173*, *174*
    mucoepidermoid carcinomas, 173–174
    squamous cell carcinoma (SCC), 170–171
MALT lymphoma, *see* Mucosa-associated lymphoid tissue lymphoma
Mammalian target of rapamycin (mTOR), 116, 117, *117*, 122, 123, 132
    mTORC2, 116–117
MAPK pathway, *see* Mitogen-activated protein kinase pathway
Marfan syndrome, **18**
MARS, *see* Mesothelioma and radical surgery
MDAD, *see* Mineral dust airway disease
MDCT, *see* Multidetector computed tomography
Mediastinal amyloidosis, 165
Mediastinal disease, 88
Mediastinal pleural thickening, *201*
Medical thoracoscopy, 196, 203
Meigs syndrome, 185, *187*
MEN1 syndrome, *see* Multiple endocrine neoplasia syndrome
Mepolizumab, 55
Mesenchymal tumors of uncertain differentiation, 205
Mesothelioma, management of, 204
Mesothelioma and radical surgery (MARS), 204
Metal-related occupational lung diseases, 105
    berylliosis, 106, *108*
    siderosis, 105
    talcosis, 105–106
Metastatic pancreatic cancer, *207*
Methylthioadenosine phosphorylase (MTAP), 203

Index

Microscopic polyangiitis (MPA), 67
MILES trial, see Multicenter International Lymphangioleiomyomatosis Efficacy of Sirolimus trial
Mineral dust airway disease (MDAD), 47
Mitogen-activated protein kinase (MAPK) pathway, 138
Mitomycin C, 35
Monoclonal gammopathy, 125
MPA, see Microscopic polyangiitis
MPE, see Malignant pleural effusion
MPM, see Malignant pleural mesothelioma
MRA, see Magnetic resonance angiography
MTAP, see Methylthioadenosine phosphorylase
mTOR, see Mammalian target of rapamycin
Mucoepidermoid carcinomas, 169, 173–174
Mucosa-associated lymphoid tissue (MALT) lymphoma, 125, 145, *146*
Mucosal sparing techniques, 35
Multicenter International Lymphangioleiomyomatosis Efficacy of Sirolimus (MILES) trial, 120, 122, 123
Multicenter randomized controlled trials, 1
Multidetector computed tomography (MDCT), 10
Multiple endocrine neoplasia (MEN1) syndrome, 155
Mycophenolate mofetil, 89
Mycoplasma pneumoniae, 45

N

National Organization for Rare Disorders (NORD), 1, 153
NE, see Neutrophil elastase
NEB, see Neuroendocrine bodies
Neuroblastoma RAS viral oncogene (NRAS) mutations, 138
Neuroendocrine bodies (NEB), 153
Neurofibromatosis (NF), 16, *17*
Neutrophil elastase (NE), 22, *23*
Newer occupational lung diseases, 106
    flavor-worker's lung, 107
    flock-worker's lung, 106–107
    indium tin oxide lung disease, 107
    lung disease in deployed military personnel, 107
NF, see Neurofibromatosis
Niemann–Pick disease, **18**
Nodular amyloidosis, *163*
Nodular pulmonary amyloidosis (NPA), 160–163
NORD, see National Organization for Rare Disorders
NPA, see Nodular pulmonary amyloidosis
NRAS mutations, see Neuroblastoma RAS viral oncogene mutations

O

Occupational lung diseases, 101
Orphan Drug Act, 1
Osler–Weber–Rendu syndrome, see Hereditary hemorrhagic telangiectasia
Ovarian hyperstimulation syndrome, 185, *187*
Oxygenation, maintaining, 66

P

PA, see Pulmonary agenesis
PAM, see Pulmonary alveolar microlithiasis
Pancreatico-pleural fistula and pancreatic pseudocyst
    cause and pathogenesis, 182
    clinical presentation and evaluation, 182–183
    management, 183
    pleural fluid characteristics, 183
Panniculitis, 25, *26*
"Pan," 47
PAP, see Pulmonary alveolar proteinosis
PAPVR, see Partial anomalous pulmonary venous return
Paragangliomas, 175
Parasite larvae, 96
Parasitic infection causing eosinophilic pneumonia, 96
Parenchymal and endobronchial lymphoma, *147*
Parenchymal disease, 86–88
Parenchymal lung disease, 103
    bronchoscopy, 104
    clinical features, 103
    establishing diagnosis, 103
    histopathology, 104
    laboratory findings, 104
    occupational exposure history, 103
    pulmonary function testing, 104
    radiographic findings, 104
    treatment
        anti-inflammatory agents, 104
        exposure, removal of, 104
        lung transplantation, 104
Partial anomalous pulmonary venous return (PAPVR), 9–10, *10*
Pathognomonic "blind-ending bronchus," 5
Patient resources, 1
PAVMs, see Pulmonary arteriovenous malformations
PCH, see Pulmonary capillary hemangiomatosis
PEEP, see Positive end-expiratory pressure
PEEVO, see Pleural effusion of extra-vascular origin
PEL, see Primary effusion lymphoma
Periodic acid-Schiff (PAS)-positive diastase-resistant globules, 23, *24*
Periodic acid-Schiff staining, 111
Peripheral eosinophilia, 53, 94, 98
PFT, see Pulmonary function testing
PH, see Pulmonary hypertension
PI*S$_{iiyama}$, 21
PIRCLAD, see Pirfenidone for Restrictive Chronic Lung Allograft Dysfunction trial
Pirfenidone for Restrictive Chronic Lung Allograft Dysfunction (PIRCLAD) trial, 81
Plasmapheresis, 68, 114
PLCH, see Pulmonary Langerhans cell histiocytosis
Pleura, tumor-like lesion of, *208*
Pleural biopsy, ultrasound-guided, *203*
Pleural disease, 88

Pleural effusion, 112, 127, 177
    in amyloidosis, 165
    dasatinib-related, *186*
    eosinophilic, 185
        drug-related eosinophilic pleural effusions, 185
        unusual causes of, 185
    pleural effusion of extra-vascular origin (PEEVO), 177
        exudative PEEVO, 177–183
        transudative PEEVO, 183–184
    related to connective tissue diseases and vasculitis, 185
    related to endocrine and reproductive systems, 185
    secondary to atypical infections, 185
    secondary to esophageal and gastric perforation
        cause and pathogenesis, 181
        clinical presentation and evaluation, 181
        management, 181
        pleural fluid characteristics, 181
    unusual causes, 188
        immunoglobulin G4 (IgG4)-related disease, 188, *189*
        yellow nail syndrome (YNS), 188
Pleural effusion of extra-vascular origin (PEEVO), 177
    exudative PEEVO, 177
        bilothorax, 181–182
        chylothorax, 177–179
        pancreatico-pleural fistula and pancreatic pseudocyst, 182–183
        pleural effusion secondary to esophageal and gastric perforation, 181
        pseudochylothorax, 179–180
    transudative PEEVO, 183
        central venous catheter (CVC)-related pleural effusions, 184
        continuous ambulatory peritoneal dialysis (CAPD)-related pleural effusion, 184
        duro-pleural fistula-related pleural effusion, 184, *185*
        glycinothorax, 184
        hepatic hydrothorax, 183–184, *183*
        urinothorax, 184
Pleural lipoma, 207
Pleural lymphoma, 205, *206*
Pleural mesenchymal tumors, 204
    fibroblastic tumors
        calcifying fibrous tumor (CFT), 205
        desmoid-type fibromatosis, 205
        malignant solitary fibrous tumor, 204–205
    vascular tumors
        mesenchymal tumors of uncertain differentiation, 205
        primary pleural angiosarcoma (PPA), 205
        primary pleural epithelioid hemangio-endothelioma, 205
Pleural mesothelial tumors, 199
    clinical presentation, 199–200
    diagnosis
        mesothelin, 204

pleural biopsy, 203–204
pleural fluid cytology, 202–204
epidemiology and pathogenesis, 199
imaging, 200
management
of malignant pleural effusion, 204
of mesothelioma, 204
Pleural plaques, 200, *200*, 208
Pleural splenosis, 208
Pleural tumors, 199
primary malignant pleural tumors, 199
pleural mesenchymal tumors, 204–205
pleural mesothelial tumors, 199–204
primary pleural tumors related to lymphoproliferative disorders, 205
secondary pleural metastasis, 205
benign pleural tumors, 207
tumor-like lesions of the pleura, 207–208
Pleurobilia, *see* Bilothorax
Pleuroparenchymal fibroelastosis (PPFE)
apical caps and, **81**
biomarkers, 81
prognosis, 81
treatment, 81–82
causes of, **78**
clinical characteristics, 79–82
diagnosis, 79–82
epidemiology, 77–78
histopathology and radiological diagnostic definitions, **79**
history, 77
imaging findings in, *80*
pathogenesis, 78–79
pulmonary function tests, 81
radiology, 79
chest x-ray, 79
high-resolution computed tomography (HRCT), 79
surgical biopsy, 79
histopathology, 79–81
vs. UIP, and NSIP patterns, **80**
Pleuroparenchymal pulmonary fibroelastosis, 77
Plexiform lesion, 71
PNECs, *see* Pulmonary neuroendocrine cells
Pneumocystis jirovecii, 66
Pneumocystis pneumonia, 111
Pneumothorax, 79, 81, 112, 116, 121, 134, 135, 194
Polymerization, 23
Positive end-expiratory pressure (PEEP), 66
Positive lung biopsy, 36
Post-transplantation lymphoproliferative disorders (PTLD), 149
epidemiology and clinical features, 149–150
pathology, 150
prognosis and treatment, 150–151
radiology, 150
PPA, *see* Primary pleural angiosarcoma
PPFE, *see* Pleuroparenchymal fibroelastosis
Prednisone therapy, 94
Primary effusion lymphoma (PEL), 149, *150*, 205
epidemiology and clinical features, 149
pathology, 149

prognosis and treatment, 149
radiology, 149
Primary malignant pleural tumors, 199
pleural mesenchymal tumors, 204
fibroblastic tumors, 204–205
vascular tumors, 205
pleural mesothelial tumors, 199
clinical presentation, 199–200
diagnosis, 202–204
epidemiology and pathogenesis, 199
imaging, 200
management of malignant pleural effusion, 204
management of mesothelioma, 204
mesothelin, 204
pleural biopsy, 203–204
pleural fluid cytology, 202–204
primary pleural tumors related to lymphoproliferative disorders, 205
diffuse large B-cell lymphoma associated with chronic inflammation (DLBCL-CI), 205
pathogenesis, 205
primary effusion lymphoma (PEL), 205
Primary pleural angiosarcoma (PPA), 205
Primary pleural epithelioid hemangioendothelioma, 205
Primary pleural tumors related to lymphoproliferative disorders, 205
diffuse large B-cell lymphoma associated with chronic inflammation (DLBCL-CI), 205
pathogenesis, 205
primary effusion lymphoma (PEL), 205
Primary pulmonary lymphoproliferative neoplasms, 145
primary pulmonary diffuse large B-cell lymphoma (P-DLBCL), 147
epidemiology and clinical features, 147
pathology, 147–148
prognosis and treatment, 148
radiographic findings, 147
pulmonary lymphomatoid granulomatosis, 148
epidemiology and clinical features, 148
pathology, 148–149
prognosis and treatment, 149
radiographic findings, 148
pulmonary mucosa-associated lymphoid tissue lymphoma, 145
epidemiology and clinical features, 145–146
pathology, 146
prognosis and treatment, 146–147
radiographic findings, 146
Primary tracheal tumors, *see* Tracheal tumors
Prophylactic treatment, for *Pneumocystis jirovecii* pneumonia, 66
Prothrombin time-international normalized ratio (PT-INR), 66
Pseudochylothorax, 179, *180*, 185
cause, 179, **179**
clinical presentation and evaluation, 180
management, 180
pathogenesis, 179
pleural fluid characteristics, 180
Pseudomonas aeruginosa, 47, 52

Pseudostratified ciliary columnar epithelial cells, 168
PT-INR, *see* Prothrombin time-international normalized ratio
PTLD, *see* Post-transplantation lymphoproliferative disorders
Pulmonary agenesis (PA), 4
Pulmonary alveolar microlithiasis (PAM), 15–16, *16*
Pulmonary alveolar proteinosis (PAP), 110
autoimmune PAP, 112
bronchoalveolar lavage in, *112*
classification of, **111**
clinical features, 110–111
diagnosis, 111–112
hereditary PAP, 112
pathogenesis and classification, 110
radiographic features, 111
secondary PAP, 112
treatment, 112, *113*
gene therapy, 114
glucocorticoids, 114
granulocyte-macrophage colony-stimulating factor (GM-CSF) supplementation, 112–113
lung transplantation, 114
plasmapheresis, 114
rituximab, 113–114
whole lung lavage (WLL), 112
unclassifiable PAP, 112
Pulmonary amyloidosis
diffuse alveolar-septal amyloidosis, 160
and light chain deposition disease, 129
nodular pulmonary amyloidosis (NPA), 160–163
tracheobronchial amyloidosis (TBA), 163, *164*, *165*
mediastinal amyloidosis, 165
pleural effusions in amyloidosis, 165
pulmonary hypertension (PH), 165–166
types of, 160
Pulmonary aplasia, *4*
Pulmonary arteriovenous malformations (PAVMs), 10, *11*, 57
angiography of, *60*
clinical presentation, 58–59
diagnostic evaluation, 59–60
hereditary hemorrhagic telangiectasia, 57–58
monitoring and management, 60–61
prevalence and risk factors, 57
Pulmonary artery sling, 9, *9*
Pulmonary capillaritis, 64
Pulmonary capillary hemangiomatosis (PCH), 16, 70
burden of, 71
clinical presentation of, 72–73
genetic risk factors, 72
imaging and diagnostic evaluation, 73–74
risk factors for the development of, 72
symptoms and physical examination findings, **72**
treatment and outcomes, 74
Pulmonary fibrosis, 16
Pulmonary function testing (PFT), 34, 36, 43, 52, 65, 92, 120, 126, 138, 156
Pulmonary hypertension (PH), 9, 10, 16, 58, 70, 165–166

Index

Pulmonary Langerhans cell histiocytosis (PLCH), 134, 137
    management, 138
    pathogenesis, 137–138
    pathology, 138
    pulmonary function tests (PFTs), 138
        diagnosis and clinical manifestations, 138
    radiology, 138
Pulmonary lymphomatoid granulomatosis, 148
    epidemiology and clinical features, 148
    pathology, 148–149
    prognosis and treatment, 149
    radiographic findings, 148
Pulmonary mucosa-associated lymphoid tissue lymphoma, 145
    epidemiology and clinical features, 145–146
    pathology, 146
    prognosis and treatment, 146–147
    radiographic findings, 146
Pulmonary neuroendocrine cells (PNECs), 42, 153, 154
Pulmonary neuroendocrine disorders, characteristics of, 157–**158**
Pulmonary vascular resistance (PVR), 71
Pulmonary vein varix, 10
Pulmonary veno-occlusive disease (PVOD), 70
    burden of, 71
    centrilobular ground glass nodules pathognomic, 73
    clinical presentation of, 72–73
    genetic risk factors, 72
    imaging and diagnostic evaluation, 73–74
    pathogenesis of, 71–72
    risk factors for the development of, 72
    symptoms and physical examination findings, 72
    treatment and outcomes, 74
    ventilation perfusion scan in, 73
PVOD, *see* Pulmonary veno-occlusive disease
PVR, *see* Pulmonary vascular resistance

Q

QALY, *see* Quality-adjusted life-years
Quality-adjusted life-years (QALY), 27

R

RA, *see* Rheumatoid arthritis
Rapamycin, 122
RAS, *see* Restrictive allograft syndrome
Ras homolog enriched in the brain (Rheb), 116
Ras proteins, 16
RB, *see* Respiratory bronchiolitis
RDD, *see* Rosai–Dorfman disease
Regulatory T cells, 85
Relapsing polychondritis (RP), 37
    clinical presentation, 38
    management, 38
Respiratory bronchiolitis (RB), 43, 44–45, *45*
Respiratory syncytial virus (RSV), 45
Restrictive allograft syndrome (RAS), 78
RHC, *see* Right heart catheterization
Rheb, *see* Ras homolog enriched in the brain
Rheumatoid arthritis (RA), 43
Right chest pulmonary venous drainage, 10

Right heart catheterization (RHC), 11, 74
Rigid bronchoscopy, 169, 170
Rigid medical thoracoscopy equipment, *196*
Rituximab, 68, 89, 113–114, 129, 164
Rosai–Dorfman disease (RDD), 141
    diagnosis and clinical presentation, 141–142
    epidemiology, 141
    imaging, 142
    management, 142
    pathogenesis, 141
    pulmonary, 142
Rosenberg/Patterson criteria, 52
Round atelectasis, *202*
RP, *see* Relapsing polychondritis
RSV, *see* Respiratory syncytial virus

S

SAFS, *see* Severe asthma with fungal sensitization
Sarcoidosis of the lower respiratory tract (SLRT), 38
SCC, *see* Squamous cell carcinoma
Schwannomas, 175
Scimitar syndrome, 11, *11*
Secondary PAP, 112
Secondary pleural metastasis, 205
    benign pleural tumors
        pleural lipoma, 207
        solitary fibrous tumor (SFT), 207, *207*
    tumor-like lesions of the pleura, 207
        diffuse pleural thickening, 208
        focal tumor-like lesions of the pleura, 208
        pleural plaque, 208
        pleural splenosis, 208
SEER study, *see* Surveillance, Epidemiology, and End Results study
Serum IgE, 53
Serum protein electrophoresis (SPEP), 20
Severe asthma with fungal sensitization (SAFS), 51
SFT, *see* Solitary fibrous tumor
SGS, *see* Subglottic stenosis
Sharp, Harvey, 20
Short telomere syndrome, 81
Siderophages, 66
Siderosis, 105
Signet ring sign, 53
Silicone stents, 35
Simple pulmonary eosinophilia (SPE), 96
Sirolimus, 123
SJM, *see* Swyer–James–MacLeod syndrome
Sjögren's disease/syndrome, 125, *126*, *128*, 129
Skin testing, 53
SLB, *see* Surgical lung biopsy
SLE, *see* Systemic lupus erythematosus
SLRT, *see* Sarcoidosis of the lower respiratory tract
Smoking cessation, 45, 138
Solitary fibrous tumor (SFT), 207, *207*
Solitary pulmonary nodules, 89
Somatostatin, 157
SP-D, *see* Surfactant protein D
SPE, *see* Simple pulmonary eosinophilia
SPEP, *see* Serum protein electrophoresis

Spindle cell neoplasm, *172*
Squamous cell carcinoma (SCC), 169, 170–171
Squamous papillomas, 174, *174*
Staphylococcus aureus, 64
Stents, 35
Steroid-sparing immunosuppressive agents, 105
Steroid-sparing therapy, 95
Streptomyces hygrocopicus, 122
Stridor, 35
Strongyloides, 96
Subglottic stenosis (SGS), 33, 36
    clinical features, 33–34
    diagnosis, 34
    etiology, 33
    pathophysiology and risk factors, 33
    treatment, 34–35
Surfactant protein D (SP-D), 81
Surfactant proteins, 110
Surgical lung biopsy (SLB), 94
Surveillance, Epidemiology, and End Results (SEER) study, 168
Swyer–James–MacLeod syndrome (SJM), 7
Systemic amyloidosis, **161**, 163
Systemic corticosteroids, 54
Systemic lupus erythematosus (SLE), 64, 68
Systemic steroids versus antifungals, 54

T

Talcosis, 105–106
Talc pneumoconiosis, *107*
TAPSE, *see* Tricuspid annular plan systolic excursion
Targeted biologics, 54–55
TB, *see* Tracheal bronchus
TBA, *see* Tracheobronchial amyloidosis
TBM, *see* Tracheobronchomalacia
TD, *see* Tracheal diverticulum
TE, *see* Thoracic endometriosis
TF, *see* Tissue factor
TGF-β1, *see* Transforming growth factor-beta 1
Th2, *see* T-helper 2 cells
T-helper 2 cells (Th2), 85, 95
Therapeutic thoracentesis, 180
Thoracic endometriosis (TE), 194
    clinical manifestations, **195**
    clinical presentation, 194
        catamenial hemoptysis, 195
        catamenial hemothorax/hemorrhagic pleural effusion, 195
        diaphragmatic rupture, 195
        lung nodules, 195
        pneumothorax, 194
    diagnosis of, 195
        bronchoscopy, 196–197
        histopathologic and immunohistochemical analysis, 197
        laboratory testing, 195
        medical thoracoscopy, 196
        radiologic studies, 195
        video-assisted thoracoscopic surgery (VATS), 195–196
    management of, 197
        medical management, 197
        surgical management, 197
    pathophysiology, 194

Index

Thoracic ultrasound, 202
Thoracobilia, *see* Bilothorax
Thoracobiliary fistula, *see* Bilothorax
Thoracoscopy, 204
Thrombin, 66
Thyroid transcription factor-1 (TTF-1), 7
Tissue biopsy, 88
Tissue factor (TF), 66
T-lymphocytes, 95
Toxocara canis, 96
TPC, *see* Tunneled pleural catheter
TPO, *see* Tracheobronchopathia osteochondroplastica
Tracheal adenocarcinoma, *172*
Tracheal anatomy and embryology, 168–169
Tracheal bronchus (TB), 8
Tracheal diverticulum (TD), 8–9
Tracheal mucoepidermoid carcinomas, 173
Tracheal mucosa, thickening of, *36*
Tracheal papillomas, 174
Tracheal tumors, 168, **171**
    benign tumors
        glomus tumors, 175, *175*
        paragangliomas, 175
        schwannomas, 175
        squamous papillomas, 174, *174*
        tracheobronchopathia osteochondroplastica (TPO), 175–176, *175*
    clinical presentation, 169
    diagnostic studies, 169–170
    malignant tumors, 169
        adenoid cystic carcinoma (ACC), 171–173, *173*, *174*
        mucoepidermoid carcinomas, 173–174
        squamous cell carcinoma (SCC), 170–171
    management and treatment, 170
    survival and follow-up, 170
    tracheal anatomy and embryology, 168–169
Tracheobronchial amyloidosis (TBA), 163, *164*, *165*
    mediastinal amyloidosis, 165
    pleural effusions in amyloidosis, 165
    pulmonary hypertension (PH), 165–166
Tracheobronchial chondritis, 37
Tracheobronchomalacia (TBM), 37
    clinical features, 37
    diagnosis, 37
    etiology, 37
    management, 37
Tracheobronchopathia osteochondroplastica (TPO), 164, 175–176, *175*
Tracheobronchoplasty, 37
Tracheoesophageal ridges, 169
Trametinib, 138
Tranexamic acid (TXA), 66
Transbronchial biopsies, *16*, *139*
Transbronchial lung biopsy, 94

Transforming growth factor-beta 1 (TGF-β1), 85
Transthoracic contrast-enhanced echocardiography (TTE), 59
Transthoracic echocardiography, 73
Transudative PEEVO, 183
    central venous catheter (CVC)-related pleural effusions
        clinical presentation and management, 184
        pathogenesis, 184
        pleural fluid characteristics, 184
    continuous ambulatory peritoneal dialysis (CAPD)-related pleural effusion
        management, 184
        pathogenesis and clinical presentation, 184
        pleural fluid characteristics, 184
    duro-pleural fistula-related pleural effusion, *185*
        clinical presentation and management, 184
        pathogenesis, 184
        pleural fluid characteristics, 184
    hepatic hydrothorax, *183*
        management, 183–184
        pathogenesis and clinical presentation, 183
    urinothorax and glycinothorax
        management, 184
        pathogenesis and clinical presentation, 184
        pleural fluid characteristics, 184
"Tree-in-bud" opacities, 43
Trichodiscomas, 133
Tricuspid annular plan systolic excursion (TAPSE), 73
Tropical pulmonary eosinophilia, 96
TTE, *see* Transthoracic contrast-enhanced echocardiography
TTF-1, *see* Thyroid transcription factor-1
Tumor-like lesions of the pleura, 207
    diffuse pleural thickening, 208
    focal tumor-like lesions of the pleura, 208
    pleural plaque, 208
    pleural splenosis, 208
Tungsten carbide, 102
Tunneled pleural catheter (TPC), 196
TXA, *see* Tranexamic acid

U

UIP, *see* Usual interstitial pneumonia
Ultrasound-guided pleural biopsy, *203*
Unclassifiable PAP, 112
Urinothorax
    management, 184
    pathogenesis and clinical presentation, 184
    pleural fluid characteristics, 184
Usual interstitial pneumonia (UIP), 18

V

Vascular anomalies, 9
    central pulmonary artery, proximal interruption of, 9
    combined pulmonary parenchymal-vascular anomalies, 11
    bronchopulmonary sequestration (BPS), 12–13, *12*
    hypogenetic lung syndrome (HLS), 11–12, *11*
    cystic hygroma (CH), 10–11
    left pulmonary artery (LPA), anomalous origination of, 9
    partial anomalous pulmonary venous return (PAPVR), 9–10, *10*
    pulmonary arteriovenous malformation (AVM), 10, *11*
    pulmonary vein varix, 10
Vascular endothelial factors C (VEGF-C), 117
Vascular endothelial factors D (VEGF-D), 117, 120–121
Vascular endothelial growth factor (VEGF), 205
Vascular tumors
    mesenchymal tumors of uncertain differentiation, 205
    primary pleural angiosarcoma (PPA), 205
    primary pleural epithelioid hemangio-endothelioma, 205
Vasculitis, 25
VATS, *see* Video-assisted thoracoscopic surgery
VEGF, *see* Vascular endothelial growth factor
Vemurafenib, 138
Venous malformation, 9
Video-assisted thoracoscopic surgery (VATS), 127, 184, 195–196, 203–204
Visceral larva migrans, 96
von Recklinghausen disease, 16, 175

W

Web resources, for RLD, **2**
Whole lung lavage (WLL), 112, 113
WLL, *see* Whole lung lavage
Wuchereria bancrofti, 96

Y

Yellow nail syndrome (YNS)
    management, 188
    pathogenesis, 188
    pleural fluid characteristics, 188
YNS, *see* Yellow nail syndrome